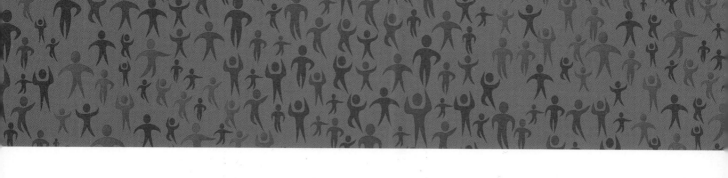

The World of the Counselor
An Introduction to the Counseling Profession

FIFTH EDITION

Ed Neukrug
Old Dominion University

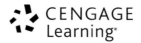

CENGAGE
Learning®

Australia • Brazil • Mexico • Singapore • United Kingdom • United States

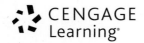

The World of the Counselor, An Introduction to the Counseling Profession, **Fifth Edition**

Ed Neukrug

Product Director: Jon-David Hague

Product Manager: Julie Martinez

Content Developer: Lori Bradshaw

Product Assistant: Kyra Kane

Media Developer: Kyra Kane

Marketing Manager: Jennifer Levanduski

Art Director: Vernon Boes

Manufacturing Planner: Judy Inouye

Photo Researcher: Veerabaghu Nagarajan

Text Researcher: Punitha Rajamohan

Production Management, and Composition: MPS Limited

Cover Designer: Cheryl Carrington

Cover Image: © Denis Cristo/Shutterstock.com

For product information and technology assistance, contact us at **Cengage Learning Customer & Sales Support, 1-800-354-9706.**

For permission to use material from this text or product, submit all requests online at **www.cengage.com/permissions.** Further permissions questions can be e-mailed to **permissionrequest@cengage.com.**

Library of Congress Control Number: 2014957654

ISBN: 978-1-305-08729-3

Cengage Learning
20 Channel Center Street
Boston, MA 02210
USA

Cengage Learning is a leading provider of customized learning solutions with office locations around the globe, including Singapore, the United Kingdom, Australia, Mexico, Brazil, and Japan. Locate your local office at **www.cengage.com/global**.

Cengage Learning products are represented in Canada by Nelson Education, Ltd.

To learn more about Cengage Learning Solutions, visit **www.cengage.com**.

Purchase any of our products at your local college store or at our preferred online store **www.cengagebrain.com**.

Printed in the United States of America

Print Number: 01   Print Year: 2015

To my mom, my first counselor

About the Author

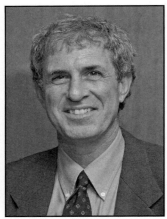

Born and raised in New York City, Dr. Edward Neukrug obtained his B.A. in psychology from SUNY Binghamton, his M.S. in counseling from Miami University of Ohio, and his doctorate in counselor education from the University of Cincinnati. Dr. Neukrug is a National Certified Counselor (NCC), Licensed Professional Counselor (LPC), Human Services Board Certified Practitioner (HS–BCP), and Licensed Psychologist.

After teaching and directing a graduate program in counseling at Notre Dame College in New Hampshire, he accepted a position at Old Dominion University, in Norfolk, Virginia, where he currently is a Professor of Counseling and Human Services and former Chair of the Department of Educational Leadership and Counseling. In addition to teaching, Dr. Neukrug has worked as a substance abuse counselor, a counselor at a crisis center, an outpatient therapist at a mental health center, an associate school psychologist, a school counselor, and as a private-practice psychologist and LPC.

Dr. Neukrug has held a variety of positions in local, regional, and national professional associations in counseling and human services. In addition, he has received a number of grants and contracts with school systems and professional associations. He has received numerous honors and awards, including being designated a University Professor at Old Dominion University in recognition of his teaching, research, and professional services. He has been a speaker on numerous radio and TV shows, including WBAI in New York City, and National Public Radio.

Dr. Neukrug has written over 70 articles and chapters in books and has presented at dozens of conferences. In addition to *The World of the Counselor*, he has published eight books: *Counseling Theory and Practice; The Sage Encyclopedia of Theory in Counseling and Psychotherapy; Experiencing the World of the Counselor: A Workbook for Counselor Educators and Students* (4th ed.); *Theory, Practice, and Trends in Human Services: An Introduction to an Emerging Profession* (5th ed.); *Skills and Techniques for Human Service Professionals; Skills and Tools for Today's Counselors and Psychotherapists; Essentials of Testing and Assessment for Counselors, Social Workers, and Psychologists* (3rd ed.); and *Brief Orientation to Counseling: Professional Identity, History, and Standards*. He has also developed a DVD that illustrates major theories of counseling and another that demonstrates important counseling skills and techniques.

In addition to his books, Dr. Neukrug has been developing Great Therapists of the Twentieth Century (www.odu.edu/~eneukrug), an interactive and animated website where you can "meet" some of the major theorists of counseling and psychotherapy and learn more about them and their theories. He has also developed an interactive survey where you can identify your view of human nature and examine which school of therapy it is closest to (http://ww2.odu.edu/~eneukrug/therapists/survey.html).

Dr. Neukrug is married to Kristina Williams Neukrug. They have two children, Hannah and Emma.

Brief Contents

---

* Chapters 13 and 16 are co-written by Christina Hamme Peterson and Emily Goodman-Scott respectively, both of whom are the lead authors.

Contents

SECTION 2
The Helping Relationship I:
Theories and Skills   97

CHAPTER 4: Individual Approaches to
Counseling   99

Preface

Purpose of Text

They brought the fireman (now firefighter) to my school. I wanted to be just like him. They brought the policeman (now police officer)—that's a pretty fun job, I thought. My father, a building contractor, came and talked about building bridges. I was very proud. Maybe I would be a building contractor. The doctor, of course, was very impressive also. But they didn't bring the counselor. In fact, few of us knew about counselors—what they did, who they were. Despite this, I became one. And now I want the world to know who they are and what they do. That is what this book is about.

After teaching for over thirty years, I have found that new students have a deep desire and longing to be counselors. I have also found that they have only a narrow knowledge of the counseling profession. It has been my experience that most students understand the importance of listening to a person who is experiencing distress, but they know little of the broad knowledge needed to be a counselor or the important professional, ethical, and cross-cultural issues that underlie so much of what counselors do. Thus, the purpose of this book is to enlighten students concerning the depth of the counseling profession so they can make an informed decision about whether they want to enter it and to help them begin their journey as a professional counselor with important knowledge and skills.

Since publication of the first four editions of *The World of the Counselor*, many reviewers, faculty, and students have remarked that the text is one of the most comprehensive, yet readable, of its kind. Often, faculty and students have suggested that it is a book that could be used when studying for comprehensive exams or when taking a certification or licensing exam. In revising the text, I have attempted to maintain its comprehensiveness. In addition, I have updated information to ensure accuracy and relevance and have increasingly added ways for you to electronically access information (e.g., URLs).

Organization of the Text

The text presents an overview of the counseling profession by offering relevant content, vignettes, and think pieces for students to ponder. The book loosely follows the common-core curriculum guidelines of the *Council for Accreditation of Counseling and Related Programs (CACREP):* (1) professional orientation and ethical practice, (2) social and cultural diversity, (3) human growth and development, (4) career development, (5) helping relationships, (6) group work, (7) assessment, and (8) research and program evaluation (see www.cacrep.org). The text also offers specific content in the specialty areas of clinical mental health counseling, school counseling, and student affairs and college counseling (postsecondary counseling). Adhering to the CACREP-accredited common-core areas ensures that the text complies with standards in the profession and offers the student a broad knowledge base.

The book is separated into seven sections and an Afterword. In writing the text, I have attempted to weave all eight common-core areas listed above into the first six sections, with the seventh section spotlighting the three specialty areas that students commonly enter: school counseling, clinical mental health counseling, and student affairs and college counseling (postsecondary counseling). The Afterword offers tips for applying to master's or doctoral programs and for applying for a job.

Sections and Afterword

Section I: Professional Orientation. The section encompasses much of the content highlighted in the CACREP common-core curriculum guideline, "Professional Orientation and Ethical Practice," and more. There are three chapters in this section:

Chapter 1:   The Counselor's Identity: What, Who, and How?
Chapter 2:   The Counseling Profession's Past, Present, and Future
Chapter 3:   Standards in the Profession: Ethics, Accreditation, Credentialing, and Multicultural/Social Justice Competencies

Section II: The Helping Relationship I: Theories and Skills. Section II loosely follows the CACREP common-core curriculum guideline "Helping Relationships," although "consultation" and "systems perspective," which are listed under this guideline, are covered in Section III. The two chapters in this section are:

Chapter 4:   Individual Approaches to Counseling
Chapter 5:   Counseling Skills

Section III: The Helping Relationship II: The Counselor Working in Systems. This section draws from a number of CACREP curriculum guidelines that address counseling within systems. This section includes couples and family counseling, which draws from the CACREP common-core guidelines on systems located in "Helping Relationships" and from the specialty guidelines on "Marriage, Couple, and Family Counseling"; group work, which is noted in the CACREP common-core curriculum guideline "Group Work"; consultation, which is addressed in the "Helping Relationships" common core area; and supervision, which is addressed in the CACREP common-core curriculum guideline "Professional Orientation and Ethical Practices." The three chapters in this section are:

Chapter 6:   Couples and Family Counseling
Chapter 7:   Group Work
Chapter 8:   Consultation and Supervision

Section IV: The Development of the Person. The broad spectrum of human development issues in counseling are examined in this section. Loosely following two of the CACREP common-core curriculum guidelines, "Human Growth and Development" and "Career Development," the following three chapters are included:

Chapter 9:   Development Across the Lifespan
Chapter 10:   Abnormal Development, Diagnosis, and Psychopharmacology

Chapter 11:   Career Development: The Counselor and the World of Work

Section V: Research, Program Evaluation, and Assessment. This section is based on the CACREP common-core curriculum guidelines "Research and Program Evaluation" and "Assessment." The two chapters in this section are:

Chapter 12:   Testing and Assessment
Chapter 13:   Research and Evaluation

Section VI: Social and Cultural Foundations in Counseling. This section loosely follows the CACREP common-core curriculum guideline "Social and Cultural Diversity." The two chapters included in this section are:

Chapter 14:   Theory and Concepts of Multicultural Counseling
Chapter 15:   Knowledge and Skills of Multicultural Counseling

Section VII: Select Specialty Areas in Counseling. This final section examines the three most popular specialty areas in counseling: school counseling, clinical mental health counseling, and student affairs and college counseling or postsecondary counseling. Each of these chapters provides history, defines roles and functions, presents theory and practice issues, and provides the counselor with specific examples of what it's like to work in each of these specialty areas. Places of employment and potential salaries are also given. The section includes the following chapters:

Chapter 16:   School Counseling
Chapter 17:   Clinical Mental Health Counseling
Chapter 18:   Student Affairs and College Counseling (Postsecondary Counseling)

Afterword. The Afterword provides students with tips on how to get into master's and doctoral programs in counselor education and related fields and how to apply for jobs in the helping professions.

A Focus on Multicultural and Social Justice Issues, Ethical, Professional, and Legal Issues, and "The Counselor in Process"

The counseling profession has zeroed in on the importance of understanding the critical knowledge and skills related to multicultural counseling and social justice and has also focused on the importance of acting ethically, professionally, and legally. Thus, at the end of each chapter, you will find a section that highlights multicultural and social justice issues and another section that focuses on important ethical, professional, and legal issues related to that chapter's content. Finally, I conclude each chapter with "The Counselor in Process," a section that stresses how the self-reflective counselor who is willing to risk changing might deal with issues related to the chapter content.

Pedagogical Aids

Filled with material that highlights the content of each chapter in the text, the *World of the Counselor* includes the following:

1. Personal vignettes from the author and co-authors concerning their experiences in the field of counseling and in related professional fields
2. Vignettes that highlight specific chapter content
3. Testimonials from individuals in the field about their work
4. Experiential exercises that are peppered throughout the text that students can do in class or at home
5. References to websites that can highlight specific course content
6. Tables and graphs that elaborate what is in the chapter content
7. For the instructor, numerous instructional aids (for more information, see the section "Ancillaries to the Text," later in this preface)

Specific Changes to This Edition

If you've seen past revisions of this text, you'll know that I do not take a revision lightly. Thus, to keep the content updated and to improve the quality of the text, there have been numerous changes to each chapter in the book; if you were to compare this text to the last edition, you would see some substantial differences between parallel chapters. The following describes some of these changes.

Since there is a section at the conclusion of each chapter in the book that addresses ethical concerns, many of these sections had to be substantially updated to reflect the new ethics code of the American Counseling Association (ACA) developed in 2014. In addition, since there have been changes to the accreditation standards of CACREP, chapters that addressed accreditation, particularly the chapters in the first section of the book ("Professional Orientation") and the chapters in the last section of the book ("Select Specialty Areas in Counseling"), needed to reflect such changes. Also, in 2013, the fifth edition of the *Diagnostic and Statistical Manual* was published (DSM-5). Since diagnosis is touched on in a number of chapters, I ensured that all material relative to DSM reflected the new DSM-5. In particular, I had to revamp a large section of Chapter 10, since it gives an overview of DSM-5.

Other important changes included revamping the section on the roles and functions of clinical mental health counselors (Chapter 17) and of postsecondary counselors (Chapter 18). With significant changes in credentialing, licensing laws, and the nature of the workplace, I thought that the roles and functions of these professionals had deepened and broadened, thus demanding important changes to these chapters.

Although years ago I had been a part-time school counselor, and even though my wife is an elementary school counselor, I felt that I was not close enough to this important specialty area to do it justice. Thus, I asked a colleague of mine, Dr. Emily Goodman-Scott, if she would revise Chapter 16. Emily has recently moved into academia and is already well networked within the school counseling professional associations. Her expertise in school counseling is admirable, and I asked her to update this important chapter. I think you will find that the chapter fully covers cutting-edge knowledge relative to school counseling, particularly the national model of the American School Counselor Association (ASCA) and the establishment of comprehensive school counseling programs (CSCPs).

With every revision, one or two chapters are always particularly challenging. For me, Chapter 8, on consultation and supervision, is one of those. Every time I revise it, I work feverishly to make this chapter a bit more cutting-edge, more readable, and somewhat less bulky—yes, I actually try to *reduce* the amount of information. I think you'll find it concise and interesting.

The other chapter that I often find challenging when revising this text is Chapter 13, which covers research and evaluation. I always struggle with presenting this chapter in a readable, focused, and interesting manner. Since writing the last edition, I have conducted research with a colleague from Ryder College, Christina Hamme Peterson. Because she is such an expert on research and evaluation, I thought she might be able to contribute a crisper viewpoint on these important subject areas. I think you'll find that she succeeded admirably, as the chapter is extremely well written and now covers some important areas that were lacking in the last edition.

The above includes some of the major changes, but in addition, many other revisions were made. For instance, I always look to streamline information; thus, when revising the text, I ask myself questions such as "Is this really important?" "Do students actually need to know about this?" and so forth. So I eliminated some information that I thought was not necessary (and, of course, added new information when needed). Needless to say, any revision entails updating references, revising and reconfiguring charts and tables, and working on making sentences, paragraphs, and chapters more readable.

Finally, at the end of each chapter, you will see a reference to CengageBrain. On CengageBrain, you'll find CourseMate tailored to this text that has assessment exercises, vignettes, and experiential exercises that reflect each chapter's content, and students can respond to these activities and later discuss them in class. If you are participating in CourseMate, you may be assigned these activities. I think you'll find them interesting, educational, and fun. Similarly, I have uploaded a workbook called Experiencing the World of the Counselor on CourseMate. This workbook has dozens of activities that correspond with each chapter's course content, and your instructor may select some exercises for you to do at home or in class.

Ancillaries to the Text
For Students

Cengage Learning's CourseMate brings course concepts to life with interactive learning, study, and exam preparation tools that support the printed textbook. CourseMate includes an integrated eBook, glossaries, flashcards, quizzes, video activities, workbook activities, downloadable PDF of *Experiencing the World of the Counselor* and more-as well as Engagement Tracker, a first-of-its-kind tool that monitors student engagement in the course. CourseMate is available with the text.

For the Instructor

1. ***Experiencing the World of the Counselor***. This companion book can be downloaded by students and faculty on CourseMate. In it, you will find dozens of exercises and activities that can enhance student learning that coincide with chapters in the text.
2. **Online PowerPoint**®. These vibrant Microsoft® PowerPoint® lecture slides for each chapter assist you with your lecture by providing concept coverage using images, figures, and tables directly from the textbook.
3. **Online Test Bank**. For assessment support, the updated test bank includes true/ false, multiple-choice, matching, short answer, and essay questions for each chapter.
4. **Online Instructor's Manual**. The Instructor's Manual (IM) contains a variety of re- sources to aid instructors in preparing and presenting text material in a manner that meets their personal preferences and course needs. It presents chapter-by-chapter suggestions and resources to enhance and facilitate learning.

II. Web Sites to Enhance Learning

Over the years, I have developed a number of websites to assist with learning various topics. These include the following:

1. *Great Therapists of the Twentieth Century:* This animated website introduces you to about twenty famous therapists of the twentieth century, with whom you can inter- act and learn important information. The site should be viewed on Google Chrome or on a Safari browser. Go to http://www.odu.edu/~eneukrug/gttc/.
2. *Survey of Your Theoretical Orientation:* This 72-item survey allows students to com- pare their theoretical orientation to a number of well-known therapeutic approaches and schools of therapy (psychodynamic, cognitive-behavioral, existential-humanistic, postmodern). Go to http://www.odu.edu/~eneukrug/therapists/booksurvey.html.
3. *Stories of the Great Therapists:* This website has short, select stories about a number of famous therapists of the twentieth century. Go to: http://www.odu.edu /~eneukrug/therapists/index.html.
4. *Galton's Board:* This website presents a version of Galton's Board, a computer- generated normal curve where students can ponder the nature of normal curves and statistical probability.

Acknowledgments

This book could not have been completed without the help of a number of people from Cengage. First, a special thanks to Julie Martinez, Product Manager for Counseling and

Human Services, who has been extremely supportive in the revision of this book and all my books. Thank you, Julie! Vernon Boes, Senior Art Director, played a critical part in the development of the wonderful new cover design and other artwork. Brittani Morgan, Intellectual Property Project Manager, was great to work with as we struggled to get all the artwork, pictures, and other materials in on time. Kyra Kane, Associate Content Developer, worked closely with me on the development of ancillaries for the book. And finally, thanks to Deanna Ettinger, Intellectual Property Analyst, and Ruth Sakata Corley, Senior Content Project Manager, both of whom ensured that the book was on schedule.

Many others associated with Cengage were also critical to the completion of this project. Teresa Christie at MPS Limited was Project Manager and worked very closely and diligently with me to finish this book. She was great. Thanks, Teresa! Lori Bradshaw, Developmental Production Editor at S4 Carlisle Publisher Services, was always there to ensure that the book was on track and that things went smoothly. Lynn Lustberg, who filled in briefly as Project Manager, was extremely helpful. Veerabhagu Nagarajan, Associate Project Manager from Image Research & Permissions for Lumina Datamatics, was critical in securing the artwork and pictures in the text. Finally, thanks to Sue McClung, the copy editor, who worked hard to make sure that *The World of the Counselor* was accurate and readable. Thanks so much.

A book like this tends to go through a number of faculty reviews, and in this case, I have the following faculty to thank for reviewing parts or all of the text. Their time and effort are sincerely appreciated. Thanks go to David Kleist, Idaho State University–Pocatello; Kristopher Goodrich, University of New Mexico; Thomas McLure, Faulkner University Birmingham; Jason K. Neill, Colorado Christian University.

A very special thanks for the hard work of Christina Hamme Peterson and Emily Goodman-Scott for their revisions to Chapters 13 and 16, respectively. Their efforts have made these chapters considerably stronger. In addition, I would like to send special thanks to Gina Polychronopoulos, whose work on the PowerPoints, Test Questions, and Glossary were essential to the final version of this book. Thanks, Gina!

Overview

The first section of this book offers an overview of important professional issues in the field of counseling. A common theme running through Chapters 1 through 3 is how the counseling profession has developed its unique professional identity. This topic is explored by looking at how we are the same, as well as how we are different from other mental health professionals. This is done by examining our unique history and by describing the standards of our profession.

Chapter 1 defines counseling and distinguishes it from related fields such as guidance and psychotherapy. This chapter compares different kinds of mental health professionals who do counseling, and it concludes by examining the characteristics of an effective counselor. Chapter 2 reviews the history of the counseling profession, tracing it from the distant past, through the beginnings of the mental health field, to the current status of the profession. It also offers us a glimpse into its future. Chapter 3 explores the development and implementation of four important standards in the counseling profession: ethics, accreditation, credentialing, and multicultural/social justice competencies.

At the conclusion of every chapter in the book, chapter content is tied in with important multicultural/social justice issues; ethical, professional, and legal issues; and, in a section called "The Counselor in Process," issues of how the counselor lives as a person and professional in the world.

CHAPTER 1

The Counselor's Identity: What, Who, and How?

. . . counseling has proven to be a difficult concept to explain. The public's lack of clarity is due, in part, to the proliferation of modern-day practitioners who have adopted the counselor label. They range from credit counselors to investment counselors, and from camp counselors to retirement counselors. Although their services share the common ingredient of verbal communication, and possibly the intention to be helpful, those services have little in common with … [psychological counseling].

(Hackney & Cormier, 2013, p. 2)

Sometimes as a child, I would have a temper tantrum, and my mother would say, "I just don't understand why you get so angry; maybe I should take you to see a counselor." This threat intimated that there was something terribly wrong with me, and perhaps, in some way, also showed her love for and desire to understand and help me.

I used to wonder what it would be like to see a counselor. It couldn't be a good thing if my mom was using it as a threat, I thought! On the other hand, maybe counseling would be a place where I could talk to someone who understood me, someone who could understand my moods, moods that felt normal to me yet were being defined as being wrong, or kind of abnormal. Maybe seeing a counselor would be okay. In fact, maybe a counselor would say I was normal! But what exactly would a counselor do, I wondered?

Thankfully, over the years I've had the opportunity to be in counseling. And, irony of all ironies, I became a counselor. Well, maybe my mom intuited early that I was going to be intimately involved in counseling in one way or another!

This chapter is about defining the words *counseling* and *counselor*. First, I will highlight the word *counseling* and distinguish it from related words such as *guidance* and *psychotherapy*. Then I will compare and contrast counselors with other mental health professionals who do counseling. Next, I will examine the characteristics of an effective helper.

As we near the end of the chapter, I will provide an overview of the various professional associations in the counseling field, with particular emphasis on the American Counseling Association (ACA). I will conclude the chapter by highlighting the importance of multicultural issues in the field of counseling and by focusing on ethical, professional, and legal issues that apply to counselors.

Guidance, Counseling, and Psychotherapy: Variations on the Same Theme?

Counseling is a professional relationship that empowers diverse individuals, families, and groups to accomplish mental health, wellness, education, and career goals.

(ACA, 2013a, para. 2)

This statement, recently endorsed by a wide range of counseling associations, took a long time coming, as over the years, the word *counseling* has not been easily defined. In fact, for years there have been differing opinions about what counseling is and how to distinguish it from guidance and psychotherapy. Let me offer some of my own associations with these words, and see if they match your own. For instance, when I hear the word *psychotherapy*, I think of the following words: *deep, dark, secretive, sexual, unconscious, pain, hidden, long-term,* and *reconstructive.* The word *counseling* makes me think of *short-term, facilitative, here and now, change, problem solving, being heard,* and awareness. And lastly, *guidance* makes me think of *advice, direction, on the surface, advocacy,* and *support.* Did these associations ring true for you? Now, let's look at how the literature has defined these words.

Over the years, counseling has been defined in a variety of ways suggesting that it could be anything from a problem-solving, directive, and rational approach to helping normal people—an approach that is distinguishable from psychotherapy (Williamson, 1950, 1958); to a process that is similar to but less intensive than psychotherapy (Nugent & Jones, 2009); to an approach that suggests that there is no essential difference between the two (Neukrug, 2011).

Some of the confusion among these words rests in their historical roots. The word *guidance* first appeared around the 1600s and was defined as "the process of guiding an individual." Early guidance work involved individuals giving moralistic and direct advice. This definition continued into the twentieth century, when vocational guidance counselors used the word to describe the act of "guiding" an individual into a profession and offering suggestions for life skills. Meanwhile, with the development of psychoanalysis near the end of the nineteenth century, came the word *psychotherapy.* Meaning "caring for the soul," the word was derived from the Greek words *psyche,* meaning spirit or soul, and *therapeutikos,* meaning caring for another (Kleinke, 1994).

During the early part of the twentieth century, vocational guidance counselors became increasingly dissatisfied with the word *guidance* and its heavy emphasis on advice giving and morality. Consequently, the word *counseling* was adopted to indicate that vocational counselors, like the psychoanalysts who practiced psychotherapy, dealt with social and emotional issues. As mental health workers became more prevalent during the mid-1900s, they too adopted the word *counseling* rather than use the word *guidance,* with its moralistic implications, or *psychotherapy,* which was increasingly associated with psychoanalysis. Tyler (1969) stated that "those who participated in the mental health movement and had no connection with vocational guidance used the word counseling to refer to what others were calling [psycho]therapy . . ." (p. 12).

In the training of counselors today, the word *guidance* has tended to take a back seat to the word *counseling,* while the words *counseling* and *psychotherapy* are generally used

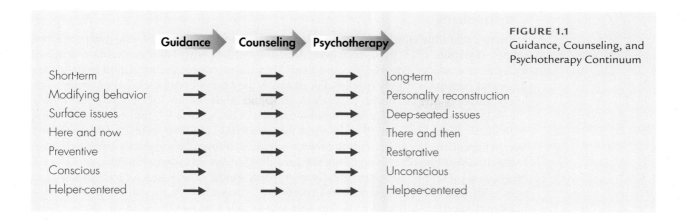

FIGURE 1.1
Guidance, Counseling, and Psychotherapy Continuum

interchangeably in textbooks. Examine most texts that describe theories of counseling and compare them to a text that describes theories of psychotherapy, and you will find them to be nearly identical. In other words, theories of counseling and psychotherapy are indistinguishable. In fact, both words often are in the title. For example, C. H. Patterson noted in his very popular text, *Theories of Counseling and Psychotherapy*, that ". . . counseling and psychotherapy are both used in the title of this book because it appears to be impossible to make any clear distinction between them" (Patterson, 1986, p. xvii). In a similar vein, Corey (2013), the author of one of the best-known text on theories of counseling and psychotherapy, simply does not address the issue, choosing to use the words interchangeably.

Despite the lack of distinction made in most texts, a differentiation between counseling and psychotherapy is likely to be made by the average person, perhaps by many counseling students, and even by professors of counseling. Acknowledging this common usage, one model of understanding these terms would place *guidance* and *psychotherapy* on opposite extremes, with *counseling* falling somewhere in the middle of the continuum (see Figure 1.1).

Comparison of Mental Health Professionals

Whether we call it *guidance*, *counseling*, or *psychotherapy*, in today's world we find a number of professionals practicing it. In fact, although differences in the training of mental health professionals exist, over the years their professional duties have begun to overlap (Todd & Bohart, 2006). For instance, many school counselors do mental health counseling; counseling and clinical psychologists do educational consultation; psychiatrists do counseling; social workers and others practice psychoanalysis; mental health counselors do family therapy; and some psychologists can prescribe psychotropic medications (Rinaldi, 2013). Let's examine some of the similarities and differences among various professionals, including counselors, social workers, psychologists, psychiatrists, psychoanalysts, psychiatric mental health nurses, psychiatrists, human service practitioners, and psychotherapists.

Counselors

For many years, the word *counselor* simply referred to any "professional who practices counseling" (Chaplin, 1975, p. 5). However, most individuals who call themselves counselors today have a master's degree in counseling. These days, counselors are found in many settings and perform a variety of roles. For instance, they may serve as school counselors, college counselors, mental health counselors, substance abuse counselors, couples and family counselors, and so forth. The counselor's training is broad, and we find counselors doing individual, group, and family counseling; administering and interpreting educational and psychological assessments; offering career counseling; administering grants and conducting research; consulting on a broad range of educational and psychological matters; supervising others; and presenting developmentally appropriate guidance activities for individuals of all ages. Although not all counselors are experts in psychopathology, they do have knowledge of mental disorders and know when to refer individuals who need more in-depth treatment.

Although there are many different kinds of counselors, all tend to have had common coursework in professional orientation and ethical practice, social and cultural diversity, human growth and development, career development, the helping relationship, group work, assessment, and research and program evaluation. In addition to these common core areas, counselors generally have had coursework in a counseling specialty area, which might include classes in the history, roles and functions, and knowledge and skills of that specialty area. Finally, all counselors have had the opportunity to practice their acquired skills and knowledge at field placements, such as a practicum or internship.

Today, most counseling programs at the master's level offer degrees in one or more of the specialty areas recognized by the accrediting body for counseling programs, the Council for the Accreditation of Counseling and Related Educational Programs (CACREP; discussed further in Chapter 3). These include school counseling; clinical mental health counseling; marriage, couple, and family counseling; addiction counseling; career counseling; and student affairs and college counseling. Rehabilitation counseling is accredited by a separate body, the Council on Rehabilitation Education (CORE), and follows similar curriculum guidelines to those above, with an added emphasis on courses related to working with individuals with disabilities. However, a joint accrediting effort between CACREP and CORE is currently underway. Not all programs use the exact names that CACREP suggests, and some programs offer specialty areas outside of those delineated by CACREP. However, most programs will offer a core curriculum and field work similar to that noted above.

All counselors can take an exam to become a National Certified Counselor (NCC) that is offered by the National Board for Certified Counselors (NBCC, 2014a, 2014b). NBCC also offers subspecialty certifications in clinical mental health counseling, school counseling, and addiction counseling. In addition, all 50 states, Puerto Rico, and the District of Columbia have established licensing laws that allow a counselor who has a master's degree in counseling, additional training, and supervision to practice as a Licensed Professional Counselor (LPC); some states use a related term (ACA, 2012a). Whereas certification is generally seen as mastery of a content area, licensure allows counselors to practice independently and obtain third-party reimbursement for their practice (an in-depth discussion of credentialing can be found in Chapter 3). The professional association for counselors, the ACA, currently has 20 divisions that focus on a variety of counseling specialty areas (a further discussion of ACA and its divisions is provided later in this chapter).

While keeping in mind that a person with a master's degree in counseling is primarily a counselor and secondarily a school counselor, mental health counselor, or a counselor in some other specialty area, the following are brief descriptions of some of the more prevalent counseling specialty areas.

School Counselors

A *school counselor* has a master's degree in counseling and a specialty in school counseling. Some states credential school counselors on the elementary, middle, and secondary levels, while other states offer credentialing that covers kindergarten through twelfth grade (K–12). Today, the majority of school counseling programs are CACREP accredited, which currently requires a minimum of 48-credit hours. The professional association for school counselors is the American School Counselor Association (ASCA), which is a division of ACA, although one can become a member of ASCA without joining ACA. In recent years, the ASCA National Model has been used as a model for the training of school counselors (see Chapter 16). In addition, over the past few decades, there has been a push by professional training programs, professional associations, and many in the field to replace the term *guidance counselor* with *school counselor*, as the latter term is seen as deemphasizing the guidance activities of the school counselor (Baker & Gerler, 2008). Individuals who go through a CACREP-accredited school counseling program can become NCCs, and in most states, with additional coursework, they can obtain their LPC as well.

Clinical Mental Health Counselors

A *clinical mental health counselor* is an individual who has obtained his or her degree in clinical mental health counseling or a closely related degree in counseling (e.g., agency counseling). Although in the recent past the CACREP standards supported a 48- and then a 54-credit clinical mental health counseling program (sometimes called *agency* or *community counseling*), CACREP's current standards support a 60-credit clinical mental health counseling degree. Although not all programs are CACREP accredited, individuals who obtain a degree in clinical mental health counseling or related degrees are generally trained to conduct counseling or psychotherapy for those who are struggling with life problems, emotional issues, or mental health disorders. They are usually found working in a wide variety of agencies or conducting counseling and psychotherapy in private practice. The clinical mental health counselors' professional association is the American Mental Health Counselors Association (AMHCA), which is a division of ACA, although one can now be a member of AMHCA without joining ACA. Individuals who have a CACREP-accredited master's degree in clinical mental health counseling often become NCCs and LPCs.

Marriage, Couple, and Family Counselors

Marriage, couple, and family counselors are specifically trained to work with couples and with family systems and can be found in a vast array of agency settings and in private practice. These counselors tend to have specialty coursework in systems dynamics, couples counseling, family therapy, family life stages, and human sexuality, along with the more traditional coursework in the helping professions. The American Association of Marriage and Family

Therapists (AAMFT) is one professional association for marriage and family counselors; another is the International Association of Marriage and Family Counselors (IAMFC, n.d.). IAMFC is a division of ACA, although one can join IAMFC without joining ACA.

Although all 50 states and the District of Columbia have some requirement for marriage and family licensure, the requirements can vary dramatically (Association of Marital and Family Therapy Regulatory Boards, 2014). While some states license marriage and family counselors who have studied from programs that follow the curriculum guidelines set forth by AAMFT'S Commission on Accreditation of Marriage and Family Therapy Education (COAMFTE), other states prefer licensing counselors who have studied from programs that follow the 60-credit CACREP guidelines for marriage, couple, and family counseling, and still others have set their own curriculum guidelines for credentialing. Most states that offer marriage, couple, and family counselor credentialing allow helping professionals with related degrees (e.g., counseling, social work, psychology) to also practice marriage and family counseling, so long as they follow the curriculum guidelines set forth by the state and abide by any additional requirements for credentialing. Individuals who go through a CACREP-accredited marriage, couples, and family counseling program can become NCCs, and in most states, with additional coursework, they can obtain their LPC.

Student Affairs and College Counselors

Student affairs and college counselors (post-secondary counseling) work in a variety of settings in higher education, including college counseling centers, career centers, residence life, student advising services, multicultural student services, and other campus settings where counseling-related activities occur. Usually, these counselors will have taken specialty coursework in college student development and student affairs practices and may have attended a 48-credit, CACREP-accredited program. There are two main professional associations of counselors in higher education settings: College Student Educators International (this organization was formerly the American College Personnel Association and has kept the acronym ACPA), which tends to focus on administration of student services; and the American College Counseling Association (ACCA), which is a division of ACA and tends to focus on counseling issues in college settings. Today, one can join ACCA without joining ACA. Individuals who go through a CACREP-accredited student affairs and college counseling program can become NCCs, and in most states, with additional coursework, they can obtain their LPC.

Addiction Counselors

Addiction counselors study a wide range of addiction disorders, such as substance abuse (drugs and alcohol), eating disorders, and sexual addiction. They are familiar with diagnosis and treatment planning, and they understand the importance of psychopharmacology in working with this population. Today, CACREP offers a 60-credit accreditation in addiction counseling. In addition to AMHCA, addiction counselors often belong to the International Association of Addictions and Offender Counselors (IAAOC), which is also a division of ACA. Many addiction counselors can become certified through their state, and NBCC offers a national certification as a Master Addiction Counselor (MAC). Individuals who go through a CACREP-accredited addiction counseling program can become NCCs, and in most states, with additional coursework, they can obtain their LPC.

Rehabilitation Counselors

Rehabilitation counselors offer a wide range of services to people with physical, emotional, and developmental disabilities. "Rehab" counselors work in state vocational rehabilitation agencies, unemployment offices, or private rehabilitation agencies. CORE is the accrediting body for rehabilitation counseling programs, although CACREP's 2016 standards may also have an accreditation process for rehabilitation programs. Currently, the curriculum in rehabilitation counseling programs largely parallels CACREP-approved programs and also includes specialty coursework in such areas as vocational evaluation, occupational analysis, medical and psychosocial aspects of disability, legal and ethical issues in rehabilitation, and the history of rehabilitation counseling. Recently, CACREP and CORE developed an agreement to allow select CORE-accredited programs to also obtain accreditation as clinical mental health counseling programs (CACREP, 2014a). Many rehabilitation counselors join the National Rehabilitation Counseling Association (NRCA), the American Rehabilitation Counseling Association (ARCA), a division of ACA, or both. Today, one can join ARCA without joining ACA. Rehabilitation counselors can become NCCs, or with additional coursework, LPCs; however, many choose to become Certified Rehabilitation Counselors (CRCs) through a certification process offered by the Commission on Rehabilitation Counselor Certification (CRCC).

Pastoral Counselors

Pastoral counselors sometimes have a degree in counseling but can also have a degree in a related social service, or even just a master's degree in religion or divinity. Pastoral counselors sometimes work in private practice or within a religious association. Pastoral counselors, religious counselors, or counselors with a spiritual orientation might join the Association for Spiritual, Ethical, and Religious Values in Counseling (ASERVIC), a division of ACA, the American Association of Pastoral Counselors (AAPC), or both. AAPC offers a certification process for those who are interested in becoming Certified Pastoral Counselors (CPC). Depending on their degree, pastoral counselors may be able to become NCCs, and in some states, LPCs.

Social Workers

Although the term *social worker* can apply to those who have an undergraduate or a graduate degree in social work or a related field (e.g., human services), the term has recently become more associated with those who have acquired a master's degree in social work (MSW). Whereas social workers traditionally have been found working with the underprivileged and with family and social systems, today's social workers provide counseling and psychotherapy for all types of clients in a wide variety of settings, including child welfare services, government-supported social service agencies, family service agencies, private practices, and hospitals.

Training as an MSW in many ways parallels training as a counselor, although differences in the history of these fields leads social work and counseling programs to emphasize different areas of the helping relationship (see Chapter 2). With additional training and supervision, social workers can become nationally certified by the Academy of

Certified Social Workers (ACSW). In addition, most states have specific requirements for becoming a Licensed Clinical Social Worker (LCSW). The professional association for social workers is the National Association of Social Workers (NASW).

Psychologists

Psychologists practice in a wide range of settings, including agencies, private practice, health maintenance organizations (HMOs), universities, business and industry, prisons, and schools. Although counselors will generally have the most contact with *counseling psychologists*, *clinical psychologists*, and *school psychologists*, there are many other types of psychologists, including cognitive and perceptual, community, developmental, educational, engineering, environmental, experimental, industrial/organizational, neuro, quantitative, social, and sports (APA, 2013a). The professional association for psychologists is the American Psychological Association (APA).

Relative to the practice of psychotherapy, all states offer licensure in counseling, clinical psychology, or both, and many states allow individuals with a "Psy.D.," a practitioner doctorate in psychology, to become licensed as clinical or counseling psychologists. Whereas clinical psychologists have historically focused more on working with individuals with severe emotional disorders, counseling psychologists have worked with relatively healthy populations. Today, however, the different foci of counseling and clinical psychologists have become increasingly blurred. To obtain a license as a counseling or clinical psychologist, one must graduate from an APA-accredited doctoral program in clinical or counseling psychology and complete additional requirements identified by state licensing boards. The professional association for clinical psychologists is Division 12 of the APA and, for counseling psychologists, *Division 17 of the APA*. Division 17 is the division of APA that is most closely aligned with the goals and mission of counselors.

School psychologists have a master's or doctoral degree in school psychology and are licensed by state boards of education. Their work involves helping children succeed academically, and to accomplish this, they work with children, families, teachers, school counselors, school administrators, community partners, and others (NASP, n.d.). A large portion of their work involves testing and assessment and helping students address their social and emotional health. Although most school psychologists work in schools, you can sometimes find them in private practice, in agencies, and in hospital settings. The professional associations for school psychologists are the National Association of School Psychologists (NASP) and Division 16 of the APA.

Psychiatrists

A *psychiatrist* is a licensed physician who generally has completed a residency in psychiatry, meaning that in addition to medical school, he or she has completed extensive field placement training in a mental health setting. In addition, most psychiatrists have passed an exam to become *board certified* in psychiatry. Being a physician, the psychiatrist has expertise in diagnosing organic disorders, identifying and treating psychopathology, and prescribing medications for psychiatric conditions. Although two states and some branches of the federal government have granted psychologists prescription privileges for psychotropic medications (Rinaldi, 2013), currently it is psychiatrists (and in some cases psychiatric nurses) who take the lead in this important treatment approach.

Because psychiatrists often have minimal training in the broad array of delivery methods of counseling offered in graduate school for counselors, social workers, and psychologists, they are sometimes not seen as experts in counseling and psychotherapeutic services. Psychiatrists are employed in mental health agencies, hospitals, private practice settings, and health maintenance organizations. The professional association for psychiatrists is the American Psychiatric Association.

Psychoanalysts

Psychoanalysts are professionals who have received training in psychoanalysis from a number of recognized psychoanalytical institutes. Although in past years, the American Psychoanalytic Association (APsaA), the professional association of psychoanalysts, would only endorse psychiatrists for training at psychoanalytical institutes (Turkington, 1985), they now allow other mental health professionals to undergo training (APsaA, 2012). Because states do not license psychoanalysts, clients who are seeing a psychoanalyst should make sure that the analyst was trained at an institute sanctioned by the APsaA and that he or she is also a licensed psychiatrist, psychologist, social worker, counselor, or related mental health professional.

Psychiatric–Mental Health Nurses

Primarily trained as medical professionals, *psychiatric–mental health nurses (PMHNs)* are also skilled in the delivery of mental health services (APNA, n.d.a). The professional association of PMHNs is the American Psychiatric Nurses Association (APNA). Most PMHNs work in hospital settings, with fewer of them working in community agencies, private practice, or educational settings. Psychiatric–mental health nursing is practiced at two levels. The Registered Nurse–PMHN does basic mental health work related to nursing diagnosis and nursing care. The Advanced Practiced Registered Nurse (APRN) has a master's degree in psychiatric–mental health nursing and assesses, diagnoses, and treats individuals with mental health problems. Currently holding prescriptive privileges in all 50 states (Von Gizycki, 2013), APRNs hold a unique position in the mental health profession.

Creative and Expressive Therapists

Creative and expressive therapists include art therapists, play therapists, dance/movement therapists, poetry therapists, music therapists, and others who use creative tools to work with individuals who are experiencing significant trauma or emotional problems in their lives (Deaver, 2015). Through the use of expressive therapies, it is hoped that individuals can gain a deeper understanding of themselves and work through some of their symptoms. Expressive therapists work with individuals of all ages and do individual, group, and family counseling. They work in many settings and are often hired specifically for their ability to reach individuals through a medium other than language. Many expressive therapists obtain degrees in counseling or social work and later pick up additional coursework in expressive therapy. However, there are programs that offer curricula in creative and expressive therapies, such as those approved by the American Art Therapy Association (AATA). Other related associations include the Association for Creativity in Counseling (ACC), a division of ACA; the American Dance Therapy Association (ADTA); the American Music Therapy Association (AMTA); and the Association for Play Therapy (APT). Although certifications exist for some kinds of creative and expressive therapies (e.g., see Art Therapy Credentials Board, 2012), states generally do not license creative and expressive therapists. However, some creative and expressive therapists can become licensed if their degree is in a field credentialed by the state (e.g., counseling or social work) or if the state licensing board of the therapist allows the individual to take additional courses so that their coursework matches the curriculum requirements of the existing state licenses (American Association of State Counseling Boards, 2009).

Human Service Practitioners

Individuals who serve as *human service practitioners* have generally obtained an associate's or bachelor's degree in human services. These programs are accredited by the Council for Standards in Human Service Education (CSHSE), which sets specific curriculum guidelines for the development of human service programs. Individuals who hold these degrees are often found in entry-level support and counseling jobs and serve an important role in assisting counselors and other mental health professionals. The professional organization for human services is the National Organization of Human Services (NOHS, n.d.). Recently, CSHSE, in consultation with NOHS and the Center for Credentialing and Education (CCE), created a certification in human services, called the Human Services–Board Certified Practitioner (HS–BCP) (Hinkle & O'Brien, 2010).

Psychotherapists

Because the word *psychotherapist* is not associated with any particular field of mental health practice, most states do not offer legislation that would create a license for psychotherapists. This means that in most states, individuals who have no mental health training can call themselves "psychotherapists." However, legislatures generally limit the scope of psychotherapeutic practice to those individuals who are licensed mental health professionals within the state (e.g., LPCs, LCSWs, or psychologists). The bottom line is that in most states, anyone can claim to be a psychotherapist, but only licensed practitioners can practice psychotherapy.

Professional Associations in the Social Services

In order to protect the rights of their members and support the philosophical beliefs of their membership, professional associations have arisen over the years for each of the social service professionals discussed in this chapter. Some benefits that these associations tend to offer include:

> ➤ National and regional conferences to discuss training and clinical issues
> ➤ Access to malpractice insurance
> ➤ Lobbyists to advocate to government officials in the interests of the membership
> ➤ Newsletters and journals to discuss topics of interest to the membership

> ➤ Opportunities for mentoring and networking
> ➤ Information on cutting-edge issues in the field
> ➤ Codes of ethics and standards for practice
> ➤ Job banks

Most of you who are reading this text are likely to be interested in joining ACA and its divisions, which will be discussed in detail shortly. However, to broaden your professional knowledge and acquaint you with related associations that you might want to join, some of the other major associations within the social service fields will also be highlighted. Keep in mind that there are dozens of professional organizations in the social services, and this section of the text features only a few of the more popular ones.

American Counseling Association

The beginnings of ACA can be traced back to the 1913 founding of the National Vocational Guidance Association (NVGA). After undergoing many changes of name and structure over the years, today's ACA is the world's largest counseling association. This 55,000-member not-for-profit association serves the needs of all types of counselors in an effort to "enhance the quality of life in society by promoting the development of professional counselors, advancing the counseling profession, and using the profession and practice of counseling to promote respect for human dignity and diversity" (ACA, 2013b, para 1).

Divisions of ACA

ACA currently sponsors twenty divisions, all of which maintain newsletters and most of which provide a wide variety of professional development activities. Many of these divisions also publish journals. ACA's divisions, along with the year they were founded and the journal(s) they publish, follow. (See http://www.counseling.org and click on "Divisions, Regions, and Branches" at the bottom of the page for more information.)

> ➤ AADA: Association for Adult Development and Aging (1986)
>   Journal: *Adultspan*
> ➤ AARC: Assessment for Assessment and Research in Counseling (1965)
>   Journals: *Measurement and Evaluation in Counseling and Development, Counseling Outcome Research and Evaluation*
> ➤ ACAC: Association for Child and Adolescent Counseling (2013)
> ➤ ACC: Association for Creativity in Counseling (2004)
>   Journal: *Journal of Creativity Mental Health*
> ➤ ACCA: American College Counseling Association (1991)
>   Journal: *Journal of College Counseling*
> ➤ ACEG: Association for Counselors and Educators in Government (1984)
> ➤ ACES: Association for Counselor Education and Supervision (1952)
>   Journal: *Counselor Education and Supervision*
> ➤ AHC: Association for Humanistic Counseling (1952)
>   Journal: *Journal of Humanistic Counseling*

➤ ALGBTIC: Association for Lesbian, Gay, Bisexual, and Transgender Issues in Counseling (1997)
Journal: *Journal of LGBT Issues in Counseling*

➤ AMCD: Association for Multicultural Counseling and Development (1972)
Journal: *Journal of Multicultural Counseling and Development*

➤ AMHCA: American Mental Health Counselors Association (1978)
Journal: *Journal of Mental Health Counseling*

➤ ARCA: American Rehabilitation Counseling Association (1958)
Journal: *Rehabilitation Counseling Bulletin*

➤ ASCA: American School Counselor Association (1953)
Journal: *Professional School Counseling*

➤ ASERVIC: Association for Spiritual, Ethical & Religious Values in Counseling (1974)
Journal: *Counseling and Values*

➤ ASGW: Association for Specialists in Group Work (1973)
Journal: *Journal for Specialists in Group Work*

➤ CSJ: Counselors for Social Justice (2002)
Journal: *Journal for Social Action in Counseling and Psychology*

➤ IAAOC: International Association of Addictions and Offender Counselors (1974)
Journal: *Journal of Addictions and Offender Counseling*

➤ IAMFC: International Association of Marriage and Family Counselors (1989)
Journal: *The Family Journal: Counseling and Therapy for Couples and Families*

➤ NCDA: National Career Development Association (est. 1952 as NVGA, name changed in 1985)
Journal: *Career Development Quarterly*

➤ NECA: National Employment Counseling Association (1964)
Journal: *Journal of Employment Counseling*

Associations Related to ACA

ACA supports a number of affiliates and organizations that contribute to the betterment of the counseling profession in unique ways. Brief descriptions follow.

➤ **The American Counseling Association Foundation (ACAF).** ACAF offers support and recognition for a wide range of projects, including scholarships for graduate students, recognition of outstanding professionals, publishing materials to for counselors and to advance the profession, partnering with others, and support counselors and others in need (see http://www.acafoundation.org/).

➤ **The Council for Accreditation of Counseling and Related Educational Programs (CACREP).** CACREP is an independent organization that develops standards and provides accreditation processes for counseling programs (see www.cacrep.org/).

➤ **The Council on Rehabilitation Education (CORE).** CORE is an independent organization that develops standards and provides accreditation processes for rehabilitation counseling programs (see http://www.core-rehab.org/).

➤ **The National Board for Certified Counselors (NBCC).** NBCC provides national certification for counselors (National Certified Counselor; NCC); mental health counselors (Certified Clinical Mental Health Counselor; CCMHC), school counselors (National Certified School Counselor; NCSC), and substance abuse counselors (Master Addiction Counselor; MAC) (see www.nbcc.org /ourcertifications).

➤ **Chi Sigma Iota (CSI).** CSI is an honor society that promotes and recognizes scholarly activities, leadership, professionalism, and excellence in the profession of counseling (see www.csi-net.org/)

Branches and Regions of ACA

In addition to its 20 divisions, ACA has 56 branches that consist of state associations, associations in Latin America, and associations in Europe. Four regional associations support counselors throughout the United States: the North Atlantic Region, Western Region, Midwest Region, and Southern Region.

Membership Benefits of ACA

Membership in ACA provides a number of unique opportunities and benefits, including the following:

➤ Subscriptions to the *Journal of Counseling and Development*, the monthly magazine *Counseling Today*, and to other professional journals based on division membership
➤ Professional development programs, such as conferences, online courses, free webinars and podcasts, and continuing education workshops
➤ A variety of discount and specialty programs (e.g., rental cars, auto insurance, hotels, discounts on books, etc.)
➤ Counseling resources, including books, ethical codes, DVDs, audiofiles, electronic news, and journals
➤ Links to ACA divisions and other relevant professional associations
➤ Assistance in lobbying efforts at the local, state, and national levels
➤ Consultation on ethical issues and ethical dilemmas
➤ Legislative updates and policy setting for counselors
➤ Links to ACA listservs and interest networks
➤ Networking and mentoring opportunities
➤ Computer-assisted job search services
➤ Professional liability insurance
➤ Graduate student scholarships
➤ A counselor directory

American Art Therapy Association

Founded in 1969, the AATA is open to any individual interested in art therapy. AATA is "dedicated to the belief that making art is healing and life enhancing. Its mission is to serve its members and the general public by providing standards of professional competence, and developing and promoting knowledge in, and of, the field of art therapy" (AATA,

2013, Mission section). The association establishes criteria for the training of art therapists, supports licensing for art therapists, maintains job banks, sponsors conferences, and publishes a newsletter and the *Art Therapy* journal.

American Association for Marriage and Family Therapy

If you have a counseling degree, you may be interested in joining the IAMFC, a division of ACA. However, in recent years, the AAMFT, with its 25,000 members, has become another important association in the field of marriage and family counseling. Founded in 1942 as the American Association of Marriage and Family Counselors, AAMFT was established by family therapy and communication theorists. Today, AAMFT "facilitates research, theory development and education . . . [and develops] standards for graduate education and training, clinical supervision, professional ethics and the clinical practice of marriage and family therapy" (AAMFT, 2002–2013a, "What We Do" section, para 1). AAMFT publishes the *Journal of Marital and Family Therapy*, sponsors a yearly conference, and offers professional activities related to family counseling and family development.

American Psychiatric Association

Founded in 1844 as the Association of Medical Superintendents of American Institutions for the Insane, today the American Psychiatric Association (which has the same acronym as the American Psychological Association, APA) has over 33,000 members. The association's main purpose is to "Promote the highest quality care for individuals with mental disorders (including intellectual disabilities and substance use disorders) and their families; Promote psychiatric education and research; advance and represent the profession of psychiatry; [and] Serve the professional needs of its membership." (APA, 2012, "Key Facts & Mission" section). The APA publishes journals in the field of psychiatry and is responsible for the development and publication of the *Diagnostic and Statistical Manual*, currently in its fifth edition (DSM-5).

American Psychiatric Nurses Association

Founded in 1986 with 600 members, today the APNA has over 9,000 members. APNA is "committed to the specialty practice of psychiatric mental health nursing, health and wellness promotion through identification of mental health issues, prevention of mental health problems, and the care and treatment of persons with psychiatric disorders" (APNA, n.d.b, "Mission" section). The association also provides advocacy for psychiatric nurses to improve the quality of mental health care delivery. APNA offers a number of continuing education and professional development activities and publishes the *Journal of the American Psychiatric Nurses Association*.

American Psychological Association

Founded in 1892 by G. Stanley Hall, the APA started with 31 members and now maintains a membership of 134,000. The main purpose of this association is to "advance the creation, communication and application of psychological knowledge to benefit society and improve people's lives" (APA, 2013b, para 2). The association has 54 divisions in various specialty areas and publishes numerous psychological journals. The Counseling

Psychology Division (Division 17) of the APA shares many of the same goals and purposes of some divisions of ACA.

National Association of Social Workers (NASW)

The NASW was founded in 1955 as a merger of seven membership associations in the field of social work. Servicing both undergraduate- and graduate-level social workers, NASW has nearly 140,000 members. NASW seeks "to enhance the professional growth and development of its members, to create and maintain professional standards, and to advance sound social policies" (NASW, 2013, "About NASW" section). The association publishes five journals and other professional publications. It has 56 chapters that include every state, as well as New York City, District of Columbia, Puerto Rico, Virgin Islands, Guam, and an International chapter.

National Organization for Human Services (NOHS)

The mission and values of NOHS, founded in 1975, support advocating for social justice, supporting clients' strengths and abilities, promoting professional development, and supporting the physical, emotional, mental, and spiritual well-being of individuals (NOHS, n.d). NOHS is mostly geared toward undergraduate students in human services or related fields, faculty in human services or related programs, and human service practitioners. NOHS publishes the *Journal of Human Services.*

Characteristics of the Effective Helper

In 1952, Hans Eysenck examined 24 uncontrolled studies that looked at the effectiveness of counseling and psychotherapy and found that "roughly two-thirds of a group of neurotic patients will recover or improve to a marked extent within about two years of the onset of their illness, *whether they are treated by means of psychotherapy or not* [italics added]" (p. 322). Although found to have serious methodological flaws, Eysenck's research did lead to debate concerning the effectiveness of counseling and resulted in hundreds of studies that came to some very different conclusions, such as the following:

> It is a safe conclusion that as a general class of healing practices, psychotherapy is remarkably effective. In clinical trials, psychotherapy results in benefits for patients that far exceed those for patients who do not get psychotherapy. Indeed, psychotherapy is more effective than many commonly used evidence-based medical practices. . . .

> (Wampold, 2010a, pp. 65–66)

But what makes counseling effective? First and foremost, factors such as readiness for change, psychological resources, and social supports may affect how well a client does in counseling (Lambert & Barley, 2001). Although such client factors are clearly important to positive outcomes, the counselor's ability to work with the client is equally critical. When looking specifically at the counselor, there has been recent emphasis on matching research-based treatment methodologies to the unique issues that the client is presenting. Called *evidence-based practice* (Thomason, 2010), this approach has become commonplace in training clinics. However, it has also become clear that specific counselor qualities, sometimes called *common factors,* seem to be at least as important as matching a treatment approach to a presenting problem (Wampold, 2010a, 2010b, 2010c; Wampold & Budge, 2012).

One common factor, the ability to build a *working alliance* (Norcross, 2011), has been alluded to by almost every counselor and therapist from Freud to the modern-day, new age counselor. Based on the research (and perhaps some of my own biases), this working alliance may be composed of the following six components: empathy, acceptance, genuineness, embracing a wellness perspective, cultural competence, and something that I call the "it" factor. Another common factor that may be important to positive client outcomes includes one's ability to deliver a theoretical approach. Here, I suggest that there may be three components: belief in one's theory, competence, and cognitive complexity. Let's take a look at all nine of these essential components, which may be related to the working alliance and one's ability at delivering a theoretical approach (see Figure 1.2).

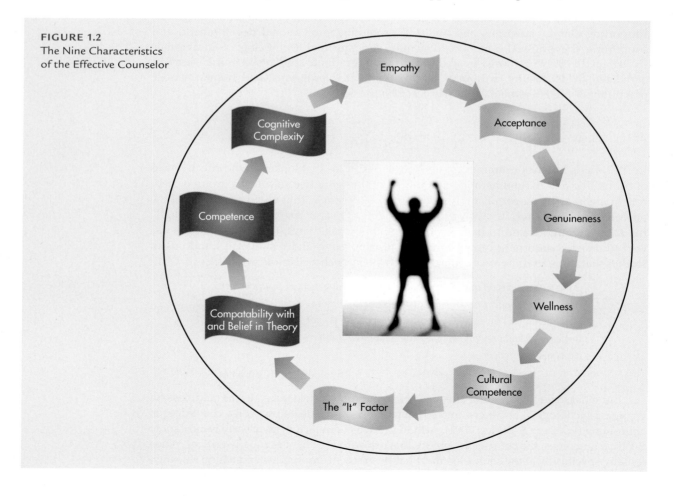

FIGURE 1.2
The Nine Characteristics of the Effective Counselor

Empathy

More than any component, *empathy* has been empirically shown to be related to positive client outcomes and is probably the most important ingredient to building a successful working alliance (Elliot, Bohart, Watson, & Greenberg, 2011; Norcross, 2010). Understanding our clients, or being empathic,

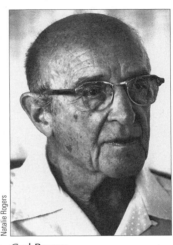

Natalie Rogers

Carl Rogers

> . . . means that the therapist senses accurately the feelings and personal mean-
> ings that the client is experiencing and communicates this acceptant under-
> standing to the client. When functioning best, the therapist is so much inside
> the private world of the other that he or she can clarify not only the meanings
> of which the client is aware but even those just below the level of awareness.
> Listening, of this very special, active kind, is one of the most potent forces of
> change that I know.
>
> (Rogers, 1989, p. 136)

Whether one can truly understand the inner world of another has been discussed for centuries and was spoken of by such philosophers as Plato and Aristotle (Gompertz, 1960). However, Carl Rogers (1957) is given credit for bringing this concept to life in the twentieth century. With respect to the counseling relationship, understanding through empathy is seen as a skill that can build rapport, elicit information, and help the client feel accepted (Egan, 2014; Neukrug, Bayne, Dean-Nganga, & Pusateri, 2013). Because empathy is seen as an important personal attribute, as well as a critical counseling skill to learn, it will be discussed in more detail in Chapter 5.

Acceptance

Acceptance, sometimes called *positive regard*, is another component likely related to building a strong working alliance (Norcross, 2010). Acceptance is an attitude that suggests that regardless of what the client says, within the context of the counseling relationship, he or she will feel accepted. Just about every counseling approach stresses the importance of acceptance (see Neukrug, 2011). For instance, person-centered counseling suggests that one of the core conditions in the helping relationship is *unconditional positive regard*, or the ability to accept clients with "no strings attached." Behavior therapists suggest that issues cannot be discussed and goals cannot be developed if clients do not feel accepted by the counselor or by themselves. Solution-focused brief therapy stresses the importance of acceptance in helping to quickly develop preferred goals. Reality therapy suggests that the suspension of judgment (acceptance!) is one of the critical "tonics," or relationship-building skills. Psychoanalysts talk about the importance of analytic neutrality and empathy in building a relationship in which all feelings, thoughts, and behaviors can be discussed. And even Albert Ellis, not a person typically known for his relationship-building skills, suggests in his rational emotive behavioral approach that clients be shown unconditional acceptance and not be berated for thinking, feeling, and acting in a certain manner.

Genuineness

Genuineness refers to the counselor's ability to be authentic, open, and in touch with his or her feelings and thoughts within the context and parameters of the helping relationship. Thus, one may not have all aspects of his or her life "together," but within the counseling relationship, the counselor is real and seen by the client as being in a state of congruence (feelings, thoughts, and behaviors are in sync). Genuineness may also be related to *emotional intelligence*, which is the ability to monitor one's emotions, a quality that counselors and counseling students seem to have more than others (Martin, Easton, Wilson, Takemoto, & Sullivan, 2004). Rogers (1957) popularized the term *genuineness* (or *congruence*) and noted that it was a core condition in the counseling relationship, along with empathy and unconditional positive regard.

Research by Gelso (Gelso, 2009; Gelso et al., 2005) suggests that regardless of one's theoretical orientation, there exists an ongoing "real relationship," in which the client will see the counselor realistically, at least to some degree. This real relationship has at its core the ability of the client to recognize the genuine (or nongenuine) self of the counselor. Genuineness has been shown to be one more quality that is sometimes related to positive outcomes in counseling (Norcross, 2010; Zuroff, Kelly, Leybman, Blatt, & Wampold, 2010).

Embracing a Wellness Perspective

Counselor stress, burnout, compassion fatigue, vicarious traumatization, and unfinished psychological issues can all hinder the counselor's ability to have a working alliance (Lawson, 2007; Norcross, 2010; Puig et al., 2012). Such concerns can prevent a counselor from being empathic, lower the ability to show acceptance, lead to incongruence, and increase *countertransference*, or "the unconscious transferring of thoughts, feelings, and attitudes onto the client by the therapist" (Neukrug, 2011, p. 50).

Counseling students, and counselors in general, all need to attend to their own wellness by *embracing a wellness perspective* if they are to be effective counselors. One method of assessing your level of wellness is by examining what Myers and Sweeney (2008) identify as the "Indivisible Self." This model views wellness as a primary factor composed of five subfactors and takes into account an individual's context. The factors (creative self, coping self, social self, essential self, and physical self) and contexts are described in Table 1.1.

TABLE 1.1   Abbreviated Definitions of Components of the Indivisible Self Model

WELLNESS FACTOR	DEFINITION
Total Wellness	The sum of all items on the 5F-Wel a measure of one's general well-being or total wellness
Creative Self	The combination of attributes that each of us forms to make a unique place among others in our social interactions and to positively interpret our world
Thinking	Being mentally active, open-minded; having the ability to be creative and experimental; having a sense of curiosity, a need to know and to learn; the ability to solve problems
Emotions	Being aware of or in touch with one's feelings; being able to experience and express one's feelings appropriately, both positive and negative
Control	Belief that one can usually achieve the goals one sets for oneself; having a sense of planfulness in life; being able to be assertive in expressing one's needs
Work	Being satisfied with one's work; having adequate financial security; feeling that one's skills are used appropriately; the ability to cope with workplace stress

TABLE 1.1   Abbreviated Definitions of Components of the Indivisible Self Model (*Continued*)

WELLNESS FACTOR	DEFINITION
Positive Humor	Being able to laugh at one's own mistakes and the unexpected things that happen; the ability to use humor to accomplish even serious tasks
Coping Self	The combination of elements that regulate one's responses to life events and provide a means to transcend the negative effects of these events
Leisure	Activities done in one's free time; satisfaction with one's leisure activities; having at least one activity in which "I lose myself and time stands still"
Stress Management	General perception of one's own self-management or self-regulation; seeing change as an opportunity for growth; ongoing self-monitoring and assessment of one's coping resource
Self-Worth	Accepting who and what one is, positive qualities along with imperfections; valuing oneself as a unique individual
Realistic Beliefs	Understanding that perfection and being loved by everyone are impossible goals, and having the courage to be imperfect
Social Self	Social support through connections with others in friendships and intimate relationships, including family ties
Friendship	Social relationships that involve a connection with others individually or in community, but that do not have a marital, sexual, or familial commitment; having friends in whom one can trust and who can provide emotional, material, or informational support when needed
Love	The ability to be intimate, trusting, and self-disclosing with another person; having a family or family-like support system characterized by shared spiritual values, the ability to solve conflict in a mutually respectful way, healthy communication styles, and mutual appreciation
Essential Self	Essential meaning-making processes in relation to life, self, and others
Spirituality	Personal beliefs and behaviors that are practiced as part of the recognition that a person is more than the material aspects of mind and body
Gender Identity	Satisfaction with one's gender; feeling supported in one's gender; transcendence of gender identity (i.e., ability to be androgynous)
Cultural Identity	Satisfaction with one's cultural identity; feeling supported in one's cultural identity; transcendence of one's cultural identity
Self-Care	Taking responsibility for one's wellness through self-care and safety habits that are preventive in nature; minimizing the harmful effects of pollution in one's environment
Physical Self	The biological and physiological processes that compose the physical aspects of a person's development and functioning
Exercise	Engaging in sufficient physical activity to keep in good physical condition; maintaining flexibility through stretching
Nutrition	Eating a nutritionally balanced diet, maintaining a normal weight (i.e., within 15% of the ideal), and avoiding overeating
Contexts	
Local Context	Systems in which one lives most often—families, neighborhoods, and communities—and one's perceptions of safety in these systems
Institutional Context	Social and political systems that affect one's daily functioning and serve to empower or limit development in obvious and subtle ways, including education, religion, government, and the media
Global Context	Factors such as politics, culture, global events, and the environment that connect one to others around the world
Chronometrical Context	Growth, movement, and change in the time dimension that are perpetual, of necessity positive, and purposeful

SOURCE: *Based on Wellness Counseling: The Evidence Base Practice; Journal of Counseling and Development, 86, p. 485.*

You may want to complete an informal assessment on each of the factors and context to determine what areas you might want to address in your life. For instance, score yourself from 1 to 5 on each of the factors, with 5 indicating you need to work on that area most. Then, find the average for each of the five factors. Next, write down the ways that you can better yourself in any factor where your scores seem problematic (probably scores of 3, 4, or 5). You may also want to consider how the contextual elements affect your ability to embrace a wellness perspective.

Finally, although many avenues to wellness exist, one that must be considered for all counselors is attending counseling themselves. Undergoing counseling can help counselors:

➤ attend to their own personal issues
➤ decrease the likelihood of countertransference
➤ examine all aspects of themselves to increase overall wellness
➤ understand what it's like to sit in the client's seat

It appears that counselors and other mental health professionals understand the importance of being in counseling, as 87% of helpers have attended counseling (Orlinsky, Schofield, Schroder, & Kazantzis, 2011).

However, some counselors resist the idea, perhaps for good reasons (e.g., concerns about confidentiality, feeling as if family and friends offer enough support, or believing they have effective coping strategies) (Norcross, Bike, Evans, & Schatz, 2008). So, have you attended counseling? If not, have you found other ways to work on being healthy and well?

Cultural Competence

If you were distrustful of counselors, confused about the counseling process, or felt worlds apart from your helper, would you want to go to or continue in counseling? Assuredly not. Unfortunately, this is the state of affairs for many diverse clients. In fact, it is now assumed that when clients from nondominant groups work with helpers from ethnic/cultural groups other than their own, there is a possibility that the client will frequently be misunderstood, misdiagnosed, find counseling and therapy less helpful than their majority counterparts, attend counseling and therapy at lower rates than majority clients, and terminate counseling more quickly than majority clients (Chapa, 2004; Evans, Delphin, Simmons, Omar, & Tebes, 2005; Sewell, 2009). Unfortunately, it has become abundantly clear that many counselors have not learned how to effectively build a bridge—that is, form a working alliance with clients who are different from them.

Clearly, the effective counselor needs to be culturally competent if he or she is going to connect with clients (Anderson, Lunnen, & Ogles, 2010; McAuliffe, 2013a). Although some rightfully argue that all counseling is cross-cultural, when working with clients who are from a different culture than one's own, the schism is often great. Therefore, cross-cultural competence is a theme that we will visit again and again throughout this text, and I will offer a number of ways for you to lessen the gap between you and your client. One model that can help bridge that gap is D'Andrea and Daniels's RESPECTFUL counseling model, which highlights ten factors that counselors should consider addressing with clients:

R – religious/spiritual identity
E – economic class background
S – sexual identity
P – level of psychological development
E – ethnic/racial identity
C – chronological/developmental challenges
T –various forms of trauma and other threats to one's sense of well-being
F – family background and history
U – unique physical characteristics
L – location of residence and language differences (Lewis, Lewis, Daniels, &
D'Andrea, p. 54)

The RESPECTFUL model offers one mechanism through which you can think about clients as you develop your skills as a counselor. Throughout this book, you will find other ways of ensuring that you have a strong sense of *cultural competence*.

The "It" Factor

I worked at a suicide crisis center where one of the counselors had an uncanny ability to make jokes on the phone that would result in suicidal clients laughing. If I had made those same jokes, it would have *driven* the caller to commit suicide! "So, is there a bridge nearby?" I would hear him say. This counselor had "it"—a way with words, a special voice intonation, and a way of being that would get the client laughing—the *suicidal* client. And, he knew he had *it* and he would use *it*. I knew I didn't have *it*—well, I didn't have his *it*, so I knew not to try to make my clients laugh. Just listening and being empathic was my way.

I believe all great counselors have their own *it factor*, although more often than not these great theorists want *us* to use their *it factor*. So, Carl Rogers, who was great at showing empathy, unconditional positive regard, and genuineness, suggested we all use these core conditions. Albert Ellis, who was a master at showing how irrational one can be, suggested we all show our clients their irrational thinking. Michael White, who believed that social injustices fueled mental illness, wanted all counselors to look at how individuals are oppressed by language. And of course Freud, who believed in the unconscious, told us to show analytic neutrality to allow the unconscious to be projected onto the therapist. I believe Salvadore Minuchin described this *it factor* best. A family counselor, Minuchin used the word *joining* to highlight the importance of each counselor finding his or her unique way of working with clients:

> The therapist's methods of creating a therapeutic system and positioning himself as its leader are known as joining operations. There are the underpinnings of therapy. Unless the therapist can join the family and establish a therapeutic system, restructuring cannot occur, and any attempt to achieve the therapeutic goals will fail.

> (Minuchin, 1974, p. 123)

So, what is your *it factor*? What do you have that's special and will enable you to bond? Is it the way you show empathy, the way you make people laugh, a tone, a look, or a way of being? Do you have *it*? (see Box 1.1)

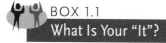

BOX 1.1
What Is Your "It"?

Write down the unique personality characteristics that allow you to build a bond with others. Then the instructor can make a master list on the board. After reviewing the list, discuss whether the characteristics are inherent and which may be learned. Is it possible for a counselor to acquire new ways of bonding with clients as he or she develops?

Compatibility with and Belief in a Theory

There are many theories to choose among when I do counseling, but most don't fit me. For one reason or another, I am simply not compatible with them. Maybe it's because they place too much emphasis on genetics, or spirituality, or early child rearing, or maybe they're a little too directive, or too nondirective. But for whatever reason, they just don't sit well with me. I am not compatible with them, and I choose not to use them. Thankfully, however, there are enough theories out there with which I am compatible. I drift toward them, and those are the ones I use. Wampold (2010a) says that helpers "are attracted to therapies that they find comfortable, interesting, and attractive. Comfort most likely derives from the similarity between the worldview of the theory and the attitudes and values of the therapist" (p. 48). Wampold (2010a, 2010b) and Wampold and Budge (2012) say that if you are drawn to a theory, and if you believe that the theory you are drawn to works, then, and only then, are you likely to see positive counseling outcomes. So, what theories are you drawn to? If you aren't sure yet, you'll have an opportunity to explore this more in Chapter 4 of this book, as well as in other courses where you will examine your own theoretical orientation to counseling. Hopefully, over time you will feel an increased sense of *compatibility with and belief in a theory*.

Competence

Not surprisingly, counselor expertise and mastery (*competence*) has been shown to be a crucial element for client success in counseling (Wampold, 2010a, 2010c, Wampold & Budge, 2012; Whiston & Coker, 2000). Competent counselors have a thirst for knowledge, and they continually want to improve and expand their expertise about their approach. Such counselors express this through their study habits, desire to join professional associations, participation in mentoring and supervision, reading of professional journals, belief that education is a lifelong process, and ability to view their own approach to working with clients as something that is always broadening and deepening. Competence also means that counselors are not only concerned about their "relationships" with their clients, but also willing to look at the evidence of what works and apply appropriate treatment strategies to client problems (Cooper, 2011). Finally, because these counselors know that they're doing, they can build expectations with their clients that what they do will help them get better. And, at least in part, these expectations help clients get better (Wampold & Budge, 2012).

Counselors have both an ethical and legal responsibility to be competent (Corey, Corey, Corey & Callanan, 2015). For instance, Section C.2 of ACA's (2014a) ethics code elaborates on eight areas of competence, including (1) practicing within one's boundary of competence, (2) practicing only in one's specialty areas, (3) accepting employment only for positions for which one is qualified, (4) monitoring one's effectiveness to ensure optimal practice, (5) knowing when to consult with others, (6) keeping current by attending continuing education activities, (7) refraining from offering services when physically or emotionally impaired, and (8) assuring proper transfer of cases when one is incapacitated or leaves a practice (see the Appendix). As Kaslow et al. (2007) highlight, the legal system reinforces these ethical guidelines because "competence is thus the touchstone by which the law will judge" (p. 488).

Finally, clients pick up on incompetence. They can see it, smell it, and feel it. Of course, clients are less likely to improve when a counselor is incompetent. And not surprisingly, incompetent counselors are sued more frequently.

Cognitive Complexity

The best helpers believe in their theory and also are willing to question it. This apparent contradiction makes sense. You have a way of working, but you are also willing to constantly examine if your way *is* working in any given instance. In other words, you are able to reflect on what you are thinking and what you are doing—you are able to consider if you approach is working well for your client (Ridley, Mollen, & Kelly, 2011). Counselors who have this capacity are often said to be cognitively complex. Not surprisingly, *cognitive complexity* has been shown to be related to being empathic, more open-minded, more self-aware, more effective with individuals from diverse cultures, better able to examine a client's predicament from multiple perspectives, and better able to resolve "ruptures" in the counseling relationship (McAuliffe & Eriksen, 2010; Norcross, 2010; Ridley, Mollen, & Kelly, 2011). Such a counselor is willing to integrate new approaches into his or her usual way of practicing counseling and is a helper who doesn't believe that his or her theory holds the lone "truth" (Wampold, 2010a). So, ask yourself: do you have this quality? Are you able to self-reflect, question truth, take on multiple perspectives, and evaluate situations in complex ways? Counselor training programs are environments that seek to expand this type of thinking (McAuliffe & Eriksen, 2010). Hopefully, in your program, you'll be exposed to such opportunities.

Now that we've looked at all nine characteristics, ask yourself: are you empathic, accepting, genuine, wellness oriented, and culturally competent? Do you have the "it" factor? Are you compatible with and do you believe in your theory? Are you competent and cognitively complex? As we start on our journey to help others, let's not forget to help ourselves—clearly, helping ourselves will significantly improve the manner in which we help others.

Multicultural/Social Justice Focus: Inclusion of Multiculturalism in the Profession

With relatively small numbers of persons from culturally diverse groups entering the counseling profession (ACA, 2009), it is imperative that the helping professions develop an environment that attracts more counselors of color. Increased cultural diversity among counselors, along with better training in multicultural counseling, are essential if culturally diverse clients are to feel comfortable seeking out and following through in counseling.

In addition, if counseling is to be an equal opportunity profession, counselors must graduate from training programs with more than a desire to help all people. As a profession, we will have achieved competence in counseling diverse clients when every graduate from each training program has (1) learned counseling strategies that work for a wide range of clients, (2) worked with clients from diverse backgrounds, (3) gained a deep appreciation for diversity, and (4) acquired an identity as a counselor that includes a multicultural perspective (see D'Andrea & Heckman, 2008b). As you read through this textbook, you will see considerable emphasis placed on multicultural and social justice issues. As you reflect on these issues, consider what the counseling profession can do to foster a more welcoming professional culture that will attract more individuals of color and what training programs can do to ensure that all individuals feel comfortable with the counseling process.

Ethical, Professional, and Legal Issues

Knowing Who We Are and Our Relationship to Other Professional Groups

Our professional identity is based on a specific body of knowledge unique to our profession. By knowing who we are, we also have a clear sense of who we are not. It is by having a strong sense of our identity that we are able to define our limits, know when it is appropriate to consult with colleagues, and recognize when we should refer clients to other professionals (Gale & Austin, 2003). The *ACA Code of Ethics* (ACA, 2014a) highlights the importance of knowing our professional boundaries in the following passages (see the Appendix):

> *Counselors practice only within the boundaries of their competence, based on their education, training, supervised experience, state and national professional credentials, and appropriate professional experience. . . .*

(Standard C.2.a.)

> *Counselors take reasonable steps to consult with other counselors, the ACA Ethics and Professional Standard Department, or related professionals when they have questions regarding their ethical obligations or professional practice.*

(Standard C.2.e.)

> *If counselors lack the competence to be of professional assistance to clients, they avoid entering or continuing counseling relationship. Counselors are knowledgeable about culturally and clinically appropriate referral resources and suggest these alternatives. . . .*

(Standard A.11.b.)

Impaired Mental Health Professionals

> *Counselors who are unwell (stressed, distressed, or impaired) will not be able to*
> *offer the highest level of counseling services to their clients…*

(Lawson, 2007, p. 20)

To avoid working on your own issues while trying to help others simply does not make sense. As already noted, mental health professionals have a responsibility, and an urgency, to be aware of the pressures and stresses that impinge on their lives and how these might affect their relationship with clients. This is stressed in the ACA (2014a) *Code of Ethics* (see the Appendix):

> *Counselors monitor themselves for signs of impairment from their own physi-*
> *cal, mental, or emotional problems and refrain from offering or providing pro-*
> *fessional services when impaired. They seek assistance for problems that reach*
> *the level of professional impairment, and, if necessary, they limit, suspend, or*
> *terminate their professional responsibilities until it is determined that they*
> *may safely resume their work. . . .*

(Standard C.2.G)

A professional who is not attending to his or her own needs is likely to be ineffective in the counseling relationship. Professional incompetence is not only unethical, it also can lead to malpractice suits (Neukrug, Milliken, & Walden, 2001; Remley & Herlihy, 2014). But, perhaps even more important, impaired practice can result in clients ending up with deeper wounds than the ones they had when they initially entered counseling.

The Counselor in Process: Personal Therapy and Related Growth Experiences

As you begin your journey in the counseling profession, I hope you have the opportunity to engage in growth experiences that will help you embody the counselor characteristics highlighted in this chapter. What kind of experiences should you seek out? First, I hope that you strongly consider undergoing your own personal counseling, for the many reasons noted earlier in this chapter. In addition to counseling, you might want to consider other related growth experiences, such as prayer, meditation, relaxation exercises and stress reduction, discussion and support groups, exercise, writing in a journal, and reading.

I also hope that you are afforded experiences in your educational program that will challenge you to grow intellectually and personally. I am hopeful that the philosophy of your program is that students need a supportive environment in which they can feel safe enough to share while being challenged to grow at the same time. This "constructive development" philosophy has become an important model for many counselor education programs, as it is built on the belief that if afforded a nurturing environment, students can develop increased flexibility and relativist thinking in their ways of understanding the world (Eriksen & McAuliffe, 2006; McAuliffe & Eriksen, 2010). Such students gain a strong sense of self, can listen to feedback about self from others, and are genuine, more empathic, and more accepting of others. (Not surprisingly, these are also the qualities to look for in an effective counselor!)

Summary

In this chapter, we have attempted to define the somewhat elusive word counseling and distinguish it from the words *guidance* and *psychotherapy*. Then some of the training, credentialing, and roles and functions of counselors, social workers, psychologists, psychiatrists, psychoanalysts, psychiatric mental health nurses, expressive therapists, human service practitioners, and psychotherapists were compared and contrasted. In addition, some of the benefits of professional associations were identified, with a special emphasis on the ACA, and identified some of the more prominent professional associations in related fields.

Next, we discussed the recent move toward evidence-based practice, but noted that even more important were the characteristics of the counselor, sometimes called the "common factors" that are critical in counseling outcomes. Six components of building an effective working alliance, followed by three components to the counselor's ability to deliver his or her theoretical approach, were highlighted. These nine components included empathy, acceptance, genuineness, embracing a wellness perspective, cultural competence, the "it" factor, compatibility with and belief in your theory, competence, and cognitive complexity.

Examining some important multicultural and social justice issues, we noted that clients of color are frequently misdiagnosed, attend counseling at lower rates, terminate counseling more quickly, find counseling less helpful, and can be distrustful of counselors who are not from their ethnic/cultural group. We talked about the importance of recruiting a more culturally diverse group of counselors to the field, as the counseling profession continues to have relatively small numbers of individuals from diverse cultures entering the profession and because clients tend to respond better to counselors of their own cultural background. Another topic of the chapter was the importance of having every counseling student graduate with knowledge of how to work with diverse clients, with experience working with diverse clients, with an appreciation for diversity, and with an identity that includes a multicultural perspective.

As the chapter concluded, the importance of a number of ethical issues were discussed, including understanding professional identity and knowing professional limits, practicing within the counselor's area of competence, consulting with other professionals, and terminating or referring clients when unable to work effectively with them. We then discussed the importance of assuring that counselors are not working while impaired. Related to this topic, the chapter ended by discussing the importance of counselors undergoing personal counseling, finding other related personal growth experiences, or both. We also expressed the hope that readers of this text are in an educational program that affords personal and intellectual growth experiences in a nurturing yet challenging environment.

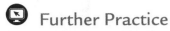 Further Practice

Visit CengageBrain.com to respond to additional material that highlight the salient aspects of the chapter content. There, you can find ethical, professional, and legal vignettes, a number of experiential exercises, and study tools including a glossary, flashcards, and sample test items. Hopefully, these will enhance your learning and be fun and interesting.

2 The Counseling Profession's Past, Present, and Future

Can you imagine a woman being hanged as a witch because she was mentally ill, or being placed in a straitjacket and thrown into a filthy, rat-infested cell for the remainder of her life? Or can you envision a man being placed in a bathtub filled with iron filings to cure him of mental illness or bled to rid him of demons and spirits that caused him to think in demonic ways? What about having a piece of your brain scraped out in order to change the way you feel? Or being placed in a box that would receive "energy" and rid you of emotional and physical problems? These examples are a part of the history of our profession.

I've taught long enough to know that when I teach history, it often is not as interesting as what you just read. Why is this so? Unfortunately, learning names, dates, and a few facts is just plain boring for some people. I used to feel the same way, but now I have a different perspective. In 1962, Thomas Kuhn wrote a book called *The Structure of Scientific Revolutions,* and reading it changed the way I understood history and the accumulation of knowledge. What intrigued me in particular was his concept that knowledge builds upon prior knowledge, and, periodically, the time is ripe for a person to synthesize this prior knowledge and develop new, revolutionary ways of understanding what has come before. He called this process a *paradigm shift.* This concept makes learning about history more exciting for me because I can now see how events unfold to bring us closer to the next paradigm shift.

We are all part of history in the making. Some of us take an active role through research and scholarly pursuits or leadership in professional organizations. Others are interested observers. Whether you assume the role of active participant or interested observer, you have been affected by the past, and, in your own unique way, you are affecting the future. And sometimes we may be riding a wave toward a paradigm shift and ironically, not even know we're on the wave. Let's look at how history has made us what we are today, and then, later in the chapter, we can consider where we might be headed in the future.

We will start our look at history by journeying into the distant past, exploring some of the precursors to the mental health field. We will then take a brief look at the history of social work, psychology, and psychiatry: three fields that dramatically affected the counseling profession.

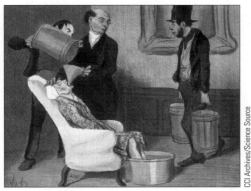

Early treatment of the mentally ill–hydrotherapy

Next, we will examine the history of our profession in detail, from its early roots in vocational guidance to modern-day counseling. The chapter will conclude by examining the relatively recent impact of ethical standards, multicultural competencies, and social justice issues.

Understanding the Human Condition: From Early Antiquity to the Present

> *The first counselors were leaders of the community who attempted to provide inspiration for others through their teachings. They were religious leaders such as Moses (1200 B.C.), Mohammed (600), and Buddha (500 B.C.). They were also philosophers like Lao-Tzu (600 B.C.), Confucius (500 B.C.), Socrates (450 B.C.), Plato (400 B.C.), and Aristotle (350 B.C.).*
>
> (Kottler & Shepard, 2015, p. 30)

Since the dawn of existence, people have attempted to understand the human condition. Myths, magic, belief in spirits, ritualism, and sacred art have been used by people as means of gaining introspection and understanding the world around us (Ellwood & McGraw, 2014). *Shamans,* or individuals who had special status due to their mystical powers, have been considered to be caretakers of the soul and thought to have knowledge of the future. Later in history, the concept of soul has often given way to the concept of psyche.

One of the first written treatises of a psychological nature can be traced back to an Egyptian papyrus of 3000 B.C. that shows a primitive attempt to understand some basic functions of the brain (Breasted, 1930). Almost 1,000 years later, also in ancient Egypt, a wise man who obviously was psychologically minded wrote:

> *If thou searchest the character of a friend, ask no questions, (but) approach him and deal with him when he is alone. . . . Disclose his heart in conversation. If that which he has seen come forth from him, (or) he do aught that makes thee ashamed for him, . . . do not answer.*
>
> (Breasted, 1934, p. 132)

Such writings show that the "counseling way" clearly preceded modern times. However, it was the Greek philosopher Hippocrates (460–377 BCE) who presented reflections on the human condition that were to greatly change the Western world's view of the person. Whereas many of his contemporaries believed that possession by evil spirits was responsible for emotional ills, Hippocrates suggested treatments for the human condition, some of which might be considered modern even by today's standards. For instance, for melancholia, he recommended sobriety, a regular and tranquil life, exercise short of fatigue, and bleeding, if necessary. For hysteria, he recommended getting married—an idea that would certainly spark the ire of many women and men in today's world!

With the advent of monotheistic religions, we see abundant examples of humankind's attempt to understand the self further. The Old and New Testaments, the Quran, and other religious writings abound with such examples (Belgium, 1992). For instance, in Buddhism, the Sanskrit term *duhkha* speaks to the ongoing disappointment, pain, and suffering inherent in most of our lives of which most of us are barely aware (Epstein, 2013), and the Old and New Testaments offer us many reflections on the concept of guilt and sin. These reflections could very well come in handy today:

> The Bible has a word for conduct unbecoming a saint. It is sin. . . . It covers everything from gossip to adultery, from impatiences to murder. Obviously, there are degrees of seriousness of sin. But in the final analysis, sin is sin. It is conduct unbecoming a saint.

> (Bridges, 2007, p. 16)

With guidance from religious texts, over the years, a number of philosophers and theologians have reflected on the nature of the person, the soul, and the human condition. For example, such philosophers as Plotinus (205–270), who believed the soul was separate from the body, had a lasting impact on the dualistic fashion in which the Western world views the mind and body.

The Renaissance in Europe, which was roughly between the fifteenth and seventeenth centuries, is considered by many to be the start of the modern era; at that time arose the invention of the printing press and the spread of scholarship throughout Europe, including the writings of modern philosophers. Individuals like René Descartes (1596–1650), who believed that knowledge and truth come through deductive reasoning, and John Locke (1632–1704) and James Mill (1773–1836), who believed that the mind is a blank slate upon which ideas become generated, set the stage for modern psychologists to study human experience. These individuals and others supplied the ingredients for modern psychology, the beginnings of modern-day social work and psychiatry, and the origins of the counseling field.

A Brief History of Related Helping Professions: Social Work, Psychology, Psychiatry

Originating in the nineteenth century, the professions of social work, psychology, psychiatry, and counseling had somewhat different beginnings, with the counseling profession evolving out of early vocational guidance activities, the social work field developing out

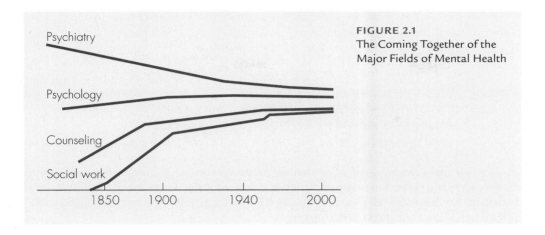

FIGURE 2.1
The Coming Together of the
Major Fields of Mental Health

of the desire to assist the destitute, psychology starting as both a laboratory science and an attempt to understand the nature of the person, and psychiatry growing out of modern medicine's attempt to alleviate mental illness through medical interventions. Despite their different origins, they all have moved slowly toward many of the same theoretical conclusions and today can be seen on slightly different yet parallel paths (see Figure 2.1).

The Social Work Profession

Historical Background

The field of social work can be traced to work with the poor and destitute in the United States and England. During the 1500s, the *Elizabethan Poor Laws* in England gave the Church of England power to oversee the raising and administering of funds for the destitute (Burger, 2014). Until then, such relief had been provided on a voluntary basis. As a carryover from this system, during the colonial period in America, local governments enacted laws to assist the poor. During this same period, organized charities (usually affiliated with religious groups) began to arise. In the 1800s, the growth of urban populations produced an increasingly large underclass whose needs could not be met by the traditional charitable organizations. Mounting political pressure thus led to the creation of specialized institutions such as reform schools, lunatic asylums, and orphanages.

To assist the underprivileged who were not institutionalized, two major approaches evolved: the *Charity Organization Society (COS)* and the *settlement movement* (Popple & Leighninger, 2011). COSs had volunteers who would visit the poor, aid in educating children, give economic advice, and assist in alleviating the conditions of poverty. Generally, the poor received advice, support, and small amounts of necessities from COS volunteers, along with a good dose of moral judgment and religious preaching. Sometimes these volunteers, who became known as "friendly visitors," would spend years assisting one family. The COSs are seen as the beginnings of *social casework*, the process in which a client's needs are examined and a treatment plan is designed.

In contrast to the COSs, the settlement movement had staff who actually lived in the poorer communities:

> *In essence it was simply a residence for university men in a city slum. . . . These critics looked forward to a society that encouraged people's social responsibility, not self-interest, to create a life that was kindly, dignified, and beautiful, as well as progressive and prosperous. Some of these thinkers rejected capitalism in favor of an idealized medieval community.*

(Leiby, 1978, p. 129)

The idealistic young staff of settlement houses believed in community action and tried to persuade politicians to provide better services for the poor. One of the best-known settlement houses was *Hull House*, established by social activist Jane Addams (1860–1935) in 1889 in Chicago (Addams, 1910/2012).

Out of this involvement with the underprivileged arose articles and books concerned with methods of adequately meeting the needs of the underclass. At the turn of the twentieth century, the first social work training programs arose. Over the next thirty years, the social work field grew in many different directions, with major areas of emphasis being social casework, social group work, and community work.

During the 1940s and 1950s, an increased emphasis on understanding the dynamics of social and family systems emerged. As social workers had already been working with social systems and families, this emphasis became a natural focus for many social work programs. Such programs stressed contextual or systems thinking, as opposed to seeing the individual as an island unto him- or herself, as had many of the early philosophers and psychologists. One social worker, Virginia Satir (1967), was particularly instrumental in reshaping the practices of the mental health profession to include a greater systems focus.

In 1955, a number of social work organizations combined to form the *National Association for Social Work (NASW)*, and in 1965, NASW established the *Academy of Certified Social Workers (ACSW)*, which sets standards of practice for master's-level social workers. Today, social workers can be found in a variety of social service settings, from hospitals to mental health centers to agencies that work with the homeless and the poor. Although many social workers today do individual psychotherapy and family therapy, others work in community settings doing advocacy work, and still others administer social service organizations.

Social Work's Influence on the Counseling Profession

The counseling profession has learned much from the field of social work. Social work, with its emphasis on understanding systems, has provided the counseling profession with an understanding of the individual from a family and social system perspective. Because many of the well-known family therapists started out as social workers, counselors have learned to apply many of their concepts with clients. Also, social work's emphasis on field experience has rubbed off on counseling, as counselor education programs have increasingly offered more field experience in their training programs. Finally, social work's emphasis on advocacy is a constant reminder to counselors that their clients are greatly affected by the culture from which they come and the larger dynamics of society. Today, a focus upon advocacy and social justice has become a major thrust of the counseling profession.

The Psychology Profession

Historical Background

The origins of the psychology profession can be traced back thousands of years. For instance, during the seventh century B.C., Greek philosophers reflected on the nature of life and the universe. A few centuries later, Hippocrates offered notions on how to treat mental illness, and Plato (427–347 B.C.) suggested that introspection and reflection were roads to knowledge, that dreams and fantasies were substitute satisfactions, and that the human condition had physical, moral, and spiritual origins. Many consider Plato's student Aristotle (384–322 B.C.) to be the first psychologist because he used objectivity and reason to study knowledge, and his writings were psychological in nature (Wertheimer, 2012).

Although Augustine (354–430) and Thomas Aquinas (1225–1274) highlighted the importance of consciousness, self-examination, and inquiry, there was a paucity of writing about "psychological thinking" during the 800-year span between their lives. This was partly due to the rise of Christianity, which at that point downplayed the role of reason and objectivity and highlighted the presence of the supernatural. However, the Renaissance saw a rediscovery of the Greek philosophies and a renewed interest in questions regarding the nature of the human condition. This interest sparked philosophical discussions regarding the nature of the person as well as the development of the scientific method.

During the nineteenth century, psychology was increasingly influenced by modern-day medicine, physics, and Charles Darwin's new theory of evolution. Wilhelm Wundt (1832–1920) and Sir Francis Galton (1822–1911), two of the first experimental psychologists, developed laboratories to examine similarities and differences in responses by individuals to sensory experiments as they attempted to understand how responses to external stimuli were related to the workings of the mind (Gillham, 2001; Green, 2009). This scientific orientation to the field of psychology quickly spread to the United States, where G. Stanley Hall (1846–1924) and James Cattell (1860–1940) opened laboratories at Harvard and the University of Pennsylvania in the late 1800s (Capshew, 1992). It was also during the nineteenth century that William James (1842–1910) published his theory of *philosophical pragmatism*, which suggested that truth or reality is continually constructed as a function of the utility or practical purpose that it has for the individual who holds that reality (Leary, 1992). Thus were seen the beginnings of two important schools of psychology: the philosophical and the scientific.

One natural outgrowth of laboratory science was the development of psychological and educational tests at the end of the nineteenth century. For instance, Alfred Binet (1857–1911) developed one of the first intelligence tests, for the Ministry of Public Education in Paris, whose purpose was to assist in classroom placement of children who were intellectually disabled. (Neukrug & Fawcett, 2014). The beginning

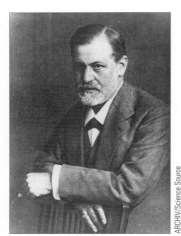

Sigmund Freud

of the twentieth century saw the first use of school achievement tests, tests for vocational assessment, and some of the first modern-day personality tests. Today, tests are used everywhere and often help provide a deeper understanding of clients.

The beginnings of the testing movement paralleled the rise of *psychoanalysis*, the first comprehensive psychotherapeutic system. Developed by Sigmund Freud (1856–1939), the development of psychoanalysis was undoubtedly affected by the new emphasis on the scientific method. Freud had been greatly influenced by Anton Mesmer (the term *mesmerize* was derived from his name) (1734–1815) and Jean Martin Charcot (1825–1893), who were practicing a new technique called *hypnosis* (Neukrug, 2011). These early hypnotists showed that suggestion could greatly influence an individual's mental state. In fact, Charcot showed that some physical disorders (e.g., some forms of paralysis), whose etiology was previously thought to be of only a physical nature, could be induced under hypnosis. Freud originally used hypnosis to uncover repressed and painful memories, but later he stopped in favor of other techniques and subsequently developed his elaborate theory to understand the origins of human behavior. Freud's views on mental health and mental illness were revolutionary and continue to have a profound effect on the conceptualization of client problems. Although Freud was trained as a physician, his concepts were quickly adopted by the psychology profession.

In addition to traditional psychoanalysis, the end of the nineteenth century saw the beginnings of other schools of psychology (Neukrug, 2015a). Ivan Pavlov (1849–1936) and his followers, in experiments with *classical conditioning* of dogs, developed *behaviorism*, deemphasized the importance of introspection, and stressed the importance of stimulus–response and environmental influences. During this same period, *phenomenological psychology* and *existential psychology* had their beginnings and stressed the nature of existence and the study of reality. Also around this time, *Gestalt psychology*, which tried to answer questions about how individuals organize experience into reality, first emerged. The early days of behaviorism, existential psychology, phenomenological psychology, and Gestalt psychology represent the roots of many of today's *cognitive–behavioral* and *humanistically oriented* therapies.

In 1892, the *American Psychological Association (APA)* was founded as an association with a membership consisting mostly of experimental psychologists (Sokal, 1992). However, starting in the 1920s, clinicians began to have a greater impact on the field and entered the association in large numbers. During the mid-1940s, the APA underwent a great revision and assimilated many new clinical associations, such as *Counseling Psychology (Division 17)* (Pepinsky, 2001; Routh, 2000; Schmidt, 2000). This division shared a common history and had similar goals as the counseling profession. Its assimilation by APA highlighted the fact that a vast majority of psychologists had begun to view themselves as clinicians, rather than as academics or scientists.

Today, we still find both *experimental psychologists*, who work in the laboratory trying to understand the psychophysiological causes of behavior, and *clinical and counseling psychologists*, who practice counseling and psychotherapy. In addition, there are other highly trained psychologists doing testing in schools, working within business and industrial organizations, and applying their knowledge in many other areas.

Psychology's Influence on the Counseling Profession

The field of psychology has affected the counseling profession more than any other related mental health profession. Although psychology was the first profession to use a comprehensive approach to therapy, the counseling field was soon to follow and borrowed many of the theories used by early psychologists. Tests developed by psychologists at the turn of the twentieth century were used by the early vocational guidance counselors and later adapted by counselors in many different settings. Research techniques developed by the early experimental psychologists became the precursors to modern-day research tools used by counselors to assess the efficacy of counseling approaches and to evaluate programs that they have developed. Finally, many modern-day counseling skills are adaptations from counseling skills developed by psychologists during the early part of the twentieth century. Psychology is truly the first cousin of counseling.

The Psychiatry Profession

Historical Background

Until the late 1700s, mental illness was generally viewed as mystical, demonic, and not treatable, but this perspective gradually gave way to new approaches to the understanding and treatment of mental diseases. In the late 1700s, in France, Philippe Pinel (1745–1826), who is credited with being the founder of psychiatry, was one of the first of many to view insanity from a scientific perspective. Administering two mental hospitals, Pinel removed the chains that bound inmates in one of the first attempts to treat inmates humanely (Weissmann, 2008).

During the 1800s, great strides were made in the understanding, diagnosis, and treatment of mental illness. Emil Kraepelin (1855–1926) developed one of the first classifications of mental diseases, and Charcot and Pierre Janet (1859–1947) both saw a relationship between certain psychological states and disorders that were formerly considered to be only of an organic nature (Solomon, 1918).

In the United States, Benjamin Rush (1743–1813), a physician and dedicated social reformer, is considered to be the founder of American psychiatry. An impassioned believer in the abolition of slavery, a signer of the Declaration of Independence, and an advocate for the establishment of a peace institute as an alternative to the U.S. Military Academy, Rush appealed for humane treatment of the poor and mentally ill. His book *Medical Inquiries and Observations upon the Diseases of the Mind*, published in 1812, became the seminal work in the field of psychiatry for the next 70 years (Baxter, 1994).

By the early 1800s, the Pennsylvania Hospital in Philadelphia and the Publick Hospital for Persons of Insane and Disordered Minds in Williamsburg, Virginia, had been established to treat the mentally insane. Early treatments for the mentally ill hardly resembled anything that we might find in today's psychiatric hospitals; however, they acknowledged that psychiatric disorders were real (see Box 2.1).

In the mid-1800s, Dorothea Dix (1802–1887) and others advocated for the humane treatment of the mentally ill and suggested supportive care, encouragement and respect, removal from stressors, and vocational training as treatments of choice

BOX 2.1
The Beginnings of the Modern Mental Hospital

In 1773, the Publick Hospital for Persons of Insane and Disordered Minds admitted its first patient in Williamsburg, Virginia. The hospital, which had 24 cells, took a rather bleak approach to working with the mentally ill. Although many of the employees of these first hospitals had their hearts in the right place, their diagnostic and treatment procedures left a lot to be desired. For instance, some of the leading reasons that patients were admitted included masturbation, "womb disease," religious excitement, intemperance, and domestic trouble—hardly reasons for admission to a mental institution. The treatment procedures included administering heavy doses of drugs, bleeding or blistering individuals, immersing individuals in freezing water for long periods of time, and confining people to straitjackets or manacles. Bleeding and blistering was thought to remove harmful fluids from the individual's

system (Zwelling, 1990). It was believed at that time that it was important to cause fear in a person, and even individuals like Dr. Benjamin Rush, known for his innovative and humane treatment of the mentally ill, wrote of the importance of staring a person down:

> The first object of a physician, when he enters the cell or chamber of his deranged patient, should be to catch his EYE. . . .The dread of the eye was early imposed upon every beast of the field. . . . Now a man deprived of his reason partakes so much of the nature of those animals, that he is for the most part terrified, or composed, by the eye of a man who possesses his reason.

(Rush, quoted in Zwelling, 1990, p. 17)

(Baxter, 1994). The spread of mental hospitals and the impetus toward more humane treatment of the mentally ill led to the founding of the Association of Medical Superintendents of American Institutions for the Insane in 1844. The forerunner of the *American Psychiatric Association,* this association sought the improvement of diagnosis, care, and the humane treatment of the mentally ill and developed standards for mental hospitals of the time.

In the first half of the twentieth century, psychiatry developed in a number of different directions. Whereas many psychiatrists became entrenched in the psychoanalytic movement, others began to drift toward psychobiology as the treatment of choice for mental disorders, while still others became increasingly involved in social psychiatry (Sabshin, 1990). During the 1950s, there was a great expansion of the use of psychotropic medications, which resulted in many individuals who had been formerly hospitalized living on their own. Then, in the 1960s, the development of community-based mental health centers greatly expanded the role of psychiatrists in community agencies. The eventual deinstitutionalization of the mentally ill as a result of the Supreme Court case *Donaldson v. O'Connor* (discussed later in the chapter) also meant that psychiatrists were needed to work at community-based agencies. Increasingly, psychiatrists became disengaged from doing psychoanalysis and more involved in exploring the psychobiology of mental illness.

During the 1950s, the APA was instrumental in developing the first *Diagnostic and Statistical Manual of Mental Disorders (DSM-I),* the forerunner of DSM-5, the current edition. One important purpose of the DSM is to provide uniform criteria for making clinical diagnoses, thereby enhancing agreement among clinicians (APA, 2013a).

Today, with research indicating that some mental illness is predominantly or partially biologically based (Chase, 2012), psychiatrists have been playing an increasingly important role in the mental health field. In addition, with the advent of new and much improved psychopharmacological drugs, psychiatrists have become very important consultants to counselors and other mental health professionals.

Psychiatry's Influence on the Counseling Profession

Psychiatry's focus on diagnosing mental illness and exploring psychopathology has assisted counselors and other professionals in the diagnosis and development of treatment plans for clients, which sometimes include psychopharmacology. In addition, the awareness that some mental health problems may be organic has helped counselors understand that at times, it is critical to make a referral to an expert in psychopharmacology and psychobiology.

The Counseling Profession: Its History and Trends

Precursors to the Counseling Profession: The 1800s

> *Counseling represents the fusing of many influences. It brings together the movement toward a more compassionate treatment of mental health problems begun in mid-nineteenth century France, the psychodynamic insights of Freud and psychoanalysis, the scientific scrutiny and methodology of the behavioral approach, the quantitative science of psychometrics, the humanistic perspective of client-centered therapy, the philosophical base of existentialism, and the practical insights and applications that evolved from the vocational guidance movement.*
>
> (Belkin, 1988, p. 19)

In the 1800s, a number of forces came together that eventually led to the early beginnings of the counseling profession. Such seemingly disparate forces as social reform movements, the early days of vocational guidance, the beginning use of assessment instruments, and the first comprehensive approach to therapy all influenced the beginning of what we now call the *counseling profession*. Let's take a brief look at each of these forces.

Social Reform Movements of the 1800s

During the 1800s, a number of reform movements occurred simultaneously that eventually influenced the development of the counseling profession. Social workers who were working with the poor and destitute, psychiatrists who were trying to change the treatment of the mentally ill, and educators such as John Dewey (1859–1952)—who insisted on more humanistic teaching methods and access to public education—all had a common desire to help people in more humane and "modern" ways (Dewey, 1956; Dykhuizen, 1973; Neukrug, 2013). The counseling profession soon bore the fruits of these reform movements, as it embraced many of their ideals and some of their basic premises. Reform movements, and their focus on caring for others, no doubt influenced the modus operandi of the first professional counselors: vocational guidance workers.

Vocational Guidance in the 1800s

Although modern-day vocational guidance activities and theory began in the latter part of the nineteenth century, interest in vocational adjustment far preceded the 1800s. For instance, as far back as the tenth century, writings in an Iraqi text addressed occupational information, while the first job classification system was developed in Spain as early as 1468 by Sanchez de Arevalo, who wrote *Mirror of Men's Lives* (Carson & Altai, 1994). At the end of the nineteenth century, dramatic shifts took place in the United States that were partially responsible for the beginnings of the vocational guidance movement and ultimately set the stage for the establishment of the counseling profession. This time in history saw the rise of social reform movements, the impact of the Industrial Revolution, and an increase in immigration, mostly to large northeastern cities. Perhaps for the first time, a large-scale need for vocational guidance arose. During the early to mid-1800s, prior to the development of vocational theory, a number of poorly written, moralistic books on occupational choice were written (Zytowski, 1972). By the end of the century, however, the stage was set for the development of the first comprehensive approaches to vocational guidance—approaches that would at least be partially based on the new science of testing (Herr, Cramer, & Niles, 2004).

The Beginnings of the Testing Movement: The Turn of the Twentieth Century

Paralleling the rise of the vocational guidance movement was the testing movement. With the development of laboratory science in Europe and the United States came an increased interest in examining individual differences. Soon people were studying differences in intelligence, as it was then defined. For instance, Binet's intelligence test, developed in 1896, signaled the beginning of the large-scale use of measurement instruments, soon to be used to assist individuals and institutions in decision making (Neukrug & Fawcett, 2014). Most significantly for the counseling profession, a number of these assessment instruments would soon be employed in vocational counseling and would earmark the beginning of the counseling profession (DuBois, 1970; Williamson, 1964).

Testing, vocational guidance theory, and the humane treatment approaches developed from the reform movements were three crucial elements involved in the formation of the counseling profession; however, the emergence of a comprehensive approach to psychotherapy may have been the most important component for the establishment of the counseling profession.

Psychoanalysis and the Development of Psychotherapy: The Turn of the Twentieth Century

Although for centuries, philosophers and shamans had reflected on the human condition and scholars had contributed treatises on psychological thought, it was not until the turn of the twentieth century that a major paradigm shift took place in the understanding of mental illness. It was at this time that many challenged the notion that mental illness was caused by demons or that it was primarily organic in nature. Instead, there evolved a consensus that at least some emotional problems were caused by unconscious psychological factors (Cautin, 2011). It is not surprising that at the end of the nineteenth century and into the early part of the twentieth century, Freud's theory of psychoanalysis, which represented the first systematic and comprehensive approach to psychotherapy, erupted into the Western world.

Freud's theory ushered in a new way of viewing the development of the person. Constructs never before discussed became commonplace and continue to be accepted in today's world. Freud and his disciples made terms like id, ego, superego, the conscious, the unconscious, and psychosexual development commonplace. Soon, these constructs permeated the Western world, and this new "psychological" way of viewing the world affected the emerging field of counseling.

Early Vocational Guidance and the First Guidance Counselors: Early 1900s

> *It is difficult even to imagine the difference of conditions now and in the early years of the century. . . . Think of what life would be without the railroad, only the stage-coach to carry our letters and ourselves across the country. Think of pulling oranges from Florida or California to Boston stores by team. Think of a city without a street-car or a bicycle, a cooking stove or a furnace, a gas jet or electric light, or even a kerosene lamp! Think of a land without photographs or photogravures, Christmas cards or color prints. . . .*

(Parsons, cited in Watts, 1994, p. 267)

It was a different world at the beginning of the twentieth century, but the rumblings of a new age were everywhere to be found. Social reformers were caring for the poor and demanding changes in education; psychiatry was changing its methods of treatment for the mentally ill; psychoanalysis and related therapies were in vogue; the modern-day use of tests was beginning; and the impact of the Industrial Revolution could be seen everywhere. In some very subtle but important ways, each of these events would affect early vocational guidance and the emergence of the field of counseling.

The first part of the twentieth century saw the beginnings of systematic vocational guidance in America. Although the concepts had been floating around in the latter part of the 1800s, the 1900s brought the first comprehensive approach to vocational guidance. Then in 1907, troubled by the attitudes of youth, Jesse Davis (1871–1955) developed one of the first guidance curricula that focused on moral and vocational guidance, which was presented during English composition classes in the school system of Grand Rapids, Michigan. At around the same time, Eli Weaver (1862–1922), a New York City principal who had written a booklet called *Choosing a Career*, started *vocational guidance* in New York. Similarly, Anna Reed (1871–1946) soon established guidance services in the Seattle school system, and by 1910, 35 cities had plans for the establishment of vocational guidance in their schools (Aubrey, 1977). Although revolutionary in their thinking, many of these early vocational guidance reformers were motivated by moralistic thinking and theories of the time, such as *social Darwinism*, that suggested individuals should fervently follow their supervisors and "fight their co-workers for advanced status"—i.e., survival of the fittest (Rockwell & Rothney, 1961, p. 352).

The person who undoubtedly had the greatest impact on the development of vocational guidance in the United States was Frank Parsons (1854–1908) (Briddick, 2009a; McDaniels & Watts, 1994). Today seen as the founder of guidance in the United States, Parsons was greatly influenced by the reform movements of the time, such as the work of Jane Addams at Hull House. Eventually establishing the *Vocational Bureau*, which assisted individuals in "choosing an occupation, preparing themselves for it, finding an opening in it, and building a career of efficiency and success" (Parsons, cited in Jones, 1994, p. 288), Parsons hoped that vocational guidance would eventually be established in the public schools—a hope that he would not see come to fruition due to his untimely death in 1908, at the age of 54. In 1909, his book *Choosing a Vocation* was published posthumously. Soon after his death, perhaps as a tribute to the energy that he gave to the vocational guidance movement, his hometown of Boston became the site for the first vocational guidance conference. This conference resulted in the founding of the *National Vocational Guidance Association (NVGA)* in 1913, which is generally considered to be the distant predecessor of the *American Counseling Association (ACA)*.

Parsons was a man with a vision (Briddick, 2009b; Pope & Sveinsdottir, 2005). He envisioned systematic vocational guidance in the schools; he anticipated a national vocational guidance movement; he foresaw the importance of individual counseling; and he hoped for a society in which cooperation was more important than competition and where concern replaced avarice (Jones, 1994). It is clear that Parsons's principles of vocational guidance greatly affected the broader field of counseling.

Parsons's main thrust toward vocational guidance was viewed as a three-part process that he described in the following manner:

> *(1) a clear understanding of yourself, your aptitudes, interests, ambitions, resources, limitations, and their causes; (2) a knowledge of the requirements and conditions of success, advantages and disadvantages, compensation, opportunities, and prospects in different lines of work; [and] (3) true reasoning on the relations of these two groups of facts.*

> (Parsons, 1909/2009 p. 5)

However, a deeper examination of his work shows that many of his principles eventually became some of the major tenets of the counseling profession (Jones, 1994). For instance, Parsons noted the importance of having an expert guide when making difficult decisions. In addition, he suggested that even an expert guide cannot make a decision *for* a person, as only the individual can decide what's best for himself or herself. He also suggested that the counselor should be frank (genuine) and kind with the client, and that it was crucial for the counselor to assist the client in the development of analytic skills. It is clear that Parsons deserves the title "founder of vocational guidance," and in many ways, he also can be seen as the founder of the counseling field.

Parsons offered the beginnings of a theoretical orientation to counseling, and with the founding of the NVGA, the vocational guidance movement was established. Although the spread of the movement did not occur as quickly as some might have liked (Aubrey, 1977), a number of acts were eventually passed to strengthen vocational education (Herr, 1985). One such act, the Depression-era *Wagner O'Day Act* of 1932, established the U.S. Employment Services and provided ongoing vocational guidance and placement to all unemployed Americans. Vocational counseling as part of the landscape of the United States was here to stay, and it would soon have an impact on all facets of counseling.

Although vocational guidance in the schools soon took hold, it was not long before individuals advocated for an approach that attended to a broader spectrum of students' psychological and educational needs. For instance, John Brewer (1932) suggested that guidance should be seen in a total educational context and that "guidance counselors" (now called *school counselors*) should be involved in a variety of functions in the schools, including adjustment counseling, assistance with curriculum planning, classroom management, and of course, occupational guidance. One tool used by the counselor was testing (Aubrey, 1982).

The Expansion of the Testing Movement: 1900–1950

It is doubtful that vocational guidance would have survived without a psychological support base in psychometrics.

(Aubrey, 1977, p. 290)

With the advent of the vocational guidance movement, testing was to become commonplace. Parsons, for instance, strongly advocated the use of tests in vocational guidance (Williamson, 1964). During World War I, some of the first crude tests of ability were used on a large-scale basis. For instance, the *Army Alpha* was used to determine placement of recruits. Although particularly crude by even standards of the time (see Box 2.2), tests of ability would soon be adapted for use in vocational guidance.

The use of tests to assist in vocational counseling was promoted by the development of one of the first major interest inventories, the *Strong Vocational Interest Blank*, in 1927 (Campbell, 1968). This test, which in its revised form is still one of the most widely used instruments of its kind, was to revolutionize vocational counseling. But the use of tests extended beyond vocational assessment. For instance, *Woodworth's Personal Data Sheet* was an early personality instrument used by the military to screen out emotionally disturbed individuals. The successful large-scale military use of tests led to the development and adoption of similar instruments in the schools, business, and industry (Neukrug & Fawcett, 2014). By the middle of the twentieth century, tests to measure achievement, cognitive ability, interests, intelligence, and personality were commonplace. Although often used in vocational counseling, many of these tests soon found their way into all kinds of counseling practices.

BOX 2.2
The Army Alpha Test

As you take the test below, consider some of the obvious cross-cultural problems that are inherent within it.

The Army Alpha was used to determine placement in the armed forces during World War I. Below is an adaptation of the test, as printed in *Discover magazine*. Take the test and discuss your thoughts about it. The average mental age of the recruits who took the Army Alpha test during World War I was approximately 13. Could you do better? You have three minutes to complete these sample questions, drawn verbatim from the original exam. (McKean, 1985)

The following sentences have been disarranged but can be unscrambled to make sense. Rearrange them and then answer whether each is true or false.

1. Bible earth the says inherit the the shall meek.
   true   false
2. a battle in racket very tennis useful is
   true   false

Answer the following questions:

3. If a train goes 200 yards in a sixth of a minute, how many feet does it go in a fifth of a second?
4. A U-boat makes 8 miles an hour under water and 15 miles on the surface. How long will it take to *cross a 100-mile channel if it has to go two-fifths of the way under water?*
5. The spark plug in a gas engine is found in the:
   crank case   manifold   cylinder   carburetor
6. The Brooklyn Nationals are called the:
   Giants   Orioles   Superbas   Indians
7. The product advertised as 99.44 per cent pure is:
   Arm & Hammer Baking Soda
   Crisco   Ivory Soap   Toledo
8. The Pierce-Arrow is made in:
   Flint   Buffalo   Detroit   Toledo
9. The number of Zulu legs is:
   two   four   six   eight

Are the following words the same or opposite in meaning?

10. vesper–matin   same   opposite
11. aphorism–maxim   same   opposite

Find the next number in the series:

12. 74,   71,   65,   56,   44,   Answer:
13. 3,   6,   8,   16,   18,   Answer:
14. Select the image that belongs in the mirror:

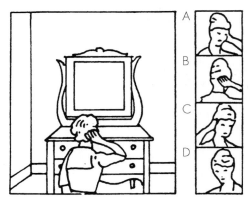

15. & 16. What's missing in these pictures?

15.

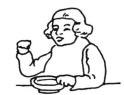

16.

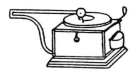

Answers: 1. true, 2. false, 3. twelve feet, 4. nine hours, 5. cylinder, 6. superbas, 7. Ivory Soap, 8. Buffalo, 9. two, 10. opposite, 11. same, 12. 29, 13. 36, 14. A, 15. spoon, 16. gramophone horn. Scoring: All item except 3, 4, 10, and 11 = 1.25 points. Items 3 and 4 = 1.875 points, Items 10 & 11 = .625 points. Add them all up, they equal your mental age.

SOURCE: *McKean, K. (1985). Intelligence: New ways to measure the wisdom of man. Discover Magazine, 6(1).*

The Spread of Psychotherapy and Its Impact on the Counseling Profession: 1900–1950

Most sane people think that no insane person can reason logically. But this is
not so. Upon reasonable premises I made most reasonable deductions, and that
at the time when my mind was in its most disturbed condition.

(Beers, 1948, p. 57)

In 1908, Clifford Beers (1876–1943), a Yale graduate who had been hospitalized for years due to schizophrenia, wrote *A Mind That Found Itself.* In 1909, he helped to establish *the National Committee for Mental Hygiene,* which lobbied the U.S. Congress to pass laws that would improve the deplorable conditions of mental institutions. Soon, this committee began to organize the first child guidance clinics, staffed by social workers, psychologists, and psychiatrists. At the same time, psychoanalysis was beginning to come out of the elite office of the psychiatrist and work its way into the community. The end of World War I saw a number of psychologists offering their services to returning doughboys who had psychological problems associated with the war (today, such problems are often diagnosed as posttraumatic stress disorder, or PTSD). Because the long-term treatment approaches of the psychoanalysts were of little use to these clinicians, they began to develop new, shorter-term approaches.

As treatment approaches to the individual changed, and as mental health clinics spread, the need for psychological assistants, often with a bachelor's or master's degree, became evident. The master's-level assistants often had degrees in social work, but increasingly there were individuals with a relatively new degree—a master's degree in counseling, which started as a degree in vocational guidance. It was a natural transition for individuals with this degree to move into the mental health field because they were trained in both counseling techniques and assessment.

The emergence of the counseling field as something other than pure vocational guidance made its greatest leap forward during the 1930s, when E. G. Williamson (1900–1979) developed what is considered to be the first comprehensive theory of counseling (as distinguished from Freud's theory of psychoanalysis). Known as the *Minnesota Point of View* (for the University of Minnesota, where Williamson was a faculty member in the psychology department), or *trait-and-factor theory*, Williamson's approach initially grew out of the ideas of Frank Parsons. Although originally vocationally oriented, the approach was modified and soon was seen as a generic approach to counseling and psychotherapy. The trait-and-factor approach involved a series of five steps, which included the following (Williamson & Darley, 1937):

1. Analysis: Examining the problem and obtaining available records and testing for the client
2. Synthesis: Summarizing and organizing the information to understand the problem
3. Diagnosis: Interpreting the problem
4. Counseling: Aiding the individual in finding solutions
5. Follow-up: Ensuring proper support after counseling had ended

With the rise of Nazism during the 1930s and 1940s, many humanistic philosophers, psychiatrists, and psychologists fled Europe for the United States and dramatically influenced the field of psychotherapy and education in their new country. One of those influenced by these humanists was Carl Rogers (1902–1987). Called one of the most influential psychologists and psychotherapists of the twentieth century (The Top 10…, 2007), Rogers initially worked from a psychodynamic perspective at the Rochester Guidance Center, but later revolutionized the practice of counseling with his client-centered approach. His nondirective approach to working with individuals was viewed as shorter-term, more humane, more honest, and more viable for most clients than the psychodynamic approaches to counseling. The early 1940s saw the publication of Carl Rogers's book *Counseling and Psychotherapy*, which eventually had a major impact on the counseling profession (Rogers, 1942). Rogers and others in the newly established field of humanistic counseling and education were a major impetus for the counseling field to move from a vocational guidance orientation to one with a much broader base. Rogers's approach was ripe for the times, as it reflected the increased focus on personal freedom and autonomy of the post–World War II years (Aubrey, 1977). Although Rogers and other humanists during the 1940s had a great impact on the field of counseling, the second half of the century would witness even more dramatic changes.

Emergence, Expansion, and Diversification: The 1950s

> *If one decade in history had to be singled out for the most profound impact on counselors, it would be the 1950s.*
>
> (Aubrey, 1977, p. 292)

During the 1950s, the counseling profession shifted increasingly toward a humanistic, nondirective orientation. This decade saw Rogers become an even greater influence on the field, as he published his second book, *Client-Centered Therapy: Its Current Practice, Implications, and Theory* (Rogers, 1951). In addition, affected by the push to depathologize individuals, this decade saw the promulgation of developmental theories in the areas of career counseling (e.g., Ginzberg, Ginsburg, Axelrad, & Herma, 1951; Super, 1953), child development (e.g., Piaget, 1954), and lifespan development (e.g., Erikson, 1950). These theories stressed the notion that individuals would face predictable tasks as they passed through the inevitable developmental stages of life, and that knowledge of these developmental tasks could greatly aid counselors in their work with clients.

Perhaps the most important event that would affect counseling during this time was the 1957 launching of Sputnik. The launching of this Russian satellite sent a chill through many Americans and provided the impetus for Congress passing the *National Defense Education Act (NDEA)* in 1958, which allocated funds for training institutes that would quickly graduate secondary school counselors. These counselors, it was hoped, would identify students gifted in math and science who could be future scientists. The obvious result of this legislation was the significant increase in secondary school counselors in the late 1950s and 1960s. The bill was extended to include the training of elementary school counselors in 1964.

Besides the dramatic increase in school counselors, the 1950s also saw the first full-time college counselors and the beginning of college counseling centers. With the GI Bill funding college expenses for World War II veterans, there was increased enrollment in colleges and an increased need for college counselors to address the needs of these soldiers, as well as other students (Kraft, 2011). As with other aspects of the counseling profession, college counseling centers quickly took on the humanistic and developmental approach to working with students and were generally staffed by counselors and psychologists. Other college student services offices (e.g., career centers) that employed counselors expanded rapidly during this time.

Community agencies also saw an influx of counselors and psychologists during the 1950s. The recognition that many mental hospitals were just holding grounds that used archaic practices, changing social mores, new medications to treat a wide variety of mental health disorders, and new laws expanding services for the mentally ill enabled the release from state hospitals of large numbers of people, who then found needed services at local community agencies (Rochefort, 1984). In addition, this decade saw counselors increasingly staffing vocational rehabilitation centers, working to address both the physical and psychological needs of individuals, especially those who had been seriously injured during World War II.

This decade saw the formation of the *American Personnel and Guidance Association* (APGA) from a merger of four counseling-related associations, and it was not long before a number of divisions representing the growing diversity of counselors in the field emerged. These included the *American School Counselor Association (ASCA)*, the *Association for Counselor Education and Supervision (ACES)*, the *National Career Development Association (NCDA)*, the *American Rehabilitation Counseling Association (ARCA)*, and *the Counseling Association for Humanistic Education and Development (C-AHEAD)*.

Changes were not only taking place in the counseling profession around this time. In 1945, the *American Association of Marriage and Family Counseling (AAMFC)*, later to be called the *American Association of Marriage and Family Therapists (AAMFT)* was formed, and the 1950s saw the formation of the *National Association of Social Workers (NASW)* and the changing of the name of Division 17 of the APA from the *Counseling and Guidance Division* to the *Division of Counseling Psychology*. Whereas Division 17 required a doctorate for full membership, APGA, AAMFT, and NASW focused on master's-level training. Differentiation and solidification of the various mental health fields was clearly occurring.

Increased Diversification: The 1960s

During the first half of the twentieth century, three approaches to counseling and therapy were particularly popular: *psychodynamic approaches* (e.g., Freud), *directive theories* (e.g., Williamson), and *client-centered theories* (e.g., Rogers) (Neukrug, 2011). However, during the late 1950s and continuing into the 1960s, a number of new (and revolutionary) approaches to counseling began to take shape, including the *rational emotive* (cognitive) approach of Albert Ellis (Ellis & Harper, 1961); the *behavioral* approaches of Bandura (1969), Wolpe (1958), and Krumboltz (1966a, 1966b); William Glasser's *reality therapy* approach (1961, 1965); the *Gestalt* approach of Fritz Perls (1969); the communication approach of *transactional analysis* (Berne, 1964); and the *existential* approaches of Frankl (1963), May

(1950), and others. These counseling approaches were at least partially developed due to the demand for counselors and therapists during this time period. Can you imagine being a young mental health professional during this time? The sheer numbers of new theories and new, thought-provoking approaches to working with clients would have been incredibly stimulating!

The need for counselors and other mental health professionals expanded as a direct result of the passage of many legislative actions related to President Lyndon B. Johnson's *Great Society* initiatives (Kaplan & Cuciti, 1986). One such law, the *Community Mental Health Centers Act of 1963*, funded the nationwide establishment of mental health centers to provide short-term inpatient care, outpatient care, partial hospitalization, emergency services, and consultation and education services. These centers made it possible for individuals with adjustment problems, as well as those with severe emotional disorders, to obtain free or low-cost mental health services. Hundreds of mental health centers were partially funded as a result of this act and was one of the reasons that the population of individuals in psychiatric hospitals was reduced from a high of about 600,000 to under 200,000 by the late 1970s (Rochefort, 1984).

Many other acts were also passed during this decade. For instance, in 1964, amendments to the NDEA expanded the training of counselors to include counselors from elementary school through junior college (Lambie & Williamson, 2004). In fact, nearly 20,000 school counselors had been trained by 1967 as a result of this act. In addition, a number of other acts provided job opportunities for counselors, such as the *Manpower Development and Training Act, Job Corps, Elementary and Secondary Education Act, Head Start*, and the *Work Incentive Program*. Other key legislative initiatives, such as the *Civil Rights Act, Economic Opportunity Act*, and *Voting Rights Act,* helped to reshape attitudes toward social problems and community service, with one result being a more accepting attitude toward the counseling profession. Clearly, the 1960s was a decade of expansion, acceptance, and diversification of the counseling profession, largely as the result of legislative actions.

With this expansion and diversification came an increased emphasis on the need for professionalism in the field. One outgrowth of this professionalization was the emergence of ethical standards of practice, such as development of the APGA's first guidelines for ethical behavior in 1961. The 1960s also saw a flurry of activity around the need for accreditation standards of counseling programs. Meetings were held throughout the country that would be the precursors to the development of the *Council for Accreditation of Counseling and Related Programs (CACREP)* in 1981. Finally, the 1960s saw the continued expansion of APGA with increased membership, the formation of what would become the *Association for Assessment in Counseling and Education* (AACE, now AARC), the *National Employment Counseling Association* (NECA), and the recommendation in 1964 by APGA to have state branches (ACA, 1995a).

Continued Proliferation of the Counseling Field: The 1970s

During the 1970s, a number of events occurred that increased the need for counselors. For instance, the 1975 Supreme Court decision in *Donaldson v. O'Connor* led to the deinstitutionalization of hundreds of thousands of state mental hospital patients who had been

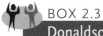

BOX 2.3
Donaldson v. O'Connor

Kenneth Donaldson, who had been committed to a state mental hospital in Florida and confined against his will for 15 years, sued the hospital superintendent, Dr. J. B. O'Connor, and his staff for intentionally and maliciously depriving him of his constitutional right to liberty. Donaldson, who had been hospitalized against his will for "paranoid schizophrenia," said he was not mentally ill, and even if he was, stated that the hospital had not provided him adequate treatment.

Over the 15 years of confinement, Donaldson, who was not in danger of harming himself or others, had frequently asked for his release, and had relatives who stated they would attend to him if he was released. Despite this, the hospital refused to release him, stating that he was still mentally ill. The Supreme Court unanimously upheld lower court decisions stating that the hospital could not hold him against his will if he was not in danger of harming himself or others (Swenson, 1997). This decision, along with the increased use and discovery of new psychotropic medications, led to the release of hundreds of thousands of individuals across the country who had been confined to mental hospitals against their will and who were not a danger to themselves or others.

hospitalized against their will (see Box 2.3). This case concluded that individuals who were not in danger of harming themselves or others could not be held against their will. With the release of individuals from these hospitals came an increased need for community mental health counselors. Thus, in 1975, Congress passed an expansion of the original Community Mental Health Centers Act and extended from five to twelve the categories of services that mental health centers were required to provide. They included:

1. Short-term inpatient services
2. Outpatient services
3. Partial hospitalization (day treatment)
4. Emergency services
5. Consultation and education
6. Special services for children
7. Special services for the elderly
8. Preinstitutional court screening
9. Follow-up care for mental hospitals
10. Transitional care from mental hospitals
11. Alcoholism services
12. Drug abuse services

The 1970s also saw the passage of legislation for individuals with disabilities. These laws increased the demand for highly trained rehabilitation counselors and expanded the role of school counselors. For instance, the *Rehabilitation Act of 1973* ensured vocational rehabilitation services and counseling for employable adults who had severe physical or mental disabilities that interfered with their ability to obtain and maintain a job. The *Education for All Handicapped Children Act of 1975 (PL94-142)* ensured the right to an education within the least restrictive environment for all children identified as having a disability that interfered with learning. PL94-142 resulted in school counselors increasingly becoming an integral part of the team that would determine the disposition of students with disabilities.

This decade also saw a major shift in the training of counseling students. The influence of the humanistic movement had fully taken hold by the 1970s, and a number of individuals began to develop what became known as *microcounseling skills training* (Carkhuff, 1969; Egan, 1975; Ivey & Gluckstein, 1974). The teaching of these microcounseling skills was based on many of the skills deemed critical by Carl Rogers and other humanistic psychologists. These packaged ways of training counselors showed that basic counseling skills such as attending behaviors, listening, and empathic understanding could be learned in a relatively short amount of time, and that the practice of such skills would have a positive impact on the counseling relationship (Neukrug, 1980). It was also during this decade that the blossoming of publications in the area of cross-cultural counseling began. Seminal works by Derald Sue, Paul Pedersen, William Cross, Donald Atkinson, and others began to make their way into counselor education curricula. In fact, it would not be long before some of the microcounseling techniques would be criticized as being too Western for some clients.

The 1970s was also the decade of increased professionalization in the field. For instance, the early 1970s saw the *Association of Counselor Educators and Supervisors (ACES)* provide drafts of standards for master's-level counseling programs. National credentialing became a reality when certification was offered for the first time by the *Council on Rehabilitation Education (CORE)* in 1973 and by the *National Academy for Certified Mental Health Counselors (NACMHC)* in 1979 (Sweeney, 1991). Finally, state licensure began in 1976, when Virginia became the first state to offer licensing for counselors.

The legislative actions of the 1970s led to increased diversification of the counseling field and resulted in large numbers of counselors settling into the mental health, rehabilitation, higher education, and school counseling specialty areas. One result of this diversification was the burgeoning membership in APGA, which reached 40,000, and the founding of a number of divisions of ACA (then called APGA), including the *Association for Multicultural Counseling and Development (AMCD*, 1972), the *International Association of Addictions and Offender Counselors (IAAOC*, 1972), the *Association for Specialists in Group Work (ASGW*, 1973), the *Association for Spiritual, Ethical, and Religious Values in Counseling (ASERVIC*, 1974), and the *American Mental Health Counselors Association* (AMHCA, 1978) (ACA, 1995a; Goodyear, 1984).

Changes During the Late Twentieth Century: 1980–2000

The 1980s and 1990s saw a continued expansion and diversification of the field of counseling, as well as a settling-in phase marked by an increased emphasis on professionalism. Counselors could now be found in almost any mental health setting, while expanded services were offered in colleges and schools. Counselors also began to practice in areas where minimal mental health services had been provided, including substance abuse agencies, agencies that worked with older persons, and business and industry. With the profession clearly having come of age, it became increasingly evident that there was an urgent need for the standardization of training and the credentialing of counselors. Therefore, in 1981, CACREP was formed to further delineate standards for the profession (CACREP, 2014b). Today, CACREP accredits master's programs in school counseling; clinical mental health counseling; marriage, couple, and family counseling; addiction counseling; career counseling; and student affairs and college counseling, as well as doctoral programs in counselor education and supervision (see Chapter 3 for a detailed discussion of CACREP).

The 1980s and 1990s saw a phenomenal increase in the types of credentials being offered and the numbers of individuals becoming certified or licensed. In 1982, APGA (now ACA) established the *National Board for Certified Counselors (NBCC)* and began to administer the first national generic certification exam for counselors (NBCC, 2014a, 2014b). In addition, in 1994, the *International Association of Marriage and Family Counselors* (IAMFC, n.d.), a division of ACA, began to offer certification for family therapists. It was also during this decade that an increasing number of states began offering licensure for counselors (Neukrug, Milliken, & Walden, 2001). Probably one of the greatest changes in the field of counseling during the 1980s and 1990s was the increased focus on multicultural counseling (Claiborn, 1991). This new emphasis was partly due to CACREP's requirement that multicultural counseling be infused into the curricula of all accredited graduate programs, the ever-increasing volumes of work being published in the field of multicultural counseling, and the 1991 adoption by AMCD of *Multicultural Counseling Competencies*, which counseling training programs were encouraged to follow (Arredondo et al., 1996; Evans & Larrabee, 2002).

The 1990s also saw an increased emphasis on the importance of ethical issues in counseling. Whereas prior to 1980, few counseling texts discussed ethical issues to any great extent, this decade saw research and publications on ethics greatly expanded, with particular focus on ethical decision making, ethics in supervision, ethics in teaching, and even the ethics of online counseling (ACA, 1995b, Attridge, 2000). It is not surprising that the 1990s brought a revision of the ACA *Code of Ethics*, as well as the development of separate ethical guidelines for online counseling by ACA and by NBCC.

In 1992, the *American College Personnel Association (ACPA)*, one of ACA's founding divisions, disaffiliated from the association. Also, in the latter part of the 1990s, the boards of the two largest ACA divisions, AMHCA and ASCA, both threatened disaffiliation from ACA. This movement toward independent functioning of the divisions was a precursor to the divisional autonomy that was to occur in the twenty-first century.

There is little doubt that the changes that took place during the 1980s and 1990s were reflected in changes in professional associations. In 1983, APGA changed its name to the *American Association for Counseling and Development (AACD)*, and in 1992, the association underwent another name change to the more streamlined *American Counseling Association (ACA)*. The 1980s and 1990s saw the founding of a number of new divisions, including the *Association for Adult Development and Aging (AADA)* in 1986, the *International Association of Marriage and Family Counselors (IAMFC)* in 1989, the *American College Counseling Association (ACCA)* in 1991, the *Association for Counselors and Educators in Government (ACEG)* in 1994, and the *Association for Gay, Lesbian, and Bisexual Issues in Counseling (AGLBIC)* in 1997. Around the same time, an affiliate organization was founded: *Counselors for Social Justice (CSJ)*, in 1999. Membership in ACA soared, and by 2000, it had surpassed 55,000, with AMHCA and ASCA representing the two largest divisions. At that point, ACA had 17 divisions and one affiliate, representing the differing specialty areas in counseling, with close to 500 counselor training programs in the United States (Hollis & Dodson, 2000).

The 21st Century: Current Issues

The first part of the new millennium has already shown us that a number of issues from the last part of the twentieth century, as well as new emerging issues, are having an impact on the counseling profession. Here are a few of the most current issues in the counseling profession.

Division Expansion and Division Autonomy

Since 2000, we have seen the addition of three divisions to ACA: CSJ, which moved from affiliate status to division status; the *Association of Creativity in Counseling (ACC)* and the *Association for Child and Adolescent Counseling (ACAC)*. With twenty divisions covering a vast array of counseling interests, it is clear that ACA is a diverse group. It also seems evident that after nearly a century of pulling together the divisions into one unified force under ACA, some divisions are asserting that their differences are too great to continue to justify this unification. Some initiatives, such as the development in 2003 of the *ASCA National Model* (ASCA, 2013), which increased the focus of school counselors on student learning (see Chapter 16), and AMHCA's increasing push toward a greater clinical focus (see Chapter 17), have made these differences deeper. Today, one can join many of the divisions without the former requirement of ACA membership. Although we are all counselors, whether we will all remain under one roof is a question that will be answered in the years to come.

A Push Toward Unity: The 20/20 Standards

Although the divisions have become increasingly independent, there has been a concurrent push for unity among all counseling professional groups that has brought forth the development of the 20/20 Standards. For three years, thirty counseling-related professional groups worked together to develop a vision of what they thought the counseling profession would want to be by the year 2020 (Kaplan & Gladding, 2011). From this, in 2010, came the *20/20: A Vision of the Future of Counseling Principles for Unifying and Strengthening the Profession* (ACA, 2013a, 2013c). This shared vision includes the following tenets (Kaplan & Gladding, 2011, p. 372):

1. Sharing a common professional identity is critical for counselors.
2. Presenting ourselves as a unified profession has multiple benefits.
3. Working together to improve the public perception of counseling and to advocate for professional issues will strengthen the profession.
4. Creating a portability system for licensure will benefit counselors and strengthen the counseling profession.
5. Expanding and promoting our research base is essential to the efficacy of professional counselors and to the public perception of the profession.
6. Focusing on students and prospective students is necessary to ensure the ongoing health of the counseling profession.
7. Promoting client welfare and advocating for the populations we serve is a primary focus of the counseling profession.

Credentialing

National counselor certification has continued to expand, and today, there are about 56,000 *National Certified Counselors (NCCs)* (NBCC, 2014b) and thousands of other counselors who are certified in related specialty areas such as clinical mental health counseling, school counseling, addiction counseling, rehabilitation counseling, supervision, and more. Meanwhile, all 50 states, as well as Puerto Rico and the District of Columbia, have state licensure for counselors, and today, there are well over 120,000 licensed counselors (ACA, 2011). As credentialing becomes increasingly important for job attainment, third-party reimbursement, and professional recognition, we will continue to see an increase in the number of certified and licensed counselors.

Changes in Ethical Guidelines

The recent 2014 ACA code of ethics represents the fifth revision since the original code was developed in 1961 (Daniel-Burke, 2014) (see the Appendix). As you might expect, the code has greatly expanded, and with each revision, it tries to keep up with current trends in the counseling profession and in society. The code is the vehicle for all professional counselors who are members of ACA, as well as licensed counselors from the twenty-one state licensing boards who have adopted it as their code of ethics. Although the code will be discussed in some detail in Chapter 3, here we will highlight some of the recent changes in the code next.

One addition to the new code is that in its preamble, the values of the counseling profession are now clearly delineated. In the new code, there is a much expanded focus on distance counseling, technology, and social media, with a whole section that focuses on this important area and infusion of these issues throughout different parts of the code. Relative to this area, the code now speaks to ensuring the security of electronic records and that such records are backed up. It also states that counselors should be knowledgeable of different laws that may exist across state lines when providing services, electronically, as one might be legally providing services in one state, but not in another. Another issue relative to this area is the importance of the client being fully informed about the risks and benefits of distance counseling and that clients have access to emergency services. This part of the code now asks counselors to find a way of ensuring that they can clearly identify the client with whom they are working. A final addition to this area is the statement that counselors should have a policy that explains their social media presence and manage their social media presence in a way that does not blur boundaries between the counseling and the client.

The current code took out the "end-of-life" exemption from the 2005 code, which allowed counselors to remove themselves from a situation in which a client may be facing end-of-life decisions (e.g., refer to another counselor). It was felt that such an exemption should not be made, and if there was a values conflict between the counselor's values and the client's values (e.g., a client considering suicide as an end-of-life decision), the counselor should seek out supervision, consultation, and or further education as opposed to exiting the situation. Also, the 2014 code specifically states that a counselor can refer someone due to incompetence or lack of training, but that it is not OK to refuse services to someone because of differences in values or personal beliefs (e.g., the sexual orientation of the client).

The new code has altered its statement about what to do if a client has a contagious and life-threatening illness and states that the counselor has a responsibility to assess if the client has placed others at risk and to act in a responsible manner to ensure that others are safe and to warn others, if necessary. The code has a statement encouraging pro bono services or having counselors refer clients to other inexpensive services if clients cannot afford their services. However, the new code also suggests that counselors consider providing other services to the public (e.g., lectures or psychoeducational groups) as a means of reaching individuals who may not be able to afford services. Finally, the new code states that when providing services, counselors should use techniques grounded in theory and research. Although counselors can use a developing theory, the code states that the counselor needs to clearly describe the risks and benefits of the theory and work to minimize any potential risks. In addition, the new code states that counselors do not use techniques that have been shown to be harmful, even if a client requests it.

Culturally Alert Counseling: Cross-Cultural Counseling and Advocacy

In recent years, the counseling profession has seen an increased focus on cross-cultural counseling and on advocacy for clients. This is evidenced by the increase in scholarship in these areas, the inclusion of these areas in the CACREP curriculum guidelines, and ACA's ethical code integrating this focus throughout. These areas have taken on such prominence that some have suggested that cross-cultural counseling has become the *fourth force* in counseling (after psychoanalysis, behaviorism, and humanism) while advocacy has become the *fifth force* (see D'Andrea & Heckman, 2008a; Ratts, 2009). Two driving forces behind this focus have been the *Multicultural Counseling Competencies* and the *Advocacy Competencies*.

Developed in 1991 by the Association for Multicultural Counseling and Development (AMCD), the Multicultural Counseling Competencies were officially adopted by ACA in 2002. These competencies delineate attitudes and beliefs, knowledge, and skills in three areas: the counselor's awareness of the client's worldview, the counselor's awareness of his or her own cultural values and biases, and the counselor's ability to use culturally appropriate intervention strategies (Arredondo, 1999; Arredondo et al., 1996). Then, in 2003, ACA endorsed the Advocacy Competencies, which encompass three areas (client/student, school/community, and public arena), each of which is divided into two levels: whether the counselor is acting on behalf of the competency area or acting with the competency area (Toporek, Lewis, & Crethar, 2009). The purpose of the competencies is to ensure that counselors are actively taking steps toward helping clients overcome some of the external and oppressive barriers they face in their lives (Niles, 2009; Snow, 2013). So important are multicultural counseling and advocacy that two chapters in this book are dedicated to working with diverse clients.

Counselor Efficacy: Evidence-based Practice and Common Factors

This century has challenged counselors to ensure that what we do is based on scientific evidence. For instance, recent research on *evidence-based practice* suggests the importance of matching research-based treatment methodologies with the presenting problem of the client (Thomason, 2010). Other research suggests there are *common factors* in all counseling relationships that counselors should strive for in order to increase the likelihood of positive treatment outcomes (Norcross, 2011; Wampold & Budge, 2012). Some of these factors include having a strong working alliance and being effective at delivering your theoretical approach, regardless of what the approach is. Whether practicing evidence-based counseling or ensuring the use of common factors, having a research base to support what one is doing is reinforced in ACA's ethical code:

> *When providing services, counselors use techniques/procedures/modalities that*
> *are grounded in theory and/or have an empirical or scientific foundation.*
>
> (ACA, 2014a, Section C.7.a)

Crisis, Disaster, and Trauma Training

The horror of the tragic shooting at Sandy Hook Elementary School in 2012, Hurricane Katrina in 2005, and the 2001 terrorist attack on the Twin Towers and the Pentagon, graphically illustrated that as a country, our readiness to react to a disaster was not always particularly good, and that many counselors were inadequately prepared to address crises, disasters, and trauma. Thus, there has been a push in recent years to have counselors trained appropriately to work with crises, disasters, and individuals in trauma (Bowman & Roysircar, 2011). One result of this focus is inclusion of crisis, disaster, and trauma counseling in the CACREP standards (Graham, 2010). The National Child Traumatic Stress Network and National Center for PTSD delineate eight steps in this process, which include (Brymer et al., 2009):

1. *Contact and engagement*
   <u>Goal:</u>   To respond to contacts initiated by survivors or to initiate contacts in a nonintrusive, compassionate, and helpful manner
2. *Safety and comfort*
   <u>Goal:</u>   To enhance immediate and ongoing safety and provide physical and emotional comfort
3. *Stabilization (if needed)*
   <u>Goal:</u>   To calm and orient emotionally overwhelmed or disoriented survivors
4. *Information gathering: Current needs and concerns*
   <u>Goal:</u>   To identify immediate needs and concerns, gather additional information, and tailor Psychological First Aid interventions
5. *Practical assistance*
   <u>Goal:</u>   To offer practical help to survivors in addressing immediate needs and concerns
6. *Connection with social supports*
   <u>Goal:</u>   To help establish brief or ongoing contacts with primary support persons and other sources of support, including family members, friends, and community helping resources

7. *Information on coping*
   Goal: To provide information about stress reactions and coping to reduce distress and promote adaptive functioning
8. *Linkage with collaborative services*
   Goal: To link survivors with available services needed at the time or in the future (p. 19)

Technology and Online Counseling

Technology has quickly changed the way that counseling is learned and practiced. Today, we see increasing numbers of online counseling programs at both the master's and doctoral levels, as well as the recognition that counseling services can now be delivered in unconventional ways, such as via the Internet (Carlisle, Carlisle, Hill, Kirk-Jenkins, & Polychronopoulos, 2013; Craigen, Cole, & Cowan, 2013). With these new delivery methods come many concerns, such as: "How will the privacy of the individual, whether student or client, be protected?" "Is the delivery of coursework or counseling as effective as in-person teaching and counseling?" "What kinds of ethical considerations do we need to consider with these new delivery systems?" and "Will our traditional delivery models of teaching and counseling work well with these new delivery modes?"

As the changes have occurred quickly, our accreditation bodies and our ethics codes have been challenged to keep up with the changing times. Thus, in the CACREP standards and in ACA's ethical codes, as well as related ethical codes, we now see attention drawn to technology—both its limitations and its advantages. As we continue into this century, no doubt there will be a continued expansion of the delivery of services using technology and a continued struggle to ensure that such services are effective.

Changes in the Health Care System

With the Affordable Care Act comes many changes to our health care system and as Obamacare becomes a reality, counselors will need to increasingly make sure that they are included as providers for all insurance companies (ACA, 2012). Similarly, in this century, counselors will be vying continually to be providers for health maintenance organizations (HMOs) and government-sponsored health insurance policies, such as Tricare and to be granted employment status for all government agencies that provide counseling, such as Veterans Administration (VA) hospitals (NBCC, 2014c; Shane, 2012).

DSM-5

Counselors have used the *Diagnostic and Statistical Manual (DSM)* to diagnose clients, plan treatment, and communicate with other mental health professionals (Neukrug & Fawcett, 2014). The recent release of the fifth edition of the DSM ("DSM-5"), with its approximately 250 diagnoses, has undergone a number of changes, including moving all diagnoses to a single-axis system (DSM-IV used two axes); eliminating, adding, and changing diagnostic descriptions; making the DSM in sync with the codes in the *International Classification of Diseases (ICD)* manual; and changing the manner in which diagnoses are reported.

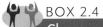

In small groups, discuss what other change you can foresee in the counseling profession during the twenty-first century. Share your ideas in class.

Although the use of DSM has always been controversial, and the ACA ethics code even allows for a counselor to "refrain from making a diagnosis" if he or she thinks that it will harm the client in some manner, it is clear that counselors will increasingly be using the DSM-5 during the coming years.

Globalization of Counseling

Counseling has gone international, and counseling programs and credentialing has emerged around the world. Most recently, the International Registry of Counselor Education Programs (IRCEP) is an organization that was created by CACREP in 2009 (CACREP, 2014c). A subsidiary of CACREP, IRCEP's mission focuses on creating standards, approving programs, maintaining a registry of approved programs, and networking counselors, students, and professionals in the field in an effort to foster excellence (CACREP, 2014d). IRCEP, as well as the independent development of programs and credentials in countries throughout the world, will challenge the manner in which counseling is understood and performed in the United States. As countries can learn much from how the United Sates has developed the counseling profession, we have a lot to learn about alternative models of counseling that have unique takes on the counseling relationship.

Other Issues

Many other issues have affected the counseling field, and still others are likely to surprise us as the twenty-first century continues (Neukrug, 2014). From life coaching, to new theories of counseling, to new drugs for the treatment of mental health issues, to genetic counseling, we will continue to face a constantly changing field—changes that we will sometimes embrace, and others that we will sometimes be wary of. What other changes do you think may arise? (An exercise to foster such exploration is given in Box 2.4.)

Do We Have to Memorize All Those Names?
A Developmental Perspective

A student of mine recently came into my office and complained about having to memorize the names of "picayune" individuals from the counseling profession's past. "What does this have to do with me being an effective counselor?" he argued. Admittedly put somewhat on the defensive, I tried to explain the importance of knowledge building, and that these individuals gave us a base of understanding that has affected the profession today. I believe that this explanation makes a justifiable argument concerning the need to learn such names. However, one thing I did not discuss with him was the concept of "roots." Most of us would agree that our past experience has shaped our development. Our experiences, whether negative or positive, relate strongly to the essence of who we are today. And the same is true in the life of a profession. We are what we are because of our past—and perhaps as important, we will become what we will become as a function of our past as well as what we do in the present. We are a profession in process—a living entity that develops over time. Yes, we could decide to forget our past, not look at our roots, and attempt to move forward. However, I believe that without our knowing it, our roots will still be directing us. Why not strive to understand from whence we came and attempt to make smart, conscious choices about the present and the future? Let's not repress what our past has been; let's be open to understanding it and to forging a new and better path for the future for our profession and ourselves. Such understanding takes courage and work. It is not easy taking a hard look at oneself, and memorizing all those names is not an easy task. Hopefully, Table 2.1 will make this a bit easier.

TABLE 2.1   Summary of Important Historical Events Related to the Field of Counseling

3000 B.C. Ancient Egypt	"Psychological" writings found on papyrus.
400 B.C. Hippocrates	Wrote first reflections on the human condition that include something like modern-day sensibilities.
350 B.C. Plato	Believed that introspection and reflection were the road to knowledge.
350 B.C. Aristotle	Considered by many to be "first psychologist"—studied objectivity and reason.
250 Plotinus	Believed in dualism—the concept that the soul is separate from the body.
400 Augustine	Examined the meaning of consciousness, self-examination, and inquiry.
1250 Thomas Aquinas	Examined the meaning of consciousness and self-examination, and inquiry.
1468 Sanchez de Arevalo	Wrote first job classification system in *Mirror of Men's Lives*.
1500s Elizabethan Poor Laws	Established legislation for the Church of England to help the destitute in England.
1650 René Descartes	Believed that knowledge and truth come through deductive reasoning.
1700 John Locke	Believed the mind is a blank slate upon which ideas are generated.
1800 James Mill	Believed the mind is a blank slate upon which ideas are generated.
1800 Philippe Pinel	Founder of the field of psychiatry; viewed insanity scientifically; advocated humane treatment.
1800 Benjamin Rush	Founder of American psychiatry;. advocated for humane treatment of mentally ill.
1800 Anton Mesmer	Discovered first uses of hypnosis.
1800s COS	Volunteers offered assistance to the poor and destitute.
1850 Jean Martin Charcot	Used hypnosis to understand disorders; saw relationship between psychological and organic states.
1850 Dorothea Dix	Advocated for humane treatment of the mentally ill; helped establish 41 "modern" mental hospitals.
1875 Wilhelm Wundt	First experimental psychologist.
1875 Sir Francis Galton	Early experimental psychologist.
1890s Sigmund Freud	Developed theory of psychoanalysis.
1890s G. Stanley Hall	Founded the APA; early American experimental psychologist.
1890s James Cattell	Early American experimental psychologist.
1890s to mid-1900s John Dewey	Educational reformer who advocated for humanistic teaching methods.

TABLE 2.1 Summary of Important Historical Events Related to the Field of Counseling (*Continued*)

1896 Alfred Binet	Developed first individual intelligence test for the French Ministry of Public Education.
1889 Jane Addams	Established Hull House in Chicago.
1900 Emil Kraepelin	Developed one of the first classifications of mental diseases.
1900 Pierre Janet	Saw a relationship between certain psychological states and organic disorders.
1900 Ivan Pavlov	Developed one of the first behavioral models of learning.
1900 William James	Originated the idea of philosophical pragmatism: reality is continually constructed as a function of its utility or practical purpose.
1906 Eli Weaver	Developed vocational guidance in New York City schools.
1907 Jesse Davis	Developed one of the first guidance curricula in the schools in Grand Rapids, Michigan.
1908 Anna Reed	Established vocational guidance in the Seattle school system.
1908 Frank Parsons	Founder of vocational guidance; developed first comprehensive approach to vocational guidance.
1908 Clifford Beers	Institutionalized for schizophrenia; wrote *A Mind That Found Itself*; advocated humane treatment.
1913 NVGA	National Vocational Guidance Association formed;. distant forerunner of ACA.
1917 Army Alpha Test	First large-scale use of test of ability.
1917 Woodworth Personal Data Sheet	One of the first structured personality tests.
1927 Strong Interest Inventory	One of the first interest inventories to assist in the career counseling process.
1930 E. G. Williamson	Developed first comprehensive theory of counseling; called Minnesota Point of View, or trait-and-factor approach.
1932 John Brewer	Suggested that guidance be seen in a total educational context.
1932 Wagner O'Day Act	Established U. S. Employment Service.
1921 American Psychiatric Association	American Psychiatric Association took current name (originally founded in 1844).
1940s Carl Rogers	Developed nondirective approach to counseling; advocate of humanistic counseling and education.
1940s Division 17 of APA	Division 17 formally became part of APA.
1945 AAMFT	AAMFT officially formed.
1950s Virginia Satir	One of first social workers to stress contextual or systems thinking.
1950s	DSM first developed.
1952 APGA	American Personnel and Guidance Association formed out of four associations;. forerunner of ACA.
1955 NASW	National Association of Social Workers founded from merger of seven associations.
1958 NDEA	National Defense Education Act; provided. training for and expansion of school counselors.
1961 Ethical Codes	Development of first APGA guidelines for ethical behavior.
1960s Great Society Initiatives	Numerous laws passed under President Johnson; development of social service agencies nationally.
1963 *Community Mental Health Centers Act*	Federal law provided for establishment of community mental health centers nationally.
1970s	Development of microcounseling skills training (e.g., Carkhuff, Ivey, Egan).
1970s Cross-cultural Issues	Seminal works published in the area of cross-cultural counseling by such individuals as Donald Atkinson, William Cross, Paul Pedersen, and Derald Sue.

(Continued)

TABLE 2.1 Summary of Important Historical Events Related to the Field of Counseling (*Continued*)

1973 *Rehabilitation Act*	Ensured access to vocational rehab services for adults;. increased need for trained rehabilitation counselors.
1973 CORE	Council for Rehabilitation Education; first credentialing for counselors.
1975 PL94-142	*Education of All Handicapped Children Act;* access to education within the least-restrictive environments; passage of this act extended need for school counselors.
1975 *Donaldson v. O'Connor*	Supreme Court decision leading to deinstitutionalization of mental hospital patients.
1979 NACMHC	National Academy for Certified Mental Health Counselors; offered national certification.
1981 CACREP	Councils for Accreditation of Counseling and Related Programs founded; established accreditation standards for counseling programs.
1982 NBCC	National Board for Certified Counselors; generic certification for counselors.
1983 AACD	APGA name changed to the American Association for Counseling and Development (AACD).
1990s Increased Emphasis	Increased focus on ethical issues, accreditation, professionalism, and multicultural issues; new divisions of ACA founded.
1992 ACA	AACD becomes the American Counseling Association.
1994 Family Therapy Certification	IAMFC offers national certification as a family therapist.
1991 Multicultural Counseling Competencies	Proposed and adopted by AMCD: Competencies suggest how to address multicultural training.
2001	New CACREP Standards.
2002	*Advocacy Competencies* endorsed by ACA.
2003	ASCA National Model.
2009	New CACREP standards; licensure for counselors in all 50 states achieved.
2010	20/20: A vision for the future of counseling; 45,000 National Certified Counselors.
2014	New ethics code.
Current issues	Division expansion and autonomy, 20/20 Standards; credentialing; changes in ethical code; cultural alertness; cross-cultural counseling and advocacy, counselor efficacy, evidenced-based practice, and common factors focus; crisis, disaster, and trauma counseling; technology and online counseling; changes in health care system; DSM-5; globalization of counseling; life-coaching; new theories; and new drugs.

Multicultural/Social Justice Focus: Learning from the Past, Moving Toward the Future

Relative to the role that social justice and cross-cultural issues play in the professional identity of the counselor, we have made great strides from where we were twenty-five years ago. However, we still have a way to go. Despite the fact that multicultural and social justice issues are now vying to be the "fourth and fifth forces" in counseling, and despite the fact that we have Multicultural Counseling Competencies and Advocacy Competencies, and even though research and scholarship on multicultural counseling pervades the counseling literature, there is much that we still must address on our journey to become social justice advocates and culturally competent counselors (Niles, 2009). Some of this includes:

1. Ensuring that all students are trained in the Multicultural Counseling Competencies and the Advocacy Competencies
2. Ensuring that all students are working on their own biases and how they might affect the counseling relationship
3. Ensuring that all students have the knowledge and skills necessary to become culturally competent counselors
4. Providing vehicles for increased scholarship, especially outcome research that provides a road map for counselor best practices relative to social justice and cross-cultural counseling

Ethical, Professional, and Legal Issues: Changing over Time

With the development of the first ACA ethical code in 1961, the counseling profession made a commitment to the conscientious and principled use of counseling approaches. As with all forward-thinking professional associations, since 1961, the ACA has revised its guidelines numerous times. Changes in ethical codes often reflect important concerns taking place in society and the profession. For instance, with the changes in technology that have quickly swept the world, the new 2014 code has an expanded section on distance counseling, technology, and social media and has incorporated information about these important areas throughout the code (see the Appendix). Other areas that the recent revision tackles are values conflicts in counseling, how to deal with life-threatening communicable diseases, and when, if ever, to use theories whose efficacy has not been supported by research (Daniel-Burke, 2014).

As values in society and in our profession evolve, and as our profession continues to develop its own professional identity, our ethical standards will continue to be revised to reflect new viewpoints. Prior ethical standards and laws tell us something about where we have been as a profession and as a country. Current standards and laws reflect the current thinking and values of our profession and country, and challenges to guidelines reflect current struggles and point in the direction of the future (Gale & Austin, 2003). Counselors need to be knowledgeable of the past, aware of the present, and speculative about the future if they are to feel thoroughly involved with the profession.

The Counselor in Process: Looking Back, Looking Ahead, and Embracing Paradigm Shifts

As we look back at our history, we saw the paradigm shifts that took place near the turn of the last century that led to the creation of our field. In the middle of the twentieth century, we saw the next paradigm shift, which led to the expansion of the profession as well as a shift toward a humanistic emphasis. And now, the impact of multicultural and social justice issues seems to be indicating that we are in the midst of another paradigm shift—a shift toward more inclusivity, increased understanding of difference, culturally competent counseling, advocacy work, and a new type of counseling that doesn't always take place in the office. Sometimes it's difficult when you're in the midst of a shift to be clear that a shift is occurring, but my best guess is that we are on the outer end of this shift—and it seems like it's here to stay. Perhaps most interesting—what do you think the next shift will be?

Summary

This chapter examined the history of counseling from its early beginnings to current-day practices. The human condition has been pondered for thousands of years, and the roots of the counseling profession can be traced to early philosophers. The helping professions of social work, psychology, and psychiatry had different beginnings from those of counseling, and over the years, all these professions have moved toward many of the same goals and objectives.

More specifically, this chapter examined the history of the field of social work and saw how its emphasis on systems and advocacy has influenced the counseling profession. We also saw how social work's emphasis on "in-the-field" experiences has had a great impact on counselor education training and its recent trends toward increasing practicum and internship hours. In addition, many of the philosophical roots of modern-day counseling theories arose from the early beginnings of psychology. We examined how laboratory science and research techniques have become important tools for counselors as they research the efficacy of programs they develop and of specific counseling techniques they use; and how tests used by many counselors today had origins in the early days of testing by psychologists. Finally, we saw how the field of psychiatry has offered ways of understanding and classifying mental health problems and how crucial it is for counselors to understand the possible organic nature of some mental health problems.

In addition to tracing the influence of other professions, this text discussed the unique history of the counseling profession. With its early focus in vocational counseling, the counseling profession has moved over the years from the somewhat moralistic, directive approach of vocational guidance to the humanistic approach it adopted starting in the 1940s. We observed how the profession expanded and diversified in the latter part of the twentieth century and how a number of legislative actions during that part of the century greatly influenced the direction and expansion of the profession. The development of ACA paralleled the expansion and diversification of the profession during the twentieth century. In addition, it is clear that the professionalism of the counseling field increased over the years, as evidenced by the creation of ethical standards, an increase in the types and numbers of individuals becoming credentialed, and the establishment of accreditation standards for counseling programs.

As the chapter shifted focus to the current century, it highlighted a number of issues that will likely be important to the counseling profession. These included continued division expansion and division autonomy, and also a push toward unity through the 20/20

Standards; expansion of credentialing; continued changes in ethical guidelines; an ever-increasing focus on being culturally alert through such things as the Multicultural Counseling Competencies and the Advocacy Competencies; an increased focus on counselor efficacy through evidence-based practice and the use of common factors in counseling; increased training in crisis, disaster, and trauma counseling; ever-changing ways of learning and performing counseling brought on by technology; changes in the health care system that will affect how and who can do counseling; changes in the ways that diagnosis is understood through DSM-5; the globalization of counseling and the expansion of IRCEP; and other issues, such as life coaching, new theories, new drugs for treatment, and more.

This chapter ended with a brief discussion of the importance of the relatively recent increased focus on multicultural counseling and social justice issues and made some suggestions regarding what still needs to be done in these areas, including having all students trained in the Multicultural Counselor Competencies and the Advocacy Competencies, ensuring that all students are working to fight their own biases, having all students learn the knowledge and skills necessary to be culturally competent, and providing vehicles for increased scholarship in these areas. The text also talked about how our ethical codes change over time and reflect changes in society and in the profession. Finally, we considered whether we are currently in another paradigm shift in counseling, focused on multicultural and social justice issues, and wondered what the future will bring.

Further Practice

Visit CengageBrain.com to respond to additional material that highlight the salient aspects of the chapter content. There, you can find ethical, professional, and legal vignettes, a number of experiential exercises, and study tools including a glossary, flashcards, and sample test items. Hopefully, these will enhance your learning and be fun and interesting.

CHAPTER 3

Ethics, Accreditation, Credentialing, Multicultural Counseling, and the Standards Associated with Them

It was 1976, and I was working at a mental health center as an outpatient therapist seeing a client who was known to have made up to 50 somewhat serious suicide attempts. I'll never forget that at the end of one session, she looked at me and said, "I'm going to kill myself," and walked out. I immediately ran to get my supervisor, who said, "Get in my car," and the next thing I knew, we were in a car chase after my client. We caught up to her, just about forced her into coming back to the center, and hospitalized her against her will. As we were doing all of this, I was wondering about the ethics of having a car chase and bringing her back to the center. I also thought about the legal ramifications if we had not done anything and risked a potential suicide, to say nothing of our moral obligation!

After receiving my doctorate in counselor education, I became a faculty member at a small college in New Hampshire. I took the national counselor certification exam and became a nationally certified counselor. A few years later, I applied for licensure as a psychologist in New Hampshire and nearby Massachusetts. Both state licensing boards gave me a hard time, saying my degree was in counseling, not psychology, and not from a school accredited by the American Psychological Association. Eventually, they did license me (which would probably be unlikely today). A few years later, I moved to Virginia, where the psychology licensing board told me I could not get licensed as a psychologist and suggested that I get licensed as a Licensed Professional Counselor (LPC). How odd, I thought, that different states view my background in different ways.

I teach at a state university in a program accredited by the Council for the Accreditation of Counseling and Related Educational Programs (CACREP). Because the program is CACREP accredited, students can take the National Counselor Exam (NCE) as they approach their graduation date. Students who have graduated from a non-CACREP-accredited university must wait until they graduate before taking the exam and must complete 3,000 hours of supervised experience within two years before they can be certified. Clearly, students from a CACREP-accredited program are at an advantage.

When I obtained my degrees, there were few, if any, courses in cross-cultural counseling. Some lip service was paid to the topic, but it was not really included in the curriculum. In fact, articles and books on cross-cultural counseling hardly existed. So, I've had to learn the old way, by reading on my own. And relative to social justice, well, that term didn't exist on nearly the scale it does today. Clearly, we didn't learn how it fit into the "counseling way." This too I had to learn the old-fashioned way. This field has certainly changed.

The examples above reflect some of the struggles and challenges associated with ethics, accreditation, credentialing, and multicultural counseling, and the development of standards related to these areas are symbols that a profession has matured and has taken a serious look at where it has been, where it is, and where it wants to go. As standards evolve, professions can reflect upon, revise, and sometimes even eliminate some of their standards. Despite the fact that the helping professions have existed for more than 100 years, the development of standards is relatively new. In this chapter, I will examine these four areas and review how professional standards related to them have influenced the delivery of counseling services today.

Ethics

Defining Values, Ethics, Morality, and Their Relationship to the Law

> *After meeting with a 17-year-old high school student who has been truant from school and has a history of acting-out behaviors, you find evidence that an uncle who is five years older than she had molested her when she was 12 years old. In addition, you believe that the young woman has been involved in some petty crimes, such as shoplifting and stealing audio equipment from the school. What are your moral, ethical, and legal obligations?*

On a daily basis, counselors are not generally faced with such difficult situations as the one just described; however, they are periodically confronted with complicated and sometimes delicate situations in their work. In these moments, they need to know how to respond. If counselors are to respond in the best manner possible, it is important that they know the difference between their moral, ethical, and legal obligations.

Morality is generally concerned with individual conduct and often reflects the values from an individual's family, religious sect, culture, or nationality. In contrast, *ethics* generally describes the collectively agreed-upon "correct" behaviors within the context of a professional group (Remley & Herlihy, 2014). Therefore, what might be immoral behavior for a minister might be ethical behavior for a counselor. For instance, relying on his or her sect's religious writings, a minister might oppose abortion. On the other hand, relying on ethical guidelines that assert a client's right to self-determination, a counselor might support a client's decision to have an abortion. Sometimes an individual's moral beliefs will conflict with his or her professional ethics (e.g., when a counselor's religious beliefs concerning abortion are in conflict with ethical obligations to preserve the client's right to self-determination). Clearly, trying to make sense of one's values, what is personally "right" or "wrong," and professional ethics can be quite an undertaking at times! And to make things even more confounding, sometimes the law will contradict one's values, sense of morality, and even professional ethics. Or, as Supreme Court Justice Potter Stewart is reported to have said, "There's a big difference between what we have the right to do and what is right." Thus, when laws are passed that are not compatible with what is stated in one's ethical code, professional associations should try to either change the law or make the code fit the law.

Finally, despite the fact that ethical codes guide our behavior, perceptions of what is or is not ethical can vary greatly. For instance, when 535 American Counseling Association (ACA) members were asked to rate whether 77 potential counselor situations were ethical, a great deal of disparity was found on a number of items, as shown in Table 3.1 (Neukrug & Milliken, 2011).

The Development of and Need for Ethical Codes

The establishment of ethical guidelines in the helping professions began at the midpoint of the twentieth century, when, in 1953, the American Psychological Association (APA) published its code of ethics. Not long after, in 1960, the National Association of Social Workers (NASW) adopted its code, and in 1961, the ACA developed its ethical code. Because ethical standards are to some degree a mirror of change in society, the associations' guidelines have undergone a number of major revisions over the years to reflect society's ever-changing values (see ACA, 2014a; APA, 2010a; NASW, 2008). Today, codes serve a

TABLE 3.1 What Is Ethically Correct Behavior?

COUNSELOR BEHAVIOR	% ETHICAL
1. Being an advocate for clients	99
2. Encouraging a client's autonomy and self-determination	98
3. Breaking confidentiality if the client is threatening harm to self	96
4. Referring clients due to interpersonal conflicts	95
5. Having clients address you by your first name	95
6. Making a diagnosis based on DSM	93
7. Using an interpreter to understand your client	89
8. Self-disclosing to a client	87
9. Counseling an undocumented worker ("illegal immigrant")	87
10. Consoling your client through touch (e.g., hand on shoulder)	84
11. Publicly advocating for a controversial cause	84
12. Keeping client records on your office computer	74
13. Attending a client's formal ceremony (e.g., wedding)	72
14. Counseling a terminally ill client on end-of-life decisions, including suicide	69
15. Providing counseling over the Internet	68
16. Hugging a client	67
17. Not being a member of a professional association	66
18. Counseling a pregnant teenager without parental consent	62
19. Telling your client you are angry at him or her	62
20. Sharing confidential information with an administrative supervisor	59
21. Guaranteeing confidentiality for couples and families	58
22. Refraining from making a diagnosis to protect a client from a third party (e.g., employer who might demote a client)	55
23. Bartering (accepting goods or services) for counseling services	53
24. While completing dissertation, using the title "Ph.D. Candidate" in clinical practice	48
25. Withholding information about minor despite parents' request	48
26. Selling clients counseling products (e.g., book, video, etc.)	47
27. Using techniques that are not theory or research based	43
28. Pressuring a client to receive needed services	43

TABLE 3.1   What Is Ethically Correct Behavior? (*Continued*)

COUNSELOR BEHAVIOR	% ETHICAL
29. Becoming sexually involved with a former client (at least 5 years after the counseling relationship ended)	43
30. Not allowing clients to view your case notes about them	43
31. Referring a client, unhappy with his or her homosexuality, for "reparative therapy"	38
32. Accepting clients who are only male or only female	37
33. Guaranteeing confidentiality for group members	37
34. Charging for individual counseling although seeing a family	35
35. Accepting clients only from specific cultural groups	32
36. Breaking the law to protect your client's rights	32
37. Reporting a colleague's unethical conduct without consulting that colleague	30
38. Sharing confidential client information with a colleague	29
39. Not reporting suspected spousal abuse	29
40. Not having malpractice coverage	28
41. Counseling a client engaged in another helping relationship	27
42. Seeing a minor client without parental consent	25
43. Viewing a client's Web page (e.g., Facebook) without consent	23
44. Counseling diverse clients with little cross-cultural training	22
45. Having sex with a person your client knows well	22
46. Setting your fee higher for clients with insurance	22
47. Counseling without training in the presenting problem	20
48. Not allowing clients to view their records	17
49. Trying to change your client's values	13
50. Kissing a client as a friendly gesture (e.g., greeting)	13
51. Accepting a client's decision to commit suicide	12
52. Accepting a gift from a client that's worth more than $25	12
53. Revealing confidential information if a client is deceased	11
54. Counseling a colleague whom you work with	11
55. Having a dual relationship (e.g., client is your child's teacher)	10
56. Telling your client you are attracted to him or her	10
57. Not having a transfer plan should you become incapacitated	9
58. Trying to persuade clients to not have an abortion	8
59. Treating homosexuality as a pathology	6
60. Making grandiose statements about your expertise	6
61. Giving a gift worth more than $25 to a client	5
62. Keeping client records in an unlocked file cabinet	5
63. Not participating in continuing education	5
64. Engaging in a counseling relationship with a friend	5
65. Terminating the counseling relationship without warning	5
66. Not offering a professional disclosure statement	3
67. Referring a client satisfied with his or her homosexuality for "reparative therapy"	3
68. Lending money to your client	3
69. Sharing confidential information with your significant other	3
70. Not reporting suspected abuse of an older client	1
71. Not informing clients of legal rights (e.g., HIPAA, FERPA, confidentiality)	1
72. Stating you are licensed when in process of obtaining it	1
73. Revealing a client's record to the spouse without permission	< 1
74. Not reporting suspected abuse of a child	< 1
75. Attempting to persuade a client to adopt a religious belief	< 1
76. Implying that a certification is the same as a license	< 1
77. Not revealing the limits of confidentiality to your client	< 1

Adapted from Neukrug, E., & Milliken, T. (2011). Counselors' perceptions of ethical behaviors. *Journal of Counseling and Development, 89*, 206–216.

number of purposes, including all of the following (Corey, Corey, Corey, & Callanan, 2015; Dolgoff, Loewenberg, & Harrington, 2009; Remley & Herlihy, 2014):

➤ They protect consumers and further the professional standing of the organization.
➤ They are a statement about the maturity and professional identity of a profession.
➤ They guide professionals toward certain types of behaviors that reflect the underlying values considered to be desirable in the profession.
➤ They offer a framework for the sometimes difficult ethical decision-making process.
➤ They can be offered as one measure of defense if the professional is sued for malpractice.

Although ethical codes can be of considerable assistance in a professional's ethical decision-making process, there are limitations to the use of such a code:

➤ Codes do not address some issues and offer no clear way of responding to other issues.
➤ There are sometimes conflicts within the same code, between the code and the law, and between the code and a counselor's value system.
➤ It is sometimes difficult to enforce ethical violations in the codes.
➤ The public is often not involved in the code construction process, and public interests are not always taken into account.
➤ Codes do not always address "cutting-edge" issues.

In the development and revision of ethical codes, deciding what might be included can be difficult. For instance, there is often a struggle between deciding which societal values should be reflected in codes (Gert, 2005; Ponton & Duba, 2009). In addition, even when societal values are included, they are not always reflective of all individuals within American culture. As an example, the idea of "self-determination," or the notion that we all should have the ability to decide for ourselves what is in our own best interest, is not a value held by all individuals in society, especially those who value the opinions of extended family or authority figures when making important decisions. In addition to societal values, universal truths are often reflected in a code. However, people also debate the universality of so-called universal truths. For example, the idea that "thou shalt not kill" seems to be universal, yet many would hold that killing is ethical if it is sponsored by the state, such as in war or in the form of capital punishment. Thus, deciding what principles to include in a code often involves a fair amount of debate among and reflection by members of professional associations as they try to develop a code that fits most counselors and can be palpable to most clients. Despite wrestling with many different values, those who developed the ethical guidelines of the three major helping professions of counseling, psychology, and social work ended up producing codes that seem fairly similar.

Codes of Ethics in the Helping Professions

ACA's Ethical Standards: A Brief Overview

ACA's ethical code has undergone a number of revisions since it was first adopted in 1961. However, because values of society and professional associations are always changing, and because codes change only periodically (e.g., every 10 years or so), the values reflected in a code sometimes lag behind the values of society and of professional associations (Daniel-Burke, 2014; Ponton & Duba, 2009). Keeping this in mind, the nine sections of ACA's ethical code are briefly summarized below (ACA, 2014a). The summary highlights aspects of the code; however, you are strongly encouraged to read the whole code in detail, which can be found in the appendix or by clicking the knowledge center tab on the ACA website: www.counseling.org.

Section A: The Counseling Relationship. Highlighting important issues within the counseling relationship, this section stresses (1) the importance of respecting the client and looking out for the client's welfare and, to this end, keeping good records, having a plan for counseling, and supporting client networks (e.g., family, community, and religious) when appropriate; (2) obtaining informed consent prior to and during treatment; (3) consulting with others who are working with your client; (4) avoiding harm and not imposing one's own values; (5) not engaging in romantic or sexual relationships or personal virtual relationships with clients and those close to them; (6) maintaining appropriate boundaries and professional relationships with clients and documenting boundary extensions (e.g., attending a graduation ceremony); (7) knowing how to advocate for clients at various levels (e.g., individual, group, institutional, and societal); (8) understanding the importance of identifying roles when working with clients who may have a relationship with one another (e.g., clients who are simultaneously in individual, group, and family counseling); (9) knowing how to screen and protect clients participating in groups; (10) knowing how to establish fees, when bartering is justified, and whether to receive or give gifts; and (11) knowing how to effectively terminate and refer clients, and not abandoning or neglecting clients in counseling (e.g., vacations, illnesses, and terminations).

Section B: Confidentiality and Privacy. Section B examines the importance of (1) respecting clients' rights to confidentiality and privacy; (2) knowing when to keep and break confidentiality (e.g., when there is "foreseeable harm," during end-of-life decision making, when a client has a contagious, life-threatening disease, or court-ordered clients); (3) knowing when and how to share confidential information; (4) understanding the nature of confidentiality relative to group and family work; (5) understanding the nature of confidentiality when working with clients who lack the capacity to give informed consent (e.g., children, incapacitated adults); (6) preserving the confidentiality of records; and (7) making reasonable efforts at protecting a client's confidentiality when consulting with a colleague about that client.

Section C: Professional Responsibility. This section discusses the importance of (1) knowing the ethical code; (2) practicing within one's professional competence and knowing what to do when one is professionally or psychologically impaired or incapacitated; (3) accurately advertising and promoting oneself; (4) accurately representing one's credentials and qualifications; (5) not discriminating against clients; (6) knowing one's public responsibilities, including not engaging in sexual harassment, accurately reporting information to third parties (e.g., insurance companies, courts), being accurate when using the media (e.g., radio talk shows), and not making unjustifiable treatment claims; (7) providing services that are empirically based or, if using a new procedure, explaining its potential risks and benefits to clients and minimizing risk and harm, and (8) ensuring the public can distinguish personal from professional statements.

Section D: Relationships with Other Professionals. This section highlights the importance of (1) maintaining mutually respectful relationships with colleagues, employers, and employees despite differing counseling approaches; forming strong, interdisciplinary relationships with others; and addressing unethical situations and negative working conditions when they might arise; and (2) when acting as a consultant, ensuring that one is competent, understands the needs of the consultee, and obtains informed consent from the consultee.

Section E: Evaluation, Assessment, and Interpretation. This section highlights the importance of (1) using assessment tools to determine client welfare and ensuring the proper use and interpretation of such assessments; (2) being competent in the use of assessment instruments and appropriately using the information gained; (3) obtaining informed consent from clients; (4) releasing data only to those identified by clients; (5) making accurate diagnoses and taking into account cross-cultural issues; (6) choosing instruments based on good reliability, validity, and cross-cultural fairness; (7) ensuring proper testing conditions; (8) ensuring nondiscrimination; (9) knowing proper ways to score and interpret instruments; (10) ensuring test security; (11) ensuring test information is up to date and not obsolete; (12) ensuring that sound, scientific knowledge is used in the construction of ssessment instruments; and (13) ensuring objective results when conducting forensic evaluations.

Section F: Supervision, Training, and Teaching. This section examines the importance of (1) supervisors being responsible for the welfare of their supervisees' clients; (2) supervisors obtaining ongoing training; (3) supervisors maintaining ethical relationships with supervisees, including respect for nonsexual boundaries; (4) supervisors obtaining informed consent from supervisees, ensuring access to consultation when they are not available, and ensuring that supervisees know standards and are familiar with proper procedures for termination; (5) students and supervisees knowing the ACA code of ethics, monitoring themselves to ensure that they are not impaired, and providing clients with a professional disclosure statement about their status as a counseling student or supervisee and how it affects confidentiality; (6) providing ongoing evaluation, assisting supervisees in securing remediation when necessary, and endorsing a supervisee only when they believe that the individual is qualified; (7) counselor educators being competent, infusing multicultural issues, integrating theory and practice, ensuring the rights of students, being careful when presenting "innovative" techniques, ensuring adequate field placements, and ensuring that students and supervisees present professional disclosure statements to clients; (8) counselor educators ensuring student welfare by offering orientations and providing self-help experiences; (9) counselor educators providing adequate program information and orientation, advising, providing self-growth experiences, and addressing personal concerns; (10) counselor educators identifying what is expected of students and working with students who may need referrals for remediation or counseling; (11) counselor educators knowing that they are prohibited from having a sexual relationship with current students or otherwise misusing the power they hold over students; and (12) counselor educators actively infusing multicultural competency into their training and working toward recruiting and retaining diverse faculty and students.

Section G: Research and Publication. A wide range of ethical areas are discussed in this section, including (1) research responsibilities, such as the appropriate use of human research participants; (2) the rights of research participants, such as offering informed consent, ensuring confidentiality, and understanding the use of deception in research; (3) standards for maintaining appropriate boundaries and relationships with research participants; (4) methods for accurately reporting results; and (5) guidelines for accurately publishing results.

Section H: Distance Counseling, Technology, and Social Media. Although issues related to distance counseling, technology, and social media are infused throughout the code, this new section highlights the importance of the following: (1) having knowledge of these areas and knowing the law; (2) conducting proper procedures for informed consent, confidentiality, and security of information; (3) making sure that the client you are corresponding with is actually the client; (4) in a distance counseling relationship, knowing the benefits and limitations, the boundaries, ensuring that clients are up to speed technologically, and knowing how to identify other services if the distance counseling services are not effective; and educating clients on misunderstandings that might arise due to distance issues (e.g., mistaken nonverbals); (5) maintaining appropriate records in light of laws and informing clients about maintenance of records; maintaining links to information about credentials; providing accessibility for individuals with disabilities or those for whom English is not their first language; and (6) maintaining separate professional and personal social media websites; explaining to clients the benefits and drawbacks of the use of social media; respecting the privacy of clients' social media unless given consent; and avoiding the disclosure of clients' confidential information on social media.

Section I: Resolving Ethical Issues. This final section of the ethical code explains the proper steps to take in the reporting and resolution of suspected ethical violations. It addresses (1) possible conflicts between ethical codes and the law and using ethical decision-making models when dealing with ethical dilemmas; (2) how to deal with suspected violations, such as first addressing the individual informally, and then, if no resolution is forthcoming or if the violation has caused harm to another, how to approach the appropriate ethics committee; and (3) the importance of working with ethics committees.

Related Ethical Codes and Standards

In addition to the ACA's ethical code, a number of the divisions and affiliated groups of ACA have established ethical codes in lieu of the codes or standards of best practices that supplement the ACA code. Highlighting just a few of these, the American Mental Health Counselors Association (AMHCA), the American School Counselors Association (ASCA), and the International Association for Marriage and Family Counselors (IAMFC) all have their own codes (AMHCA, 2010; ASCA, 2010; Hendricks, Bradley, Southern, Oliver, & Birdsall, 2011). Also, the Association for Specialists in Group Work (ASGW) has a best practices guideline that supplements the ACA code (ASGW, 2007). In addition, the National Board for Certified Counselors (NBCC) and the Commission on Rehabilitation Counselor Certification (CRCC) both have separate codes for counselors (CRCC, 2010; NBCC, 2012). Clearly, sometimes one must choose which code to adhere to. For instance, if one is a member of ASCA and ACA and is also a National Certified Counselor (NCC), which of the three codes does one follow? Although all three are fairly similar, there are some differences, and bouncing among codes to decide which one to follow when faced with a difficult ethical dilemma may not be the best way to make a decision. However, if time permits, reflecting on the different codes and debating the knowledge held in each might be smart when faced with a difficult situation.

Besides ACA and its divisions, related mental health fields have ethical codes. Thus we find ethical codes from the American Psychological Association (APA, 2010a), the National Association of Social Workers (NASW, 2008), the American Association of Marriage and Family Therapists (AAMFT, 2012), the American Psychiatric Association (2013b), and the National Organization of Human Services (NOHS, 1996). Although there is certainly much in common among the various ethical standards, differences do exist. Of course, it is important to have a clear sense of one's professional affiliation and be particularly familiar with that association's guidelines when making difficult ethical decisions.

Ethical "Hot Spots" for Counselors

By examining complaints filed against counselors, inquiries made by helpers regarding ethical problem areas, and research that examines ethical concerns with which counselors most struggle (Herlihy & Dufrene, 2011; Neukrug & Milliken, 2011), we can begin to look at those areas with which counselors are most likely to face difficult ethical decisions. Table 3.2 highlights some areas that may be ethical "hot spots" for many counselors now and in the near future.

TABLE 3.2   Ethical "Hot Spots" Grouped into Logical Categories

The Counseling Relationship

➤ Bartering (accepting goods or services) for counseling services
➤ Counseling a terminally ill client about end-of life decisions
➤ Using techniques that are not theory or research based
➤ Pressuring a client to receive needed services
➤ Trying to have a client adopt the counselor's values
➤ Dealing with client issues related to medical advances (e.g., genetic testing for diseases)
➤ Diagnosing clients
➤ Working with a client in danger of harming self or others

Legal Issues

➤ Refraining from making a diagnosis to protect a client from a third party (e.g., employer who might demote a client)
➤ Breaking the law to protect your client's rights
➤ Whether to report child abuse
➤ Whether to report spousal abuse
➤ Whether to report elder abuse

TABLE 3.2   Ethical "Hot Spots" Grouped into Logical Categories (*Continued*)

Social and Cultural Issues
➤ Referring a gay or lesbian client for sexual orientation change treatment (e.g., reparative or conversion therapy)
➤ Based on personal preference, accepting clients who are only male or only female
➤ Based on personal preference, accepting clients only from specific cultural groups
➤ Being competent in multicultural counseling
➤ Serving emerging populations with little knowledge of those groups

Boundary Issues
➤ Attending a client's wedding, graduation ceremony, or other formal ceremony
➤ Hugging a client
➤ Selling a product to your client related to the counseling relationship (e.g., book, audiotape, etc.)
➤ Becoming sexually involved with a current client
➤ Having sex with a former client
➤ Self-disclosing your feelings to your clients
➤ Counseling a client (e.g., individual counseling) while the client is in another helping relationship (e.g., family counseling)

Confidentiality
➤ Understanding and managing the nature of confidentiality
➤ Guaranteeing confidentiality for groups, couples, and families
➤ Withholding information about a minor despite a parent's request for information
➤ Not allowing clients to view case notes about them
➤ Sharing confidential client information with a colleague who is not your clinical supervisor

Informed Consent
➤ Seeing a minor client without parental consent
➤ Not obtaining informed consent
➤ Counseling a pregnant teenager without parental consent

Professional Issues
➤ Not being a member of a professional association in counseling
➤ Inappropriate fee assessment
➤ Managing the changing nature of mental health
➤ Reporting a colleague's unethical conduct without first consulting the colleague
➤ Not having malpractice coverage (on your own or through your agency/setting)
➤ Measuring the effectiveness of counseling
➤ Misrepresenting credentials

Technology
➤ Supervising over the Internet
➤ Counseling over the Internet
➤ Security of client records on computers
➤ Transmitting client information over the Internet

SOURCE: Adapted From ACA Code of Ethics.

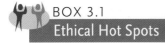
BOX 3.1
Ethical Hot Spots

Distribute the ethical concerns in Table 3.1 or Table 3.2 to students in the class and then have students form small groups to discuss each one that a student was given. In your group, try to come up with some scenarios related to the ethical concern and discuss how the issue might be dealt with. Then, present the salient points of your discussion to the larger class.

Resolving Ethical Dilemmas: Models of Ethical Decision Making

In view of the practical limitations of ethical guidelines noted earlier, and in search of a more flexible and comprehensive approach to resolving ethical dilemmas, models of ethical decision making have been devised (Cottone & Claus, 2000; Welfel, 2013). This section of the chapter examines four types of models: problem-solving, moral, social constructionist, and developmental. These models are not exclusive of each other; that is, they can be used in conjunction with one another. Regardless of the model used, the cultural, religious, and worldview (CRW) of the counselor and of the client should be taken into account when the counselor is faced with a difficult ethical decision (Luke, Goodrich, & Glibride, 2013).

Problem-Solving Models

Problem-solving models provide the clinician with a step-by-step approach to making ethical decisions. They are practical, hands-on approaches that are particularly useful for the beginning clinician. One such approach, developed by Corey et al. (2015), is an eight-step practical model that consists of (1) identifying the problem or dilemma; (2) identifying the potential issues involved; (3) reviewing the relevant ethical guidelines; (4) knowing the applicable laws and regulations; (5) obtaining consultation; (6) considering possible and probable courses of action; (7) enumerating the consequences of various decisions; and (8) deciding on the best course of action. Corey's and other similar models can be a great aid to the clinician in the sometimes thorny ethical decision-making process.

Moral Models (Principle and Virtue Ethics)

While Corey's model emphasizes pragmatism, other models stress the role of moral principles in ethical decision making. Two *moral models* have grown to prominence in recent years: *principled ethics* and *virtue ethics*. These models stress inherent principles or virtues to which the counselor should subscribe when making ethical decisions (Hill, 2004). Kitchener's (1984, 1986; Urofsky, Engels, & Engebretson, 2008) principle ethics model is often described as the foundation or core of ethical codes. Her model describes the role of six moral principles that individuals should consider in the process of ethical decision making: (1) *autonomy* has to do with protecting the independence, self-determination, and freedom of choice of clients; (2) *nonmaleficence* is the concept of "do no harm" when working with clients; (3) *beneficence* is related to promoting the good of society, which can be at least partially accomplished by promoting the client's well-being; (4) *justice* refers to providing equal and fair treatment to all clients; (5) *fidelity* is related to maintaining trust in the counseling relationship (e.g., keeping conversations confidential) and being committed to the client within that relationship, and (6) *veracity* has to do with being truthful and genuine with the client, within the context of the counseling relationship. The clinician who employs this model will use these principles to guide his or her decision-making process.

Kleist and Bitter (2009) note that whereas the focus of principle ethics is on what should be done when making ethical decisions, the focus of virtue ethics is on the character of the counselor who is making the ethical decision. For instance, Meara, Schmidt, and Day (1996) suggest that virtuous helpers are *prudent* or careful and tentative in their decision making, maintain *integrity*, are *respectful*, and are *benevolent*. In addition, virtuous counselors strive to make ideal decisions based on their understanding of their profession and the community. They do this by being self-aware, being compassionate, understanding cultural differences, being motivated to do good, and by having a vision concerning decisions that are made.

Social Constructionist Perspective

One of the more recent additions to ethical decision making, the *social constructionist perspective* sees knowledge (e.g., information in codes about how to make wise ethical decisions) as intersubjective, changeable, and open to interpretation (Guterman & Rudes, 2008). This perspective suggests that realities are socially constructed, constituted through language, organized and maintained through narrative (stories), and that there are no essential truths (Freedman & Combs, 1996). Taking a *postmodern* perspective, they believe that traditional ways of viewing ethical dilemmas could, at times, be problematic and is often the result of the language used and embedded in one's culture and in society. Such language, they suggest, is often subtly (and sometimes not so subtly) oppressive of others, particularly those from nondominant groups. They question what we often take for granted (e.g., diagnosis, theoretical assumptions) and look for dialogue with others to develop new ways of understanding situations.

Although fully aware of ethical guidelines, those who embrace a social constructionist perspective don't expect "answers" to come from a code, within themselves, or within other people. They view solutions to problems as coming out of dialogue between counselors and their clients and others (e.g., supervisors, others in the clients' world). The social constructionist approaches clients with humility, as equals, with wonder, and as collaborators with whom solutions to ethical problems can be jointly worked out.

Developmental Models

Developmental models, created by individuals like Lawrence Kohlberg (1984), William Perry (1970), and Robert Kegan (1982, 1994), suggest that individuals at "lower" levels of development have less of some qualities that are considered positive for counselors than those who are at "higher" levels (Lambie, Hagedor, & Ieva, 2009; Lambie, Smith, & Ieva, 2010; Linstrum, 2005). Although not specifically developed for ethical decision making, their models would suggest that counselors at lower levels of development would want "the answer" to complex questions that might face them, such as those involved in difficult ethical decisions. These counselors often adhere to a rigid view of the truth, and expect (or, at the very least, hope) that such formal documents as ethical codes hold the answer to complex ethical dilemmas. They are also likely to look at those in positions of authority and power (e.g., supervisors) as being able to quickly tell them the correct answer when faced with thorny ethical dilemmas. These counselors can be said to be making meaning from what Perry calls a *dualistic* perspective, in that they view the world in terms of black and white thinking, concreteness, rigidity, oversimplification, stereotyping, self-protectiveness, and authoritarianism. In contrast, higher-level counselors, sometimes called individuals *committed in relativism*, would be more complex thinkers, open to differing opinions, flexible, empathic, sensitive to the context of the ethical dilemma, and nondogmatic (Cottone, 2001; Lambie, Hagedor, & Ieva, 2009; Lambie, Smith, & Ieva, 2010; McAuliffe & Eriksen, 2010). Although few adults (or counselors) reach the highest levels of this development, these models suggest that, if afforded the right opportunities, most can.

You can see that individuals who are at lower levels would make ethical decisions in very different ways than individuals at higher levels. Counselor education programs often offer opportunities to support and challenge students to move toward these higher levels of development.

Summarizing and Integrating the Models

Often, the models just presented are not used in isolation. After reviewing the different models in Table 3.3, read the ethical dilemma presented in Box 3.2. First, consider separately how the problem-solving, moral, and social constructionist models would approach the ethical dilemma faced in the vignette. Then, when working on the developmental model, consider how a person of higher development could integrate all the models in responding to the dilemma.

 BOX 3.2
Using the Ethical Decision-Making Models

John, 82, is seriously depressed and feels that he has no reason to continue living after being recently diagnosed with pancreatic cancer and given less than one year to live. Although he has been seeing you, his counselor, for several months, his outlook on life has not changed, and he is determined to end what he considers to be an "empty existence" before death overtakes him. John's partner of 45 years, Jim, died two years ago, and he now believes that the reality of his own mortality has become apparent. John lives in a retirement complex but has few close friends. He and Jim had isolated themselves from others, and in order to safeguard their privacy, severed all social ties years ago. John has no support system and is not interested in trying to develop one now. He tells you that he has lived long enough and has accomplished most of what he wished to do in life. He is now ready to die and wants only to get it over with as quickly and painlessly as possible. He asks you to help him decide upon the most efficient means of achieving this goal. As his counselor, what should you do?

TABLE 3.3   Summary of Ethical Decision-Making Models

	THEORETICAL ASSUMPTIONS	PRINCIPLES/KEY POINTS	ROLE OF COUNSELOR
Problem-Solving Model	Step-by-step, practical, pragmatic hands-on approach.	Eight steps (see p. 74)	Go through the steps, one by one.
Moral Models			
Principle Ethics	Moral principles play a major role in ethical decision making. Six principles are the foundation of ethical codes. Decisions are based on these principles and on what should be done.	*Six principles:* Autonomy, nonmaleficense, beneficence, justice, fidelity, and veracity.	Consider the six principles in making an ethical decision.
Virtue Ethics	Moral principles play a major role in ethical decision making. The focus is on the character of the counselor, who strives to make ideal decisions based on an understanding of profession and community.	*Four virtues:* Prudence, integrity, respectfulness, and benevolence.	Counselor needs to be self-aware, compassionate, culturally astute, consider doing good, have a vision, and embrace the four virtues in making an ethical decision.
Social Constructionist Model	Knowledge in codes is intersubjective, changeable, and open to interpretation. Realities are socially constructed, constituted through language, organized, and maintained through narrative (stories). There are no essential truths. Ethical dilemmas may be result of inequities in society subtly supported through language.	Solutions to ethical dilemmas come out of dialogue between counselor, his or her clients, his or her supervisor, and others.	Approaches client with humility, as an equal, with wonder, and as a collaborator with whom solutions to ethical problems can be jointly worked out.
Developmental Model	Counselors at "lower" levels of development have less of some qualities effective in ethical decision making than those who are at "higher" levels. All individuals can increase their levels of development.	*Dualistic counselors:* Black and white thinking, concreteness, stereotyping, oversimplification, self-protectiveness, and authoritarianism. *Relativistic counselors:* Complex thinkers, open to differing opinions, flexible, empathic, sensitive to the context of the ethical dilemma, and nondogmatic.	Embody qualities of the relativist in an effort to work through ethical dilemmas.

Reporting Ethical Violations

The ACA Ethical Code (2014a), Section I, provides guidelines on how to proceed if one suspects that a counselor is violating an ethical guideline. Unless substantial harm has occurred or is likely to occur to another, the code first encourages complainants to try and resolve the issue informally by discussing the situation directly with the counselor who is suspected of violating the guideline (see Box 3.3). If no resolution is found, or if

BOX 3.3
The Importance of an Informal Resolution of an Ethical Violation

A friend of mine reported a psychologist to the licensing board for writing "inferior assessment reports." However, she did not go directly to the psychologist. She, who was also a psychologist, ended up being reprimanded by the licensing board because she had not first gone to the professional she was accusing. The accusations against the professional were never addressed.

substantial harm is suspected, then counselors are asked to take "further action," which could include any or all of the following: "referral to state or national committees on professional ethics, voluntary national certification bodies, state licensing boards, or appropriate institutional authorities" (ACA, 2014a, Standard I.2.b).

When a complaint is received, ethics committees will first examine whether they have the jurisdiction to address the complaint. For instance, if a complaint comes to the ACA ethics committee concerning a licensed counselor, and the counselor in question is not a member of ACA, then the ethics committee would likely refer the complainant to the ethics committee of the state in which the counselor is licensed. One study that examined complaints made against licensed professional counselors found that of those complaints made to licensing boards nationally, only 10% were acted upon, with the following consequences: 36% of those had their licenses revoked, 19% had their licenses suspended, 5% were sent letters of reprimand, 4% were required to receive supervision, and 1% were assessed a fine. Another 35% had some other action taken against them, such as community service, further education, or voluntary surrender of license (Neukrug, Milliken, & Walden, 2001).

Legal Issues Related to Ethical Violations
Civil and Criminal Liability

Because some complainants consider potential suspension or expulsion from a professional group too mild a punishment, they may opt to commence a civil lawsuit, or if they suspect a possible criminal act, report it to the authorities in hopes of a criminal prosecution of the counselor. Whereas, "*Criminal liability* is the responsibility under the law for a violation of federal or state criminal statute, *civil liability* is the responsibility one has as a result of having violated a legal duty to another" (personal communication, C. Borstein, Esq. February 6, 2014). As was widely recognized in the O. J. Simpson legal travails, the burden of proof in a criminal case is quite different from that in a civil case. In a criminal matter, the burden is on the state to prove guilt "beyond a reasonable doubt." In a civil matter, the burden is on the plaintiff to prove the case by a "preponderance of the evidence." To highlight these differences, imagine the scale of justice. In a criminal case, the scale needs to sharply drop to one side to establish the defendant's guilt beyond a reasonable doubt; in a civil suit, where the penalty is money rather than potential incarceration, the scale need tilt only slightly in the plaintiff's favor to obtain a verdict and a potential judgment.

In instances of alleged malpractice, complainants most often initiate civil suits against counselors, although counselors could also be charged with criminal violations in the criminal courts. For example, if a counselor is alleged to have had sex with a client in violation of a state statute, a prosecuting attorney (e.g., district attorney) could bring criminal charges against the counselor in criminal court while the client (the alleged victim) pursues a civil court action against the counselor for monetary damages. Anyone can bring a civil lawsuit alleging virtually anything; however, outlandish cases are generally dismissed in a timely manner, and some states have even set up procedures to penalize an individual for arbitrary and capricious acts of malicious prosecution and abuse of process in filing unwarranted lawsuits.

The Role of Ethical Codes in Lawsuits

Although ethical guidelines are not legal documents, whether a counselor is involved in a criminal or civil suit, a professional association's code of ethics can be an important piece of evidence. For instance, a counselor would have a difficult time defending having had sex with a client because the ethical guidelines clearly assert that sex with a client is inappropriate behavior. However, cases are often not clear-cut. For example, a counselor has sex with a former client she had seen six years earlier. The former client feels abused, brings the case to a prosecutor who determines that the statute is unclear about when a client stops being a client, and decides to file criminal charges against the counselor. The counselor then brings the most recent version of the ACA ethical guidelines to court, which states that "Sexual and/or romantic counselor–client interactions or relationships with former clients, their romantic partners, or their family members are prohibited for a period of 5 years following the last professional contact" (ACA, 2014a, Standard A.5.c.). On the other hand, the prosecutor would undoubtedly retort with the following statement, also found in the ethical guidelines: "Counselors, before engaging in sexual and/or romantic interactions or relationships with former clients, their romantic partners, or their family members, demonstrate forethought and document (in written form) whether the interactions or relationship can be viewed as exploitive in any way and/or whether there is still potential to harm the former client; in cases of potential exploitation and/or harm, the counselor avoids entering into such an interaction or relationship" (ACA, 2014a, Standard A.5.c.). Finally, because ethical guidelines are not legal documents, they are likely to carry more weight in a civil court than in a criminal court because the burden of proof is less demanding in a civil case.

Malpractice Insurance

In today's litigious society, there is little doubt that counselors need to be particularly careful—even when they are doing everything correctly, they might still get sued. Remember, anyone can be sued by anybody! Certainly, this does not mean that a counselor will lose a frivolous suit. However, if a counselor finds himself or herself in the dubious position of not having *malpractice insurance* and subsequently loses a civil suit, that counselor may be haunted by the monetary settlement for the rest of his or her life. There is little question that, in today's world, malpractice insurance is almost a necessity. Although most schools and agencies generally purchase an umbrella malpractice insurance policy, it is still prudent to own additional insurance protection. Also, if you work in a setting that has purchased a malpractice policy, review it carefully, study its monetary limits, and examine any possible exclusion to the policy. For instance, are you covered if you work after hours? What if your employer lets you run a workshop for your own personal profit at the agency on the weekend? Are you still covered?

Although colleges and universities almost always carry malpractice insurance for students doing practicum and internship, again, it is always best to check and see if the school does indeed have a policy and the monetary limits of such a policy. The ACA insurance trust has partnered with Healthcare Providers Service Organization (HPSO) to offer professional liability insurance. As of the writing of this text, depending on the state where one practices, HPSO offers $1,000,000 worth of malpractice insurance at $37 per year for students and between $247 and $358 per year for self-employed licensed professional counselors (HPSO, personal communication, February 5, 2014). In addition, new ACA members receive 50% off the price, and for master's-level students, insurance is complimentary (ACA, 2014b).

Avoiding Lawsuits: Best Practices

As one can see from the discussion on ethics and on the importance of malpractice insurance, making ethical decisions can be an arduous and potentially career-threatening process. It is, therefore, essential that clinicians are equipped with the clinical knowledge and tools necessary to make the best decisions when working with clients. Showing a court that you have followed *best practices* in your profession can be critical in winning a lawsuit. Although ethical guidelines are not legal documents, following your professional association's code of ethics can be one important piece of evidence showing that you have adhered to best practices. Gerald Corey and his colleagues describe additional ways in which a clinician can ensure that he or she has been following best practices (Corey et al., 2015). Highlighting some of these ways, they note that clinicians should:

- ➤ Know relevant laws
- ➤ Maintain good records
- ➤ Keep your appointments
- ➤ Ensure security of records
- ➤ Stay professional with clients
- ➤ Document treatment progress
- ➤ Have a sound theoretical approach
- ➤ Maintain the confidentiality of records
- ➤ Preserve appropriate confidentiality
- ➤ Obtain informed consent from clients
- ➤ Report cases of abuse as required by law
- ➤ Treat only within your area of competence
- ➤ Avoid imposing your values or influence on clients
- ➤ Obtain written permission when working with minors
- ➤ Refer when it is in the best interest of your client to do so
- ➤ Be attentive to your clients' needs and treat them with respect
- ➤ Avoid engaging in sexual relationships with current or former clients

➤ Make sure that clients understand information that you present to them

➤ Obtain permission from a client to consult with others, whenever possible

➤ Ensure that clients understand that they can terminate counseling at any point

➤ Assess clients and explain diagnoses and treatment plans and their risks and benefits

➤ Monitor your reactions to clients, especially when countertransference is involved

➤ Know cultural and clinical issues related to bartering and accepting or giving gifts

➤ Keep appropriate boundaries and know limitations of multiple relationships (e.g., counseling a person who is a neighbor)

➤ Provide a professional disclosure statement and obtain informed consent regarding course of treatment

➤ Know how to appropriately assess for clients who may pose a danger of harming self or others, and know what to do if you think a client poses a threat

Accreditation

The History and Development of Professional Preparation Standards

> *Unfortunately, the United States is cluttered with bogus "institutions of higher learning" that issue master's and doctor's "degrees" that are not worth the paper they are printed on and that can even get you into legal trouble if you attempt to proffer them as legitimate credentials. . . . Avoid these rip-offs as you would the plague.*

> (Keith-Spiegel & Wiederman, 2000, p. 53)

Mental health professionals often have responsibilities that heavily affect the lives of others, many of whom are exceptionally vulnerable. Shoddy or inept training could cause counselors to harm people. One mechanism of ensuring good training is through the accreditation of programs. Some of the first programs to offer training standards that would eventually lead to accreditation were in social work during the early part of the twentieth century—soon to be followed by psychology programs in the mid-1940s (Morales, Sheafor, & Scott, 2012; Sheridan, Matarazzo, & Nelson, 1995). Few then realized that today, there would literally be hundreds of accredited programs offering graduate training in counseling, social work, couples and family therapy, and psychology. Although starting a little later than the fields of psychology and social work, the counseling field has made great strides in its efforts toward accreditation within the past 35 years.

The Council for Accreditation of Counseling and Related Educational Programs (CACREP)

CACREP is the accrediting body for counseling programs. The following offers a short history of CACREP, advantages to an accredited program, and a quick overview of the CACREP Standards.

A Short History

> *The acronym CACREP is a mouthful to say. . . . In fact, without the Council for Accreditation of Counseling and Related Educational Programs, counseling would be far less credible as a profession compared to other human service fields that have such an agency.*

(Sweeney, 1992, p. 667)

Although the idea of having standards for counselor education programs can be traced back to the 1940s (Sweeney, 1992), it was not until the 1960s that such standards began to take form with the adoption of training standards for elementary school counselors, secondary school counselors, and student personnel workers in higher education (Altekruse & Wittmer, 1991). Soon, the Association for Counselor Education and Supervision (ACES) merged these standards into one document entitled the *Standards for the Preparation of Counselors and Other Personnel Service Specialists* (Bobby, 2013). Although the Standards were being unofficially used as early as 1973, it was not until 1979 that APGA (now ACA) officially adopted them; and in 1981, APGA created CACREP, a freestanding, incorporated legal body that would oversee the accrediting process. Adoption of the CACREP standards started slowly, and they have gone through a number of revisions prior to taking on their most recent form, which went into effect in January 2009. Today, they are considered *the* standard to which all counseling programs should strive (Urofsky, Bobby, & Ritchie; 2013).

In addition to U.S. based counseling programs, CACREP recently established the International Registry of Counselor Education Programs (IRCEP, 2014), whose focus is to foster excellence in training programs internationally. Finally, CACREP and the Council on Rehabilitation Education (CORE) have recently reached an agreement so that CORE-accredited programs can also become CACREP accredited (CORE, 2014a).

Advantages of CACREP

Considering the vast number of changes that most programs have to make and the amount of time that it takes to implement such changes, it is a tribute to CACREP that nationally, 279 CACREP institutions offer 634 accredited programs in the various specialty areas (Y. Peña, personal communication, February, 6, 2014). With New York State and California fairly recently obtaining licensure for counselors, it is likely that there will be a push in those states to accredit additional counseling programs. As you might guess, all evidence seems to indicate that there will be continued expansion of the number of CACREP-accredited programs. It is probably not surprising that accreditation of counseling problems has quickly spread, as the benefits are many (Urofsky, Bobby, & Ritchie, 2013):

> ➤ Accredited programs produce students who tend to be more knowledgeable about core counseling issues
> ➤ Accredited programs tend to offer longer field placements and practical, hands-on experience
> ➤ Accreditation is often a factor in determining eligibility for credentialing, and students in accredited programs can take the NCE prior to graduation, whereas others have to wait to complete postgraduate experience

➤ Those who graduate from accredited programs generally have better job opportunities
➤ Accredited programs often attract better students and better faculty
➤ Some organizations hire only students who have graduated from CACREP-accredited programs
➤ Those who graduate from accredited programs are sanctioned less frequently for ethical violations

Although some have argued that accredited programs can stifle creativity, are too costly, and limit what can be offered, it is clear that the advantages of CACREP are many.

A Quick Overview of the CACREP Standards

Today, CACREP offers standards for the doctoral degree in counselor education and for the master's degree in clinical mental health counseling (60 credits), school counseling (48 credits), student affairs and college counseling (48 credits), career counseling (48 credits), addiction counseling (60 credits), and marriage, couple, and family counseling (60 credits) (CACREP, 2009). The 2016 standards, which are now being developed, are likely to require 60 credits for all programs.

For all master's programs seeking CACREP accreditation, the standards delineate a variety of requirements within three primary areas. *Learning Environment*, which sets minimal standards for structure and evaluation of the institution, the academic unit, faculty, and staff; *Professional Identity*, which specifies foundations of the program (e.g., mission statement and objectives) and delineates content areas that should be learned by students (i.e., professional orientation and ethical practice, social and cultural diversity, human growth and development, career development, helping relationships, group work, assessment, and research and program evaluation); and *Professional Practice*, which specifies supervisor qualifications and requirements for field work experience that include 100 hours of practicum and 600 hours of internship. Similar types of guidelines are also given for doctoral-level programs in counselor education. In addition to these common standards, each specialty area has other standards that must be met. For instance, clinical mental health counseling requires student learning in the following areas: foundations; counseling, prevention, and intervention; diversity and advocacy; assessment; research and evaluation; and diagnosis. School counseling requires all the same areas, with the exception of diagnosis, and with the addition of academic development, collaboration and consultation, and leadership.

To meet the accreditation standards, most programs find that they need to undertake at least moderate changes. Following the changes, and often while they are being made, a self-study report is written that spells out how the program meets each of the sections of the program standards. This report is then sent along with an application to the CACREP office, which has independent readers review the report. If the report is accepted, then a CACREP team is appointed to visit and review the program and make a final recommendation for or against accreditation.

The CACREP accreditation process tends to be long and arduous. Despite this fact (or perhaps because of it), CACREP has become a major force in the preparation of highly trained counselors and will no doubt continue to have an impact on the counseling field.

Other Accrediting Bodies

Several other accreditation bodies set standards in related fields. For instance, the Council on Rehabilitation Education (CORE, 2014b) accredits rehabilitation counseling programs, and as just mentioned, CORE and CACREP have reached an agreement where CORE-accredited programs can become accredited with CACREP as well. In another related field, we find training centers being approved by the American Association of Pastoral Counselors (AAPC, 2005–2012). These centers do not offer degrees, but they do offer training in pastoral counseling. Usually, a pastoral counselor already has obtained his or her degree in counseling or a related field prior to going to one of these training centers.

In the field of psychology, the American Psychological Association (APA) currently sets standards for doctoral-level programs in counseling and clinical psychology (APA, 2014a). The Council on Social Work Education (CSWE, 2014) is responsible for the accreditation of both undergraduate and graduate social work programs, while AAMFT's Commission on Accreditation for Marital and Family Therapy Education (COAMFTE, 2002–2013) is the accrediting body for marriage and family therapy programs. Although somewhat in conflict with CACREP's accreditation of marriage and family therapy counseling programs, this commission has accredited 116 marriage and family therapy programs in the United States and Canada to date.

Credentialing

> *It is the year 1224 in the city of Sicily, and a young physician gathers his credentials to file for a medical license. He collects proof that he has studied for over eight years in physick, surgery, and logic. He proudly adds a letter from his master physician mentor extolling his extraordinary skill in leech placement and uncanny facility in astrology. The young physician nervously heads off, credentials in hand, to be examined in public by a committee of master physicians. If he passes, the emperor himself will issue a medical license. If he fails, he will be jailed if he attempts to practice medicine again.*

> (Scoville & Newman, 2009, para. 1)

As you can see from the above quote, credentialing in the allied health professions can be traced back to the thirteenth century, when the Holy Roman Empire set requirements for the practice of medicine (Hosie, 1991). Interestingly, the process of obtaining a credential today is not dissimilar to the process in 1224 Sicily. First, you study for a number of years. Then you demonstrate that a mentor (e.g., supervisor) deems you ready, and finally, you take a credentialing exam. However, unlike the young physician in the quote above, you won't get jailed if you fail your credentialing exam.

Credentialing in the helping professions is a relatively new phenomenon; it was not until the 1900s that it became common, and it was not until the 1970s that credentialing in the counseling field first started to become a reality. Today, credentialing cuts across many professions and can be found in many different forms. Usually, credentialing offers many benefits to the profession, the consumer, and the counselor (Bloom, 1996; Corey et al., 2015), including the following:

➤ *Increased professionalization.* Credentialing increases the status of the members of a profession and clearly identifies who those members are.
➤ *Parity.* Credentialing helps counselors achieve parity in professional status, salary, insurance reimbursement, and other areas with closely related mental health professions.
➤ *Delimiting the field.* The process of passing legislation to enable counselors to obtain credentials assists the profession in clearly defining who we are and where we are going.
➤ *Protection of the public.* Credentials help identify to the public those individuals who have the appropriate training and skills to do counseling.

Although credentialing takes many forms, the three most common forms of credentialing include registration, certification, and licensure.

Registration

Registration is the simplest form of credentialing and involves a listing of the members of a particular professional group (Sweeney, 1991). Registration, which is generally regulated by each state, implies that each registered individual has acquired minimal competence, such as a college degree or apprenticeship in his or her particular professional area. Registration of professional groups usually implies that there is little or no regulation of that group. Generally, registration involves a modest fee. Today, few states provide registration for professionals, opting instead for the more rigid credentialing standards of certification, licensure, or both.

Certification

Certification involves the formal recognition that individuals within a professional group have met certain predetermined standards of professionalism (ACA, 2014c). Although more rigorous than registration, certification is less demanding than licensure. Generally, certification is seen as a protection of a title (Remley & Herlihy, 2014); that is, it attests to a person's attainment of a certain level of competence but does not define the scope and practice of a professional (what a person can do and where he or she can do it). A yearly fee must usually be paid to maintain certification.

Certification is often overseen by national boards, such as the NBCC (2014a, 2014b). Although national certification suggests that a certain level of competence in a professional field has been achieved, unless a state legislates that the specific national certification will be used at the state level, such certification carries little or no legal clout. Many individuals will nevertheless obtain certification because it indicates that they have mastered a body of knowledge, which can sometimes be important for hiring and promotion. Certification often requires ongoing continuing education for counselors to maintain their credentials.

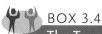

BOX 3.4
The Topsy Turvy World of Credentialing

Professional school counselors are required by law and/or regulation in every state to obtain a state-issued credential in order to be employed in public schools. In some states this credential is called "certification"; others term it "licensure" or "endorsement."

(Lum, 2003, p. 5)

There are many caveats to the above definitions of registration, certification, and licensing. For instance, although I was a licensed psychologist in Massachusetts and New Hampshire, when I moved to Virginia, the psychology licensing board would not license me. I was, however, quite content to obtain my license as a professional counselor. You see, state licenses are often not reciprocal.

Also, state boards of education often use the words *certification* or *licensure* for school personnel (e.g., teachers, school counselors, and school psychologists). This means that individuals have successfully graduated from a state-approved program in their respective area. However, there is no rhyme or reason why one state will use the word "certified" school counselor while another will use "licensed" school counselor. And in these cases, the words do not carry the same meaning as the national certifications or state licenses described earlier.

Finally, you will find other idiosyncratic usages of the words *certification* and *licensure* depending on the state you live in. Therefore, check your state regulations to be sure that you know how credentialing operates where you live.

Licensure

The most rigorous form of credentialing is *licensing*. Generally regulated by states, licensure denotes that the licensed individual has met rigorous standards and that individuals without licenses cannot practice in that particular professional arena (ACA, 2014c). Whereas certification protects only the title, licensure generally defines the scope of what an individual can and cannot do. For instance, in Virginia, the counselor licensing law not only defines the requirements that one must meet to become licensed, but also defines what is meant by counseling, who can do it, the limits of confidentiality and privileged communication (see Chapter 4), legal regulations related to suspected violations of the law (e.g., child abuse), and other various restrictions and regulations (Virginia Board of Counseling, 2013).

In terms of day-to-day professional functioning, the most important aspect of counselor licensure has become the fact that in most states, licensure carries with it legislation that mandates *third-party reimbursement* privileges. Such legislation requires insurance companies to reimburse licensed individuals for counseling and psychotherapy. As with certification, licensure generally involves a yearly fee, and often continuing education requirements are mandated (see Box 3.4).

Credentialing in Related Helping Professions

It is recognized that there is competition for clients among professionals providing mental health services and that there is also concern about the degree of preparation and expertise of a number of professions to deliver those services.

(Garcia, 1990, p. 495)

Although written almost twenty-five years ago, this quote is still relevant today. Competition between credentialed mental health professionals is real, and whether a professional is credentialed will make a huge difference in one's ability to obtain clients. Let's take a look at some of the different credentials in our cousin professions.

Master's Degree in Social Work Credentialing

On the national level, a number of credentials exist for the many types of master's-level social workers. Experienced social workers can hold a credential as an ACSW from the Academy of Certified Social Workers (ACSW). Those who have more clinical experience can become a Qualified Clinical Social Worker (QCSW), and advanced clinicians can become a Diplomate in Clinical Social Work (DCSW). In addition, many clinical social workers become licensed in their states and become Licensed Clinical Social Workers (LCSWs) (Association of Social Work Boards, 2013).

Doctoral-Level Credentialing as a Psychologist

The first push for credentialing of doctoral-level psychologists came during the 1950s (Cummings, 1990). Today, every state offers licensure for doctoral-level psychologists, generally in the areas of counseling and clinical psychology. In addition, many states now offer hospital privileges for *licensed psychologists*. Such privileges afford psychologists the right to treat those who have been hospitalized with serious mental illness. Not surprisingly, psychologists have recently sought to gain the right to prescribe medication for emotional disorders, but so far with very limited success (Rutkow, Vernick, Wissow, Kaufmann, & Hodge, 2011).

Marriage and Family Therapy Credentialing

Today, every state in the United States has enacted some credentialing laws for marriage and family counselors or therapists. In some cases, state marriage and family licensure boards are independent and have followed the guidelines set by the AAMFT. In other cases, such marriage and family licensure has been subsumed under the counseling board or the boards of other related mental health professions. In addition to licensure, in 1994 the International Association of Marriage and Family Counselors (IAMFC), a division of ACA, developed a certification process through the National Credentialing Academy (NCA) that enables a marriage and family therapist to become a Certified Family Therapist (CFT) (NCA, n.d.).

Credentialing as a Psychiatrist

Because licensure is a state responsibility and is not specialty specific, individuals are licensed as medical doctors, not pediatricians, psychiatrists, surgeons, and so forth. Therefore, a physician who obtains a license within a state can theoretically practice in any area of medicine. However, because the ability to be paid by insurance companies and hospital accreditation standards generally requires the hiring of board-certified physicians, almost all physicians today are board certified in a specialty area. Board certification means that the physician has had additional experience in the specialty area and has taken and passed a rigorous exam in that area. Thus, most psychiatrists are not only licensed physicians within the state where they practice, but are generally board certified in psychiatry (B. Britton, M.D., personal communication, February 6, 2014).

Credentialing as a Psychiatric–Mental Health Nurse

There are two levels of *psychiatric–mental health nurses*—the basic and the advanced. Basic psychiatric–mental health nurses generally do not have advanced degrees and can work with clients and families doing entry-level psychiatric nursing. In contrast, advanced psychiatric–mental health nurses are generally registered nurses (RNs) with a master's degree in psychiatric–mental health nursing. These Advanced Practice Registered Nurses (APRNs) can offer a wide-range of mental health services, prescribe medication, and receive third-party reimbursement in many states (APNA, n.d.).

Credentialing for Counselors

Although the first credentialing of counselors can be traced to the certification of school counselors in the 1940s (Bradley, 1995), counselor credentialing in the form of certification and licensure did not take off until the 1970s. Below is a brief examination of some of the certification and licensure gains within the past 40 years.

Certified Rehabilitation Counselors (CRCs)

In 1974, the field of rehabilitation counseling became one of the first counseling specialty areas to obtain certification for its members through the *Commission on Rehabilitation Counselor Certification* (CRCC, 2014; Livingston, 1979). Since its inception, CRCC has credentialed over 35,000 Certified Rehabilitation Counselors (CRCs).

National Counselor Certification (NCC)

The NBCC was established in 1982 to "monitor a national certification system, to identify those counselors who have voluntarily sought and obtained certification, and to maintain a register of those counselors" (NBCC, 2014b, para. 1). Today, over 55,000 counselors have become NCCs. Students who have graduated from a CACREP-approved program may take the *National Counselor Exam (NCE)* prior to their graduation and, assuming they pass, are certified upon graduation. Those who have not graduated from a CACREP-approved program may take the NCE immediately following graduation; however, they become an NCC only after they have successfully completed a minimum of two years of post-master's experience with 100 hours of supervision and 3,000 hours of work experience. Finally, most licensing boards have adopted the NCE, or some of its specialty certifications (see next section), as part of their licensing process (NBCC, 2014a, 2014b).

Specialty Certifications in Counseling

In addition to the NCC, NBCC offers three specialty certifications: *Certified Clinical Mental Health Counselor (CCMHC)*, *National Certified School Counselor (NCSC)*, and the

Master Addiction Counselor (MAC). The NCC is a prerequisite or co-requisite to these specialties (NBCC, 2014a, 2014b). Finally, as noted earlier, the IAMFC, through the NCA, has developed a process of national certification for marriage and family counselors (NCA, n.d.). In the past 30-odd years, the certification process has done much for the professionalization of the counseling field. Signifying competence in our field, the NCC and the specialty certifications demonstrate a unifying force within the profession that links all specialties. Similar to physicians, where one is first a physician and secondarily a cardiologist, pediatrician, psychiatrist, and so forth, a counselor is first a counselor and secondarily a school counselor, clinical mental health counselor, college counselor, addiction counselor, and so forth.

Counselor Licensure

The movement toward professional counselor licensure began slowly in the 1960s but picked up steam in 1976, when Virginia became the first state to pass a licensing law for counselors. Today, all 50 states, Puerto Rico, and the District of Columbia offer licensing, and there are approximately 120,000 licensed counselors nationally (see ACA, 2014c; NBCC, 2014a). Although usually called *Licensed Professional Counselors (LPCs)*, some states use alternative names (e.g., licensed counselor). As some densely populated states like New York and California have just recently approved counselor licensure, this number will surely rise quickly. As noted earlier, the NCC or its subspecialty certifications are often used by states as the licensing exam. In addition to an exam, licensure generally includes a minimum of two years of post-master's-degree supervision, sometimes additional coursework, and other requirements depending on the state.

Lobbying for Credentialing and Counseling-Related Issues

Political action committees, lobbyists, and offering free lunches to legislators— certainly these are not within the realm of counselors (or are they)? In fact, lobbying and grassroots efforts that counseling associations take to introduce or defeat legislation have become crucial to the survival of the profession (see ACA, 2014d). For instance, if counselors hadn't lobbied for the establishment of elementary and middle school counselors, they would not be in existence today. Similarly, counselors had to push continually to obtain licensure in all 50 states. Today, we must continue to lobby to ensure that we are included as providers for various health insurance plans. If counselors are not included, the counselor as private practitioner might no longer exist.

In today's world, the public wants to see proof that the counselor's role is necessary. Lobbyists and our grassroots efforts help to show the importance of counseling. Credentialing helps to show the public that we are experts at what we do. Who pays for these efforts? We do! A portion of our professional association membership fees goes to pay for lobbyists and legislative initiatives in which counselors find ways to support our own interests. When you refrain from joining your professional association, you reap the benefits for which others are paying!

Multicultural/Social Justice Standards: Multicultural Counseling Competencies and Advocacy Competencies

> *Both the multicultural and social justice counseling perspectives acknowledge the importance of diversity and recognize that oppression has a debilitating effect on mental health. Together, both perspectives promote the need to develop multiculturally and advocacy competent helping professionals.*
>
> (Ratts, 2011)

Increasingly, *multicultural counseling* and *social justice advocacy* are viewed as one broad effort to reduce or eliminate injustice in the helping professions (Pieterse, Evans, Butner, Colins, & Mason, 2009). However, in many ways, social justice advocacy is a subset of multicultural counseling. Whereas multicultural counseling is mostly focused upon the development of counselor competencies in an effort to maximize the ability of counselors to work with all clients, social justice advocacy focuses on taking action to effect change in an effort to help marginalized clients. Although the main focus of the counseling profession was initially on multicultural competence, social justice advocacy has taken a prominent role more recently. Thus, it is not surprising that in 1991, Sue, Arredondo, and McDavis (1992) developed a set of skills they called the *Multicultural Counseling Competencies*, and it was not until 2002 that the *Advocacy Competencies* were developed. Let's take a look at both sets of competencies.

Multicultural Counseling Competencies

The original Multicultural Counseling Competencies were developed by Sue et al. (1992), and later expanded and operationalized to help guide educators in the training of counselors (Arredondo, 1999; Arredondo et al., 1996). The competencies were subsequently adopted by the Association for Multicultural Counseling and Development (AMCD) and then by ACA (Roysircar, Arredondo, Fuertes, Ponterotto, & Toporek, 2003). Today, the competencies reflect the minimum standards needed by all counselors if they are to work effectively with diverse clients. The competencies delineate attitudes and beliefs, knowledge, and skills in three areas: the counselor's awareness of the client's worldview, the counselor's awareness of one's own cultural values and biases, and the counselor's ability to use culturally appropriate intervention strategies (see Figure 3.1). Operational definitions of the competencies can be found at the ACA website (go to www.counseling.org and click "knowledge center," then "competencies"). Today, most counselor education programs focus on these strategies to help students increase multicultural competence.

Advocacy Competencies

The development of Advocacy Competencies grew out of a number of parallel processes occurring within the broader counseling community (Toporek, Lewis, & Crethar, 2009).

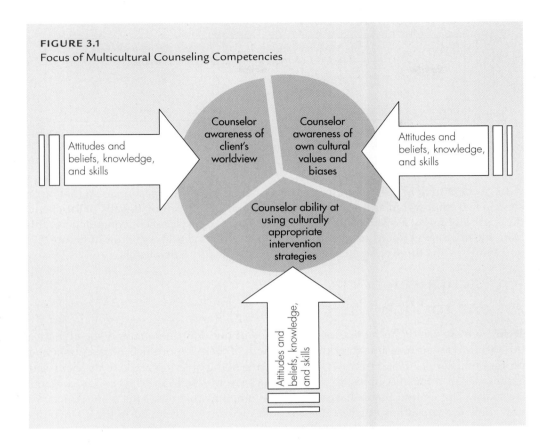

FIGURE 3.1
Focus of Multicultural Counseling Competencies

First, the *Transforming School Counseling* initiative, which sought to change the way school counselors practiced (see Chapter 16), was developed during the 1990s and had advocacy as one of its major concentrations. Also, counselors were increasingly becoming more at ease with advocacy as they took on advocacy roles to obtain counselor licensure in each of the 50 states and fought for parity with other mental health professions. Third, a number of counselors gathered during the 1990s to discuss social justice issues. Out of these discussions arose the Counselors for Social Justice (CSJ) division of ACA, which found itself in a particularly good position to conduct research and disseminate information about social justice and advocacy. Finally, during the 1990s and early part of the 2000s, ACA presidents became particularly focused on advocacy issues and a new task force was formed to examine the possibility of developing Advocacy Competencies. Soon the competencies were developed, and in 2003, they were endorsed by ACA.

The Advocacy Competencies encompass three areas of competence (client/student, school/community, public arena), each of which are divided into two levels: whether the counselor is "acting on behalf" of the competency area or "acting with" the competency area (see Figure 3.2). For instance, with the client competency, a counselor might "act

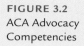

FIGURE 3.2
ACA Advocacy
Competencies

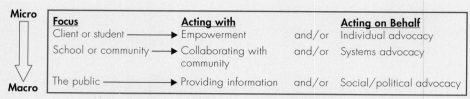

Micro	Focus	Acting with		Acting on Behalf
	Client or student ──────▶	Empowerment	and/or	Individual advocacy
	School or community ──▶	Collaborating with community	and/or	Systems advocacy
Macro	The public ──────────▶	Providing information	and/or	Social/political advocacy

Adapted from: Toporek, R. L. Lewis, J. A., & Crethar, H. C. (2009). Promoting systemic change through the ACA advocacy competencies. Journal of Counseling and Development, 87, p. 267.

with" a client to help the client identify his or her strengths and resources so that he or she can feel empowered and advocate for himself or herself; or, "on behalf" of the client, the counselor might assist the client in accessing needed services. The competencies run from the microlevel (focus on client) to the macrolevel (focus on system). In Figure 3.2, you can view the three competency areas, each divided into two levels.

Multicultural/Social Justice Focus: A Lens to View the Profession

Today, we are seeing an increasing acceptance of multiculturalism and social justice throughout our culture and an acknowledgment of their importance to the counseling profession (Ratts, 2011). From gays and lesbians being able to marry, to an increased acceptance of biracial couples, to the TV shows we watch, to the day-to-day contacts we make. The United States has clearly changed, and this new lens from which we now view the world has affected the standards we have developed in the counseling field. In fact, some suggest that multicultural and social justice orientation represent the fourth and fifth transformation of the counseling profession, and they have taken on the same importance of the first three transformations: psychoanalysis, behavior therapy, and humanistic counseling (Chang, Crethar, & Ratts, 2010).

Having a multicultural "eye" is now expected when we develop our ethical codes, when we view the ethical decisions we make, when we develop our accreditation standards, when we assess whether a program is ready to be accredited, and when we consider the skills needed for becoming credentialed. Today, we are expected to be well versed in multicultural cultural competencies and on social justice issues. In some ways, it took a long time getting here, but in other ways, our field has moved quickly in the past few years. There is still more to do, but it is clear, we have turned a corner on our push to become a professional that addresses multicultural issues.

Ethical, Professional, and Legal Issues: A Plethora of Standards?

Years ago, when asked if he believed in licensure, Carl Rogers would often respond "No," because he thought that many good counselors and therapists would be left out of the exclusive club that was slowly being developed. And, as turf battles have erupted over the years among the various professions, and as each profession has vowed to keep the other professions "out," you've got to wonder sometimes if he was right.

Today, we have counselor licensure and counselor certification, psychology licensure and psychology certification, social work licensure and social work certification, and more. We have multiple ethical codes, and sometimes we don't know which one we should follow, and we have accreditation bodies that increasingly tell programs that they will not be accredited if they hire someone outside of their discipline. And now we have the Multicultural Counseling Competencies and Advocacy Competencies, and I can tell you, I've seen many a person get shunned for not being an advocate for those competencies.

There's little doubt that we have become, in a way, our own exclusive professional club. Maybe in some ways that is not such a good thing, as we sometimes viciously vie for a position of power against our mental health cousins (e.g., psychologists and social workers), and as we proudly keep out those who do not meet or support the many standards that we have developed. On the other hand, maybe our standards play a critical role for us, as they provide our profession with a strong sense of where we have been, who we are, and where we are going. Look at the good and the bad, and decide—has it been worth it?

The Counselor in Process: A Lifelong Commitment to Professionalism

Embracing a professional lifestyle does not end once one finishes graduate school, obtains a job, becomes credentialed, has ten years of experience, or becomes a "master" counselor. It is a lifelong commitment to a way of being—a way that says that you are constantly striving to make yourself a better person, a more effective counselor, and a counselor committed to professional activities and to excellence in the field. Our profession has come a long way since the turn of the last century, as is evidenced by the increasing number of standards highlighted in this chapter. It is our job and our obligation to stay current with the most recent efforts to better ourselves as counselors and as professionals. And, despite all our efforts, 100 years from now, our successors will undoubtedly say, "How naive they were." We have come very far, and yet we still have far to go.

Summary

This chapter examined four broad standards in the field of counseling: ethics, accreditation, credentialing, and multicultural/social justice standards. Starting with ethics, we distinguished morality from professional ethics. We spoke of the relatively brief history of the development of ethical codes and identified a number of the purposes and limitations of codes. The chapter summarized the eight sections of the ACA code (Sections A through H), and we also identified other codes in the counseling profession, including those of AMHCA, ASCA, NBCC, CRCC, and IAMFC. We also identified related professional codes (e.g., AAMFT, APA, NASW, and NOHS), and then discussed a number of ethical "hot spots" and grouped them into several categories: the counseling relationship, legal issues, social and cultural issues, relationship and boundary issues, confidentiality, informed consent, and professional/practice issues. Next, we presented ethical decision-making models, including a problem-solving model; two types of moral models, principle ethics and virtue ethics; a social constructionist model; and a developmental model. Next, the discussion detailed how to report ethical violations and highlighted the consequences to licensed professional counselors who violated an ethical guideline. This section concluded with a discussion of legal issues related to ethical violations, including distinguishing between civil and criminal liability, the role of ethical codes in lawsuits, the importance of malpractice insurance, and using best practices in counseling to avoid lawsuits.

The chapter next moved to a discussion of accreditation. We presented the history of counseling program accreditation and noted that CACREP's original standards were ad-opted in 1981. We talked about the rapid spread of programs that are accredited and high-lighted some of the benefits and drawbacks to accreditation, and also noted that IRCEP was developed by CACREP to work with international programs and that CORE and CACREP have developed a policy where CORE-accredited programs can also become CACREP-accredited. We noted that the 2009 CACREP standards address accreditation for clinical mental health counseling, school counseling, student affairs and college counsel-ing, career counseling, addiction counseling, and marriage, couple, and family counsel-ing. Next, the chapter gave a quick overview of what is required for a program to become CACREP accredited. This section concluded by noting a number of accrediting bodies in related mental health professions, including CORE, AAPC, APA, CSWE, and COAMFTE.

Credentialing was covered next. We mentioned some of the benefits of credential-ing, such as increased professionalization, parity, delimiting the field, and protection of the public. We distinguished registration from certification and from licensing, and also noted that there continues to be some confusion and cross-use of these concepts. We then examined some of the credentials in related mental health fields. For instance, for social workers, we highlighted the ACSW, QSCW, DCSW, and LCSW. For psychologists, we noted that all states license doctoral level counseling, clinical psychologists, or both. We also noted that marriage and family counselors can be licensed in many states, although regulations vary, and IAMFC offers a national certification in this area. We pointed out that psychiatrists are physicians who specialize in psychiatry, and psychiatric–mental health nurses can be credentialed at a basic or advanced level. For counselors, we identified many types of credentials, including CRC, NCC, CCMHC, NCSC, MAC, and counselor licensure (usually called LPC). We concluded with a discussion about the importance of lobbying as an influence on credentialing and other counseling-related issues.

The last main focus of the chapter was on multicultural/social justice standards, in-cluding the Multicultural Counseling Competencies and the Advocacy Competencies. We noted that the Multicultural Counseling Competencies were developed in the early 1990s and have become used more frequently over the years. They delineate attitudes and beliefs, knowledge, and skills in three areas: the counselor's awareness of the client's worldview, the counselor's awareness of one's own cultural values and biases, and the counselor's ability at using culturally appropriate intervention strategies. The Advocacy Competencies, developed recently, encompass three areas: client/student, school/com-munity, and the public arena, each of which are divided into two levels: whether the counselor is "acting on behalf" or "acting with" the competency area.

The chapter ended by highlighting how multicultural counseling and social justice issues have become a lens through which the counseling field examines all of what it is doing. We concluded the chapter with some reflections on the advantages and disadvantages of having so many standards, and the importance of having a commitment to the field and to the profession.

 ## Further Practice

Visit CengageBrain.com to respond to additional material that highlight the salient aspects of the chapter content. There, you can find ethical, professional, and legal vignettes, a number of experiential exercises, and study tools including a glossary, flashcards, and sample test items. Hopefully, these will enhance your learning and be fun and interesting.

CHAPTER 4 **Individual Approaches to Counseling**

CHAPTER 5 **Counseling Skills**

Overview

This section of the text provides an orientation to the theories and skills used in individual counseling. Chapter 4 describes four broad conceptual orientations and select theories associated with them, as well as a number of extensions, adaptations, and spinoffs of these approaches. Near its conclusion, it will look at integrative therapy (eclecticism). Chapter 5 examines some of the basic skills necessary for a successful counseling relationship, many of which are common to all the theoretical approaches we use. Additional topics covered in Chapter 5 include case conceptualization, the stages of the counseling relationship, and some of the skills associated with these stages. As with all the chapters, some important ethical, professional, and legal issues will be highlighted, as well as some cutting-edge multicultural and social justice issues related to each chapter's content.

As you read through Chapter 4, consider the similarities and differences among theories and whether it is feasible to combine theories. Later, as you examine the many skills discussed in Chapter 5, reflect on the theories and consider which skills might be more applicable to each of the theories you have studied.

Individual Approaches to Counseling[1]

I've attended counseling a lot. My first counselor was able to hear the deepest parts of my being. He helped me work through some entrenched pains and hurts. He helped me look at myself and open myself up to my feelings. He was grounded in person-centered counseling but would periodically use other techniques from the existential–humanistic tradition.

My next counselor challenged me. He would ask me to close my eyes; get in touch with my thoughts, feelings, and sensations; and discuss them. He would point out inconsistencies, such as noticing that I would smile when I was angry. He would challenge me to go deeper into myself. He was a Gestalt therapist.

The third counselor I saw used to sit in his chair and listen to me, rarely responding. I would accuse him of being a psychoanalyst; he wouldn't say anything. I rarely, if ever, received feedback. I think he was a psychoanalyst, or at least psychodynamically oriented. Perhaps I didn't work with him long enough to hear some of his insights into my behaviors.

My next counselor was a good listener and would point out the choices I had in my life. He would try to understand what was important to me and helped me to redefine myself through the choices I made. He was a very well known existential therapist.

I saw a behaviorist for a short while. He helped me work on some very focused issues. He took a long history, and then we got down to work.

In recent years, a couple of counselors I saw practiced from a postmodern perspective. They were most interested in helping me understand how I come to make meaning out of my life and helped me see how certain stories, or narratives in my life, tend to be the cornerstone for how I define who I am. They have also helped me see that I can build new narratives to redefine who I am.

I've seen male counselors, female counselors, short counselors, tall counselors, bad counselors, and good counselors. I believe that counseling has helped me become a better person. I know it has deepened me, and I am pretty sure it has helped me become a better counselor.

This chapter will begin by defining *theory* and looking at the close relationship between one's view of human nature and the theoretical orientation to which one ultimately adheres. After this discussion, we will present an overview of twelve counseling theories that are subsumed within four broad conceptual orientations, including the psychodynamic approaches of psychoanalysis, analytical therapy, and individual therapy; the existential–humanistic approaches of existential therapy, Gestalt therapy, and person-centered

---

[1] Although some distinguish between the words *counselor* and *therapist* and *counseling* and *therapy,* throughout this chapter, these words are used interchangeably.

counseling; the cognitive–behavioral approaches of behavior therapy, rational emotive behavior therapy, cognitive therapy, and reality therapy; and the postmodern approaches of narrative therapy and solution-focused brief therapy. Next, we will provide a brief overview of a number of extensions, adaptations, and spinoffs of these approaches and then discuss what it means to be eclectic or integrative in our own theoretical approach. The chapter will conclude with an examination of the cross-cultural biases inherent in some of the more common theories of counseling and then highlight some aspects of the American Counseling Association (ACA) ethical code related to the counseling relationship.

Why Have a Theory of Counseling?

. . . theory is the road map that guides the therapist from Point A to Point B. Indeed, there can be no therapy without therapeutic actions, and the therapeutic actions emanate from theory. A cogent treatment is a fundamental element of psychotherapy. Choice of a theory involves multiple considerations on the part of the therapist and the client. . . .

(Wampold, 2010b, p. 59)

A former professor of mine would refer to the discovery of new knowledge as "the virgin branch on a tree." Past knowledge leads to new discoveries, and new discoveries are only the result of all that has come before. So it was with the discovery that the Earth was round, and with Einstein's theory of relativity, and so it will be when a cure for AIDS is found or a new counseling theory is developed. New knowledge is based on sound scientific hunches, connected to all of what has come before and only later accepted as scientific proof. As noted in Chapter 2, knowledge periodically leads to paradigm shifts. Such shifts occur infrequently and mark a change in the perception of scientific knowledge. Using the tree analogy, a paradigm shift represents a bud of the tree sprouting into a new branch. These shifts in our understanding of knowledge radically change perceptions of reality (see Box 4.1).

BOX 4.1

Paradigm Shifts and the Changing Nature of Reality?

What we have come to know as "truth" is probably our best guess of what might be truth and founded in knowledge that has come before. For instance, consider how different our world would seem if one of the newest paradigms in physics, superstring theory, was validated, and we no longer viewed the atom as a tiny "solar system."

> Superstring theory: The universe is composed, not of subatomic particles. . . but of tiny strings tied together at the ends to form loops. These strings exist in a ten-dimensional universe, which some time before the Big Bang cracked into two pieces, a four-dimensional universe (ours; that's three dimensions plus time) and a six-dimensional universe that [is] so small we haven't been able to see it. What physicists have been thinking of as subatomic particles are actually vibrations of the strings, like notes played on a violin.

(Jones & Wilson, 2006, p. 508)

In the arena of counseling theories, it was not until Freud put forth his theory of psychoanalysis that the first comprehensive theory of psychotherapy was formulated. Freud's theory created a shift in thinking—it brought forth a new way of understanding the person:

> . . . his theories influence how we interpret human behavior, not only in biography, literary criticism, sociology, medicine, history, education, and ethics, but also in law. We now take for granted the basic psychoanalytic concept that our early life experiences strongly influence how we think, feel, and behave as adults. Because of the unmistakable impact of his thought, some scholars refer to the twentieth century as the "century of Freud."

(Nicholi, 2002, p. 2)

However, Freud's theory was not developed in a vacuum; it evolved because others before him pondered similar questions. Over the years, we have learned that we can discard some of Freud's theory, accept other aspects of it, and continue to examine the rest. Whether it's psychoanalysis or new age therapy, theory provides a framework to conduct research to see if the theory is effective with clients.

A counseling theory offers us a comprehensive system of doing counseling and assists us in conceptualizing our clients' problems, knowing what techniques to apply, and predicting client change (Neukrug & Schwitzer, 2006). In addition, by examining what we say to our clients, we are able to evaluate whether we are acting congruently with our theory. Theories are heuristic; that is, they are researchable and testable and ultimately allow us to discard those aspects shown to be ineffective (Wampold, 2010a, 2010b). Having a theory indicates that we are not practicing chaotically; rather, that there is some order in the way we approach our clients.

Probably the most important aspect of any theory is its *view of human nature,* which is critical to the formation of the theory's template. Typically, the view of human nature held by each theorist takes into account the effects of biology, genetics, and environment on the personality development of the individual. Therefore, if I believe that an individual's behavior is determined by genetics, my theory will reflect this notion. On the other hand, if I believe that the environment holds the key to personality formation, then my theory will reflect this belief. Prior to reviewing the theories in this chapter, you may want to reflect on your view of human nature and personality formation. Then, read the chapter and consider which of the theories best aligns with your beliefs (see Box 4.2).

Today, it is generally agreed that there are hundreds of different kinds of psychotherapies, each with its own unique view of human nature, techniques, and process (Neukrug,

 BOX 4.2
Your View of Human Nature

To determine your view of human nature and theoretical orientation, take the instrument at http://www .odu.edu/~eneukrug/therapists/survey.html. Hopefully, you'll have time to discuss your results in class.

2015a). Based on their views of human nature, most of these theories can be categorized into four conceptual orientations: psychodynamic, existential–humanistic, cognitive–behavioral, and postmodern. This chapter is organized around these orientations and will provide a brief overview of a few theories within each of these classifications.

Four Conceptual Orientations to Counseling and Associated Theories[2]

In this section of the chapter, we will examine the psychodynamic approaches of psychoanalysis, analytical therapy, and individual therapy; the existential–humanistic approaches of existential therapy, Gestalt therapy, and person-centered counseling; the cognitive–behavioral approaches of behavior therapy, rational emotive behavior therapy, cognitive therapy, and reality therapy; and the postmodern approaches of narrative therapy and solution-focused brief therapy.

Psychodynamic Approaches

Beginning with Freud's theory of psychoanalysis in the late 1800s, many approaches to counseling and psychotherapy have been developed that are broadly considered to be in the psychodynamic school. Sigmund Freud (1856–1939), who developed quite a following early in the twentieth century, dominated the psychodynamic field for almost half a century. However, because Freud tolerated little divergence from his viewpoints, many of his disciples eventually split from his rigid views and developed their own related theories. Today, psychodynamic approaches vary considerably but contain some common elements. For instance, they all suggest that an *unconscious* and a *conscious* affect the functioning of the person in some deeply personal and *dynamic* ways. They all look at early *child-rearing* practices as being important in the development of personality. They all believe

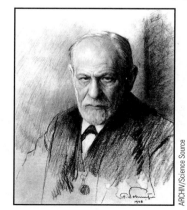

Sigmund Freud

that examining the *past*, and the dynamic interaction of the past with conscious and unconscious factors, are important in the therapeutic process. Although these approaches have tended to be long term, some have been adapted and used in relatively brief treatment modality formats in recent years. Let's take a quick look at three of the more popular psychodynamic approaches: *psychoanalysis, analytical therapy* (Jungian therapy), and *individual psychology* (Adlerian therapy).

Psychoanalysis

The first comprehensive psychotherapeutic approach, psychoanalysis dramatically changed the Western world's understanding of the individual's psychological makeup. Developed by Freud, who was trained as a physician, psychoanalysis is steeped in *biological determinism*, or the notion that instincts and drives greatly affect behavior. However, Freud's explanation for personality formation was far more complex than just the notion that biology causes behavior, for he also

ARCHIV/Science Source

---

[2] Sections of this chapter are based on Neukrug, E. (2011). *Counseling theory and practice.* Belmont, CA: Cengage.

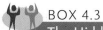

BOX 4.3
The Hidden Nature of Man (and Woman)

In the film *The Hidden Nature of Man* (Kemeny, 1970), a young man and woman are having lunch. The young man's ego is represented by him sitting at the table as he tells her how pretty she looks. His id and superego stand behind him and exert pressure on the ego (the young woman hears only the ego talking). The id, dressed in red, is saying, "I want, I want! Warm. Breasts." The superego, dressed in white, is saying, "Honor thy mother. Be a good boy." The young man makes suggestive remarks concerning them going back to her apartment, and ultimately, the young woman notes that her roommate is away and suggests they go back to her apartment. Thus, we see the complex interaction of the id, ego, and superego. Clearly, what is not shown in this film is the woman's id and superego!

believed that parenting styles within the first five or six years of life interact in a complex fashion with instincts and inherent personality structures to produce one's personality.

Freud suggested that we are born with raw *psychic energy* called *instincts*. The *life instinct (Eros)*, said Freud, meets our basic need for love and intimacy, sex, and survival for the individual and the species. It is associated with cooperation, collaboration, and harmony with others. Believing that "the aim of life is death" (Freud, 1920/1961, p. 32), Freud said the *death instinct (thanatos)* seeks our own demise and dissolution and that fear, hate, self-destructive behaviors, and aggression toward others (death instinct projected outward) is a reflection of this instinct. All psychic energy that drives the life and death instincts is called the *libido*.

Freud believed three structures are involved in one's personality formation: the *id*, *ego*, and *superego*. The id houses our instincts, operates from raw, irrational impulses, and is fueled by the *pleasure principle*, whose aim is to reduce tension through the simplest means possible. The ego develops soon after birth and is ruled by the *reality principle* as it tries to deal logically and rationally with the world. The superego develops during and soon after ego development and is responsible for the development of one's moral code and conscience. The ego must contend with the irrationality of the id and the morality of the superego as it attempts to mediate behaviors (see Box 4.3).

Freud postulated that all of one's psychic energy becomes focused on differing *erogenous zones* that correspond to the unfolding biological development of the child. When a child is *overindulged* or *frustrated* during a stage, his or her libido becomes locked or *fixated*, resulting in unfinished psychological issues and behaviors that are reflective of what Freud called the *psychosexual stages*. The five stages include the following:

1. *Oral stage.* Between birth and 18 months, the infant's erogenous zone is the mouth, and pleasure is received through sucking and eating. Withholding the breast and/or bottle and food greatly affects the child's sense of self and sense of trust and security in the world.
2. *Anal stage.* Obtaining control over bowel movements is the major task of this stage, which occurs between 18 months and 3 years. Here, children learn that they can control their bodies as well as their environment. How parents deal with toilet training and the broader experience of how the child learns to control his or her world is crucial during this stage (think of the "terrible twos," when the child is attempting to control his or her world).

3. *Phallic stage.* Experiencing pleasurable genital sensations is the major focus during this stage, which occurs between ages 3 and 5 or 6 years. Here, children self-stimulate, have a fascination with bodily functions, and are particularly affected by the moral imperatives of their parents. Relative to the phallic stage, it should be noted that Freud's ideas about childhood sexuality were revolutionary and controversial at the time and set the stage for ongoing debates about the role of sexuality in personality development.

4. *Latency stage.* Strictly speaking, not a psychosexual stage, the latency stage occurs between the ages of 5 or 6 years and puberty, when there is a repression of the libido. During this holding pattern, children focus on peer relationships and other age-appropriate activities, such as athletics and school.

5. *Genital stage.* Resulting patterns of behavior from the oral, anal, and phallic stages become evident as the young adult and adult exhibit behavior, which is influenced by conscious and unconscious motivations.

Based on how one is parented, the *structures of personality* (the id, ego, and super-ego) become established in the child as he or she traverses the first three psychosexual stages. In this process, the ego is in a difficult position as it attempts to mediate between the ongoing urges of the id and demands from the superego to act in a "proper" (moral) fashion. Fears of the id or superego taking over can wreak havoc and create anxiety for the individual. To manage the pressures from the id and the superego, children create *defense mechanisms*. For instance, consider a child in the phallic stage who is self-stimulating (the id). Seeing the child masturbate, the parent slaps his or her hand and says, "Don't do that" (development of the superego). Subsequently, the child unconsciously fears *annihilation* and *castration* by the parent and develops a defense mechanism to deal with the impulse to masturbate in the future (e.g., sublimating the desire by getting very involved in sports or through compulsive hand-washing).

Freud, and later his daughter Anna Freud (1936–1966), identified a number of defense mechanisms that unconsciously help the individual cope with anxiety (A. Freud, 1966). Although there are many defense mechanisms, some of the more common ones are *repression*, the pushing out of awareness of threatening or painful memories; *denial*, the distortion of reality in order to deny perceived threats to the person; *projection*, viewing others as having unacceptable qualities that the individual himself or herself has; *rationalization*, the explaining away of a bruised or hurt ego; *regression*, reverting to behavior from an earlier stage of development; *sublimation*, channeling impulses into socially accepted forms of behavior; *identification*, identifying with groups or others in an effort to improve one's sense of self-worth; *compensation*, exaggerating certain positive traits in an effort to mask weaker traits; and *reaction formation*, replacing a perceived negative feeling with a positive one.

Psychoanalysis is considered a *deterministic* approach because consciousness is considered the "tip of the iceberg," which implies that most of our motivations are unconscious and are the result of the intricate relationship among how the structures of personality (id, ego, and superego) are developed as a function of different parenting styles, as children traverse the stages of development (see Figure 4.1). At best, we can become a little more conscious as small parts of the iceberg are revealed.

Traditional psychoanalysis is a long-term, in-depth process in which the client may meet with a therapist three or more times a week for five or more years. In this process,

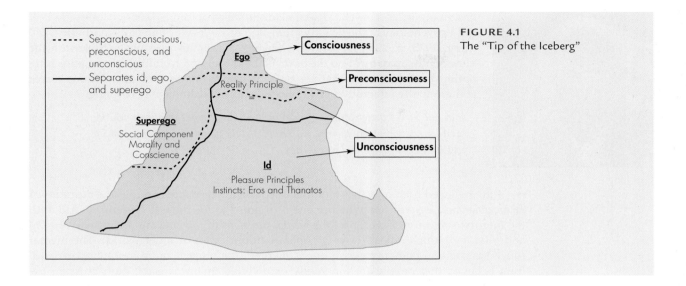

FIGURE 4.1
The "Tip of the Iceberg"

the therapist attempts to build a *transference relationship,* in which the client projects past patterns from significant early relationships onto the counselor. To encourage this relationship, the counselor remains relatively aloof from the client. Psychoanalysts initially use a fair amount of *empathy* while encouraging clients to share their deepest thoughts. Revelations by clients are responded to in a nonjudgmental manner, which encourages more revelations. Fairly early in the relationship, they will use *free association,* where clients are encouraged to say anything that comes to their minds to allow for the uninhibited expression of unconscious desires and repressed memories. Later, the therapist will incorporate *dream analysis,* where both the *manifest* (obvious) content of dreams and the *latent* (hidden) meaning of dreams are interpreted in an effort to understand unconscious desires and repressed memories (Freud, 1899/1976a, p. 769). *Interpretation of client resistance, interpretation of defense mechanisms,* and *interpretation of parapraxes* (errors of speech, slips of tongue, or misspeaks) are also used to reveal unconscious meanings that may be symbolic of repressed wishes and desires (Freud, 1905/1976b). And, of course, *analysis of the transference relationship,* where the therapist interprets client projections, including client projections onto the therapist, are examined in terms of how they relate to past patterns in early relationships (e.g., relationships with parents) (Freud & Breuer, 1895/1974). Ultimately, the relationship ends when the client has gained increased knowledge and awareness of underlying dynamics and how this gets expressed through his or her patterns and symptoms, and when the client has made some changes based on these insights.

Analytical Psychology (Jungian Therapy)

Originally a colleague of Freud's, Carl Jung (1875–1961) was trained in the psychoanalytical tradition. However, as he developed, he became disheartened by psychoanalysis,

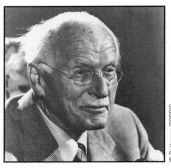

© Bettmann/CORBIS

Carl Jung

describing it "as a psychology of neurotic states of mind, definitely one-sided . . . not a psychology of the healthy mind, and this is a symptom of its morbidity . . . " (Jung, 1975, p. 227). Departing from Freud over his pessimistic, deterministic view of human nature and the psychoanalytic views on childhood sexuality, Jung optimistically believed that we could become conscious of unconscious forces and gradually integrate such knowledge into a healthier way of living.

For my part, I prefer to look at man in the light of what in him is healthy and sound, and to free the sick man from just that kind of psychology which colours every page Freud has written.

(Jung, 1975, p. 227)

Jung believed each of us has a unique *psychological type* that includes the attitudes of *extraversion* and *introversion* (whether one is oriented to the outside objective world *or* to the internal subjective world) and the *mental functions* of *thinking* and *feeling* and *sensing* and *intuiting* (which reflects how we operate in our outer or inner world). The mental functions come in pairs because if one is favored, the other is more in the background. Jung believed that people are inherently extraverted or introverted; thus, crossing extraversion or introversion with the predominant mental function that one could favor produces eight possible combinations or "types" (AFS, AFI, ATI, ATS, EFS, EFI, ETI, ETS). Thinking types evaluate information from a detached perspective and use logic, reason, and the examination of data and causal relationships in this process (consider the stereotypic scientist or behaviorist). Feeling types make decisions by evaluating situations through the use of empathy, by understanding relationships, and by considering the needs of people (think of the humanistically oriented counselor stereotype). Feeling types should not be confused with individuals who make decisions based on feelings or affect. Sensing types make sense of information through the use of the five senses: hearing, seeing, smelling, touching, and tasting, whereas intuitive types make sense of the world by listening to one's "gut" and unconscious (e.g., Sensing type: "I can smell your lover's perfume" versus Intuitive type: "I just know that you're having an affair—I just have that gut feeling").

Jung believed that our psychological type mediates our conscious experience. For instance, the extraverted person who is predominantly a Thinking and Sensing type would tend to see the world from those frames of reference, with other experiences being pushed into what Jung called the *personal unconscious*. In addition to the personal unconscious, Jung believed that each of us has a *collective unconscious*. Almost mystical in its nature, the collective unconscious is a depository of ancient experiences—an entity from the early beginnings of civilization that has been passed down to each of us.

The deepest we can reach in our exploration of the unconscious mind is the layer where man is no longer a distinct individual, but where his mind widens out and merges into the mind of mankind, not the conscious mind, but the unconscious mind of mankind, where we are all the same. . . . On this collective level we are no longer separate individuals, we are all one.

(Jung, 1968, p. 46)

Jung believed that the collective unconscious is inherited, identical in all of us, and contains *archetypes*, which provide the psyche with its tendency to perceive the world in certain ways that we identify as "human." Evidence for archetypes, said Jung, can only be inferred and is found in the similar behaviors, artwork, images, and myths that are recognized in all cultures. Some of the more well-known archetypes include the *persona*, or the mask we wear in public life; the *anima* and *animus*, which represent the feminine and masculine characteristics that all of us have; and the *shadow*, which represents the most hidden and scariest parts of ourselves that we are afraid to reveal to the self. Jung also believed that archetypes provide the energy for the development of complexes. A *complex* is created, according to Jung, when repressed experiences get pushed into the personal unconscious and become bound with one or more archetypes. For instance, a young child who is abused by his or her parents might repress the resulting feelings of hurt and shame into the personal unconscious. In an effort to gain protection from these experiences, the child becomes bound with the trickster and power archetypes, creating a bully complex. In the end, this person becomes a bully.

Believing that we could become "conscious of almost anything" (Jung, 1968, p. 48), Jung suggested that awareness of all parts of ourselves is the first step to integration, self-acceptance, and wholeness (e.g., the bully could become aware of his or her hurt and pain and how the archetypes serve a survival function for him or her). Thus, understanding our personal unconscious (e.g., our repressed attitudes and mental functions; our complexes) and our collective unconscious (our archetypes) are critical goals in analytical therapy and are achieved by examining our *dreams*, amplifying the meaning *symbols* have in our lives, participating in *creative techniques* (e.g., working with clay), and a process Jung called *active imagination*.

Individual Psychology (Adlerian Therapy)

Alfred Adler believed that every child was born with innate and unique capabilities and is inherently moving toward the future, not determined by the past. Using the word *teleology*, from the Greek *teleos* (meaning "goal-directed process"), Adler suggested that we move toward the future to makes ourselves whole and complete and to fulfill our one true drive, our *striving for perfection*. If unimpeded, this path would bring out our uniqueness and natural creativity, leading us toward connection and cooperation with others, a sense of wholeness and completion, and meaningfulness in life (Sweeney, 2009). Adler stated that all other drives, including our sexual or aggressive instincts, are subsumed by this drive. However, he also warned that if one's natural striving for perfection was diverted, the individual would develop neurotic or even psychotic behaviors.

Part of being human, said Adler, was dealing with inevitable *feelings of inferiority*. In attempting to overcome those feelings, Adler believed that we all develop unconscious beliefs, or *private logic*. Private logic leads to what Adler originally called a *fictional final goal*, later referred to as a *subjective final goal*, to emphasize its subjective nature (Watts & Holden, 1994). He also asserted that the picture in one's mind of what the individual would like to be, which was shaped by the subjective final goal, could drive a person throughout his or her life. Adler stated that the child's experiences by age 5, and the subsequent memories of those

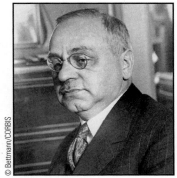

Alfred Adler

experiences, were critical factors in the development of one's *private logic* and subjective final goal. Thus, birth order and other factors in early childhood could play critical roles in the development of the person. However, Adler also believed that a child is not determined by his or her early experiences. Rather, he believed that the child could change if afforded a corrective education. And if the child can change, so too can the adult!

Adler suggested that our drive toward our subjective final goal often results in the development of behaviors that *compensate* for feelings of inferiority (a "100-pound weakling" becomes an obsessed bodybuilder). Ultimately, Adler stated that a person believes that his or her subjective final goal will bring a sense of mastery, superiority, and eventually, perfection, completion, and wholeness. For instance, Adler himself had feelings of inferiority as the result of a number of ailments he had had as a young child. This led him to develop a subjective final goal of conquering death, and thus he was driven to become a doctor in this unconscious quest (Hoffman, 1994). Similarly, due to being bullied as a child, Olympic star Michael Phelps developed his own private logic and compensated for his feelings of inferiority by putting his all into his natural ability at swimming. Sometimes, however, feelings of inferiority can lead to a subjective final goal that results in maladaptive behaviors. For instance, consider the child who feels bad about his or her body, ends up as an adult with a body dysmorphic disorder, and becomes bulimic in his or her attempt to have the perfect body. (Subjective final goal: "If I could have the perfect body, my life would be fine.") Finally, Adler suggested that the individual develops a *style of life* that is reflective of the person's movement toward his or her subjective final goal. Whether our subjective final goal results in a lifestyle that is reflected by healthy or maladaptive behaviors, it is deeply rooted in the past, affects our present, and leads us toward our future.

Considered by some a psychodynamic theorist, Adler hypothesized that an individual's drive toward perfection could best be understood through in-depth counseling. In such work, the therapist helps the client understand how early experiences, and the memories of those experiences, have led to private logic that affects the development of one's subjective final goal and is reflected in one's style of life. However, there are also clear existential and humanistic leanings in Adler's approach as he stressed the importance of *social interest* (*Gemeinschaftsgefühl*) and because he believed that if unimpeded by feelings of inferiority, one would naturally move toward meaningful relationships, empathy toward and cooperation with others, the betterment of society, and an understanding of our place in the universe (Ansbacher, 1964; Watts, 1996). Called by some the first humanist, Adler came up with a theory that was optimistic and anti-deterministic, and it has impacted the development of subsequent humanistic theories of counseling.

Adler's influence over the years was widespread, with Rudolf Dreikurs (1897–1972) and Don Dinkmeyer (1924–2001) becoming particularly well known for adapting individual psychology to work with children. Dinkmeyer and Dreikurs (1963) theorized that children have an inherent desire to belong and feel part of their peer groups (similar to Adler's concept of "social interest"), but due to feelings of inferiority and maladaptive parenting, some exhibit maladaptive behaviors in an unsuccessful attempt to gain this sense of belonging. Typical behaviors that such children exhibit include *attention seeking* (e.g., interrupting), *the use of power* (e.g., bullying), *revenge seeking* (e.g., playing nasty practical jokes), and displaying *inadequacy* (e.g., withdrawing). Like Adler, Dinkmeyer and Dreikurs believed that children can be taught new behaviors by significant others in their lives, such as parents, counselors, and teachers (Wolfgang, 2008).

The purpose of the therapeutic relationship in individual psychology is to help clients gain insight into how their current style of life is not working for them and develop new behaviors that will lead to healthier relationships highlighted by empathy, a sense of belonging, and cooperation (Carlson, Watts, & Maniacci, 2006). For children and adults, Adlerian therapy can be viewed through a series of four phases: *building the therapeutic relationship; assessing and understanding the lifestyle; insight and interpretation;* and *reeducation and reorientation* (Neukrug, 2011). As clients move through the phases, they are encouraged to give up their misguided private logic, dysfunctional subjective final goals, deleterious compensatory behaviors, and dysfunctional styles of life, and adopt new values and behaviors that reflect a healthier style of life that increasingly focuses on the importance of others and the broader community. Dinkmeyer, Dreikurs, and Adler developed a wide range of techniques to help accomplish this with some of the more common ones being *exploring the family constellation, examining early recollections, encouragement, democratically held discussion groups, limit setting, acting "as if"* (in other words, "fake it 'til you make it"), *spitting in the client's soup* (showing the client how behaviors are not working), and *setting logical and natural consequences.*

Existential–Humanistic Approaches

At the turn of the twentieth century in Europe, the writings of such existential philosophers as Søren Kierkegaard, Paul Tillich, Jean-Paul Sartre, and Albert Camus became particularly well known (Neukrug, 2015b). American counselors and psychotherapists began to see the value in some of these thinkers' explorations of the *struggles of living* and how people *construct meaning* in their lives, eventually embracing some of their concepts and adapting them to the counseling relationship. The new theories that evolved tended to be far more *optimistic*, less *deterministic*, and more *humane* than the earlier psychodynamic approaches and became known as existential–humanistic approaches to counseling.

Today, existential–humanistic approaches embrace a *phenomenological perspective* by stressing the subjective reality of the client, deemphasizing the role of the unconscious, and focusing on the importance of *consciousness* and *awareness*. Deeply opposed to the reductionistic, impersonal tradition of psychoanalysis, existential–humanistic therapy stresses the counselor's personal qualities and how the counselor uses himself or herself in *the relationship* to effect change. In addition, most existential–humanistic approaches believe in an inborn tendency for individuals to *self-actualize*, or fulfill their potential, if they are afforded an environment conducive to growth (Maslow, 1968, 1970). Although many modern-day approaches to counseling and psychotherapy have borrowed from the existential–humanistic schools, a few are particularly based in this tradition. Thus, in this section of the chapter, we will look at *existential therapy*, which is presented here as an integration of a number of well-known, existentially based therapies; examine the *person-centered counseling* approach of Carl Rogers; and then discuss *Gestalt therapy*, originally founded by Fritz Perls.

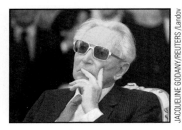

JACQUELINE GODANY/REUTERS /Landov

Viktor Frankl

Existential Therapy

Although Ludwig Binswanger (1881–1966) is generally acknowledged as being the first existential therapist (Cain, 2002), Viktor Frankl is seen as the person who popularized this approach through his form of existential therapy called *logotherapy* ("meaning therapy"). Frankl, who spent years in a Nazi concentration camp, wrote his theory on scraps of paper as he watched others around him lose hope and fall into the depths of despair (see Frankl, 1968; 1946/2004; 1946/2006). Eventually deciding that we can choose how we decide to exist in the world even when faced with horrendous circumstances, he developed his approach. Frankl was to influence others, including such famous existential therapists as Rollo May (1909–1994) (May, Angel, & Ellenberger, 1958), James Bugental (1976), and Irvin Yalom (1980). May is often considered the father of American existential therapy, while Yalom is often looked to as the person who popularized the existential approach in the United States, partly because of his bestselling novels, *Love's Executioner* and *When Nietzsche Wept* (the latter was also turned into a movie in 2007).

Existential therapists believe that people are born into a world that has no inherent meaning or purpose. People are not born good or bad; they are just thrust into the cosmos. Because life has no inherent meaning, each of us is charged with the responsibility of making it meaningful through the choices we make. Existential therapists reject the notion that we are determined by early childhood development, instincts, or intrapsychic forces, although talking about the past is not avoided if the client believes that it would help him or her understand the self in a more meaningful way.

Central to existential therapists' beliefs is the notion that, consciously or unconsciously, people struggle throughout their lives with basic questions related to what it is to be human. Some of this struggle has to do with a few core issues, such as the fact that we are born alone, will die alone, and except for periodic moments when we encounter another person deeply, we live alone; death constantly looms over us and reminds us of the relatively brief amount of time we have; we alone are responsible for making our lives meaningful; and meaning, as well as a limited sense of freedom, come through consciousness and the choices we make (Yalom, 1980).

Existential therapists believe that most people live a life of limited self-reflection as they put energy into avoiding the core issues related to their humanness. Such avoidance is the result of trying to maneuver around the anxiety and dread that we will feel if we examine these issues head on. After all, it is not easy to accept one's aloneness in the world, it can be frightful to be cognizant of one's ultimate demise (death), it can be humbling to examine whether one is living a meaningful existence, and it takes focused self-discipline to change the way that one has been living. And the result of living with limited self-awareness and steering clear of the inherent struggles of living is the development of neuroses and psychopathology, which from the existential perspective is the result of living inauthentically. In essence, we can live authentically, with a life that sometimes includes anxiety and dread, if we face our core issues squarely, but are doomed to an inauthentic, neurotic existence if we do not.

Existential therapists suggest that in dialogue with others, people can gain a greater awareness of the choices they have made and can begin to direct their lives toward a more personally meaningful and authentic existence by making new choices that involve facing

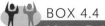

BOX 4.4
Major Points of Existential Therapy

1. We are born into a world that has little inherent meaning.
2. We are born alone and we will die alone.
3. We alone make our lives meaningful.
4. We bring meaningfulness into our lives through the choices that we make.
5. Meaningful choices occur only if we are conscious of our aloneness and our limited time on Earth.
6. Anxiety, feelings of dread, and having struggles are a natural part of living and are important messages about how we live and relate to others.

7. Limited freedom is experienced through the realization that we choose our existence.
8. With the recognition that we choose our existence comes the responsibility to choose wisely for ourselves and to recognize how those choices affect those close to us and all people.

life's struggles honestly and directly. With this awareness, however, comes a great sense of responsibility, as we come to realize that every choice we make affects ourselves, those close to us, and to some degree, the entire planet, as each decision we make has a ripple effect throughout the world. Some of the major points of existential therapy can be found in Box 4.4.

Although there are no preset techniques that existential therapists use in applying its core philosophy, most existential therapists will stress the importance of the relationship between the therapist and the client, discuss the philosophy of existential psychotherapy and how it might apply to the individual's particular life circumstances, be authentic with the client, and view the therapeutic process as a *shared journey*. This journey is significant, as it is only through a genuine relationship that change can occur. Therapy is not seen as a process of applying techniques; instead, it is viewed as a joint discussion concerning the meaning of life and how one can make constructive change to alter one's sense of fulfillment and meaningfulness. Therefore, inherent in existential therapy is the assumption that the client can change, has the capacity for deepening self-awareness, and can build a meaningful and real relationship with the therapist—a relationship that can have an impact on the client, the therapist, and the world.

Person-Centered Counseling

Trained as a clinical psychologist, Carl Rogers (1902–1987) greatly changed the face of psychotherapy with the development of his nondirective approach to counseling (Rogers, 1942). First called *client-centered therapy* (Rogers, 1951), and later *person-centered counseling*, his approach was seen not only as a means of assisting clients, but also as a way of living (Rogers, 1980). Considered the most influential psychotherapist of the twentieth century (Cook, Biyanova, & Coyne, 2009; Kirschenbaum & Henderson, 1989), Rogers believed that people had an *actualizing tendency* (Rogers, 1951), and if placed in a nurturing environment, they would develop into fully aware, fully functioning selves. However, Rogers postulated that all too often, an individual's natural growth process is thwarted as others place *conditions of worth* on the person. Because the person has a strong *need to be regarded positively* by others, he or she may act in unnatural, unreal ways and develop a distorted sense of self in order to meet these conditions of worth. Therapy, Rogers said, offers the

BOX 4.5
The Core Conditions

Rogers believed that congruence, unconditional positive regard, and empathy were the three core components of an effective counseling relationship and carefully described them. The following are based on Rogers's descriptions:

Congruence or genuineness. Rogers believed that the counselor needs to be in touch with his or her feelings toward the client, regardless of what they may be (Rogers, 1957). The level of self-disclosure that the therapist shows the client, however, may vary depending on the session and whether the feeling was persistent, keeping in mind the impact that expression of the feeling might have on the client. Although Rogers had negative feelings toward some clients during a session, almost invariably he found that the feelings dissipated as the client opened up and unraveled his or her inner self. Thus, he warned therapists against using excessive self-disclosure. Finding the ideal balance between awareness of feelings and the expression of those feelings is one of the challenges facing the person-centered counselor.

Unconditional positive regard. Rogers believed that counseling relationships should be highlighted by a sense of acceptance, regardless of what feelings are expressed by the client. This unconditional acceptance allows the client to feel safe within the relationship and to delve deeper into himself or herself. As the client begins to take steps toward understanding this deepening self, the client will begin to recognize those aspects of self that have been lived for others as the result of conditions of worth that were placed upon him or her. Rogers viewed unconditional positive regard as an ideal to strive for during the totality of the session, but not always successfully achieved.

Empathic understanding. Perhaps the most researched and talked-about element of the counseling relationship, empathy, or deep understanding, was Rogers's third crucial element. Such understanding can be shown in a number of ways, including accurately reflecting the meaning and affect of what the client expressed; using a metaphor, analogy, or visual image to show the client that he or she was accurately heard; or simply nodding one's head or gently touching the client during the client's deepest moments of pain. Such acknowledgment of the client's predicament tells the client that the therapist experiences the client's world "as if it were [his or her] own, but without ever losing the 'as if' quality" (Rogers, 1957, p. 99). In other words, the therapist is "with" the client, "hears" the client, understands the client fully, and is able to communicate such understanding to the client.

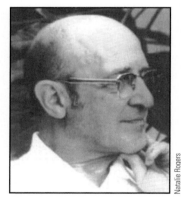

Carl Rogers

Natalie Rogers

individual an opportunity to realize an increased sense of *congruence* with one's true self and achieve a more realistic sense of what Rogers called the *ideal self*, or the self that we strive to be (Neukrug, 2015c; Rogers, 1959).

Rogers felt that people can get in touch with their true selves if they are around others who are *real* (*congruent* or *genuine*), *empathic*, and exhibit *unconditional positive regard*, which he collectively called the *core conditions*, believing that these attributes alone are enough to facilitate change (Rogers, 1957; also see Box 4.5). Applying the core conditions to the therapeutic relationship, Rogers believed that personality change would occur if the therapeutic framework included what he called the *necessary and sufficient conditions*:

1. Two persons are in psychological contact.
2. The first, whom we shall term the client, is in a state of incongruence, being vulnerable or anxious.
3. The second person, whom we shall term the therapist, is congruent or integrated in the relationship.
4. The therapist experiences unconditional positive regard for the client.
5. The therapist experiences an empathic understanding of the client's internal frame of reference and endeavors to communicate this experience to the client.
6. The communication to the client of the therapist's empathic understanding and unconditional positive regard is to a minimal degree achieved (Rogers, 1957, p. 96).

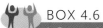

BOX 4.6
I Guess Nobody Is Perfect—Not Even Dr. Rogers

In the late 1970s, I went to hear Carl Rogers talk for my second time. I was excited—Rogers was my hero. There were thousands of people in the audience, and as he fielded questions, I shyly raised my hand. Suddenly, he was pointing to me. I stood up and blurted something out, at which point he asked me to repeat myself. I again tried to formulate my question, and he said something like, "I can't understand what you're talking about." He moved on to another question. I was shattered, hurt, and felt like rolling up into a ball. And he—yes, Carl Rogers—had not been very caring to this young counselor. I then discovered that even our heroes are not perfect.

Hear this story (entitled "Oh My God, He Doesn't Like Me") and other stories about Carl Rogers by clicking "Carl Rogers" at the "Stories of the Great Therapists" website (see http://www.odu.edu/sgt).

If the counselor could exhibit the core conditions to the client, the client would begin to open up and understand past pains and hurts that were caused by conditional relationships in the client's life. In fact, such a therapeutic relationship would assist the client in his or her movement from living a life marked by nongenuineness to a life highlighted by realness and would also result in the client changing specific behaviors. Other results of therapy could include increased openness to experience, more objective and realistic perceptions, improved psychological adjustment, increased congruence, improved self-regard, movement from an external to an internal locus of control, more acceptance of others, better problem solving, and a more accurate perception of others (Rogers, 1959).

Because Rogers felt that the attributes of empathy, congruence, and unconditional positive regard were important in all interpersonal relationships, he spent much time later in his life advocating for social change and helping people understand differences among themselves (Kirschenbaum, 2009). Working with such people as Protestants and Catholics in Northern Ireland, Blacks and Whites in South Africa, and individuals in what was then the Soviet Union, he attempted to get people who held widely disparate political and philosophical points of view to hear one another and form close, long-lasting relationships (see Box 4.6).

When originally developed, person-centered counseling was considered a short-term therapy, at least in comparison to the then–widely popular psychodynamic methods. However, with recent changes in the health care system and the movement toward brief treatment, what was traditionally considered short term is now seen as long term. Although the principles of person-centered counseling can be applied if you meet with a client one time or for five years, generally, person-centered counseling lasts from a few weeks to a year or more. Probably the most important determining factors in the length of treatment are the level of incongruence in the client and the kinds of issues that the client is bringing to treatment. However, it should be noted that many counselors today have integrated the core skills of congruence, unconditional positive regard, and empathy with techniques from some of the shorter-term approaches currently used.

Gestalt Therapy

Gestalt therapy was created by Fritz Perls (1893–1970), a German Jew who fled Nazi Germany. Trained as a psychoanalyst, Perls quickly became disheartened with the

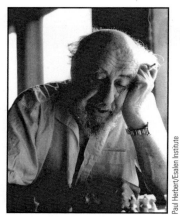

Fritz Perls

Paul Herbert/Esalen Institute

approach. Borrowing ideas from *Gestalt psychology*, *phenomenology*, and *existentialism*, Perls developed a highly directive approach that pushes clients to confront their unfinished business and live a more real and sane life.

Today, most Gestalt therapists believe that from birth, the individual is in a constant state of *self-regulation* through a process of *need identification and need-fulfillment*. They believe that the individual's pressing need dictates his or her perceptual field (what the person sees), or, as Gestalt therapists state, the individual is only aware of the need that is in the *foreground*. Because needs can vary dramatically, this theory contrasts with the psychoanalytic view, which suggests that a limited number of instincts drive behavior (e.g., hunger, thirst, survival, sex, aggression), or the Maslowian (humanistic) idea that basic needs (e.g., hunger, thirst) are addressed prior to higher-order needs (love and belonging, self-esteem).

> *You can believe in two instincts . . . or you can believe in two million instincts, or unfinished situations, like I like to do. I believe that our organism is so complicated, that every time something happens to it, is experienced by it, we are thrown out of balance and at each moment we have to regain this balance.*
>
> (Perls, 1978, p. 58)

For the Gestalt therapist, how the individual makes contact with his or her environment in an attempt to satisfy needs is reflective of the individual's way of being in the world and determines the *self* (Perls, Hefferline, & Goodman, 1951; Polster & Polster, 1973). The healthy individual has a semipermeable boundary that allows the individual to maintain a sense of self, while also allowing material from the environment to be engulfed, "chewed," and taken in as it becomes assimilated (Yonteff, 1976). This person has a constant free-flowing exchange between self and *other* (all that is outside of self), and this exchange causes the self, or *ego*, to be constantly changing; that is, as needs are met, the self changes. For instance, when "falling in love," the boundary extends to include the essence of the other person. At that moment, the person's sense of self—indeed the person's ego itself—has changed.

Although satisfaction of needs is a natural process, need satisfaction can be thwarted by such things as parental shoulds, social and cultural dictates, and peer norms. Such influences result in the development of mechanisms that resist the experience of that pressing need. These mechanisms yield individuals who are fake, incongruent, false to their nature, and "playing" at being a self-created image, all in an effort to avoid the experience of the need. Such false behaviors result in *impasses* or *blockages* that prevent experiencing and are revealed through dysfunctional and neurotic behaviors that are called *unfinished business* by Gestalt therapists. Breaking free from these influences and the resulting impasses and dealing with one's unfinished business is one of the goals of Gestalt therapy. Successfully doing so allows individuals to live more authentic lives in which they are fully in touch with themselves and are able to have open and honest communication with others. Because unfinished business prevents a person from experiencing oneself fully, one goal of Gestalt therapy is to help the client once again experience *the now*. Experiencing fully is the basis for seeing one's reality clearly. In fact, one of Perls's famous quotes is, "To me, nothing exists except the now. Now = experience = awareness = reality. The past is no more and the future not yet. Only the now exists" (Perls, 1970, p. 14).

Because Gestalt theorists believe that we can free ourselves from our impasses and blockages, the Gestalt approach is considered *anti-deterministic*. In fact, one of the greatest contributions of Gestalt therapy is that it circumvented the years of therapy that were needed in psychoanalysis to get to the raw, unconscious, hidden parts of the self. Whereas psychoanalysts believed defense mechanisms should be dealt with gingerly because of their importance in maintaining ego integrity, Gestalt and related therapies viewed defenses as something that one should break free of in an effort to fully experience the present and become sane (Hart, Corriere, & Binder, 1975).

You would probably not be surprised that Gestalt therapists use a variety of techniques to help clients access all their feelings, thoughts, and experiences, as they are pushed to increasingly experience the now, quickly identify and understand their impasses, and work on their unfinished business. After specific unfinished business is worked through, it leaves the foreground and allows room for new issues to arise. This process is akin to the peeling-of-an-onion metaphor: "We can open one door at a time and peel off one layer of the onion at a time. Each layer is part of the neurosis. . . " (Perls, 1973, p. 84). Some of the more popular techniques that Gestalt therapists use include the following:

Awareness Exercises.   With this technique, therapists ask clients to close their eyes and experience all their feelings, thoughts, and senses. This allows clients to quickly get in touch with hidden feelings or thoughts that are defended against when one uses the external world to avoid inner senses.

Use of "I" Statements.   One frequently used defense is the projection of issues onto people or things. Thus, therapists will encourage clients to take ownership of such projections through the use of "I" statements. For example, "This world sucks," becomes "I suck; I don't take responsibility for my happiness."

The Exaggeration Technique.   Here, therapists have clients exaggerate a word, phrase, or nonverbal behavior that is believed to hold some hidden meaning. For instance, a client who is slouched over might be asked to slouch more and to attach words to what it feels like to be so slouched. One client might say, "I feel as though the world is on my shoulders," and then soon realize that the "world" represents demands the client feels placed upon him. Further exploration may reveal how the client blames others for his inability to stop taking on tasks.

Empty-Chair Technique.   This popular technique has clients imagine that a person, or a part of the client's self, is sitting in an empty chair. The therapist then facilitates a dialogue between the client and this "other person" in order to uncover underlying issues within the client. For instance, a therapist might ask a client who feels as if she has the world on her shoulders to have a conversation with the world, eventually getting to the hidden meanings that "the world" holds.

Playing the Projection.   When an individual has strong feelings about other persons or things, a therapist may ask the client to make an "I" statement about that person or thing. Here, it is assumed that the client's strong feelings about the "other" are really a projection of strong feelings about the client's self. Imagine a client who has stated that she doesn't trust men in relationships saying, "I don't trust myself in relationships with men."

Turning Questions Into Statements About the Self.   Gestalt therapists assume that all questions hide a statement about the self. Therefore, the therapist asks the client to change questions into statements about the self. Imagine a client changing: "Why don't people care more about others?" to the following statement about the self: "I feel that people don't care about me."

Other Techniques.   Assuming that individuals will often avoid responsibility, project onto others, and try to find ways of not dealing with hidden feelings, Gestalt therapists use a wide variety of other techniques to confront clients into awareness. For instance, they encourage clients to "stay with the feeling," to play out different parts of their dreams, to make statements asserting that they take responsibility for their behaviors, or to act out the opposite behavior of the one they are exhibiting.

In summary, the Gestalt therapist is an *active, directive* therapist who has an existential–humanistic orientation. Although this type of therapist shares many similar goals with the existential and person-centered therapists, the ways of reaching those goals vary dramatically.

Cognitive–Behavioral Approaches

Around the turn of the century, the Russian scientist Ivan Pavlov (1848–1936) found that a hungry dog that salivated when shown food would learn to salivate to a tone if that tone were repeatedly paired or associated with the food. In other words, eventually the dog would salivate when it heard the tone, regardless of whether food was present. Pavlov discovered what was later called *classical conditioning*. John Watson (1925; Watson & Raynor, 1920) and later Joseph Wolpe (1958) would eventually take these concepts and apply them in clinical settings.

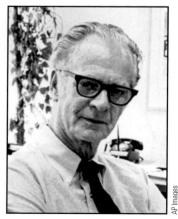

During the 1930s, the psychologist B. F. Skinner (1904–1990) showed that animals would learn a specific behavior if they were *reinforced* (Bjork, 2015; Skinner, 1938, 1971). His *operant conditioning* procedures demonstrated that *positive reinforcement*, the presentation of a stimulus that yields an increase in behavior, or *negative reinforcement*, the removal of a stimulus that yields an increase in behavior, could successfully change behavior. Skinner also found that *punishment* was not a particularly effective means to change behavior (see Box 4.7).

During the 1940s, Albert Bandura found that children who viewed a film in which an adult acted aggressively toward a Bobo doll would act out more aggressively than did children who had not seen the film when all the children were placed in a room together (Bandura, Ross, & Ross, 1963). This third behavioral approach, known as *social learning* or *modeling*, has shown that although we often do not immediately enact behaviors we have observed, we have the capacity to do so at a later date (Bandura, 1977).

In recent years, cognitive therapists have focused on how deeply embedded *cognitive structures*, or *illogical and irrational ways of thinking*, can be conditioned in

AP Images

B.F. Skinner

BOX 4.7

Can a Behaviorist Be a Humanist?

During the defense of my doctoral dissertation, my advisor (who was a behaviorist) asked me if "a behaviorist can be a humanist." I went on to give what I thought at the time to be a rather esoteric response, noting that the basic orientations of the approaches were philosophically different and therefore incompatible with one another. A few years later, I had the opportunity to hear B. F. Skinner talk at a church in New Hampshire. Following his talk, I went up to him and asked, "Can a behaviorist be a humanist?" Waiting a moment, he turned to me, and with a deeply reflective look, he said, "Well, I don't know about that, but he can surely be humane."

You can hear this and other stories by clicking on "B. F. Skinner" at the "Stories of the Great Therapists" website (see http://www.odu.edu/sgt).

a similar way as behaviors. And, like behaviors, old dysfunctional cognitions can be *extinguished* and new, more functional cognitions can be adopted through *counter-conditioning*. Because behavior therapists and cognitive therapists tend to believe that there is an intimate, sometimes seamless relationship between cognitions and behaviors, there has been a tendency for these individuals to merge the tenets of both approaches into what has become known as the *cognitive–behavioral school*. Some of the common assumptions underlying these approaches include the following:

1. The individual is born capable of developing a multitude of personality characteristics.
2. Significant others and cultural influences play a particularly important role in how the individual is conditioned.
3. Genetics and other biological factors may play a significant role in who we become.
4. Despite the fact that the past plays an important role in how a person is conditioned, long periods of time do not need to be spent on examining the past. Instead, one needs to determine what behaviors and thoughts need to be changed and focus on changing them.
5. Behaviors and cognitions are generally conditioned in very complex and subtle ways.
6. The kinds of behaviors and cognitions that are conditioned play a central role in the development of normal and abnormal behavior.
7. By carefully analyzing how behaviors and cognitions are conditioned, one can understand why an individual exhibits his or her current behavioral and cognitive repertoire.
8. By identifying what behaviors have been conditioned, one can eliminate undesirable behaviors and set goals to acquire more functional ways of behaving and thinking.
9. By actively disputing dysfunctional thinking and through counterconditioning, change is possible in a relatively short amount of time.

This section of the chapter will provide an overview of four cognitive–behavioral approaches: *modern-day behaviorism, rational emotive behavior therapy (REBT), cognitive therapy*, and *reality therapy*.

Modern-Day Behavior Therapy

Based on an understanding of classical conditioning, social learning or modeling, and operant conditioning, modern-day behaviorists have at their disposal a wide range of techniques that they can apply with clients. However, choosing and applying techniques effectively is a careful and deliberate process that occurs through a series of stages that includes building the relationship, clinical assessment, focusing on problem areas and setting goals, choosing techniques and working on goals, assessment of goal completion, and closure and follow-up. Let's take a brief look at each of these stages.

Stage 1: Building the Relationship.   During this stage, the major goal is to build a strong relationship with the client and to begin to clearly define the goals of therapy. Building the relationship is done by showing an accepting attitude to the client, and today it is usual to find behavior therapists demonstrating good listening skills and being empathic, showing concern and positive regard, and informing the client that any issue can be discussed in counseling. As a supportive, trusting relationship is developed, the therapist increasingly inquires about the how's, where's, and what's of the presenting problem.

Stage 2: Clinical Assessment.   Critical to choosing the most effective technique for client change is to make a thorough assessment of client needs. Sometimes called a *functional behavior analysis (FBA),* such an assessment should minimally include an in-depth structured interview that examines a broad range of predetermined areas in the client's life and particularly focuses on events that occur prior to and directly after the problematic behavior (Alberto & Troutman, 2012; Wolpe & Lazarus, 1966). In addition, it is often wise to incorporate the use of personality instruments, observation by the clinician, interviews with significant others, and self-monitoring by the client, who will later report back observations to the clinician (Neukrug & Fawcett, 2015).

Stage 3: Focusing on Problem Areas and Setting Goals.   During the second stage, the therapist has completed a thorough assessment and defined potential problem areas. Now, identified areas are further examined by obtaining a baseline of the frequency, duration, and intensity of the behaviors. Often, this is accomplished by having the client complete a journal or ledger of the behaviors in question. A careful analysis of problem behaviors can help to reveal their magnitude, sets parameters for how and when to change the behaviors, and is useful when assessing progress made. Completion of the baseline is also helpful in setting goals for treatment. From an examination of the baseline, clients can better understand the magnitude of various problem behaviors, decide upon which they want to focus, and collaboratively set goals with the therapist.

Stage 4: Choosing Techniques and Working on Goals.   By drawing from social learning theory, operant conditioning, and classical conditioning, therapists have a large array of techniques to assist the client through the change process (see Box 4.8). At this stage in the therapeutic process, the therapist must carefully explain various techniques to the client and collaboratively choose those techniques that would be most efficacious for the problem at hand. Now the work begins, as the client and therapist together devise a plan to use the techniques to reach decided-upon goals.

BOX 4.8
Select Techniques Used in Behavior Therapy

Modern-day behavior therapy uses a wide variety of techniques from operant conditioning, classical conditioning, and modeling in an effort to help the client change behaviors and feel better about himself or herself. Just a few of the dozens of popular behavior techniques that are used today include:

➤ *Reinforcement*, where basic positive and negative reinforcement contingencies are applied (e.g., using sticker charts, saying "good job," etc.)

➤ *Modeling*, where the client observes a model and then practices the model's behaviors on his or her own

➤ *Relaxation and systematic desensitization*, where clients learn basic relaxation techniques and apply them to the alleviation of specific phobias (e.g., fear of elevators)

➤ *Token economies*, where tokens are given to clients when they exhibit specific targeted behaviors and are later exchanged for a reward

➤ *Flooding and implosion techniques*, where clients are exposed to a feared stimulus for an extended amount of time until the stimulus no longer evokes the fear response

➤ *Aversion therapy*, where a stimulus that is perceived to be highly noxious by a client is associated with a targeted behavior (e.g., a pedophile receives electric shock when aroused by pictures of children)

➤ *Stimulus control*, where a stimulus is altered or removed and a new, healthier behavior is reinforced (e.g., a binge eater places a lock on the refrigerator)

➤ *Self-management techniques*, where clients learn how to apply any of a number of behavioral techniques on their own and monitor their own progress

Stage 5: Assessment of Goal Completion.   Now that goals have been decided upon, techniques chosen, and work begun, it becomes important to assess whether clients are reaching their stated goals. Because a baseline of the intensity, frequency, and duration of the problem behavior has usually been recorded, it is a relatively easy task to assess whether there is a lessening of the problem behavior. If no such progress is seen, it is important to reassess the problem and the techniques chosen (or recycle from stage 3). If the problem was originally diagnosed accurately, and if appropriate techniques were chosen, the client should begin to see an amelioration of the problem.

Stage 6: Closure and Follow-Up.   Reinforcement theory suggests that *extinction* of most behaviors will usually be followed by a resurgence of the targeted behavior called *spontaneous recovery* (Jozefowiez & Staddon, 2015). Therefore, it is important to remain with the client long enough to ensure success and to prepare the client for a possible resurgence of the problem after therapy has ended. Therefore, many behaviorists build in follow-up sessions to the course of therapy. Of course, as in any therapy, when success is reached, it is important that the client experiences a sense of closure as he or she nears the end of therapy.

Behavior therapy today is a far cry from the deterministic, objectivistic, scientific behavior therapy of years ago. Whereas classical behaviorists viewed the client as an object to be experimented upon, the modern-day behaviorist understands the importance of building a relationship so that he or she can better understand the client's problem and so the client will be more amenable to the therapeutic process. The stages just described are an example of how such a process might occur.

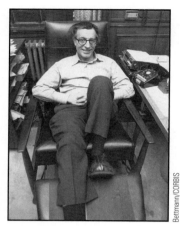

Albert Ellis

Rational Emotive Behavior Therapy (REBT)

. . . if you have right opinions, you will fare well; if they are false, you will fare ill. For to every man the cause of his acting is opinion. . . .

(Epictetus, c. 100 CE)

Developed by Albert Ellis (1913–2009) during the 1950s, rational emotive behavior therapy (REBT) asserts that we are fallible human beings who have the potential for rational or irrational thinking. *Rational thinking*, say REBT therapists, leads to healthy ways of living and results in people who show unconditional acceptance of self, of others, and of the way things are. In contrast, *irrational thinking* leads to emotional distress, dysfunctional behaviors, and neurotic ways of living, as well as people who tend to be critical of others and of themselves. Although early child-rearing practices, family dynamics, societal influences, and innate biology tend to be the basis for the development of rational or irrational thinking, REBT therapists believe that it is the individual who sustains his or her unique way of thinking (Ellis & MacLaren, 2005).

REBT therapists believe that there is a complex interaction between one's thinking, feeling, and behavioral states, and they view the interpretation of cognitive processes as being mostly responsible for self-defeating emotions and dysfunctional behaviors. Reactions to events, say REBT therapists, are filtered through one's belief system, and the individual responds consciously or unconsciously to the belief system, not to the event. If the belief system is irrational, the individual responds with self-defeating emotions and self-perpetuating dysfunctional behaviors. If the belief system is rational, the individual responds with emotions that perpetuate healthy ways of functioning in the world. Thus, strong emotions, such as grief after the loss of a dear friend or sadness if one's house is flooded from a hurricane, would be considered a reasonable response, whereas a deep depression after the ending of a relationship or road rage at a fellow driver would be seen as unreasonable responses and a reaction to an irrational belief system.

Although REBT therapists view an individual's belief system as generally being created early in life, they also believe that it can be challenged and systematically changed by analyzing its philosophical basis and helping the individual gain awareness into the irrational beliefs that fuel maladaptive ways of living. Long-winded examination of the past is not necessary; indeed, it could be harmful and inhibit progress toward change.

Freud was full of horseshit. He invented people's problems and what to do about them. Tell me one thing about the past. I'll prove it's not what upset you. It's how you philosophized about it that made you disturbed.

(Ellis, as cited in Aviv, 2005, para. 2)

As you can see from the preceding quote, the insight-oriented approach of REBT has a strong *anti-deterministic* philosophy suggesting that we can choose new ways of thinking and ultimately feel better and act in healthier ways. This optimistic view of change has an existential flavor to it, although REBT is rarely placed within the existential schools. Perhaps REBT can best be seen as a philosophy that is a mixture of learning theory and existential–humanistic philosophy: learning theory in the sense that we learned a way of

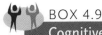

BOX 4.9
Cognitive Distortions and Three Core Irrational Beliefs

Cognitive Distortions

Absolutistic musts and shoulds occur when an individual believes that he or she must or should act a certain way in life (e.g., "I must be the best parent," or "I should always be polite").

Awfulizing occurs when an individual exaggerates events by making them horrible, terrible, awful, or catastrophic (e.g., "If I don't get into that graduate program, my life will be shattered," or "It's so horrible, I can't even tell you what happened—OK, my husband abused me—I can't go on!").

I-can't-stand-it-itis occurs when an individual continually sees events as being unbearable and exaggerates the event through his or her irrational belief system (e.g., "I just can't stand my daughter's behavior any more—she's going to drive me crazy!" or, "Those immigrants are taking jobs away from us; they're going to eventually take my job!").

Demands on oneself add unnecessary stress to an individual because they assume that a person should, must, or ought to act in a certain manner ("I need to find love or my life will be ruined").

People-rating (damning oneself and others) occurs when an individual rates or views oneself, or another person, as having all or none of a quality (good, bad, worthless) (e.g., "My boss is a no-good idiot; I hate him," or "I loved that woman, she was perfect. Why did she do this to me?").

Three Core Irrational Beliefs

1. "I absolutely must, under all conditions, do important tasks well and be approved by significant others, or else I am an inadequate and unlovable person!"
2. "Other people absolutely must, under all conditions, treat me fairly and justly, or else they are rotten, damnable persons!"
3. "Conditions under which I live absolutely must always be the way I want them to be, give me almost immediate gratification, and not require me to work too hard to change or improve them; or else it is awful, I can't stand them, and it is impossible for me to be happy at all!" (Ellis & MacLaren, 2005, pp. 32–33)

---

thinking, feeling, and acting that is self-perpetuating, and existential–humanistic because we can choose to learn new and healthier ways of thinking, feeling, and behaving.

Basic to REBT philosophy is the idea that we have adopted certain *cognitive distortions* in our lives that have led to one or more of 3 core *irrational beliefs* (see Box 4.9; Ellis originally suggested *11 irrational beliefs* that he eventually pared down to 3). As you might expect, the techniques used in REBT are based on helping the client identify and stop using cognitive distortions while also replacing irrational beliefs with rational beliefs. In addition, because the REBT therapist sees an intimate connection between thinking, behaving, and feeling, other techniques will be used to encourage new ways of responding and feeling that are aligned with the new rational way of thinking.

The REBT therapist tends to be *active* and *directive* and not overly concerned about the building of caring, empathic relationships when working with clients as he or she shows the client how cognitive distortions and irrational beliefs have led to dysfunctional ways of living in the world (see Box 4.10). They do this by demonstrating the *ABCs of feeling and behaving*. Here, the therapist shows the client how it is not the *activating event* ("A") that has caused the *consequential* negative feelings ("C") but the *irrational belief* ("iB") about the event that has led to those feelings. For instance, look at the following scenario:

Activating event (A): My lover has left me.

Cognitive self-statement or belief: I must have a lover, otherwise I am worthless.

Underlying core irrational belief (iB): Conditions under which I live absolutely must always be the way I want them to be, give me almost immediate gratification, and not require me to work too hard to change or

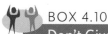

A few years after finishing my doctorate, I considered doing a postdoctoral fellowship at the Rational Emotive Behavior Institute in New York City. I sent in my resume and was called for an interview. At first, I interviewed with one of the directors; then I was told I would have to do a role-play with "Al." I was brought in to see Al, who was sitting in a big, comfortable armchair. He proceeded to ask me to role-play a counselor. He was the client, playing a male college student who had difficulty dating. I began to listen and respond with empathy, thinking that after hearing about the problem, I would move

into an REBT style of response. After about three empathic responses in a row, Al said to me, something like, "Don't give me any of that Rogerian ___! I want to see a rational emotive counselor." I proceeded to give him what he wanted, thinking to myself, "He sure is serious about the unimportance of the 'necessary and sufficient conditions.'" I decided not to pursue the fellowship.

You can hear this and other stories by clicking on "Albert Ellis" at the "Stories of the Great Therapists" website (see http://www.odu.edu/sgt).

---

improve them; or else it is *awful,* I *can't stand* them, and it is impossible for me to be happy *at all!*

Possible consequence (C):

> *Feelings consequence:* depression, panic

> *Behavioral consequence:* need to immediately seek out another person, even if the relationship may not be healthy or positive; or isolation if depression is particularly bad.

After the client learns the basic ABCs, he or she is taught how to *dispute* ("D") the irrational belief by replacing the irrational belief with a rational belief (rB).

Activating event (A): My lover has left me.

Rational belief (rB): This is unfortunate, and things don't always work out in life the way that I want them to. However, I'll move on in my life and perhaps even meet someone I like more.

Possible consequence (C): Feeling "okay" and actively trying to meet new people.

In addition to the "ABC" method, several other techniques are used in REBT to ensure a new cognitive, behavioral, and emotional outlook. These include *cognitive homework,* where the client practices disputing irrational beliefs at home; *bibliotherapy,* where clients can read about REBT philosophy; *role-playing,* to try new behaviors consistent with a rational view; *shame-attacking exercises,* where clients practice unconventional social behaviors (dressing unusually) to learn how to rid themselves of their conventional ways of being; *imagery exercises,* where clients imagine healthier ways of acting; *behavioral techniques,* where clients practice new behaviors; and *emotive techniques,* where clients are encouraged to get in touch with their feelings to help understand their underlying belief system.

The actual practice of REBT is relatively short term and can be viewed through the following five steps:

> *Step 1:* Assessing the client's situation and hypothesizing how the ABCs apply
> *Step 2:* Teaching the REBT philosophy

Step 3: Demonstrating how the client's situation fits the REBT model
Step 4: Directing the change process through a variety of techniques
Step 5: Reinforcing change and terminating the relationship

REBT is an active and directive therapy in which clients are challenged to take on a more rational way of living. Although REBT therapists don't tell people how to live, they do help them look at how current thinking and associated behaviors and feelings may be related to specific cognitive distortions and irrational beliefs.

Cognitive Therapy

Cognitive therapy was developed during the 1960s by Aaron Beck (1921–). Although similar to Ellis's approach in many ways, Beck believed more strongly than Ellis that the relationship was critical to positive therapeutic outcomes and disagreed with Ellis's use of the word *irrational*. Beck's writings suggest that there is a genetic and evolutionary predisposition toward certain emotional responses. Although adaptive in the distant past, their expression in today's world can sometimes be maladaptive (e.g., excessive anxiety and anger) (Beck, A., 1967, 1976, 1999, 2005). Called the *continuity hypothesis*, these older, emotional responses are seen as "continuing" into the modern world (Weishaar, 1993), and when an individual today exhibits these emotional responses frequently, he or she is often viewed as having a mental disorder. Beck also suggests that individuals who have a tendency toward exhibiting these maladaptive emotional responses will not express them if taught effective skills by parents and others. And taking a rational, pragmatic, and some say "constructivist" perspective, which suggests that one can "reconstruct" their sense of who they are, Beck assumes that those who do exhibit maladaptive responses can change through therapeutic discourse with others (Beck, J., 2005; Leahy, 2003). Thus, cognitive therapy is seen as an *anti-deterministic, active, educative,* and *empirical* approach to counseling that suggests that in a relatively short amount of time, people can effect changes in their lives.

Courtesy of the Beck Institute of Cognitive Therapy and Research
Aaron Beck

Beck posits a *diathesis–stress model* of mental disorders that suggests that genetics, biological factors, and experiences combine to produce specific *core beliefs*, some of which may lie dormant and then suddenly appear as the result of stress and other conditions impinging on the person. Core beliefs are embedded, underlying beliefs that provide direction toward the manner in which one lives in the world (Beck, A., 1967, 1991), with negative core beliefs leading to negative feelings and dysfunctional behaviors, and positive core beliefs leading to healthy ways of living. Three broad categories of negative core beliefs are listed in Box 4.11.

Beck believes that most individuals are not aware of their core beliefs. Instead, such beliefs become the underlying mechanism for the creation of *intermediate beliefs*, which set the *attitudes, rules* and *expectations,* and *assumptions* we live by. These attitudes, rules and expectations, and assumptions can be understood by looking at how situations lead to what are called *automatic thoughts,* which result in a set of behaviors, feelings, and physiological responses that end up reinforcing core beliefs. Beck found that automatic thoughts are often related to one of a number of *cognitive distortions,* which are similar to Ellis's 3 core irrational beliefs, as well as his original 11 irrational beliefs (see Box 4.12). Beck also found that certain diagnoses are related to specific core beliefs. Thus, when a client comes in presenting with certain symptoms, if an accurate diagnosis is made, the counselor can make

BOX 4.11
Negative Core Beliefs

Helpless Core Beliefs
"I am inadequate, ineffective, incompetent; I can't cope."
"I am powerless, out of control; I can't change; I'm stuck, trapped, a victim."
"I am vulnerable, weak, needy, likely to be hurt."
"I am inferior, a failure, a loser, not good enough; I don't measure up to others."

Unlovable Core Beliefs
"I am unlikable, undesirable, ugly, boring; I have nothing to offer."
"I am unloved, unwanted, neglected."

"I will always be rejected, abandoned; I will always be alone."
"I am different, defective, not good enough to be loved."

Worthless Core Beliefs
"I am worthless, unacceptable, bad, crazy, broken, nothing, a waste."
"I am hurtful, dangerous, toxic, evil."
"I don't deserve to live."

SOURCE: Beck, J. (2005). *Cognitive therapy for challenging problems.* New York, NY: Guilford Press, p. 22.

BOX 4.12
Cognitive Distortions

1. *All-or-nothing thinking:* Seeing the world categorically, rather than in a more complex fashion
   Examples: "I am never good at my job." "You are always happy."
2. *Catastrophisizing:* Assuming that something will go wrong rather than looking at situations more realistically
   Examples: "I shouldn't have said that to my boss, I know I'll get fired." "If I fly, the plane will crash."
3. *Disqualifying or discounting the positive:* Even when a positive event occurs, assuming that it means little
   Example: "That award I won at work is meaningless—everybody wins awards."
4. *Emotional reasoning:* Assuming that feelings are always correct, even when there is evidence to the contrary
   Example: "My wife and kids may tell me they love me, but I know no one can love me."
5. *Labeling:* Defining oneself in terms of a "label" or "type" instead of more nuanced ways
   Examples: "I'm just a negative person." "I'm always introverted."
6. *Magnification/minimization:* Magnifying the negative or minimizing the positive
   Example: "I might have done well on that one test, but I know I'm not good in that subject."
7. *Mental filter:* Focusing on one negative aspect of oneself, of another, or of a situation
   Example: "I know why people stay away from me: They always see my disability."
8. *Mind-reading:* Making assumptions about what other people are thinking and discounting other possibilities.
   Example: "She thinks I'm ugly."
9. *Overgeneralization:* Making large generalizations from a small event
   Example: "That dinner for my kids was horrible; I'll never be a good parent."
10. *Personalization:* Assuming that you are the cause for another person's negative behavior
    Example: "My colleague, James, was in a bad mood today because I didn't get that project to him in time."
11. *"Should" and "must" statements:* Believing if one does not act in a specific manner, it is horrible
    Example: "My grandmother never should have acted so boldly in front of the company."
12. *Tunnel vision:* Only seeing the downside or negative aspect of a situation
    Example: "Her expressing her opinion is uncalled for. We'll never make friends that way."

Adapted from: Beck, J. (1995). *Cognitive therapy: Basics and beyond.* New York, NY: Guilford Press.

a fairly good guess at the core belief that fuels the client's intermediate beliefs, automatic thoughts, and cognitive distortions.

Cognitive therapists initially focus on the client's automatic thoughts, as they are easily "caught" and are a more natural starting point (e.g., a core belief of "I am inadequate" is much more difficult for a client to initially grasp than an automatic thought of "I never will get this report done right"). Slowly and methodically, the therapist, in collaboration with the client, works his or her way up toward the client's core beliefs. As the client increasingly understands the relationships between symptoms, automatic thoughts, cognitive distortions, intermediate beliefs, and core beliefs, he or she can begin to change. Figure 4.2 shows

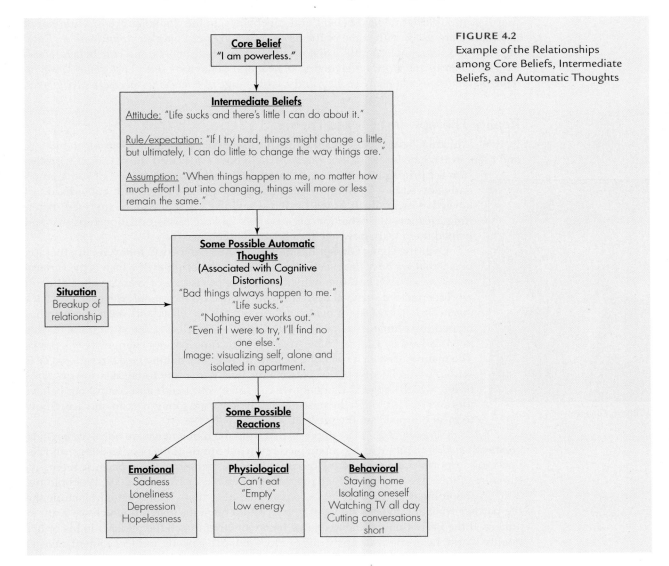

FIGURE 4.2
Example of the Relationships among Core Beliefs, Intermediate Beliefs, and Automatic Thoughts

a graphic representation of this for a client who comes in after a breakup of a relationship and initially presents with a variety of emotional, behavioral, and physiological responses. Fairly quickly, the client can begin to "catch" his or her automatic thoughts and over time can see the relationship between those thoughts and the more embedded cognitive distortions, intermediate beliefs, and ultimately, core beliefs.

In working with clients, counselors initially build a strong therapeutic alliance by being *collaborative*, demonstrating *empathy*, being *caring*, and being *optimistic*. Fairly quickly, the counselor uses *Socratic questioning* to help clients understand their thought processes while at the same time educating them about the cognitive model. Soon clients are able to identify and challenge automatic thoughts and later can identify and challenge cognitive distortions, intermediate beliefs, and core beliefs. In the change process, a number of techniques are used, with some of the more common ones being *identifying and challenging* automatic thoughts, cognitive distortions, intermediate beliefs, and core beliefs; *homework assignments,* to work on changing beliefs and behaviors; *thought-stopping; imagery-changing; rational–emotional role-play*; and a wide range of *behavioral and emotive techniques*.

Reality Therapy and Choice Theory

In 1960, William Glasser (1925–2013) wrote his first book, *Mental Health or Mental Illness,* and then, in 1965, he wrote *Reality Therapy*. These books criticized the psychiatric profes-

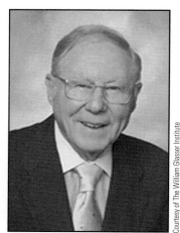

sion for propagating the belief that mental illness was the result of some inherently flawed biological brain functioning. Instead, he suggested that individuals labeled as mentally ill, as well as those having daily living problems, were exhibiting irresponsible behaviors because they had not formed relationships that had helped them learn how to effectively meet their needs.

Over the years, Glasser has greatly refined his theory. Today, reality therapy posits that we have *five genetically based needs*, the original of which is the *survival or self-preservation need* that helped us endure thousands of years ago in a difficult world. From the survival need spun off the needs for *love and belonging, power* (or *inner control*), *freedom* (or *independence*), and *fun* (or *enjoyment*), each of which has helped the human species thrive in distinct ways. Today, the strength of all five needs is said by Glasser to be "fixed at birth and does not change" (1998, p. 91). The manner in which each of us learns to meet our unique *need-strength profile* is said to be a reflection of our personality. Reality therapy today is based on *choice theory*, which suggests that only we can satisfy our needs and control our behaviors and that although the past affected who we are today, we can only learn how to meet our needs in the present.

William Glasser

Glasser (1998, 2001) suggests that from the moment we are born, we begin to create our *quality worlds*, which contain pictures in our minds of the people, things, and beliefs most important to us in meeting our unique need-strength profiles. Because these pictures are unique, they represent each person's take on reality (Brickell, 2007; Wubbolding, 2010; Wubbolding & Brickell, 1999). As some examples, these pictures might include the life partner we want, the car we want to buy, and a religious belief to which we want to adhere. If the individual is able to choose behaviors that match the pictures in his or her quality world, he or she will satisfy one or more of the five needs and feel content, at least

Courtesy of The William Glasser Institute

for a short period of time. These pictures can change throughout one's lifetime; however, sometimes pictures that previously satisfied us can remain in our minds for long periods of time and can become a source of pain if we can no longer satisfy them. For instance, it can take a long time to rid oneself of the image of a lover who has left.

Central to reality therapy is the idea that our *total behavior* is chosen and generated from within in an effort to match the pictures in our quality worlds. By "total behavior," Glasser means our actions, our thinking process, our feelings, and our physiological responses. Glasser goes on to state that we can only *choose our actions and thoughts*, which are jointly called *doing*, and that our feelings and our physiology result from those choices.

Glasser suggests that language usage is reflective of how individuals make choices in their attempts to meet their needs (Glasser & Glasser, 1999). *Internal-control language* is accepting, respectful, and supportive of others, and it reflects a person who is clear about the choices that will best meet his or her needs. On the other hand, *external control language* is blaming, critical, and threatening of others, and it reflects a person who sees his or her life controlled by others and by events. Along these lines, Glasser suggests that instead of saying: "My depression is making me sleep all the time," or "I have a mental illness that has stopped me from working," or "My anger makes my blood pressure go up," individuals say: "I am depressing myself and choosing to sleep much of the time," "I make myself mentally ill and choose not to work," and "I anger myself and make my blood pressure rise." Language such as this shows that the individual is in control of his or her state of being and differs with the mainstream psychiatric view, which suggests that mental disorders are the result of intrinsic, organically based problems (e.g., genetic differences in brain function) or that individuals are determined by such things as early childhood experiences.

As you can probably tell, Glasser's approach is anti-deterministic, because at any point in life, a person can evaluate his or her total behaviors, adopt internal control language, and make new choices that better match one's need-strength profile and quality world. And because Glasser believes that needs can only be satisfied in the here and now, the approach is focused mostly on the *present*. Even if an individual had been traumatized and learned maladaptive ways of behaving in an attempt to meet his or her needs, that person can learn new ways of choosing that can lead to more effective satisfaction of needs. Generally, people can learn these new ways through the development of relationships that are accepting, loving, and caring, like one might find in counseling. Such relationships teach internal-control language, how to make better choices, and how to best match one's quality world.

Today, a common method of training reality therapists is the *WDEP system* developed by Bob Wubbolding (Wubbolding, 2000; Wubbolding & Brickell, 1999). The acronym WDEP stands for *wants* of the client, what the client is *doing* in his or her life's direction, *evaluating* if what the client is doing is working, and developing a *plan* of action that can be implemented. This system allows clients to look at what their needs are, what they are doing to get their needs met, examine if what they are doing is working for them, and decide on what they need to do differently to better get their needs met. Wubbolding suggests that for a client to effectively involve himself or herself in the WDEP cycle, there must be a strong therapeutic relationship based on trust and hope. This is accomplished by the counselor's demonstrating and embodying the techniques

FIGURE 4.3
Wubbolding's WDEP Model

SOURCE: Developed by Robert E. Wubbolding, Ed.D from the works of William Glasser, MD. Copyright 1986 Robert E. Wubbolding, EdD. 17th Revision 2010.

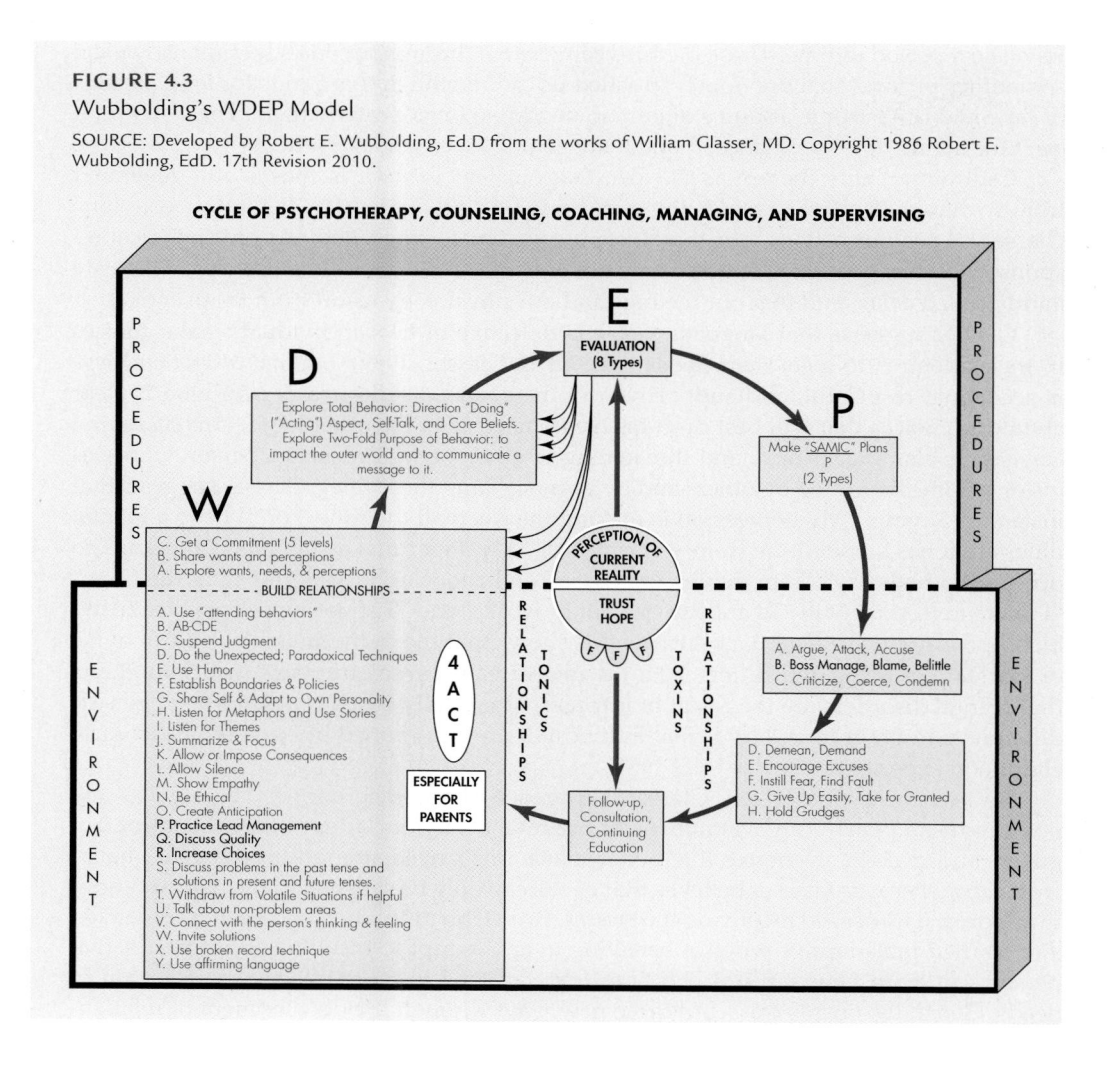

CYCLE OF PSYCHOTHERAPY, COUNSELING, COACHING, MANAGING, AND SUPERVISING

the attitudes of what Wubbolding calls the *environmental elements,* which include exhibiting the *tonics of creating the counseling relationship* and avoiding the *toxins of creating the counseling relationship* (see Figure 4.3).

Postmodern Approaches

Narrative therapy and *solution-focused brief therapy,* the two approaches examined in this section, are recent additions to the therapeutic milieu and are based on the philosophies of *postmodernism, social constructionism,* and *poststructuralism.* Postmodernists question modernism and the many assumptions and beliefs that are taken for granted as a result of the use of empiricism and the scientific method. Postmodernism suggests that there is no one way to understand the world, no foundational set of rules to make sense of

who we are, and no one approach to communication in understanding a person. Social constructionism has to do with how values are transmitted through language by the social milieu (e.g., family, culture, and society) and suggests that the person is constantly changing with the ebb and flow of the influences of significant others, culture, and society. Poststructuralism questions the inherent "truth" of such things as intrinsic psychological structures to which many psychological theorists point in explaining their view of human nature. Those with this philosophy doubt many of the basic assumptions of past popular therapies, which suggest that certain structures cause mental health problems (e.g., id, ego, superego, core beliefs, lack of internal locus of control, etc.). Rather than harp on past problems that tend to be embedded in oppressive belief systems, postmodern approaches suggest that clients can find exceptions to their problems and develop creative solutions. Postmodern therapies tend to be short term, with solution-focused brief therapy being considered a particularly brief approach, sometimes lasting fewer than five sessions.

Narrative Therapy

One of the newest forms of therapy, narrative therapy was developed by Michael White (1948–2008) and David Epston (1948–), among others. Greatly affected by the philosophy of social constructionism and postmodernism, White and Epston began to develop a new means of working with clients based on such premises as *realities are socially constructed, realities are constituted through language, realities are organized and maintained through narrative,* and *there are no essential truths* (Freedman & Combs, 1996). The narrative therapist's belief in there being no essential truths is closely associated with issues of power and inequity in society because "truths" from the dominant culture are often accepted and subtly forced upon us. And, say the narrative therapists, it is these same truths that tend to maintain the power structure in society that is responsible for the oppression of nondominant groups. For the narrative therapist, *dominant stories* from society are internalized by individuals, cause people to live out and believe stories that tend to oppress the underclass, and blind clients to other possible stories and opportunities (Freedman & Combs, 1996; White, 1993, 1995; White & Epston, 1990). Thus, stories about how certain individuals or groups of people are "lazy," "stupid," "rebellious," and so on are often subtly, and sometimes openly, passed down. These constructions become part of the dominant stories of those in power and are even sometimes internalized and "believed" by the very people whom the stories are about. For these reasons, narrative therapy is often referred to as an approach that has a very strong *social justice orientation.*

From the narrative point of view, individuals are constantly in discourse with others within their social milieu, and it is through such interactions that they develop their sense of self. Although people are deeply affected by the language used in their social spheres, narrative therapy is *anti-deterministic* because it assumes that people can understand the realities that have been created, *deconstruct* their foundations (take them apart), and develop or *reauthor* new stories that are empowering. Because the major focus of narrative therapy is "where people want to go" rather than "where they have been" (Hoyt, 1994, p. 1), narrative therapy is more optimistic than other approaches. In fact, narrative therapists are considered *anti-objectivists,* which means that they oppose those approaches that develop a theoretical model that explains reality and then uses that hypothetical

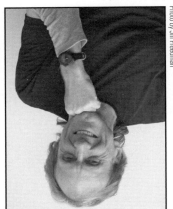

Michael White

Photo by Jill Freedman

model to define the experience of others (e.g., psychodynamic approaches, the DSM). This objectification of others, which almost always focuses on the client's past, often re- sults in the disdain for or oppression of the client:

The objectivists and monumentalists, on the other hand, prefer to stand above the fray, where they can assume a position of omniscience, and work in the "clean" realm of detachment and ethical neutrality. To me, the attitudes em- bodied in their "standing above it all" range from mild condescension through active surveillance to brute domination . . .

(Rosaldo, 1993, p. 221)

Narrative therapists suggest that we are all *multistoried* and that some stories are help- ful, while others are unhelpful, such as the dominant, *problem-saturated stories* with which clients often present. They suggest that it is important to help clients deconstruct their problem-saturated story and begin to look at other stories (or narratives) that are also an aspect of an individual's life. In doing this, they suggest that clients will move from what they call *thin stories* toward *thick stories*, or more complex ways of seeing their lives, which is not based on the problem-saturated dominant story. Narrative therapists help clients find *exceptions* to their problem-saturated dominant stories and have them look at the multiple stories that are present in their lives. In this way, clients can begin to reauthor their lives or identify with new stories that are not problem saturated (Figure 4.4).

Narrative therapists approach clients with *mystery, respectful curiosity, and awe.* They will often ask a lot of *questions* in an effort to have clients talk about their dominant, problem-saturated stories and help them look at other, less dominant, but potentially em- powering stories. They tend to be *collaborative* and *encouraging* to clients in their attempts to help them look at the stories that sprinkle their lives. Often the narrative therapist will

FIGURE 4.4
Identification of New, Alternative Stories

The line with the triangles is symbolic of times John remembers being verbally abused by his father for being sensitive—his dominant story. The line with the ovals represents times John remembers being a content, sensitive child or man. And the line with stars reflects times John remembers being a content, "strong" child or man. John is now beginning to reauthor or redefine who he is, and the problem-saturated story is beginning to become less meaningful.

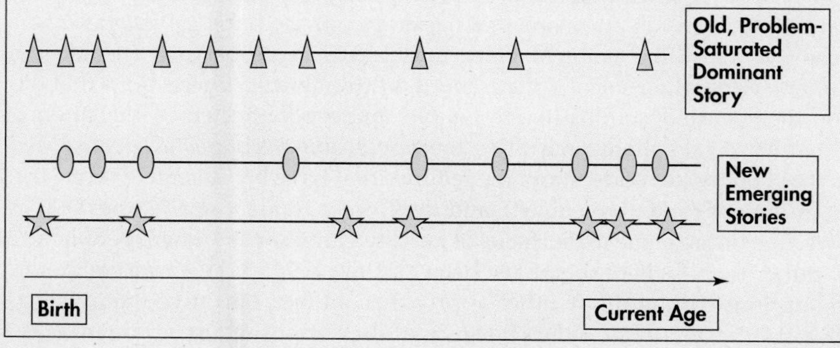

have clients name and externalize the dominant problem so that they will not see the problem as something inherent. They will help clients see how dominant, problem-saturated stories have affected their lives and help them identify unique outcomes or exceptions to these stories. In this way, they can begin to examine new stories and reauthor their lives. To reinforce these new stories, they will sometimes have clients *journal*, have outside *witnesses* listen to their new stories, and have clients *retell* their new stories to reinforce the new, more positive way of being. Sometimes *symbols* might be used to reinforce the new stories (e.g., handing a client who has lived a story that she is "dumb" a certificate of "brightness").

Narrative therapy can be viewed in four phases. *Phase 1, the joining phase*, occurs when the therapist meets the client, begins to build a relationship, and invites the client to share his or her problem-saturated story; *Phase 2, examining patterns*, is when the client is invited to examine stories that contradict, deny, or oppose the problem-saturated story; *Phase 3, reauthoring*, is when the client begins to build new, more positive stories; and *Phase 4, moving on*, is when the client has developed a new, more positive outlook on life and is ready to leave therapy. An exciting and relatively new type of therapy, narrative therapy is quickly becoming an approach that challenges many of the existing therapies' understandings of client problems and of mental illness.

Solution-Focused Brief Therapy

> *Suppose that one night, while you were asleep, there was a miracle and this problem was solved. How would you know? What would be different?*
>
> (de Shazer, 1988, p. 5)

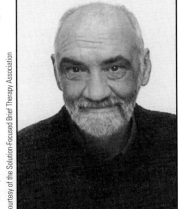

Steve de Shazer

Developed by the husband and wife team of Steve de Shazer (1940–2005) and Insoo Kim Berg (1934–2007), *solution-focused brief therapy (SFBT)* was greatly influenced by John Weakland and others from the *Mental Research Institute* (MRI) at Palo Alto, CA.

After taking part in training at MRI, de Shazer and Berg, as well as three other colleagues, decided to start the *Brief Family Therapy Center (BFTC)* of Milwaukee, which initially mirrored what was happening at MRI. As the team began to treat large numbers of clients, they noticed that solution-focused interventions, in contrast to problem-focused ones, seemed to have better and quicker results. In fact, the group realized that the average number of sessions that clients spent in therapy was six, yet most therapists, with their insight-oriented approaches, expected clients to be in therapy for months, if not years (Gingerich, 2006). They also realized that most therapists saw clients as diseased and were continually hypothesizing about their clients as if the therapist knew something about them that they did not know about themselves (Cade, 2005).

Deciding that clients were their own best resources, and confident that clients could be helped quickly, they decided to use videotapes and live observation to determine which techniques seemed to have the quickest and best results. In fact, this is how de Shazer (1988) came up with his famous *miracle question* that is quoted at the beginning of this section. Confident they could quickly and effectively work with clients, the team decided to contract with one health insurance

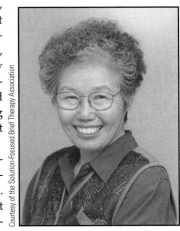

Insoo Kim Berg

company for a flat fee of $500 per client, regardless of how long treatment took (Riding the. . . , 2006). Using informal follow-up studies of their clients, de Shazer was able to show that his new approach to counseling was effective in a short amount of time (Gingerich, 2006).

Today, SFBT is a *pragmatic, optimistic, anti-deterministic,* and *future-oriented* approach that believes in the ability of the client to change. SFBT rejects the notion that individuals have an inherent tendency toward mental health problems or illnesses and focuses almost exclusively on solutions and on client strengths, not on client deficits or problems (Fernando, 2007). Trusting that change can occur quickly, this approach asserts that individuals can find *exceptions* to their problems and build on those exceptions to find new ways of living in the world (O'Hanlon & Weiner-Davis, 2003).

Although de Shazer and Dolan (2007) have suggested that SFBT is "not theory-based" (p. 1), most modern-day solution-focused therapists would likely identify themselves as *social constructionists* and *postmodernists,* and it is clear that this is where solution-focused therapy has its philosophical home (Bidwell, 2007; Guterman, 2006). The postmodern, social-constructionist position asserts that pathology, for all practical purposes, does not exist because one cannot prove that it is inherently found within the person. Thus, this perspective assumes that problems can be viewed as challenges that are inherent in a language-based system. Seen from this viewpoint, how the counselor brings himself or herself into the relationship is critical to helping the individual overcome his or her problems. If the counselor believes that pathology exists within the person, he or she will find this pathology; if the counselor believes that the problems are system-based (e.g., residing within the family), he or she will find this to be the case; but if the counselor assumes that problems are a function of the language used by the client within his or her social sphere (including the counselor's office!), opportunities for change through the use of new language are plentiful. With this in mind, "SFBT eschews the 'medical model' perspective and takes a nonpathological approach" (Watts & Pietrzak, 2000, p. 443).

Given the pragmatic and future-oriented focus, as well as the philosophical assumptions inherent in social constructionism and postmodernism, solution-focused therapists believe that clients can change quickly; are the experts; have strengths that can be expanded upon; should focus on solutions, not problems; should focus on the future; and in dialogue with the counselor, can create problem-free language as they move toward a new reality (O'Hanlon & Weiner-Davis, 2003). To work quickly and effectively with clients, SFBT uses a variety of techniques that can be seen through the following six stages:

Stage 0: Pre-Session Change.   Knowing that clients are generally ready to change when they seek counseling, prior to the first session the therapist and client decide on an appointment time, and the therapist asks the client to become cognizant of any changes that are made prior to their first meeting.

Stage 1: Forming a Collaborative Relationship.   Instead of presenting oneself as an expert at knowing a particular theory that posits why the client might respond in a certain manner, the solution-focused therapist focuses on downplaying power differentials and helping the client identify his or her own strengths and resources. Thus, the counselor builds a *trusting, collaborative, and equal relationship* by being an *ambassador (showing curiosity, respect, and acceptance),* being a *good listener, using empathy, and being tentative.*

Stage 2: Describing the Problem.   Although the focus of therapy is almost exclusively on solutions, it is important that clients feel heard when they first enter counseling, so many of the same skills that are used to form the collaborative relationship are initially used to listen to clients' problems. However, De Jong and Berg (2002) suggest that problems need to be listened to for only about 15 minutes before the therapist begins to use other techniques that will move clients toward focusing on preferred goals.

Stage 3: Establishing Preferred Goals.   One of the first steps toward helping clients focus on *preferred goals* is to have them begin to respond to questions about what they would like to see in the future (Bannink, 2010). Letting go of the problem-saturated way of viewing the world is critical for clients if they are to make progress quickly. O'Connell (2003) suggests asking the following types of questions to facilitate this movement toward preferred goals:

- ➤ How will you know that coming here has been worthwhile for you?
- ➤ What are your best hopes for this session?
- ➤ What will be the first sign for you?
- ➤ How will you know when things are getting better?
- ➤ How long do you think it will take before things get better?
- ➤ How will you know when things are getting better? (p. 7)

Stage 4: Problem-To-Solution Focus.   To help clients increasingly focus on solutions instead of problems, a number of different types of questions are employed, including the following:

- ➤ *Evaluative questions*, which help clients distinguish behaviors that have led to preferred goals from those that have not
- ➤ *Coping questions,* which help clients focus on past behaviors that have been successful in dealing with problems
- ➤ *Exception-seeking questions,* which help clients examine when they haven't had the problem in their lives to explore how they previously lived a problem-free life
- ➤ *Solution-focused questions,* which are future-oriented and offer clients the opportunity to develop new, positive ways of reaching their preferred goals

Therapists support clients' solution focus in a number of ways, including *amplification,* which encourages clients to detail how they have used their strengths and resources so that they can increasingly employ these strategies as they work toward their preferred goals; *reframing,* which provides a different take on past behaviors in an effort to normalize and depathologize how clients view themselves (e.g., a client who sees himself or herself as a procrastinator, may be reframed as a person who reflects deeply before making decisions); and *complimenting,* in an effort to reinforce clients' efforts toward reaching their preferred goals.

Stage 5: Reaching Preferred Goals.   By the end of the first session, clients have shifted from focusing on problems to focusing on solutions. Between their first session and subsequent meetings, they work on implementing and reaching their preferred goals. Therapists help clients evaluate the effectiveness of their new solution focus by using *scaling*, which involves a rating scale to measure progress, and can tweak goals in future sessions, with the focus being on working quickly. Therapists reinforce clients by being good listeners, showing empathy, and by complimenting them on their efforts.

Stage 6: Ending Therapy.

> . . . [B]rief therapy means, among other things, "as few sessions as possible and not one more than necessary."
>
> (de Shazer, as cited in Hoyt, 1996, p. 61)

Because therapy is brief, as soon as the preferred goals are reached, therapy is finished. Follow-up can be conducted to ensure that clients are continuing their solution-focused orientation. As in stage 5, the chief techniques include listening and empathy, complimenting, and scaling.

SFBT is one of the newest and most popular forms of counseling and seems to fit in well with the fast-paced world and the demands by some insurance companies to help clients quickly. Its solution-focused, constructionist and postmodern bent is in stark contrast to many of the more traditional approaches examined in this chapter.

Extensions, Adaptations, and Spinoffs of the Major Theories

With hundreds of approaches to counseling and psychotherapy out there (Neukrug, 2015a), even if we spent the rest of our lives in therapy, we could only participate in a small number of them. But why do some theories become the standard bearers while others do not? A combination of factors is probably at play. First, the standard bearers usually have some history to them—they've been used and people believe that they are helpful. Second, these approaches usually have some research, if not significant clinical experience, to back them up. Third, the theorists who created these theories have generally written a great deal, thus publicizing their theories. Fourth, many of the theorists were entrepreneurs, in the sense that they wrote, developed institutes, initiated journals, and were out on the road giving workshops about their theories. Finally, the public seems to have a thirst for certain theories at specific times in history. For some theories, it's just the right time.

In this section of the chapter, we will look at a number of extensions, adaptations, and spinoffs of the theories already discussed. Some of these theories have had staying power and appear to have much to offer. Others are very new and riding a wave of popularity, and still others are just interesting and are the newest "breakthrough" theories. The following offers only a sample of these approaches. As you read through them, you may find that you are drawn to one or more. If so, read about it, study it, and maybe embrace that theory as one of your main approaches to counseling and therapy. However, try to stay open to many approaches, as you may find other ways of working with clients helpful in your therapeutic journey.

Let's take a look at Erik Erikson's psychosocial theory, object–relations theory, relational and subjectivity therapy, dialectical behavior therapy, acceptance and commitment therapy, constructivist therapy, eye movement desensitization therapy, motivational interviewing, gender-aware therapy, positive psychology and wellness therapy, and complementary, alternative, and integrative approaches (see Neukrug, 2011, for a broader description of these theories).

Erikson's Psychosocial Theory

Erik Erikson (1902–1994) suggested that individuals pass through *eight stages of psychosocial development* and that social forces play a bigger role in development than Freud or earlier psychoanalysts had suggested. He believed that the influence of instincts and the unconscious were not as great as many had suggested and that as individuals pass through the stages, they face a task that could be seen as representing opposing forces (e.g., trust versus mistrust; autonomy versus shame and doubt). He also believed that the development of a healthy ego is contingent on the individual's ability to master the stages and is highlighted by a particular *virtue* or *strength* that is associated with successful passage through each stage. For more on this theory, see Chapter 9.

Object–Relations Theory

The purpose of *object–relations therapy* is to resolve early traumatic experiences so the individual can build a new self-structure. In contrast to the instincts of sex and aggression driving behavior, object–relations theory stresses the importance of relationships in motivating people. Object–relation theorists talk about *good-enough mothering* and providing positive holding environments for children in the development of the self through a series of stages that tend to move from *symbiosis* to *separation of self*. These theorists also suggest that the *splitting* of others (e.g., into a good and bad "other") plays an important role in the development of the self and needs to be overcome for the successful development of the ego. In object–relations therapy, clients are reparented by taking in new *objects* (e.g., the therapist), which then serve as a new blueprint for the self. Some of the better-known object–relations theorists include Melanie Klein, Margaret Mahler, and Harry Stack Sullivan.

Relational and Subjectivity Therapy

One of the more recent additions to the psychodynamic approach, *relational and subjectivity therapy* speaks to the importance of an ongoing dialogue between the client and the therapist. These therapists suggest that we have internalized images of significant, early relationships (e.g., parents), and those images affect how individuals relate. However, they also argue that personality and the patterns of understanding and relating do not develop in isolation from others, but rather within the mutually influencing subjectivities of people in relationships. They highlight the *myth of the independent mind*, suggesting that it is through interactions that the "self" is formed. Those who practice this perspective develop a deep, intimate, self-disclosing relationship with their clients and give attention to transference and to carefully timed self-disclosures of the therapist's countertransference as well. Mutual sharing can then be understood in terms of past patterns in relationships and how it affects current relationships. Some of the more well known theorists include Robert Stolorow and Daniel Stern.

Dialectical Behavior Therapy

Developed by Marsha Linehan, dialectical behavior therapy (DBT) was designed to treat borderline personality disorders, but is now used for other disorders. Based on a *biosocial theory of personality development*, DBT assumes that some people are born with heightened emotional sensitivity. These individuals not only are in particular need of acceptance but also need to be encouraged to change. DBT therapists are accepting by demonstrating empathy, genuineness, caring, warmth, and understanding, and by teaching *mindfulness*. They show commitment and realness to clients by being willing to do some self-disclosure and by being open to such things as receiving telephone contacts between sessions. Such therapist behaviors discourage self-destructive patterns and encourage new, healthier behaviors.

Acceptance and Commitment Therapy

Acceptance and commitment therapy (ACT) is based on *relational frame theory*, which explains behaviors and cognitions as a complex web of relational associations. Developed by Steven Hayes and others in the late 1980s, ACT uses a mixture of cognitive techniques, behavioral techniques, and Eastern philosophy and applies it in novel ways. The goal of ACT is to help create a rich and meaningful life while accepting the pain that inevitably goes with it, and this is achieved by applying six core principles of psychological flexibility: *defusion, acceptance, contact with the present moment, self as context, values*, and *committed action*. ACT can be viewed through three stages: *accepting thoughts and feelings, choosing direction*, and *taking action*.

Constructivist Therapy

Developed by Michael Mahoney, *constructivist therapy* suggests that people are continually creating and recreating their understanding of reality. Constructive therapists believe that deep underlying schemata are more difficult to change than surface structures. They suggest that there is a complex and inseparable interaction between one's thoughts, feelings, and actions; we do not simply have thoughts and interpretations of the world; we are our thoughts and interpretations. Such thoughts and interpretations are constantly undergoing reconstruction as we interact with others. Using a *dialectical process* to examine the client's meaning-making system, the goal of therapy is to assist the client in understanding how he or she makes sense out of the world and to help the client create new constructions that may work better for him or her.

Eye Movement Desensitization and Reprocessing

Developed by Francine Shapiro in the late 1980s, eye movement desensitization and reprocessing (EMDR) has clients focus on *rapid eye movements*, or some other *rhythmic stimulation* (e.g., tapping), while imagining a traumatic or troubling event. In addition, new, positive core beliefs are substituted for older, negative ones, and new behaviors are encouraged. EMDR suggests that past traumas become embedded in our psyche; core beliefs maintain negative experiences; new cognitions and behaviors can help a person adopt new ways of being in the world; and there are neural pathways that store traumatic memories that can become *depotentiated* or blocked during treatment. Using these core ideas, EMDR treatment involves eight phases that sometimes can be completed within a few sessions.

Motivational Interviewing

Originally used with substance abuse, gambling, anxiety disorders, eating disorders, chronic disease management, and health-related disorders, in recent years motivational interviewing has been applied to a vast array of client issues. Motivational interviewing assumes that motivation is a key to change, is multidimensional, is dynamic and fluctuating, is influenced by social interactions, can be modified, and is influenced by the clinician's style. The main task of clinicians is to be *collaborative, evocative,* and *honoring of their clients.* At the same time, clinicians try to elicit and enhance motivation by adhering to four basic principles (Miller & Rollnick, 2013): (1) *expressing empathy* in an effort to build a relationship and hear the client; (2) *developing discrepancies,* to help clients hear how their behaviors and values may not always be in sync (a gambling-addicted father who values saving money for his child to go to college); (3) *rolling with resistance,* in an effort to understand the importance of the client's resistance and what purpose it serves (the gambler gets a "rush" because he or she has no meaning in life); and (4) *supporting self-efficacy,* or believing and supporting that the client has the necessary skills to make changes and is the final decider in the change process.

Gender-Aware Therapy

Encompassing feminist therapy and counseling men, gender-aware therapy includes the following common elements: gender is central to counseling, problems are viewed within a societal context, counselors actively address gender injustices, collaborative and equal relationships are developed, and clients choose their gender roles regardless of their political correctness. Feminist therapy has its origins in the feminist movement and recognizes the impact of gender, the oppression of women, and the influence of politics. The goal of feminist therapy is empowerment of female clients through the use of a wellness model. To help understand how to work with women, the *American Psychological Association's Guidelines for Psychological Practice with Girls and Women* (APA, 2007) are often used. Men too have unique issues that impinge on them and affect their way of viewing the world. When working with men, it is important to accept the feelings men tend to be comfortable with (e.g., anger, competitiveness) and not to push men too quickly to focus on what have been called "traditionally female feelings." In addition, counselors need to know common issues related to the male experience and should have empathy for the male perspective. (See Chapter 15 for a more in-depth look at gender-aware therapy.)

Positive Psychology and Well-Being Therapy

A relatively recent addition to the field of therapies, officially launched in 1998 by Martin Seligman, then-president of the APA, positive psychology can be traced to the humanistic therapies. However, in contrast to humanistic therapies' tendency to believe in an inherent good self, positive psychology suggests that humans are capable of good and bad but helps clients focus on the positive aspects of self. This optimistic, wellness-oriented approach suggests that individuals can learn how to increase their positive cognitions and emotions and change their behaviors to match this new positive focus. Such a focus, they suggest, can result in longer life, increased creativity, increased sense of engagement and meaningfulness, resilience to diversity, and a decrease in health problems (Rankin, 2013; Seligman, Ernst, Gilham, Reivich, & Linkins, 2009).

One positive psychology therapeutic model recently developed by Giovanni Fava (2012), *well-being therapy*, suggests that clients be viewed through three phases along *Ryff's six dimensions of well-being*: *autonomy, personal growth, environmental mastery, purpose in life, positive relations*, and *self-acceptance*. This approach attempts to replace negative thoughts and behaviors with positive ones by identifying the problematic areas of the six dimensions and then helping the client develop positive aspects in his or her life in those areas.

Complementary, Alternative, and Integrative Approaches

Although recently gaining in popularity, the many different types of complementary, alternative, and integrative approaches are based on some of the oldest forms of healing (U.S. Department of Health and Human Services, 2014a). *Complementary medicine or therapy* includes using unconventional practices in conjunction with conventional methods to treat biological and mental health problems. *Alternative therapy* is when alternative approaches are used instead of conventional methods. An *integrative approach* suggests that conventional practice may integrate complementary or alternative approaches within its practice, such as when a person is receiving mainstream cancer treatment is also given acupuncture and medical marijuana to treat side effects. The overall emphasis of these approaches is to focus on a client's overall wellness, such as what Myers and Sweeney (2004, 2005) describe as one's *creative self, coping self, social self, essential self,* and *physical self* (see Chapter 1).

Integrative Counseling and Psychotherapy (Eclecticism)

The idea that a helper might be able to combine varying theoretical approaches into his or her own way of working with clients is not new (Marquis, 2015). In fact, today, about one-fourth of mental health professionals identify themselves as using a purely *integrative approach* (Norcross, Bike, & Evans, 2009). In many ways, as most of us mature as professionals, we take on a more integrative approach as our adherence to one theoretical orientation becomes less rigid and we incorporate other ideas into our way of doing counseling and psychotherapy.

Formerly called *eclecticism*, an integrative approach is when the helper develops a core theory by integrating elements from different theories into his or her approach. Unfortunately, some counselors who think they are using an integrative approach are actually practicing a mishmash of techniques that have little or no underlying theoretical basis. This type of a theoretical eclecticism is counterintuitive and is considered by many to be "shooting-from-the-hip" therapy. Integration of this kind is not based on systematic research and is detrimental to the goals of our profession and, more important, to the successful treatment of clients. Effective helpers, on the other hand, know that an integrative approach involves a deliberate effort to integrate techniques into the helper's repertoire. Although different models attempt to explain this process (Corey, 2015; Marquis, 2015), most of them address some common elements that lead me to view an integrative approach as a developmental process that moves from *chaos*, to *coalescence*, to *multiplicity*, and ends with a *commitment to a metatheory*.

Stage 1: Chaos. This initial stage of developing an eclectic approach is based on a limited knowledge of theory and involves moment-to-moment subjective judgments of the helper. Often practiced while students are still in training programs, this approach is the helper's first attempt to pull together different theoretical orientations, and if used with clients, is likely to be of limited help.

Stage 2: Coalescence. As theory is learned, most helpers begin to drift toward adherence to one approach. Although they ascribe mostly to one theory, they are beginning to use some techniques from other approaches when they believe that it would be helpful to clients.

Stage 3: Multiplicity. During this stage, helpers have thoroughly learned one theory and are beginning to gain a solid knowledge of one or more other theories. They are also now beginning to realize that any of the theories may be equally effective for many clients. This knowledge presents a dilemma for the counselor: "What theoretical perspective should I adhere to, and how might I combine, or use at different times, two or more theoretical perspectives so that I could offer the most effective treatment?" Ultimately, this helper is able to feel facile with different approaches and is sometimes willing to integrate other approaches into his or her main approach.

Stage 4: Metatheory. At this point, the helper has become a master therapist and has settled into a theoretical orientation based on his or her work with clients and the gathering of knowledge about theories over the years. This master therapist has a metatheory that drives what he or she does. This metatheory is a thought-through approach that defines the theoretical nature of the therapist's work (e.g., psychodynamic, humanistic, cognitive–behavioral, postmodern, systems, etc.), and usually incorporates a number of different elements from many theories into the helper's way of doing counseling and therapy. However, the elements chosen from other approaches have a "flavor" that reflects the helper's unique style. For instance, the "humanist" will use behavioral techniques, but from the framework of the humanistic perspective.

The ability to assimilate techniques from varying theoretical perspectives takes knowledge, time, and finesse. If you are just beginning your journey as a counselor, you should expect eventually to pass through these four stages as you begin to sort through the various theoretical approaches and develop your own unique style of counseling.

Multicultural/Social Justice Focus: Bias in Counseling Approaches

Almost every predominant theory of counseling and psychotherapy has been developed by White men. Now, not every White male is prejudiced, but they do tend to carry with them values based on their heritage. And since their heritages are, for the most part, from a Western European framework, it is not surprising that many of the approaches stress Western values. Some of the values that are embraced by many of these approaches include the following (Neukrug, 2011; Sue & Sue, 2013):

1. The importance of individualism and being able to work things out on one's own.
2. It is healthier to express feelings than not express them.

3. One must search within "self" to discover the truth of one's existence.
4. If one works hard enough, he or she will meet with success when working on problems.
5. Mind–body dualism, or the sense that there is a separation of our thinking selves and our physical selves.
6. Truth can be found, or uncovered, through scientific inquiry.
7. Facts can be found, values are opinions.
8. External factors are of little impact on internal psychological states.

For some clients, the above values work. These clients want to search within their selves, get in touch with their feelings, uncover the "truth," and work hard, on their own, to feel better. Other clients do not hold these values and may be labeled by some therapists as resistant, defensive, or lacking in insight. These are the clients who view expression of feelings as a weakness. They are the clients who defer to family or community for answers to life's questions. These are the clients who find it strange to think of the mind and body as separate. These are the clients who feel comfortable in the mystical, nonscientific world, believing that answers don't always come from empirical evidence. These are the clients who believe that fate is in God's hands, and these are the clients who believe that prejudice and racism are the reasons for their hardships. Who are these clients? Mostly, they are minority clients, the immigrant, and the American with roots outside the dominant culture, for they have not historically experienced life in the United States in the same way as those in the dominant culture, they might not share the same values as the majority culture, and they have not, for the most part, had the same privileges as most White Americans.

So, imagine a world where symbols often reflect male phalluses, and if you don't see them, you're hiding from your feelings of inadequacy (e.g., psychoanalysis). Or, imagine a world where you're told that your defensiveness is your conscious and unconscious minds struggling with one another (psychodynamic theories). Imagine a world where you were marginalized for not crying after the death of a loved one (Gestalt therapy and some other humanistic approaches), or a world where you were made to feel as if you were acting irrationally because you spoke out loud to God to find the answers to your life's questions (REBT). Imagine a world where you were told that you alone control your own fate (existential therapy), or a world where you were given the message that every negative feeling you have, you *chose* to have, and that only you can choose to act and feel differently (reality therapy). And imagine a world where you were told that you're thinking irrationally or distorting reality and you can adopt a more rational or sane way of living (REBT and cognitive therapy). Well, many clients have been subtly (and sometimes not so subtly) given these messages. If you're a client from a nondominant group, you're more likely to feel at odds with many of the above assumptions. This means you are more likely to be labeled as defensive, be misdiagnosed, drop out of therapy, and find counseling less helpful than clients from the dominant culture. These are the clients that don't follow the Western values that many hold as "truth."

Finally, in recent years, just about every approach to counseling and psychotherapy has acknowledged that it is somewhat cross-culturally biased due to the fact that it is based on Western values. And many, if not most, of these approaches have tried to address some of these biases. Let's at least give these professionals credit for trying to respond to the bias that is inherent in many of their practices.

Ethical, Professional, and Legal Issues

Theory and the ACA Code

As noted in previous chapters, the ACA (2014a) ethical code highlights a large number of issues critical to the counseling relationship, and you are encouraged to review the code which can be found in its entirety in the Appendix. More specifically related to the knowing and practice of theory, a few items in the code stand out. For instance, the code suggests that counselors should practice only in an area for which they have been trained. Also, the code highlights the importance of using theory that is based on sound scientific evidence. The code also suggests that ongoing continuing education be obtained if counselors are to practice new techniques. In addition, the code highlights the importance of obtaining supervision so that counselors can practice their theory at optimal levels. Finally, the code notes that knowledge of multicultural/diversity issues is critical if counselors are to be effective when they practice their theories.

Working Effectively with All Clients

What happens when counselors don't practice at optimal levels? In these cases, the door is opened for poor client outcomes and for being sued for malpractice. Over the years, some critical cases have highlighted the importance of being well trained, knowing when to take action, and knowing when one should refer and when one should not.

The Tarasoff Case and Foreseeable Harm

In a well-known legal case concerning client confidentiality, a man named Prosenjit Poddar, who was being seen at the counseling center at the University of California at Berkeley, told his psychologist that as a result of his girlfriend's recent threats to break up with him and date other men, he intended to kill her. As a result, his psychologist informed his supervisor and the campus police of his client's threat, at which point the campus police detained Poddar. The supervisor reprimanded the psychologist for breaking confidentiality; and, finding no reason to detain Poddar further, the campus police released him. Two months later, he did kill his girlfriend, Tatiana Tarasoff. Tarasoff's parents sued the university, the therapist, the supervisor, and the police, and won their suit against all but the police. The decision, which was seen as a model for "duty to warn" (now called "foreseeable harm") was interpreted by courts nationally to mean that a therapist must make all efforts to prevent danger to another or to self.

Julea Ward v. Board of Regents of Eastern Michigan University (EMU)

Julea Ward, a graduate student in counseling at EMU, discovered that she would be counseling a client who had been in a same-sex relationship (Rudow, 2013). Believing that she could not counsel him due to her religious beliefs, she asked her supervisor to refer him to another counselor. At that point, the supervisor scheduled an informal review of Ward, and the faculty informed her that she would have to set aside her religious beliefs, as the 2005 ACA ethics codes stated that "counselors do not condone or engage in discrimination based on age, culture, disability, ethnicity, race, religion/spirituality, gender, gender identity, sexual orientation, marital status/partnership, language preference, socioeconomic status or any basis proscribed by law" (ACA, 2005, Section C.5). She was asked to complete a remediation program or have a formal hearing with the faculty. She requested a formal hearing, which eventually led to her dismissal from the program. Ward sued EMU, and after years of litigation, the courts upheld the school's decision and the ACA code. Although the case was appealed and eventually was settled out of court, it marked an important challenge to the ACA code and impacted ACA's 2014a code. ACA's current code now stipulates that "[c]ounselors refrain from referring prospective and current clients based solely on the counselor's personally held values, attitudes, beliefs, and behaviors" (ACA, 2014b, section A.11.b). Although the case was appealed and eventually was settled out of court, it marked an important challenge to the ACA code and impacted ACA's 2014a code.

Sexual Orientation Change Efforts (Conversion and Reparative Therapy)

In recent years, there have been important guidelines developed by our professional associations regarding the practice of sexual orientation change efforts, referred to in the past as *conversion therapy* or *reparative therapy* (Goodrich, 2015). As there has been evidence that referring a client to change his or her sexual orientation is rarely if ever successful and can often be harmful, the ACA and other professional associations have made strong statements that counselors should not refer clients to such therapies unless the client insists that he or she wants such a practice. However, even in these cases, the ACA suggests that clients who seek to change their sexual orientation should be clearly told of the lack of scientific evidence of such counseling practice, the potential harm it can do, and questions to ask any practitioner who might be practicing this approach. Also, counselors who practice such treatments are ethically bound to inform clients of the lack of scientific evidence, the purpose of practicing the approach, the potential harm it can cause, and offer referrals to gay-, lesbian-, and bisexual-affirming counselors (Whitman, Glosoff, Kocet, & Tarvydas, 2013).

The Counselor in Process: Embracing a Theory but Open to Change

For a few years after obtaining my master's degree, I remember dogmatically adhering to an existential–humanistic approach in my counseling style. I staunchly argued against a psychodynamic approach, even though I had minimal knowledge about this orientation. Although I was barely aware of it at that time, the views I had were at least partly based on some of my own unfinished issues.

As I have grown older, I have acquired a deep appreciation for all counseling approaches. I believe each of them offers something. No doubt, as you have read through the various theories, you have identified more with some than others. Probably this is due to some personal style and perhaps some unfinished business of your own. Although I encourage you to practice and learn more about the theory or theories with which you feel an affinity, I also strongly suggest that you not stubbornly adhere to only one approach;

I hope that you will gain some knowledge from all theories. As your professional life as a counselor proceeds, and as you read new research about differing theories, I hope that you will remain open to changing your theoretical views and adapting your theory accordingly (see Spruill & Benshoff, 2000). Those who are closed to this ongoing process are stuck in one view of the helping relationship, and this rigidity is likely to hinder client growth, as well as one's own growth as a counselor.

Perhaps we can learn something from Hoyt (1994), who suggests that counselors, like clients undergoing solution-focused therapy, might want to answer the following "miracle" question:

> *Suppose tonight, while you're sleeping, a miracle occurs . . . and when you awaken you find you are helping clients in a more positive and effective way than before! How will you notice your practice has changed? What new skills will you be using? (p. 8)*

Summary

This chapter focused on a number of major theories of counseling and psychotherapy. It began by explaining the concept of paradigm shifts, and then it reviewed how familiarity with past knowledge is crucial for an understanding of current knowledge. Relating this concept to counseling theories, we explained that such theories are our best current conception of what is effective in the counseling and psychotherapy process. We noted that by their very nature, theories are heuristic, or researchable and testable, and can be modified over time, and also discussed the intimate relationship between one's view of human nature and the theory to which it adheres. We encouraged you to examine your view of human nature.

As the chapter continued, it offered a quick overview of twelve theories that encompassed four conceptual orientations. In the psychodynamic arena, we examined psychoanalysis, analytical therapy, and individual therapy. From the existential–humanistic perspective, we explored existential therapy, Gestalt therapy, and person-centered counseling. With the cognitive–behavioral focus, we reviewed behavior therapy, rational emotive behavior therapy (REBT), cognitive therapy, and reality therapy, and the postmodern perspective highlighted narrative therapy and solution-focused brief therapy. Next, the chapter offered a very brief look at a number of extensions, adaptations, and spinoffs of these approaches, including Erikson's psychosocial theory, object–relations theory, relational and subjectivity therapy, dialectical behavior therapy, acceptance and commitment therapy, constructivist therapy, eye movement desensitization and reprocessing (EMDR), motivational interviewing, gender-aware therapy, positive psychology and wellness therapy, and complementary, alternative, and integrative approaches.

The chapter next explored a recent trend in counseling and psychotherapy: the adaptation by many counselors of an integrative approach to therapy (eclecticism). We noted that an integrative approach tends to progress in complexity from chaos to coalescence to multiplicity and metatheory as counselors learn more about different theories and become more willing to integrate other ideas into their existing ways of practicing counseling.

This chapter examined how most of the counseling theories used today were developed from a European perspective that stresses a number of Western values such as individualism; expression of feeling; searching for "self" within; hard work will meet with success; mind–body dualism; truth through scientific inquiry; facts are findable whereas values are opinions; and the notion that external factors have little impact on internal psychological states. We pointed out that the counseling theories examined in this chapter were developed largely by White men from Western heritages and suggested that counselors may need to be particularly vigilant in ensuring that they can adapt their approaches to nondominant clients. In addition, we noted that many of the approaches have tried to make some adaptations as a result of these value differences.

The chapter neared its conclusion by reviewing a number of ethical, professional, and legal issues related to counseling theory and the counseling relationship. Relative to the ACA ethics code and theory, we noted that counselors should practice only in an area for which they have been trained, the importance of using theory based on scientific evidence, that continuing education is critical for optimal client outcomes, the importance of supervision and of having knowledge of multicultural/diversity issues. To work effectively with all clients, we highlighted a few cases and situations. For instance, we discussed the Tarasoff case relative to foreseeable harm and knowing when one must break confidentiality. The chapter also discussed the importance of counselors being able to work with all different kinds of clients, as highlighted by the outcome of the *Julea Ward v. Board of Regents of Eastern Michigan University* case, where a counselor was not willing to work with a gay client. Ultimately, she was dismissed from her program, and the courts upheld her dismissal. Finally, we noted that relative to sexual orientation change efforts (conversion and reparative therapy), counselors should not refer clients for such practices unless the client insists, and that they should tell clients that evidence suggests that referring a client to change his or her sexual orientation is rarely if ever successful and can even be harmful. A counselor who practices such an approach is ethically bound to inform his or her clients of the lack of scientific evidence to support its practice, the purpose the counselor has for practicing the approach, its potential for harm, and to have at hand referrals to gay-, lesbian-, and bisexual-affirming counselors for clients. Finally, the chapter discussed the importance of being open to different theoretical approaches throughout one's career.

Further Practice

Visit CengageBrain.com to respond to additional material that highlight the salient aspects of the chapter content. There, you can find ethical, professional, and legal vignettes, a number of experiential exercises, and study tools including a glossary, flashcards, and sample test items. Hopefully, these will enhance your learning and be fun and interesting.

Counseling Skills

The first time I counseled was at a drug crisis clinic in college. I had little training, but somehow I instinctively knew that it was probably best to listen and have a caring attitude. I had never had a course in counseling theories or counseling methods, and I knew little about the "correct" way to respond to a drop-in at the center. Looking back, I hope that I did more good than harm as I tried to help students who had overdosed or were on a "bad trip."

In graduate school, I learned the way to counsel. I became an ardent existential–humanist and believed that it was best to help people express their feelings. After obtaining a job at a crisis center, I began to practice my skills on my unsuspecting clients. Although my counseling approach had become somewhat focused, my old untrained self, which sometimes would get very advice oriented, periodically raised its ugly head.

Over the years, I have had numerous jobs, obtained my doctorate, attended continuing education workshops, and read the professional journals. Experience, education, and reading have all helped me fine-tune my skills. Although there are some whom I believe to be natural counselors, I have come to suspect that most of us are not born with an ability to counsel—we all must learn how to apply counseling skills. In fact, even those with natural ability need training to become masters at what they do. Much like riding a bicycle or learning how to use a skateboard for the first time, learning counseling skills at first feels awkward. However, you will find that the more you practice, the more natural and at ease you will feel. In my own life, I now approach the learning and refinement of my skills as a never-ending process.

To help you move from being a natural but untrained helper to becoming a professional counselor, this chapter will examine the importance of the counseling environment and some of the techniques that have been shown to be effective in working with clients. We will also explore one model of client case conceptualization, which is a method of organizing one's thinking around working on client problems. In addition, we will identify six stages of counseling and review how the case conceptualization process can be understood related to these stages. The chapter will also present important issues related to record keeping and the writing of case notes.

The Counseling Environment

. . . alliance formation, as understood by clients, actually begins before the counselor fully engages the client, as clients may develop predispositions or impressions on the basis of the counselor's attire, the counselor's nonverbal gestures, the counselor's greeting the office environment, and the reception staff . . .

(Bedi, 2006, p. 33)

A client who walks into a counselor's office immediately encounters the world of the counselor, as reflected in his or her work environment. Soon, this client will be asked to look at his or her inner world. Although we have no control over the defensiveness that the client brings to the session, through a careful assessment of the *counseling environment*, we can reduce or eliminate any external irritation that could potentially increase defensiveness. Thus, that first experience of the counselor's environment is crucial to building an effective counseling relationship.

What creates the counseling environment? Three components are particularly important: the office itself, the use of nonverbal behaviors, and how the counselor presents himself or herself to the client. Let's look at how each of these factors plays an important role in the success or failure of the counseling relationship.

The Office

Whether in an agency, business, or school setting, the practice of counseling requires that one has a place to go to establish a relationship. Almost always, this will be one's office. The counseling relationship requires the quiet, comfort, safety, and confidentiality that the *office* provides. Although counselors sometimes have to build the helping relationship outside the office (e.g., school counselors; counselors who work with clients who are uncomfortable in a traditional office), an office can be key to deepening the relationship. This is partly because a successful counseling relationship requires the quiet, comfort, safety, and confidentiality that the office provides.

The arrangement of one's office can be crucial to eliciting positive attitudes from people and to building the therapeutic alliance (Bedi, 2006; Nassar & Devlin 2011). How should the office be designed? There is little question that it should be soundproofed, have soft lighting, be relatively uncluttered, have client records stored appropriately, be free from distractions such as the phone ringing or people knocking on the door, and have comfortable seating. As we create our offices, each of us will try to find a balance between having it reflect our taste and making sure that it is appealing to the vast majority of our clients (see Box 5.1).

No matter how you arrange your office, it is difficult, or even impossible, to not offend somebody. Thus, it is probably best if one tries to arrange one's office in a manner that is likely to offend the fewest people. Of course, it may be that you will want to attract a certain clientele who would feel comfortable with a particular ambiance. For instance, a Christian counselor might include articles of a religious nature in his or her office, while a person dealing with mostly gay, lesbian, and bisexual issues might include related literature in his or her office.

BOX 5.1
What Should Your Office Look Like?

Review the items below and reflect on whether you think any of them would be offensive to you if you walked into a counseling office. Then think about the most liberal and the most conservative person you know and imagine how he or she might feel about each of the following:

➤ Feminist literature
➤ A bear rug
➤ Gay literature

➤ A cluttered desk
➤ Information on abortion
➤ A leather chair
➤ Fundamentalist religious literature
➤ A compulsively clean desk
➤ An AIDS pin
➤ A desk between you and your client
➤ Information on female and male sexuality
➤ A brochure supporting a politician

How one dresses and the language one uses with clients are two additional components of the office environment. Should you wear jeans at work? What about an expensive suit? Are your clothes revealing? What does your jewelry or hairstyle say about you? Do you call your client by his or her first name? Should you change the way you talk for the client, such as using less complex language for a client who is less educated? Ultimately, each counselor must determine the importance of these factors and how he or she will be addressed.

Nonverbal Behavior

> *If you do **not** pay attention to the nonverbal behavior there is a great chance that you are missing much of what is actually being communicated by the other person. Thus, while active listening is always good, active observation is also necessary.*

> (Matsumoto, Frank, & Hwang, 2013, p. 12)

The importance of our nonverbal interactions with clients is vastly underrated. In fact, *nonverbal behavior* is involved in an ongoing, elaborate interaction with verbal behavior that leads people to send and interpret complex messages (Knapp & Hall, 2010). With conservative estimates indicating that more than twice the amount of communication is nonverbal rather than verbal (Guerrero & Floyd, 2006), the implications for counselors are great, as they must be able to accurately read messages from clients and be clear about the messages they are sending.

A number of nonverbal behaviors can affect our relationship with our clients. For instance, *posture*, *eye contact*, or *tone of voice* that communicates "Don't open up to me" will obviously affect clients differently from the counselor who is nonverbally communicating "I'm open to hearing what you have to say."

Personal space is an additional nonverbal factor that affects the counseling relationship (Guerrero & Floyd, 2006; Zur, 2007). Mediated at least somewhat by culture, age, and gender, individuals vary greatly in their degree of comfort with personal space. Therefore, the counselor must allow enough personal space so that the client feels comfortable, yet not so much that the client feels distant from the counselor. When necessary, the counselor should take the lead in respecting the client's need for personal space.

Touch is a final aspect of nonverbal behavior important to the counseling relationship (Calmes, Piazza, & Laux, 2013). Touching at important moments is quite natural. For instance, when someone is expressing deep pain, it is not unusual for us to hold a hand or embrace a person while he or she sobs. Or when a person is coming to or leaving a session, one might find it natural to place a hand on a shoulder or give a hug. However, in today's litigious society, touch has become a particularly delicate subject, and it is important for each of us to be sensitive to our clients' boundaries, our own boundaries, and limits as suggested by our professional ethics.

Some have become so touchy over this issue that a therapist in Massachusetts, branded "the hugging therapist," was fired from his job at a mental health agency because he hugged his clients too much. Brammer and MacDonald (2003) suggest that whether one has physical contact with a client should be based on (1) the helper's assessment of the needs of the helpee, (2) the helper's awareness of his or her own needs, (3) what is most likely to be helpful within the counseling relationship, and (4) risks that may be involved as a function of agency policy, customs, personal ethics, and the law.

Traditionally, counselors have been taught to lean forward, make good eye contact, speak in a voice that meets the client's affect, and rarely touch the client. However, even though many nonverbal behaviors appear to be universal, culture can mediate the expression of nonverbal behaviors (Bonitz, 2008; Matsumoto, 2006; Matsumoto et al., 2013; Stenzel & Rupert, 2004). Therefore, it is now suggested that counselors be acutely sensitive to client responses to nonverbal behaviors. Counselors must understand that some clients will expect to be looked at, while others will be offended by eye contact; that some clients will expect you to lean forward, while others will experience this as an intrusion; and that some clients will expect you to touch them, while others will see this as offensive. With respect to nonverbal behavior, effective counselors keep in mind what works for the many while remaining sensitive to what works for the few.

Counselor Qualities to Embrace and to Avoid

How we bring ourselves into the counseling relationship can have a positive or negative effect on the outcome of counseling, and the qualities highlighted in Chapter 1 are crucial to the establishment of an effective counseling relationship. As a quick reminder, they include the six factors related to building an effective working alliance (empathy, acceptance, genuineness, embracing a wellness perspective, cultural competence, and the "it" factor) and the three factors related to effectively delivering your theoretical approach (ability with and belief in your theory, competence, and cognitive complexity). The counselor who continually makes empathic failures is not hearing the client. The counselor who seems false, judgmental, and closed-minded will create an atmosphere of defensiveness during the session. The counselor who struggles with his or her own issues will attend poorly to the client, and the counselor who cannot understand cultural differences will have difficulty relating to his or her client. The counselor who is not cognitively complex will view the client's situation in a limited way, and the counselor who lacks knowledge of and commitment to a theory will proceed awkwardly with his or her clients.

Not only must the counselor be able to demonstrate the personal characteristics that will nurture a healthy counseling relationship, but he or she also must avoid attitudes and behaviors that will foster a destructive relationship. The many common attitudes that would be detrimental to a counseling relationship (and need little explanation as to why) include being critical, disapproving, disbelieving, scolding, threatening, discounting, ridiculing, punishing, and rejecting of one's client (Wubbolding, 2011). Clearly, these attitudes and behaviors, as well as others of a similar nature, are to be avoided. Let's now look at some of the specific skills that will foster a productive counseling relationship.

Counseling Skills

Ask a room filled with counselors to agree on the time of day, and you're most likely to have a room filled with counselors arguing that the time of day would depend on one's time zone and discussing the subjective nature of time. In the same way, arriving at any consensus regarding the most important skills to use within the counseling relationship would be difficult, to say the least. However, I have attempted to categorize skills into four broad categories with which many counselors might agree: foundational skills, commonly used skills, commonly used advanced skills, and advanced and specialized skills. Certainly, regardless of what skills are used, the misuse or abuse of counseling skills can quickly have a deleterious effect on the outcome of counseling.

Foundational Skills

Regardless of the theoretical orientation to which you adhere, some skills are essential to establishing the relationship, building rapport and trust, setting a tone with the client, and beginning the client's process of self-examination. Although these skills remain important throughout the counseling relationship, they are generally most crucial as counseling begins and should be continually revisited, especially when an impasse is reached. They include the ability to listen, show empathy, and use silence effectively.

Listening Skills

> . . . *First there is the hearing with the ear, which we all know; and the hearing with the non-ear, which is a state like that of a tranquil pond, a lake that is completely quiet and when you drop a stone into it, it makes little waves that disappear. I think that [insight] is the hearing with the non-ear, a state where there is absolute quietness of the mind; and when the question is put into the mind, the response is the wave, the little wave.*
>
> (Krishnamurti, cited in Jayakar, 1986/2003, p. 328)

We have all been in the situation when someone close to us has said, "You're not listening to me" or "You're not hearing me," and we have also probably been in the situation when we have accused others of the same. Although we all have a general sense of what *listening* is, this skill is particularly difficult to implement, as Americans are rarely

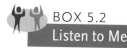

BOX 5.2
Listen to Me

When I ask you to listen to me and you start giving me advice, you have not done what I asked.

When I ask you to listen to me and you begin to tell me why I shouldn't feel that way, you are trampling on my feelings.

When I ask you to listen to me and you feel you have to do something to solve my problem, you have failed me, strange as that may seem.

Listen: All that I ask is that you listen, not talk or do—just hear me.

When you do something for me that I can and need to do for myself, you contribute to my fear and inadequacy.

But when you accept as a simple fact that I do feel what I feel, no matter how irrational, then I can quit trying to convince you and get about this business of understanding what's behind these feelings.

So, please listen and just hear me.

---

taught how to hear another person. In fact, ask an untrained adult to listen to another, and usually he or she ends up interrupting and giving advice. Listening helps to build trust, convinces the client you understand him or her, encourages the client to reflect on what he or she has just said, ensures that you are on track with your understanding of the client, and is an effective way of collecting information from a client without the potentially negative side effects of using questions (Neukrug & Schwitzer, 2006) (see Box 5.2). You can see why good listening is intimately related to positive client outcomes.

A good listener:

➤ talks minimally,
➤ concentrates on what is being said,
➤ does not interrupt,
➤ does not give advice,
➤ gives and does not expect to get,
➤ accurately hears the content of what the helpee is saying,
➤ accurately hears the feelings behind what the helpee is saying,
➤ is able to communicate to the helpee that he or she has been heard (through head nods, "uh-huhs," or reflecting back to the client what the helper heard),
➤ asks clarifying questions such as, "I didn't hear all of that. Can you explain that in another way so I'm sure I understand you?" and
➤ does not ask other kinds of questions.

Hindrances to Listening.   A number of factors can impede the counselor's ability to listen effectively. Some of these include (1) having preconceived notions about the client that interfere with the counselor's ability to hear the client, (2) anticipating what the client is about to say and not actually hearing the client, (3) thinking about what you are going to say and therefore blocking what the client is saying, (4) having personal issues that interfere with your ability to listen, (5) having a strong emotional reaction to your client's content and therefore not being able to hear the client accurately, and (6) being distracted by such things as noises, temperature of the office, or hunger pangs (Neukrug & Schwitzer, 2006).

Preparing to Listen. When you are ready to listen, the following practical suggestions should assist you in your ability to hear a client effectively (Egan, 2014; Ivey, Ivey, & Zalaquett, 2014):

1. Prior to meeting your client, calm yourself: meditate, pray, jog, or blow out air to calm your inner self.
2. Maintain appropriate eye contact with the client (being sensitive to cultural differences).
3. Have an open body posture that invites the client to talk (being sensitive to cultural differences).
4. Be sensitive to the personal space between you and the client.
5. Clear your mind of extraneous thoughts that are not relevant to hearing the client (e.g., personal issues or interpretations of client behavior).
6. Concentrate on the client and be prepared to focus on the meaning of and feelings behind what the client is discussing.
7. Do not talk except to gently encourage the client to talk.
8. Listen.

Whereas basic listening is a crucial skill for counselors, empathic understanding, the next essential skill, takes listening to new depths.

Empathy and Deep Understanding: A Special Kind of Listening

Highlighted as one of the nine personal qualities to embrace in Chapter 1, *empathy* is also one of most important counseling skills to develop. The importance of listening to a person from a deep inner perspective was extolled by many early Greek philosophers and has been recognized for centuries for its healing qualities (Gompertz, 1960). At the turn of the twentieth century, Theodor Lipps (1960/1903) coined the word *empathy* from the German word *Einfuhlung*, "to feel within," but probably the person who has had the greatest impact on our modern understanding and use of empathy is Carl Rogers.

> *The state of empathy, or being empathic, is to perceive the internal frame of reference of another with accuracy and with the emotional components and meanings which pertain thereto as if one were the person, but without ever losing the "as if" condition.*

> (Rogers, 1959, pp. 210–211)

The popularity of Rogers in the 1950s and 1960s naturally led to a number of operational definitions of empathy. For instance, Truax and Mitchell (1961) developed a nine-point rating scale to measure empathy, which was later revised by Carkhuff (1969) into a five-point scale. A scale to measure empathy had important implications. For the first time, researchers could measure the empathic ability of counselors and determine whether there was a relationship between good empathic responses and client outcomes in therapy. Indeed, numerous research studies indicated that good empathic ability was related to progress in therapy (Elliott, Bohart, Watson, & Greenberg, 2011; Wampold & Budge, 2012).

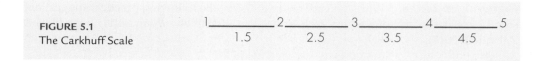

FIGURE 5.1
The Carkhuff Scale

The *Carkhuff scale* became a mainstay of counselor training during the 1970s and 1980s, and although it is no longer used as extensively, it set the stage for similar microcounseling skill training methods in counselor education (Santiago-Rivera, 2009). The scale ranged from a low of 1.0 to a high of 5.0 with 0.5 increments. Any responses below 3.0 were considered subtractive or nonempathic, while responses of 3.0 or higher were considered empathic, with responses over 3.0 considered additive responses (see Figure 5.1).

The original Carkhuff scale is reproduced in Table 5.1. Dramatically changing the manner in which empathic responding was taught, this scale allowed professors, students, and counselors to assess one another's ability at making an empathic response. As reflected in Table 5.1, a Level 1 or Level 2 response in some ways detracts from what the person is saying (e.g., giving advice, not accurately reflecting feeling, and not including content), with a Level 1 response being way off the mark and a Level 2 only slightly off. For instance, suppose that a client said, "I've had it with my dad; he never does anything with me. He's always working, drinking, or playing with my little sister." A Level 1 response might be, "Well, why don't you do something to change the situation, like tell him what an idiot he is?" (giving advice and being judgmental). A Level 2 response might be, "You seem to think your dad spends too much time with your sister" (does not reflect feeling and misses content). On the other hand, a Level 3 response, such as "Well, it sounds as though you're pretty upset at your dad for not spending time with you," accurately reflects the affect and meaning of the client.

TABLE 5.1   Carkhuff's Accurate Empathy Scale

Level 1	The verbal and behavioral expressions of the first person either do not attend to or detract significantly from the verbal and behavioral expressions of the second person(s), in that they communicate significantly less of the second person's feelings than the second person has communicated himself.
Level 2	While the first person responds to the expressed feelings of the second person(s), he does so in such a way that he subtracts noticeable affect from the communications of the second person.
Level 3	The expressions of the first person in response to the expressed feelings of the second person(s) are essentially interchangeable with those of the second person in that they express essentially the same affect and meaning.
Level 4	The responses of the first person add noticeably to the expressions of the second person(s) in such a way as to express feelings a level deeper than the second person was able to express himself.
Level 5	The first person's responses add significantly to the feeling and meaning of the expressions of the second person(s) in such a way as to (1) accurately express feelings below what the person himself was able to express or (2) in the event of ongoing, deep self-exploration on the second person's part, to be fully with him in his deepest moments.

SOURCE: Carkhuff, 1969, p. 121.

Level 4 and Level 5 responses reflect feelings and meaning beyond what the person is outwardly saying and add to the meaning of the person's outward expression. For instance, in the above example, a Level 4 response might be, "It sounds as though you're pretty angry at your dad because he doesn't pay any attention to you" (expresses a new feeling, anger, which the client didn't outwardly state). Level 5 responses are usually made in long-term therapeutic relationships by expert counselors. They express to the helpee a deep understanding of the pain that he or she feels, as well as recognition of the complexity of the situation.

Usually, it is recommended in the training of helpers that they attempt to make Level 3 responses, as a large body of evidence suggests that such responses can be learned in a relatively short amount of time and are beneficial to clients (Carkhuff, 2009; Cormier, Nurius, & Osborn, 2012; Lam, Kolomitro, & Alamparambil, 2011). Effective empathic responses not only accurately reflect content and feelings but do so at a moment when the client can hear this reflection. For instance, you might sense a deep sadness or anger in a client and reflect this back to him or her. However, if the client is not ready to accept these feelings, then the timing is off and the response is considered subtractive.

Often, when first practicing empathic responding, it is suggested that beginning counselors make a formulaic response, which generally starts with reflection of feeling followed by paraphrasing of content. Look at the example below:

Client: I'm at my wit's end. I'm as depressed as ever. I keep trying to change my life and nothing works. I try communicating better, I change my job, I change my looks. I even take antidepressants, but nothing helps.

Counselor: You feel frustrated because you try making all of these changes and things are not any better.

As counselors become more comfortable with formulaic responses, they can begin to use more natural conversational tones when making empathic responses. For instance, to the client above, a counselor might say:

Counselor: Your frustration really shows—you've tried so many different things yet nothing seems to work. I can see your frustration and sadness in your eyes.

Master therapists become very creative with empathic responding and will use metaphors, analogies, and self-disclosure in an attempt to tell the client that he or she has been heard accurately (Neukrug, 1998; Neukrug, Bayne, Dean-Nganga, & Pusateri, 2013):

Counselor: It's kind of like you're rearranging deck chairs on the *Titanic*.

or

Counselor: When you just told me what you're going through, I felt my stomach twist and turn. I imagine this is how you must be feeling.

As noted in Chapter 4, empathic responses sometimes have been confused with "active listening" or "reflection of feeling" over the years. Although Carl Rogers was instrumental in encouraging the use of empathy, he warned against the mechanistic, stilted, and wooden response to clients that is sometimes found when helpers practice reflection of feeling. Usually with practice, however, a helper's response to clients becomes more naturally empathic, as in some of the more advanced examples given above.

Silence

> *That I do not say something does not mean that nothing has been said. That I do not hear something does not mean that there is nothing to hear. I listen to silence and it speaks. I cannot, ever, say nothing at all.*

> (Linnell, Bansel, Ellwood, & Gannon, 2008, p. 305)

When   is   empty   space   facilitative,   and   when   does it   become   a   bit   much? Silence is a powerful tool that can be used advantageously by the counselor for the growth of clients (Levitt, 2001; Sommers-Flanagan & Sommers-Flanagan, 2014). It allows clients to reflect on what has been said and gives the counselor time to process sessions and to formulate the next responses. It shows clients that communication does not always have to be filled with words and that words sometimes can be used as a diversion from feelings. Silence is powerful. Sometimes it will raise anxiety within clients—anxiety that on the one hand could push them to talk further about a particular topic, and on the other hand could cause them to drop out of treatment.

A former professor of mine suggested waiting 30 seconds before making a response. During a counseling session, 30 seconds is a veeeeeeeeeery looooonng tiiiiiiiiiiiiiiiiiiime. There have been times when I've had a student role-play a client, and I've waited 30 seconds before responding. Trust me—this is a *very* long time. I would have difficulty waiting this long during a counseling session. Silence is powerful; however, the effective amount of silence may vary depending on the situation. For instance, during these 30 seconds, you could see my former professor thinking about the client's last statement, moving in his chair, and thinking about what he was to say next. This worked for him, but it might not for others.

Finally, the use of silence may be somewhat culturally determined. For instance, some research has found that the *pause time* for different cultures varies. Therefore, one's natural inclination to talk—to respond to another—will vary as a function of culture (Levitt, 2001; Zur, 2007). As a counselor, you may want to consider your pause time to discover your comfort level with silence, and when working with clients, you might consider a client's pause time. In fact, Native Americans have at times been labeled reticent and resistant to treatment, when in fact they just have long pause times (Hendrix, 2001). If they had been treated by Native American therapists, they most likely would not have been labeled in this fashion.

Commonly Used Skills

Although foundational skills are the bedrock of the counseling relationship, a number of additional skills are employed that counselors should understand. Some of these *commonly used skills* should be used judiciously and cautiously, as their overuse or misuse can lead to client defensiveness or create client dependency issues. These skills include the use of questions, self-disclosure, modeling, affirmation giving and encouragement, offering alternatives, providing information, and advice giving.

Questions

What purposes do *questions* serve? Can you tell me more about the use of questions? Is a question really a question or a hidden statement about self? When should questions be questioned? Would you prefer the use of short or long questions? Why do you question questions? A question can come in many different forms, can't it? Would you prefer a question that gives you two options from which to choose, or one that offers an open-ended response?

Questions can serve a multitude of purposes, including finding historical patterns, revealing underlying issues, gently challenging the client to change, encouraging the client to deepen his or her self-exploration, and helping clients move toward preferred goals. Although many different kinds of questions exist, some of the more important ones to the counseling relationship include open and closed questions, tentative questions, solution-focused questions, and "why" questions.

Open Versus Closed Questions.

Open questions allow clients to respond in a myriad of ways, whereas *closed questions* focus on a particular topic or point of view and force them to pick among the choices given (Neukrug & Schwitzer, 2006). Open questions offer a client greater options in the kinds of responses he or she can make and are generally considered more facilitative than closed questions, which limit client response (Langewitz, Nübling, & Weber, 2003; Sommers-Flanagan & Sommers-Flanagan, 2014). For instance, one could ask the closed question, "Do you feel you had a good or bad childhood?" An even more limiting question would be, "What made your childhood so bad?" Instead, one could ask the open question, "What was your childhood like?" which allows for unlimited responses. Although open questions are generally considered more expansive than closed ones, there are times, such as when you need to gather information quickly, when you want to zero in on a couple of responses rather than leaving the question wide open.

Tentative Questions.

Benjamin (2001) notes that a question can be made even more open if it is asked indirectly or tentatively. For instance, I could ask an open question directly: "What feelings did you have concerning your wife leaving you?" However, to make the question even more palatable, I might ask it in the following manner: "I would guess you must have had many feelings concerning your wife leaving?" In fact, this *tentative question* is more akin to making an empathic response. Open questions that are tentative tend to sit well with clients. They're easier for clients to hear, help the session flow, help to create a nonjudgmental and open atmosphere, are expansive rather than delimiting, and are easily responded to by clients. However, if you need to get some information quickly, you may want to stay away from these kinds of questions.

Solution-Focused Questions.

In contrast to the more traditional ways of conducting counseling, in which open, closed, and tentative questions might be used, with the advent of brief treatment, questions have played an increasingly important role and constructivist understanding of counseling (Strong & Nielsen, 2008). If you find yourself in a setting where brief treatment is being used, you might want to consider the kinds of questions that follow. Borrowing from solution-focused brief counseling (as noted in Chapter 4), we find the following:

> *Preferred goals questions:* These are questions which are generally asked near the very beginning of counseling to assess what the goals or hope of counseling can be. For instance, one might ask, "How will you know that coming to counseling has been worthwhile for you?"

> *Evaluative questions:* These questions help clients distinguish behaviors that have led to preferred goals from those that have not. For instance, "Has that new behavior worked for you?"

> *Coping questions:* Coping questions focus on past behaviors that have been successful in dealing with problems. For instance, "So, you've had this problem in the past; how did you tend to cope with it then?"

> *Exception-seeking questions:* These questions help clients examine when they haven't had the problem in their lives so that they can explore how they previously lived a problem-free life. For instance, "So what was going on in your life when you were not feeling this way?"

> *Solution-focused questions:* Future-oriented, these questions offer clients the opportunity to develop new, positive ways of reaching their preferred goals. For instance, "What kinds of things do you think you can do to help reach your preferred goals?"

The Use of "Why" Questions.   "Why do you feel that way?" Ever been asked that question? Did it make you feel defensive? In actuality, if one could honestly answer "why," the *why question* would be one of the most powerful questions used in counseling. However, clients are in counseling to find the answer to "why"; if they knew, they wouldn't be in your office. Because "why" questions tend to make a person feel defensive, it is generally recommended that counselors use other kinds of questions or empathic responses. I have found that after I've formed an alliance with a client, I might periodically slip in a soft "why" question and say something like, "Why do you think that is?" However, during sessions I use this type of question sparingly, if at all.

When to Use Questions.   Questions can be helpful in uncovering patterns, gathering information quickly, inducing self-exploration, challenging the client to change, and moving a client along quickly to preferred goals. However, their overuse can create an authoritarian atmosphere in which clients feel humiliated and dependent, expecting the counselor to come up with the solution (Benjamin, 2001; Sommers-Flanagan & Sommers-Flanagan, 2014). In addition, a question is generally not as facilitative as an empathic response that empowers clients to discover answers on their own (Neukrug, 2002; Neukrug & Schwitzer, 2006; Rogers, 1942). In fact, often an empathic response can be made in place of asking a question. For instance, suppose that the client said the following:

Client: You know, I can't stand talking about my parents' destructive attitude toward me and my siblings any longer.

A counselor could respond with an open question, such as:

Counselor: What is it about discussing your parents' destructive attitude that is so disturbing to you?

However, probably a more effective response would be:

Counselor: I hear how upset you get when you begin to talk about your parents' destructive attitude toward you and your siblings.

In short, those counselors who view themselves as less directive, less authoritarian, and more client-centered would tend to avoid questions. Those who are more directive, involved in brief treatment, and see themselves as more counselor-centered may be at ease with the use of some questions. Keeping this in mind, and adapting what Benjamin (2001) suggests, one might want to consider the following prior to the use of questions:

➤ Are you cognizant of when you are using a question?
➤ Are you aware of why you have decided to use a question?
➤ Do you have limited time with the client and thus are deciding that questions might be useful?
➤ Are you aware of the impact that a question has on the counseling relationship?
➤ Are there better alternatives to the use of questions?

Self-Disclosure and Immediacy

A former student of mine was in therapy with a psychiatrist, who, over time, increasingly began to disclose *his* problems to *her*. One day, she heard that he had committed suicide. Following his death, she revealed to me that she felt intense guilt that she hadn't saved his life. What a legacy to leave this client! Clearly, the psychiatrist's *self-disclosure* was unhealthy and unethical. However, under some circumstances, certain amounts of therapist self-disclosure may facilitate a client's ability to open up and may also serve as a model of positive behaviors.

Self-disclosure has been broadly defined as "anything that is revealed about a therapist verbally, nonverbally, on purpose, by accident, wittingly, or unwittingly . . ." (Bloomgarden & Mennuit, 2009, p. 8). As a counseling skill, counselor self-disclosure is a mixed bag and is best conducted intentionally and judiciously (Bloomgarden & Mennuit, 2009; Farber, 2006; Maroda, 2009). However, the positive results of such self-disclosure can be many, including showing your client that you are "real," thus creating a stronger alliance; developing deeper intimacy in the helping relationship, which ultimately could foster deeper client self-disclosure; and offering behavior that your client can model. Sometimes client actions may necessitate self-disclosure on the part of the therapist (see Box 5.3).

Sometimes counselors and clients will share their moment-to-moment experience of themselves in relation to each other (Mayotte-Blum et al., 2012). When done by the counselor, this type of self-disclosure, called *immediacy*, can help a client see the impact that he or she has on the therapist and, ultimately, on others in his or her life; help a client see how moment-to-moment communication can enhance relationships; and act as a model for a new kind of communication that can be generalized to important relationships in the client's life. Similar to the Rogerian concept of genuineness, immediacy suggests that the counselor be real with his or her feelings toward the client (Rogers, 1957). However, it is important not to share transient feelings toward clients because as clients increasingly share deeper parts of themselves, the counselor's feelings toward them change—and usually in a positive direction. Thus, instead of sharing moment-to-moment feelings, it is often suggested to share persistent feelings, as these are more meaningful to the relationship (Rogers, 1970).

BOX 5.3
Awkward Self-Disclosure with a Client

A former client of mine who was in a dysfunctional relationship with her boyfriend was struggling with feelings of attraction toward me. We had discussed these feelings and noted that perhaps they were being exaggerated as she contrasted her feelings toward an "idealized" me with her feelings toward her verbally abusive boyfriend. She was a runner, as I was, and during one session, she informed me that she was interested in going to the Bahamas to run in an international race. I had already planned on running in this same race and was planning on going to the island with the woman I was dating. I suddenly was faced with a number of dilemmas. Do I disclose my plans and reveal an intimate aspect of my life, or do

I wait, and almost assuredly run into my client on the island? Or I could decide not to go. I quickly assessed the situation, and it seemed obvious to me that I needed to reveal my plans to her. I believe it would have been a mistake for me to change my plans, yet I didn't want to create an awkward situation for my client when on the island. Revealing as little information as possible about my life, I said to my client that I was planning on going to the race with a woman friend. Having this information, my client eventually decided not to go.

When do you think it is appropriate to disclose something personal about your life to a client? What ramifications can such a disclosure have?

Self-disclosure needs to be done sparingly, at the right time, and as a means for promoting client growth rather than satisfying the counselor's needs (Zur, 2009). A general rule of thumb that I use is: If it feels good to self-disclose, don't. If it feels good, you're probably meeting more of your needs than the needs of your client. Hill & Knox (2002) suggest a number of guidelines for counselor self-disclosure:

1. Therapists should generally disclose infrequently.
2. The most appropriate disclosure is about professional issues, and the least appropriate is about sexual issues.
3. Disclosure is best used to normalize situations, validate reality, build the relationship, or offer alternatives.
4. Avoid disclosures for own needs or disclosures that are intrusive, blur boundaries, interfere with the flow, or confuse the client.
5. The best disclosures are probably ones that match the client's disclosure.
6. Some clients respond better to disclosures than others, so it is important to see how the client reacts to disclosures and back off of them when necessary.

Finally, I agree with Kahn (2001), who states:

> I try not to make a fetish out of not talking about myself. If a client, on the way out the door, asks in a friendly and casual way, "Where are you going on your vacation?" I tell where I'm going. If the client were then to probe, however ("Who are you going with? Are you married?") I would be likely to respond, "Ah . . . maybe we'd better talk about that next time."

(p. 150)

Modeling

Clients can learn a wide variety of new behaviors by observing desired behaviors in others and later *modeling* these behaviors by practicing them on their own. Sometimes called *social learning, imitation,* or *behavioral rehearsal,* modeling can be a significant part of the change process as one imitates the behaviors of others and rehearses those behaviors that he or she intends on integrating (Cooper, Heron, & Heward, 2007; Naugle & Maher, 2003).

Modeling can occur in a number of ways, such as (1) when a therapist decides to highlight certain clinical skills with the hope that the client will learn from example (e.g., expressing empathy, being nonjudgmental, being assertive); (2) through the use of role-playing during the session (e.g., the counselor might role-play job-interviewing techniques for the client); and (3) by teaching the client about modeling and encouraging him or her to find models outside the session to emulate (e.g., a person who has a fear of speaking to a large group might choose a speaker he or she admires and view the specifics of how that person makes a speech).

With modeling, targeted behaviors that the client wishes to acquire need to have a high probability for success (Bandura, 1977). Thus, it is important to accurately identify desired behaviors that want to be changed, pick appropriate models from which one can emulate the identified behavior, ensure that the client can remember the model and has the ability to repeat what was observed, and be motivated to practice the new behaviors within and outside of the session. For instance, an individual who has a fear of making speeches would first need to find a model to emulate. After observing this model, a hierarchy could be devised whereby the client would make a speech—first to the counselor, then to some trusting friends, then to a small group, and so forth, perhaps asking for feedback along the way in order to sharpen his or her performance.

Modeling has been used to help clients develop a wide range of new behaviors. Imagine how one might use modeling to help clients become more assertive, communicate more effectively, eat more slowly, or relax more easily. Finally, modeling occurs all of the time, even when one does not purposefully seek to model another person's behaviors. And the more perceived power the model holds, the more likely modeling will occur. As you might expect, counselors who are often looked up to (and sometimes even idealized) by their clients can be very powerful models, even unintentionally (Brammer & MacDonald, 2003). Thus, regardless of the theoretical approach of the counselor, he or she should consider that the very skills being demonstrated during a session will likely be modeled to some degree by the client.

Affirmation Giving and Encouragement

> *The need for supporting core self-esteem doesn't end in childhood. Adults still need "unconditional" love from family, friends, life partners, animals, perhaps even an all-forgiving deity. Love that says: "no matter how the world may judge you, I love you for yourself."*

> (Steinem, 1992, p. 66)

Although *affirmation giving* and *encouragement* are not generally considered techniques, it is the rare counselor who does not affirm and encourage clients. Fleeting statements such as "good job," "I'm happy for you," "I know you can do it," or strong handshakes, warm hugs, and approving smiles are just a few of the ways in which counselors affirm and encourage their clients. Whereas affirmations are seen as a genuine positive response to a client's behaviors, encouragement is focused more on helping a client achieve a specific goal.

Whether called "reinforcement" or "a genuine response to our client's hard work," such responses may greatly affect our clients, and perhaps not always in positive ways (Orlinsky, Ronnestad, & Willutzki, 2004). Therapists must reflect upon whether affirmations and subtle encouragement of client progress are assisting in the formation of a higher degree of self-worth, or if they may actually be doing little to discourage (or even may be fostering) dependency and the continuation of a higher degree of externality (Kinnier, Hofsess, Pongratz, & Lambert, 2009). In my practice, I aim to genuinely affirm the client while taking care not to inadvertently foster a dependent relationship.

Offering Alternatives, Providing Information, and Giving Advice

Like affirmations and encouragement, *offering alternatives*, *providing information*, *and giving advice* are not typical counselor responses because they tend to place the counselor in the role of expert and can result in leading the client toward certain behaviors (often based on the counselor's values). As with affirmation giving and encouragement, these types of responses can encourage externality and foster dependency (Benjamin, 2001; Sommers-Flanagan & Sommers-Flanagan, 2014). It is therefore not surprising that some research has shown that these types of responses are not particularly effective (Orlinsky et al., 2004). Nevertheless, there may be times when these responses are helpful, such as when a client and counselor have agreed upon a specific course of action and the client wants suggestions on how to move in that direction (e.g., a client who is committed to working on her social skills is advised by the counselor to join a local community group), or when it appears obvious that the actions of a client will be harmful to the client or others.

Although offering alternatives, providing information, and giving advice are similar in the sense that they are all "counselor-centered" and not "client-centered," each has a different potential for being destructive to the counseling relationship. Clearly, of the three possible leading responses, offering alternatives would be least likely to have destructive influences on the counseling relationship (see Figure 5.2). As we move toward advice giving, the counselor's responses tend to become more value laden and more

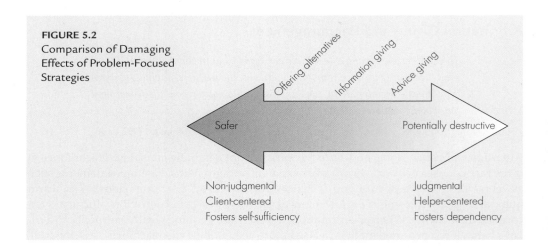

FIGURE 5.2
Comparison of Damaging Effects of Problem-Focused Strategies

Offering alternatives Information giving Advice giving

Safer   Potentially destructive

Non-judgmental   Judgmental
Client-centered   Helper-centered
Fosters self-sufficiency   Fosters dependency

counselor-centered (Van Rooyen, Durrheim, & Lindegger, 2011). Whether any of these responses are used should be based on a careful understanding of your client's needs and whether an alternative response could be more effective for the client. Finally, if counseling is optimal, the counselor is less likely to consider one of these responses because an atmosphere has been created where the client is already considering any of the alternatives or advice that could be offered, or already finding on his or her own the information that is needed to help resolve the situation at hand.

Commonly Used Advanced Skills

In addition to the commonly used skills we just discussed, other skills that involve a little more sophistication on the part of the counselor are often employed at different points of the counseling relationship. These include confrontation, interpretation, and collaboration.

Confrontation: Support, then Challenge

People generally define *confrontation* as some type of hostile challenge when attempting to overcome an obstacle. However, within the context of the counseling relationship, confrontation is usually thought of as a much softer challenge to the client's understanding of the world, which invites the client to gain an alternative perspective to his or her current situation; or, as Strong and Zeman (2010) suggest, a conversational process whereby clients are invited to partake in a discussion about how they are living their lives. To be effective, this gentle challenge needs to be preceded by the building of a trusting and caring relationship, thus lessening the likelihood that any harm to the client will occur (Egan, 2014; Neukrug & Schwitzer, 2006; Polcin, 2006). The use of good listening skills and empathy is generally considered to be the most effective way to develop a relationship that can successfully process a challenge and potentially change the client's perception of reality. In short, confrontation requires accurate timing, tact, and gentleness on the part of the counselor (see Box 5.4).

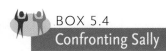

BOX 5.4
Confronting Sally

Sally made close to $60,000 a year and was in a verbally abusive relationship. Even though she had no major bills to pay, she insisted that she could not leave the relationship and live on a "meager" $60,000 a year. Clearly, her verbal statement that she could not leave the relationship did not match the reality that one could live on this amount (certainly, most of us would be happy to live on this amount). After building a relationship using empathy, I gently challenged this perception. I did this by using many of the techniques described above. Using "you/but" statements, I pointed out the obvious discrepancy between her salary and her perceived inability to live on her own. Also, I gently asked her to justify to me how she could feel this way. This assisted her to see that her logic did not hold up. Using higher-level empathy, I reflected back a deeper issue that I experienced

her saying—that she felt as if she was a failure in the relationship and was scared to be alone (she was a recovering alcoholic and was concerned she would start drinking again if alone). I encouraged her to work on communication issues with her lover. At the same time, I assisted her in reframing her situation so that she could believe that she could live on her own—if she chose eventually to do so. I did not use irony with her, as I felt it would be too disturbing for her. The result for this client was that she became a more assertive woman who improved her communication with her lover and could realistically see her choices about staying in the relationship or finding a place on her own.

When do you think it's appropriate to challenge a person's perception of the world? How vigorously do you think a counselor should challenge a client, if at all?

Some have suggested that challenging a client gently can be accomplished by helping the client see discrepancies among words, feelings, and behaviors (Hackney & Cormier, 2012; Hill, 2014; Neukrug et al., 2013). For instance, discrepancies can exist between a client's (1) values and behavior (e.g., a client says she believes in honesty in relationships, yet won't express her anger toward her lover because she is afraid he will leave her); (2) feelings and behavior (e.g., a man who says he loves his wife deeply and then tells the counselor about the affair he is having); (3) self-descriptions and other verbal statements (e.g., a client who states that she wants to communicate more effectively but finds excuses for not doing so: "If only I had more time to work on my communication problems"); and (4) verbal expression of feelings and the underlying feelings to which a client won't admit or of which he or she is not currently aware (e.g., a person who states that she feels fine about her marriage and yet seems to be holding back tears; you note this, and she begins to sob). Following the building of a trusting and caring relationship, there are a number of ways a discrepancy can be confronted:

1. *You/but statements.* Such statements point out client incongruities by reflecting them back in a "you/but" framework (Hackney & Cormier, 2012). For instance, to a client who states that he believes in honesty but is having an affair, the counselor might say:

   Counselor: On the one hand, you say that you believe in honesty, but you seem to be hiding a serious matter from your wife.

2. *Asking the client to justify the discrepancy.* This kind of response has the counselor gently asking the client to explain how he or she justifies the discrepancy. For example, in the above example, the counselor might say:

   Counselor: Based on your knowledge of who you are, tell me how you make sense of the fact that you say you are honest, and yet you are hiding an affair from your wife?

3. *Reframing.* This way of highlighting the discrepancy challenges the client to view his or her situation differently by offering an alternative reality:

   Counselor: What you're telling me is that in some cases, honesty is not always the best way to go.

4. *Using irony or satire.* Using irony or satire highlights the absurdity of the discrepancy and is more confrontational than the other techniques. This technique should be used carefully. For instance, in the above example, you might say:

   Counselor: Well, I guess it's okay in this instance to be dishonest; after all, you are saving your wife from those painful feelings, aren't you?

5. *Higher-level empathy.* Higher-level empathy, the final way of challenging a client's discrepancy, reflects to the client any underlying, out-of-awareness feelings and conflicts and challenges the client to expose deeper parts of the self. For instance, in the above example:

   Counselor: You must be feeling quite conflicted. On the one hand, you say you believe in honesty; on the other hand, you are hiding an affair. I guess I sense there is more to this story for you.

Interpretation

A client offers details to you, his counselor, about his current lover. Later, he shares details about his relationship with his parents. You hear similar themes and feelings running through these relationships and reveal your analysis to the client. The client nods his head in agreement. Is this *interpretation* or is this empathy? Although some may consider this interpretation, I consider this a high-level empathic response (above Level 3.0 on the Carkhuff scale) for a number of reasons. First, it is a result of deep listening and concentration on the part of the counselor. Second, it is based on a deep understanding of the client's framework of reality. Third, you have reflected back your understanding of the client's predicament without adding material from an external source, such as a counseling theory, that might suggest certain conclusions about your client. And finally, the client agrees with your assessment. You are on target with your response. This definition of empathy is a profound response to the client that reaches deep inside the client's soul and speaks to the imaginary line between facilitating and leading a client (Neukrug et al., 2013).

On the other hand, true interpretation is the analysis of a client's behaviors and meaning-making system from the perspective of the counselor, usually with a preset model of counseling and psychotherapy in mind that makes assumptions about how a person would react under certain circumstances.

> To interpret another's experience means to claim privileged access to its underlying meaning. Interpreting another's experience also means claiming the right to transform, to convert, to translate it into something different, and to relate to this meaning as its "real" meaning.
>
> (Willig, 2011, p. 263)

Psychoanalysis uses interpretation as a major therapeutic intervention. For instance, many psychodynamic therapists believe that our dreams hold symbols to unresolved conflicts from our psychosexual development and can provide the client with understanding of his or her development (Brill, 1921/2010). In this vein, a dream about a goat being your pet in an immaculate apartment could represent an underlying need to rebel against a repressive upbringing, the goat representing the archetypal oppositional animal. Similarly, interpretations about the transference relationship are used in many psychodynamic therapies to explain how a person's current relationships are reflections of past relationships. Some cognitive therapists also use interpretation when they assume that individuals with specific diagnoses would be expected to have certain kinds of underlying cognitive structures, which can be explained (interpreted) to the client (Beck, 2005). For example, it would be assumed that a person with an anxiety disorder has underlying cognitive beliefs that the world is a fearful and dangerous place. Whether we are psychodynamically oriented, cognitively oriented, or relying on some other theoretical approach, the timing of the interpretation is crucial, with the desired result being a deeper understanding of why the client responds the way he or she does—an understanding that may lead to client change.

When on target, interpretations can assist a client in making giant leaps in counseling. However, there are risks involved in using this technique. For instance, interpretation sets the counselor up as the "expert" and lessens the realness of the relationship (Willig, 2011). In addition, it detracts from the here-and-now quality of the therapeutic relationship while increasing the amount of intellectualizing that occurs as both the counselor and client discuss the interpretive material. Finally, research done on the use of interpretation seems mixed, at best, relative to successful client outcomes (Høglend et al., 2008; Orlinsky, Ronnestad, & Willutzki, 2004).

For these reasons, Carl Rogers and others (e.g., Benjamin, 2001; Kahn, 2001) warn that the use of interpretation can be detrimental to the counseling relationship.

> . . . To me, an interpretation as to the cause of individual behavior can never be anything but a high-level guess. The only way it can carry weight is when an authority puts his experience behind it. But I do not want to get involved in this kind of authoritativeness. "I think it's because you feel inadequate as a man that you engage in this blustering behavior," is not the kind of statement I would ever make.

> (Rogers, 1970, pp. 57–58)

Collaboration

Collaboration in the counseling relationship involves communicating to your client that you value his or her feedback and that you want to come to a mutually agreed-upon decision about the next phase in treatment (Sommers-Flanagan & Sommers-Flanagan, 2014). Here, the counselor is asking for feedback from the client as to his or her assessment of the counseling relationship and uses techniques that lead to a mutual decision about the future of treatment. Effective collaboration implies that one has built a strong therapeutic alliance and is increasingly used in a wide variety of counseling approaches (see Neukrug, 2011). Generally, collaboration includes the following:

1. Using one's foundational skills to offer a summary of what has been discussed thus far
2. Asking the client, through the use of questions, how he or she feels about the course of treatment thus far
3. Asking the client, through the use of questions, about the direction he or she would like to take in treatment
4. Sharing with the client one's own thoughts about which areas might be important to focus upon
5. Having an honest discussion concerning any discrepancies between actions 3 and 4, which leads to a mutual decision about the course of treatment

Collaboration can, and often does, occur throughout the helping relationship and is often most useful at transitional points, such as (1) after rapport building and prior to problem identification, (2) after problem identification and prior to the development of treatment goals, (3) after the development of treatment goals and prior to treatment planning, and (4) during the closure stage prior to ending counseling. These stages of the relationship will be discussed later in this chapter.

Advanced and Specialized Counseling Skills

We have examined in this chapter a number of common skills used by most counselors, whether they are beginning students or advanced master therapists. Although not within the purview of this text, there are literally dozens of other skills that can be attained through additional training by an interested and astute counselor. Many of these skills are unique to specific counseling approaches. Mentioning just a few, they include the use of metaphor, hypnosis, strategic skills, cognitive restructuring methods, narratives and storytelling, therapeutic touch, paradoxical intention, role-playing, visualization techniques, and a wide variety of cognitive and behavioral techniques (Neukrug, 2011; Rosenthal, 2011a, 2011b). Suffice it to say that use of these skills may often take training beyond the master's degree. Today, many institutes nationally and internationally offer such advanced training. Such training can also be obtained through the attainment of an advanced degree, participation in workshops at conferences, and good supervision.

Conceptualizing Client Problems: Case Conceptualization

Case conceptualization is a method that allows the counselor to understand a client's presenting problems and subsequently apply appropriate counseling skills and treatment strategies based on the counselor's theoretical orientation. Whereas experienced counselors develop their own systematic method of conceptualizing client problems, beginning counselors, who are often still struggling with their theoretical orientation, have a more difficult time conceptualizing client problems (Neukrug & Schwitzer, 2006; Schwitzer, MacDonald, & Dickinson, 2008). One model of case conceptualization is Schwitzer's (Schwitzer & Rubin, 2012) *inverted pyramid method (IPM)*.

IPM is a step-by-step method that can be used to identify and understand client concerns while offering a visual guide for counselors in how to organize client information; see connections among client concerns, symptoms, and behaviors; and consider different areas to focus on in counseling. The IPM includes four steps in clinical problem formulation (see Figure 5.3):

1. Broadly identifying client concerns and symptomatic behavior
2. Organizing client difficulties into logical groupings or constellations
3. Tying symptom groups to one's theoretical orientation
4. Narrowing these symptom groups to the client's most basic difficulties in development or adjustment based on one's theoretical orientation

Using this method, a beginning counselor would start at the top of the inverted pyramid and attempt to identify problem behaviors. Going down the inverted pyramid, the counselor would, in step 2, attempt to organize the information obtained in step 1 into groups called "thematic groupings." During step 3, the groupings developed in the two previous steps are related to the counselor's theoretical perspective. In step 4, inferences from step 3 are further distilled into deeper difficulties in functioning or deeper personality traits, when present.

FIGURE 5.3
Inverted Pyramid Method of Case Conceptualization

SOURCE: Adapted from "Using the Inverted Pyramid Heuristic," by A. M. Schwitzer, 1996, *Counselor Education and Supervision, 35*, p. 260. Copyright © 1996 ACA. Reprinted with permission. No further reproduction authorized without written permission of ACA.

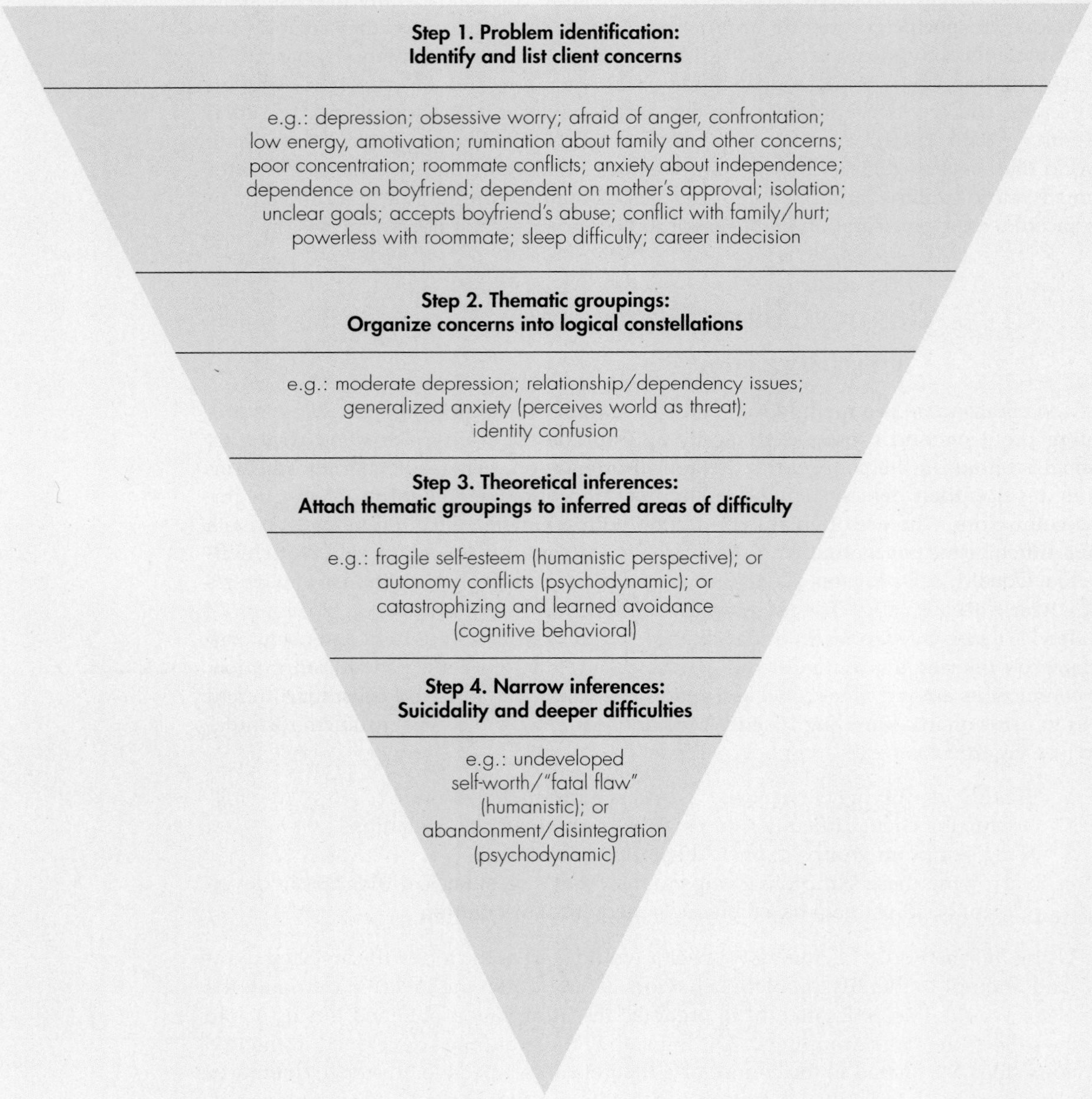

Step 1. Problem identification:
Identify and list client concerns

e.g.: depression; obsessive worry; afraid of anger, confrontation;
low energy, amotivation; rumination about family and other concerns;
poor concentration; roommate conflicts; anxiety about independence;
dependence on boyfriend; dependent on mother's approval; isolation;
unclear goals; accepts boyfriend's abuse; conflict with family/hurt;
powerless with roommate; sleep difficulty; career indecision

Step 2. Thematic groupings:
Organize concerns into logical constellations

e.g.: moderate depression; relationship/dependency issues;
generalized anxiety (perceives world as threat);
identity confusion

Step 3. Theoretical inferences:
Attach thematic groupings to inferred areas of difficulty

e.g.: fragile self-esteem (humanistic perspective); or
autonomy conflicts (psychodynamic); or
catastrophizing and learned avoidance
(cognitive behavioral)

Step 4. Narrow inferences:
Suicidality and deeper difficulties

e.g.: undeveloped
self-worth/"fatal flaw"
(humanistic); or
abandonment/disintegration
(psychodynamic)

The pyramid provides a conceptual map of working with clients. It begins by offering a broad presentation of client concerns, and slowly integrates those concerns with the theoretical framework of the counselor. Thus, this model can work with any of a number of theoretical orientations, and the same presenting issues can ultimately be worked on in very different ways by different counselors. It is clear that decisions concerning treatment approaches can be greatly aided through the use of the case conceptualization process.

Stages of the Counseling Relationship

The application of counseling skills can vary considerably as a function of the counselor's job role, setting, and theoretical orientation. Despite these differences, there are many commonalities within the counseling relationship. For instance, all counselors have to address technical issues unique to the first session (e.g., meeting times, length of session, billing issues, and frequency of sessions). All counselors will face issues of trust. All counselors will need to identify client concerns, develop goals, and assist the client in working on the identified goals. And all counselors will have to deal with termination. These commonalities tend to be displayed in a series of stages of the counseling relationships through which clients pass (Neukrug & Schwitzer, 2006). Let's examine these stages and see how our conceptual model may be applied within them. Refer back to Figure 5.3 as you consider this material.

Stage 1: Rapport and Trust Building

When clients initially see a counselor, they are wondering whether they can trust their counselor enough to discuss the concerns they have. The counselor, on the other hand, is dealing with a number of issues that are crucial to the development of an effective working relationship. For instance, the counselor is concerned about using basic skills to build trust in the relationship, ensuring that the physical environment feels safe, and informing the client of the basic framework and concerns of the counseling relationship:

> Counselors explicitly explain to clients the nature of all services provided. They inform clients about issues such as, but not limited to, the following: the purposes, goals, techniques, procedures, limitations, potential risks, and benefits of services; the counselor's qualifications, credentials, relevant experience, and approach to counseling; continuation of services upon the incapacitation or death of the counselor; the role of technology; and other pertinent information.

> (ACA, 2014a, Section A.2.b)

Often, these *professional disclosure statements* are provided in written form for both the client and counselor to sign and may be considered legal documents to which the counselor should adhere (Remley & Herlihy, 2014).

During the *rapport and trust building stage*, the development of a comfortable, trusting, and facilitative relationship can be accomplished through the use of listening skills, empathic understanding, cultural sensitivity, and a fair number of good social skills (Hackney & Cormier, 2012). During these beginning sessions, it is usual to discuss superficial items with clients or common interests in an effort to establish camaraderie. However, always keep in mind that the one major purpose of counseling is to assist the client toward disclosure of self-identified problems. Therefore, it is probably wise not to make the session too chatty.

As this stage continues, the counselor will begin to mentally identify and eventually delineate the issues presented by the client. This is the first step of the case conceptualization model. The counselor should review and evaluate the accuracy of this list with the client by reflecting back to the client those problems thought to be highlighted during this stage, or by asking the client directly if the list is accurate.

Stage 2: Problem Identification

The building of a trusting relationship and the ability to do an assessment of client problems are signs that you are moving into the second stage, where you and your client will validate your initial identification of the problem(s). It may be that what the client initially came to counseling for was masking other issues. Or additional issues may arise as you explore the client's situation—perhaps even issues of which the client was not fully aware. In either case, during these sessions, you validate your original assessment and make appropriate changes as necessary. Validation of original concerns or reassessment and identification of new issues in the *problem identification stage* allow you to move into step 2 of the conceptual model, the grouping of identified problems into broad themes.

Stage 3: Deepening Understanding and Goal Setting

Although your basic counseling skills are still important, because trust has been built in the earlier stages, other skills can now be added—skills that will allow you to understand your client in deeper ways. For instance, in the *deepening understanding and goal setting stage*, the client will now allow you to confront him or her, ask probing questions, and give advanced empathic responses. You can increasingly push the envelope and move into the inner world of the client. However, it is always crucial to maintain sensitivity to your client's needs and to maintain a supportive and nurturing base. Move too fast, and the client will rebuff your attempts to expose his or her inner world. Move at the right pace for the client, and the counseling relationship will deepen, and advanced skills based on your particular theoretical orientation can be used.

As you begin to understand your client in deeper and broader ways, you move into step 3 of the conceptual model, where you begin to make inferences based on your theoretical orientation about underlying themes. These may be shared with your client, and at this point, clients are likely to begin to work on some of these identified themes. If given enough time, you will move into step 4 of the conceptual model with some clients. In this step, based on your theoretical orientation, you can now identify specific underlying themes that permeate the client's life and affect many aspects of his or her functioning.

Now that themes have been identified from step 3 or step 4 of the conceptual model, goals can be established based on these themes. The counselor, in collaboration with the client, can determine how the client would like to reach these goals. This will be based partly on the practicality of the relationship (e.g., the number of sessions available for counseling), the desires of the client (e.g., the client may want short-term counseling), and the theoretical orientation of the counselor. The result of this collaboration should be anything from an informal verbal agreement concerning goals to a written contract that is signed by both the client and counselor.

Stage 4: Work

During the fourth stage, the client is beginning to work on the issues that were identified in stage 3 and agreed upon between the counselor and client. The counselor will use his or her counseling skills to facilitate progress, and, if necessary, the counselor and client may want to revisit and reevaluate some of the goals set.

In the *work stage*, the client increasingly takes responsibility for and actively works on his or her identified issues and themes. For instance, if the counselor is humanistically oriented, the client is pushing himself or herself to work on identified existential–humanistic themes (e.g., issues related to self-esteem). If the counselor is cognitive/behavioral, the client will be actively working on changing cognitions and behaviors (e.g., self-statements like "I am worthless" are worked upon, and self-affirming behaviors are practiced). If the counselor is psychodynamic, the client will be exploring identified analytical themes in the session (e.g., what impact past overdependency on his or her mother is having on current relationships). Advanced skills based on the counselor's theoretical orientation are used in this stage. As clients work through their issues, they move closer to the termination of counseling.

Stage 5: Closure

The main issues of the *closure stage* are termination and the loss associated with it. As the client has successfully worked through some of his or her issues, it becomes increasingly clear that there is little reason for counseling to continue. Counseling is one of the few intimate relationships that is time-limited, which consequently means that clients (and counselors) will have to work through their feelings of loss (Murdin, 2000).

When is a client ready to terminate a counseling relationship? Probably, termination should be considered when (1) the client is close to reaching the agreed-upon number of sessions; (2) there is a reduction or elimination of symptoms; (3) the client has gained enough insight and skills to deal with future recurring symptoms; (4) there is a resolution of transference issues; (5) the client has the ability to work effectively, enjoy life, and play; and (6) continued services are not likely to be helpful (ACA, 2014a, Section A.11.C; Vasquez, Bingham, & Barnett, 2008).

Termination should be a gradual process in which the client and counselor have time to deal with the loss involved and discuss whether stated goals have been met.

As with many issues that carry a heavy emotional burden, many clients will attempt to defend against or resist the termination process (Emanuel, 2014; Murdin, 2000; Sommers-Flanagan & Sommers-Flanagan, 2014). This can happen in a number of ways:

➤ The client may insist that he or she needs more time to work on the problem(s).
➤ New issues may suddenly arise.
➤ The client may miss sessions in an effort to avoid discussing termination.
➤ The client may suddenly become angry with the therapist in an effort to distance himself or herself.
➤ The client may prematurely end therapy in an effort to avoid discussing termination.

Because counselors also may find themselves resisting termination (Sommers-Flanagan & Sommers-Flanagan, 2014), it is important that they be vigilant about working through their own loss issues while, at the same time, be sensitive to the loss issues of their clients. Of course, consultation with colleagues and supervisors can be invaluable at this point in the therapeutic relationship.

Finally, successful termination is more likely if (1) clients discuss termination early, (2) goals are clear so clients know when counseling is near completion, (3) the counselor respects the client's desire to terminate yet feels free to discuss feelings that termination may be happening too soon, (4) the relationship remains professional (e.g., does not move into a friendship), (5) clients know they can return, (6) clients are able to review the success they had in counseling, and (7) clients can discuss feelings of loss around termination.

Stage 6: Post-Interview Stage

We believe that patients can and should return as needed.

(Budman & Gurman, 1988, p. 20)

The end of counseling may not be the end. Clients may return with new issues, may want to revisit old ones, or may desire to delve deeper into themselves. In fact, it is not unusual for clients to return to the same counselor or seek out another counselor at some later date.

The *post-interview stage* involves ensuring that you have completed your case management tasks, such as paperwork, billing tasks, and eventual follow-up with clients. Follow-up with clients can function as a check to see if clients would like to return for counseling or would like a referral to a different counselor, and it also allows the counselor to assess if change has been maintained. Usually done a few weeks to six months after counseling has been completed, it enables the counselor to look at which techniques have been most successful, gives the counselor the opportunity to reinforce past change and is one way in which the counselor can evaluate services provided (Neukrug, 2002; Neukrug & Schwitzer, 2006). Some counselors follow up by making a phone call, others send a letter, and still others do a more elaborate survey of clients.

Theory, Skills, Stages, and Case Conceptualization: A Reciprocal Relationship

The application of our counseling skills deepens our relationship with our clients and moves them into the next counseling stage (see Figure 5.4). Movement into the next stage requires the use of new skills and brings forth a deeper understanding of our clients from our unique theoretical orientation. Concurrently, as we apply the case conceptualization model, we gain a deeper understanding of our clients from our particular theoretical perspective. In other words, our case conceptualization model informs our theoretical model. As we understand our clients in new and deeper ways, we move into later stages of the counseling relationship that require the use of new counseling skills. After the counseling relationship has ended, counselors should follow up, at which point they may find that a client wants to recycle through the stages of the relationship or be referred to a new counselor. Thus, we see a deepening reciprocal relationship among the skills that we use, the case conceptualization model, our theoretical orientation, and the stages of the counseling relationship.

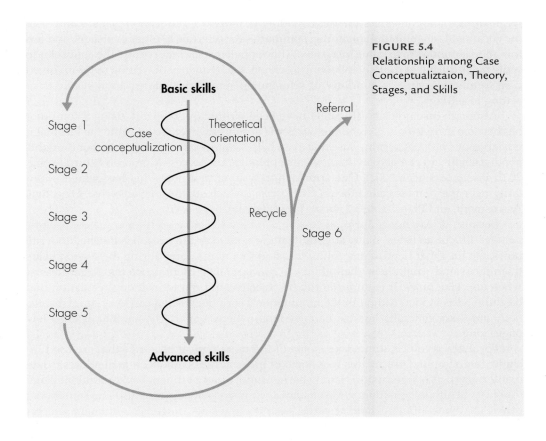

FIGURE 5.4
Relationship among Case Conceptualiztaion, Theory, Stages, and Skills

Case Notes

With the increasing number of people reading and writing *case notes*, note taking has become particularly important in the life of the counselor (Prieto & Scheel, 2002; Wiger, 2009). Regardless of the setting in which you work, there are numerous reasons why the writing of careful case notes has become so critical:

> ➤ They are important in the case conceptualization process.
> ➤ They can help us pull together our thoughts when making a diagnosis.
> ➤ They are a measure of our standard of care and subsequently can be used in court, if necessary, to show adequate client care.
> ➤ They assist in our understanding of whether our clients have made progress.
> ➤ They can be useful when we obtain supervision.
> ➤ They can help us remember what our clients say.
> ➤ They are needed by insurance companies, agencies, and schools to support the treatment we are providing to our clients.

Today, there are many kinds of case report writing, including process notes (aka "psychotherapy notes"), progress notes, intake summaries, quarterly summaries, summaries for insurance companies, summaries for students' individual education plans, summaries for vocational rehabilitation planning, summaries for referrals to other clinicians, and termination summaries, to name just a few. Although many settings require the counselor to write notes during or directly following a session, the frequency of writing more-involved case summaries, such as quarterly or semiannual summaries, varies dramatically from setting to setting.

Although case notes traditionally have been written out by hand, using a computer has become increasingly common today. Some argue, however, that despite the fact that it is a laborious process, writing case notes can help a counselor organize his or her thoughts about a client and can help in the case conceptualization process (Cameron & turtle-song, 2002; Prieto & Scheel, 2002). One approach to writing case notes that has gained popularity over the years is called the *S.O.A.P. format*, which stands for Subjective, Objective, Assessment, and Plan. Table 5.2 shows how such notes are used.

Because taking notes during a session can be distracting and, for some counselors, make it difficult to listen, many suggest waiting until after the session is finished to write notes. On the other hand, some counselors find that note taking during the session helps them focus and strengthens their ability to conceptualize client problems. Regardless of when you take notes, it is important to be objective and not to include speculation that has little basis in fact. Although the requirements for note writing can vary dramatically, daily notes are generally less than a page long, whereas quarterly summaries are a few pages long.

For more involved summaries, some of the more typical headings that are used include demographic information (e.g., date of birth, address, phone, e-mail address, date of interview), reason for report, family background, other pertinent background information (e.g., health information, vocational history, history of adjustment issues/emotional problems/mental illness), mental status, assessment results, diagnosis, summary, conclusions, and recommendations.

TABLE 5.2   S.O.A.P. Case Notes

	SUBJECTIVE-DESCRIPTION	SUBJECTIVE-EXAMPLES	SUBJECTIVE-POINTERS
S	➤ What the client tells you (feelings, concerns, plans, goals, and thoughts) ➤ How the client experiences the world ➤ Client's orientation to time, place, and person	➤ Client reports . . . ➤ Client shares . . . ➤ Client describes . . . ➤ Client indicates . . .	➤ Avoid quotations. ➤ Full names of others are generally not needed. ➤ Be concise. ➤ Limit adjectives.
	OBJECTIVE-DESCRIPTION	**OBJECTIVE-EXAMPLES**	**OBJECTIVE-POINTERS**
O	➤ Factual: What the helper personally observes, witnesses, or both ➤ Quantifiable: What was seen, heard, smelled, counted, or measured (may include outside written materials)	➤ Appeared as evidenced by . . . ➤ Test results indicate . . . ➤ Client's hair uncombed; clothes unkempt	➤ Avoid words like client"appeared" or"seemed" when not supported by objective examples. ➤ Avoid labels, personal judgments, or opinionated statements.
	ASSESSMENT-DESCRIPTION	**ASSESSMENT-EXAMPLES**	**ASSESSMENT-POINTERS**
A	➤ Summarizes the helper's clinical thinking ➤ Includes diagnoses or clinical impressions and reasons for behavior	➤ Behavior/attitude consistent with individuals who . . . ➤ DSM-5 diagnosis ➤ Rule out . . .	➤ Note themes or recurring issues. ➤ Remain professional. ➤ Remember that others may view assessment.
	PLAN-DESCRIPTION	**PLAN-EXAMPLES**	**PLAN-POINTERS**
P	➤ Describes parameters of treatment ➤ Includes action plan, interventions, progress, prognosis, treatment direction for next session	➤ Counselor established rapport, challenged, etc. ➤ Client progress is indicated by . . . ➤ Next session, counselor will . . . ➤ Client and counselor will continue to . . .	➤ Give supporting reasons for progress. ➤ "Progress is fair due to client's inconsistent attendance at sessions."

Adapted from Cameron, S., & turtle-song, i. (2002). Learning to write case notes using the SOAP format. *Journal of Counseling & Development, 80*, 286–92.

Finally, a wide range of ethical, professional, and legal issues accompanies the case note process and will be addressed shortly in the section of this chapter entitled "Ethical, Professional, and Legal Issues."

Multicultural/Social Justice Focus: Applying Skills Cross-Culturally

It must be stressed that while the application of specific counseling skills discussed in this chapter may be beneficial to some clients, they may not be helpful and even may be harmful to the counseling relationship when used in a cross-cultural counseling relationship (McAuliffe, 2013b). For instance, a Native American client may feel uncomfortable with prolonged eye contact; many Latin American clients are comfortable with less personal space than other clients and may interpret counselor distance as aloofness; a Muslim may consider being touched by the left hand of a counselor as obscene (because the left hand is seen as unclean and used as an aid in the process of elimination, while the right hand is seen as clean and used for eating); and an African American client may be put off by a White counselor who is nondirective and aloof.

In a similar vein, some clients may feel defensive with the use of questions, while other clients may feel uncomfortable because the counselor uses an abundance of empathy. Some clients may feel as though they are being pushed to self-disclose—a quality that may be viewed as weak in their culture—while other clients may feel offended that the counselor has not allowed them to talk more, as their culture tends to feel comfortable with the expression of feeling. And members of some cultures may be embarrassed by counselor self-disclosure, while for others, such disclosure may bring a counselor and client who are from two different cultures closer together.

Clearly, counselors need to have knowledge of the cultural background of the client and how a specific client's values, beliefs, and customs will play a part in the counseling relationship. At the same time, it must be remembered that each client is unique. For instance, although many Latin American clients may be turned off by too much counselor–client personal space, some will feel uncomfortable with little space. Or an African American client may be offended by the intentional lack of eye contact from his or her White counselor as a result of the counselor's belief that African Americans prefer less eye contact from White counselors.

Ethical, Professional, and Legal Issues

Listed as one of the most important issues relative to the client's welfare, maintenance of client records encompasses a broad range of ethical, professional, and legal issues. The following addresses some of the more salient issues that have arisen over the years, including the *confidentiality of records* and *privileged communication; client's rights to records; progress notes, process notes,* and the *Health Insurance Portability and Accountability Act (HIPAA);* and *security of records.*

Confidentiality of Records and Privileged Communication

As noted in the American Counseling Association (ACA) ethical code (ACA, 2014a), client records should be kept confidential except when legal concerns supersede confidentiality (as discussed in the next section of this chapter, "The Clients' Rights to Records"). For instance, in cases where there is danger to a person or society, when a court has the legal right to obtain records, or when clients want access to their records, counselors would likely need to yield their records.

A 1996 Supreme Court ruling, *Jaffee v. Redmond,* involving the case records of a social worker, upheld the right for licensed professionals to maintain the confidentiality of their records. Describing the social worker as a "therapist" and "psychotherapist," the ruling suggested that all licensed therapists who hold privileged communication have a right to withhold information about their clients (Remley, Herlihy, & Herlihy, 1997) (see Box 5.5). *Privileged communication* is the right of the client to expect that communication with the counselor is confidential as defined by state or federal statute.

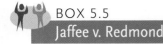

BOX 5.5
Jaffee v. Redmond

Mary Lu Redmond, a police officer in a village near Chicago, responded to a "fight in progress" call at an apartment complex on June 27, 1991. At the scene, she shot and killed a man she believed was about to stab another man he was chasing. The family of the man she had killed sued Redmond, the police department, and the village, alleging that Officer Redmond had used excessive force in violation of the deceased's civil rights. When the plaintiff's lawyers learned that Redmond had sought and received counseling from a licensed social worker employed by the village, they sought to compel the social worker to turn over her case notes and records and testify at the trial.

Redmond and the social worker claimed that their communications were privileged under an Illinois statute. They both refused to reveal the substance of their counseling sessions even though the trial judge rejected their argument that the communications were privileged. The judge then instructed jurors that they could assume that the information withheld would have been unfavorable to the policewoman, and the jury awarded the plaintiffs $545,000 (Remley et al., 1997, p. 214). After a series of appeals, the case was heard by the Supreme Court on February 26, 1996. The Court decided that the licensed therapist did indeed hold privilege and that the judge's instruction to the jury was therefore unwarranted.

Despite this ruling, licensed counselors should continue to act cautiously, as the definition of privileged communication varies dramatically as a function of the state in which one is licensed, and there are many exceptions to privilege (Younggren & Harris, 2008). For instance, the following excerpt shows how limiting the privileged communication statute is in Virginia. It starts out by asserting privileged communication and ends by stating that the court, for almost any reason, can nullify such privilege:

> . . . no duly licensed practitioner of any branch of the healing arts shall be permitted to testify in any civil action, . . . [except] when a court, in the exercise of sound discretion, deems such disclosure necessary to the proper administration of justice. . . .

(Virginia Code, 2009, para. A, B)

The Clients' Rights to Records

Clients generally have a legal right to view their records, and increasingly they have been exercising these rights in schools and agencies (Corey, Corey, & Callanan, 2015; Remley & Herlihy, 2014). Along these same lines, it has generally been assumed that parents have the right to view records of their children (C. Borstein, personal communication, March 20, 2014). ACA's ethical standards support these assumptions by stating that clients should generally be provided access to their records:

> Counselors provide reasonable access to records and copies of records when requested by competent clients. Counselors limit the access of clients to their records, or portions of their records, only when there is compelling evidence that such access would cause harm to the client.

(ACA, 2014a, Standard B.6.4.)

In terms of federal law, the *Freedom of Information Act (FOIA)* allows individuals access to any records (except in special circumstances), maintained by a federal agency that contain personal information about the individual, and every state has complied with similar laws governing state agencies (U.S. Department of Justice, 2011). Similarly, the *Family Education Rights and Privacy Act (FERPA)* ensures parents the right to access their children's educational records (U.S. Department of Education, 2014a). Although FERPA generally excludes counseling notes from the category of educational records (Merlone, 2005). Finally, the *Health Insurance Portability and Accountability Act (HIPAA)* ensures the privacy of client records and limits the sharing of such information (Zuckerman, 2008). In general, HIPAA restricts the amount of information that can be shared without client consent and allows for clients to have access to their records, except for process notes used in counseling (see the next section of this chapter).

In a more practical vein, clients generally do not ask to view their records. However, if a client did make such a request, I would first explore with the client why he or she wants to see the records. Next, I would want to talk with the client about what is written in the records. If this was not satisfactory to the client, I would suggest that I might write a summary of the records. However, if a client steadfastly states a desire to view his or her records, generally, this is his or her right.

Process Notes, Progress Notes, and HIPAA

Although clients generally have a right to access information about themselves, HIPAA states that psychotherapy notes, or what we commonly call *process notes*, are protected from the client's right to access them.

> *The Privacy Rule defines psychotherapy notes as notes recorded by a health care provider who is a mental health professional documenting or analyzing the contents of a conversation during a private counseling session or a group, joint, or family counseling session and that are separate from the rest of the patient's medical record.*

> (U.S. Department of Health and Human Services, n.d.)

Process notes are generally written notes that are used to help the counselor remember salient points of a session, and they should be distinguished from progress notes, which clients do have a right to access and include such things as type of treatment plan, diagnosis, medications, prognosis, and frequency of treatment.

Security of Record Keeping

The security of your records is vital, as clients have the ethical and often legal right to have information they share with others kept confidential (Remley & Herlihy, 2014). Therefore, it is critical that information obtained both verbally and in writing be kept confidential, secured, and not shared with others without client permission. This rule may not apply in certain instances, such as when you share client information with your supervisor, if the court subpoenas your records, and, in some cases, if parents request information regarding their children. If you are going to share information with other agencies who might also be working with your client, it is essential that you obtain permission in writing from your client or your client's parent(s) if the client is a minor. This ensures your client's right to privacy and affords you legal protection.

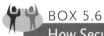

BOX 5.6
How Secure Are Records?

When I worked as an outpatient therapist at a mental health center, a client of another therapist had apparently obtained his records, which had been left "lying around." As his records tended to be written in psychological jargon, he was understandably quite upset by what he found. Therefore, he would periodically call the emergency services at night and read his records over the phone to the emergency worker, making fun of the language used in the records.

Another time, while taking a class in my doctoral program, we reviewed an assessment of an adolescent that had been done a number of years prior. Suddenly, one of the students in the class yelled out, "That's me!" Apparently, although there was no identifying name on the report, he recognized it as himself (he had been given a copy of the report previously).

Written client records need to be kept in secured places such as locked file cabinets (see Box 5.6). If records are kept on computers, then access to those files needs to be limited to you (and possibly your supervisor). Clerical help should be instructed about the importance of confidentiality when working with records. In fact, today's agencies sometimes will have nonclinical staff who have access to client information sign statements acknowledging that they understand the importance of confidentiality and that they will not discuss client issues outside the office. Obviously, the importance of hiring nonclinical staff whom you can trust with client information is paramount.

The Counselor in Process: The Developmental Nature of Counseling Skills

When you first learn specific counseling skills, you may want to adhere rigidly to the techniques you are taught. I believe this is good because the counselor who practices skills repeatedly will learn them well. However, giving responses in a mechanistic manner can lead to stiltedness in the helping relationship. Thus, one needs to try to find a balance between offering the "right" responses and being genuinely oneself in the relationship. Finding this balance is often not easy, but once you do, you will begin to feel more comfortable within the relationship, and you are likely to find your voice as a counselor.

As you continue through your career, you will refine your skills, learn new skills, become more proficient at case conceptualization, and adjust and maybe even change your theoretical orientation. Slowly, you will become more grounded in your approach. It's as though you're continually finding yourself—rediscovering your voice and making it a little clearer. Carl Rogers used to say that as an individual goes through his or her self-discovery process, choices become clearer—almost as if one does not have a choice because his or her path in life becomes obvious (Rogers, 1989b). I believe that a similar process occurs as we develop ourselves as counselors. Our skills, abilities, and who we are within the relationship become increasingly more refined and focused. It's as if we have little choice in how we should act within the relationship—we become the master counselor.

Summary

This chapter examined the basic skills necessary for a successful counseling relationship and began with an overview of the importance of having an environment that can optimize the use of these basic skills. Thus, we first examined the counseling environment, including having a comfortable office that ensures confidentiality, understanding nonverbal behaviors, and embracing counselor qualities that will lead to effective client outcomes, such as the nine personal qualities highlighted in Chapter 1.

The chapter next examined counseling skills, starting with foundational skills. Here we looked at how to listen effectively and how to make an effective empathic response; in particular, we emphasized the Carkhuff scale. We concluded this section with a short discussion concerning the importance of silence and pause time. We next examined a number of commonly used skills that are employed throughout the counseling relationship, including the use of questions, such as open and closed questions, tentative questions, solution-focused questions, and why questions; self-disclosure, sometimes called immediacy; modeling; affirmation giving and encouragement; and offering alternatives, providing information, and giving advice. We then went on to review some commonly used, albeit more complex skills, such as confrontation (support and challenge) that assist clients in seeing discrepancies; interpretation; and collaboration. We pointed out the pitfalls of many of these counselor responses, including the creation of defensiveness or dependency needs on the part of the client. We concluded this section by noting that, with advanced training, there are many advanced and specialized skills that a counselor can adopt.

Counseling skills are important to a successful counseling relationship; however, they become even more powerful when placed within the context of case conceptualization. Looking at the inverted pyramid method (IPM) of case conceptualization, we discussed how this process can assist the counselor in understanding the client's symptomatic behaviors, feelings, and thoughts and how it can help the counselor decide treatment planning and intervention strategies. We then identified six stages of the counseling relationship, including the rapport and trust-building stage, the problem identification stage, the deepening understanding and goal-setting stage, the work stage, the closure stage, and the post-interview stage. We also showed how case conceptualization, counseling skills, and one's theoretical orientation can be applied across the stages of the counseling relationship.

Next, we highlighted the importance of case notes, talked about the many different kinds of case notes and case records, and highlighted one frequently used system of case note taking called the S.O.A.P. format.

As the chapter continued, we examined the importance of knowing the values, beliefs, and customs of clients from diverse backgrounds in the application of counseling skills. We highlighted the fact that in the cross-cultural counseling relationship, some clients from diverse backgrounds may be turned off by what the counselor might consider to be common counseling skills. At the same time, we encouraged counselors not to jump to conclusions and assume that because a client is from a certain culture, he or she will respond in a prescribed manner.

We next highlighted some of the ethical and legal issues related to client records. For instance, we noted that records should be kept confidential except when legal concerns supersede confidentiality. We noted that relative to confidentiality, in the *Jaffee v. Redmond* Supreme Court decision, licensed therapists do have privileged communication that protects their right to withhold information about their clients. We warned, however, that full privilege currently is not offered in many states. We also noted that such laws as the *Freedom of Information Act (FOIA)*, the *Family Education Rights and Privacy Act* (FERPA), and the *Health Insurance Portability and Accountability Act* (HIPAA), as well as ethical codes, generally assert the right of client access to their records, except for process notes. We then contrasted process and progress notes and noted that process notes are used to help the counselor remember the salient points of a session. We also highlighted the importance of case note security and how critical it was to ensure the confidentiality of records by counselors, the security of file cabinets and computers, and the confidentiality of records when nonclinical staff (e.g., clerical help) have access to them.

Finally, this chapter ended with a discussion of the importance of continually developing one's counseling skills and ability at case conceptualization. These evolving skills and formulations allow the counselor to feel more capable about his or her ability and move the counselor toward ever-increasing self-assurance and effectiveness.

 ## Further Practice

Visit CengageBrain.com to respond to additional material that highlight the salient aspects of the chapter content. There, you can find ethical, professional, and legal vignettes, a number of experiential exercises, and study tools including a glossary, flashcards, and sample test items. Hopefully, these will enhance your learning and be fun and interesting.

CHAPTER 6   Couples and Family Counseling

CHAPTER 7   Group Work

CHAPTER 8   Consultation and Supervision

Overview

The three chapters of Section III examine how knowledge of the complex interactions of systems is crucial to working effectively with families and groups, and when consulting or supervising.

Chapter 6 starts with a brief history of couples and family counseling. This is followed by a discussion concerning the views of human nature held by most marriage and family counselors. The remainder of the chapter will examine key concepts of marriage and family counseling, followed by an examination of different models of couples and family work. In Chapter 7, the reader is reminded that groups, like families, follow many of the same system rules as families. Here we examine some advantages and disadvantages of group work compared to other forms of counseling, present a brief history of group counseling, and discuss the kinds of groups that are conducted by counselors. Chapter 8 will examine two important aspects of the helping relationship: consultation and supervision. In this chapter we will note that knowledge of systems is important for both the consultant and the supervisor and define and offer different models of consultation and supervision.

As you read through these chapters, consider how a contextual (systems) approach to the work of the counselor offers a different way of conceptualizing client issues and adds a new dimension to the counseling relationship.

Couples and Family Counseling

When I was in private practice, I received a call from a woman who wanted me to see her 12-year-old son; his grades in school had dropped precipitously and he was having behavioral problems. Having had training in family counseling, I asked the whole family to come to the first session, rather than just seeing the boy alone. During the first session, I obtained basic information about the family. The boy was the older of two children; his sister was one year younger. The family was middle class, and there was no significant family history that could explain any problems. Both mom and dad had some difficulties in childhood, but nothing out of the ordinary.

I decided to see the parents and the boy in family sessions. Although some family counselors would insist on seeing the whole family, I did not work like that. The parents saw no reason to have the daughter in the sessions, and I didn't want to resist their resistance. My style is to go with the family's wishes in order to build rapport. At a later date, if I felt the daughter should come in, I would request that of the family.

I saw the family, without the daughter, for approximately two months. Other than the school problems, there seemed to be no significant issues—at least any that I could get a handle on. I did, however, notice that most of the sessions were centered around the boy. Suddenly, during one session, the father blurted out, "I'm really depressed." Next thing I knew, he was talking about wanting to kill himself. Then the mother started saying that she was bulimic, throwing up a few times a day; then she started alluding to having an affair.

As the parents continued to talk about their problems, I looked at the boy and saw that, for the first time, he was relaxed. It was becoming clear: The parents were using the boy to distract them from the pain of their own problems. I asked them to begin to look at their issues and lay off their son a little. Within a week, the boy's grades started to improve and his acting out ceased. Now the real work was to begin—helping the couple deal with their issues! This is family counseling.

This chapter will start with a brief history of couples and family counseling and then describe some common elements of the view of human nature to which most couples and family counselors adhere. Next, we will describe key concepts to couples and family counseling, followed by an examination of some of the more prominent models of couples and family work, including the human validation process model, structural family therapy, strategic family therapy, multigenerational approaches, experiential family therapy, psychodynamic family therapy, cognitive–behavioral family counseling, narrative family counseling, and solution-focused family therapy. The chapter then will focus on multicultural and social justice concerns and then examine some ethical, professional, and legal issues related to couples and family counseling. As usual, we will conclude with a statement about "the counselor in process" relative to couples and family counseling.

Couples and Family Counseling: A Brief History

Although the emergence of couples and family counseling as a profession began around the middle part of the twentieth century, there were a number of events that led up to its birth. For instance, during the 1800s, two approaches to working with families and communities evolved (Burger, 2014). *Charity Organization Societies (COSs)* had volunteers visiting the poor to assist in alleviating conditions of poverty. These *friendly visitors* would often spend years assisting one family by helping to educate the children, giving advice and moral support, and providing necessities. At about the same time, the *settlement movement*, which had staff who lived in the poorer communities, began to develop (Leiby, 1978). These idealistic staff believed in community action and tried to persuade politicians to provide better services for the poor. One of the best-known settlement houses was Hull House, established by social activist Jane Addams (1860–1935) in 1889 in Chicago (Addams, 1910/2012). Out of involvement with the underprivileged, articles and books appeared that were concerned with finding methods of meeting the needs of the poor and how to work with destitute families within the larger social system. Here, we see the beginnings of *social casework* and one of the first times that the "system" is acknowledged as an important component to consider when helping individuals and families overcome their difficulties.

Paralleling the work of early social workers was the psychotherapeutic approach of Alfred Adler, who believed that external forces greatly affected personality development and that through education, one could help to alleviate problems. In fact, Adler's approach to working with children is often cited as an early precursor to family therapy models (Goldenberg & Goldenberg, 2013; Sherman, 1999). At Adler's child guidance clinics, parents would often meet with therapists to discuss problems with their children, although generally the parents and children were not in the same room together (Bottome, 1957). This family counseling approach, for the first time, had counselors suggesting that problems with one family member had a significant effect on the whole family.

Despite these early efforts at working with families, because psychoanalysis and other individual-oriented approaches were firmly embedded as the treatments of choice for counselors and psychotherapists, there was little room for novel therapeutic approaches to take hold (McAdams, 2015). Thus, until the late 1940s and early 1950s, counselors who saw value in working with the whole family often felt pressure to see the "patient" separately from the family. Soon, however, this new approach to psychotherapy began to take shape.

> [At first, s]ome hospitals had a therapist to deal with the carefully protected intrapsychic process, another psychiatrist to handle the reality matters and administrative procedures, and a social worker to talk to relatives. In those years this principle was a cornerstone of good psychotherapy. Failure to observe the principle was considered inept psychotherapy. Finally, it became acceptable to see families together in the context of research.
>
> (Bowen, 1985, p. 287)

As increasing numbers of therapists believed it was useful to see the "whole" family together, a variety of approaches to family counseling developed during the 1950s

(McAdams, 2015). Although some of these evolved independently, there was a core group of early therapists and family therapists who influenced one another and whose training often overlapped (see Bitter, 2014).

Although treating the whole family slowly became accepted, the continued popularity of psychoanalysis influenced many of the early pioneers of couples and family counseling, and it was common for early family approaches to combine systems theory with basic psychoanalytic principles. Probably the best-known of these was developed by Nathan Ackerman (1958, 1966), a child psychiatrist. Another psychoanalytically trained therapist, Ivan Boszormenyi-Nagy (1973, 1987), stressed the importance of ethical relationships in families and highlighted the notion that one's sense of fairness and loyalties are unconsciously passed down through generations and create a specific view of the world that may, or may not, match the view of one's partner or spouse. Establishing the Eastern Pennsylvania Psychiatric Institute (EPPI), Boszormenyi-Nagy's *contextual family therapy* sometimes would include grandparents and other significant individuals when examining these cross-generational issues, with the goal of helping families develop healthier and more loving ways of communicating. At around the same time, Murray Bowen (1976, 1978) developed what some would later call *multigenerational family counseling*. Working initially at the Menninger Clinic in Kansas and later at the National Institute of Mental Health (NIMH) in Washington, D.C., Bowen was interested in understanding the communication of families in which one member was schizophrenic. Working with all members of a family, one member at a time, his experiences with these families, and later with families struggling with "normal" problems, resulted in new ideas about how family dysfunction is passed on through generations.

The group that was to have the most profound influence on the evolution of couples and family counseling was led by an anthropologist named Gregory Bateson in Palo Alto, California (Bitter, 2014; Mental Research Institute, 2008). Fascinated by human communication, in the early 1950s Bateson hired Jay Haley (1997–2014), John Weakland, Don Jackson, and William Fry to look at how individuals communicate in systems, particularly families who had schizophrenic members. Their *double-bind theory* attempted to explain how schizophrenics are often caught in a web of mixed messages from family members who hold power. Applying principles of *general systems theory* and *cybernetics* to help understand family communication, their ideas fueled the manner in which a generation of couples and family counselors would work and continue to influence them today. Out of this project came the Mental Research Institute (MRI) at Palo Alto. Led by Jackson, and joined by Haley, Virginia Satir (Banmen, 2015), and later Cloé Madanes (2015a), this group focused on communication and family process. Satir's work at MRI, an earlier collaboration with Bowen, and influences from humanistic psychology eventually led to the development of her *human validation process model*, which focused upon communication and self-esteem in couples and families (Satir, 1967, 1972a, 1972b). Meanwhile, Haley (1973, 1976, 1997–2014) and Madanes (1981) would take a different route. Concentrating mostly on making strategic behavioral changes, their *strategic therapy* became one of the most popular and intriguing approaches to couples and family counseling.

At around the same time that the Palo Alto group was formulating their ideas, Carl Whitaker started to become popular. Influenced by individuals as varied as Gregory

Bateson, Carl Jung, psychoanalyst Melanie Klein, and Buddhist philosopher Alan Watts, Whitaker was unconventional and willing to freely experiment with his responses during sessions (Keith, 2015; Napier & Whitaker, 1972, 1978; Whitaker, 1976). With the concurrent spread of humanistic psychology during the 1950s and 1960s, his *experiential approach* to couples and family work evolved at this time.

Influenced by his work with families in Israel, low-income and minority families in New York City, and the work of Bateson and others at Palo Alto, Salvador Minuchin (1974, 1981; Colapinto, 2015) developed one of the most widely respected approaches to couples and family counseling during the 1960s. An Argentine-born psychiatrist, Minuchin became known for his work with minorities and the poor at the Philadelphia Child Guidance Clinic, where he applied his *structural family therapy* approach, which demonstrated how family problems are related to problems in family structure. Eventually, Haley joined Minuchin, and the two shared their ideas on working with families. It is also here that Jay Haley and Cloé Madanes met and eventually married.

In 1966, the Brief Family Therapy Center (BFTC) was established within MRI. Led by Paul Watzlawick, Dick Fisch, and John Weakland, BFTC focused solely on helping families solve their problems, as opposed to spending an inordinate amount of time on "underlying" issues, communication sequences, or systemic patterns (Cade, 2007; Goldenberg & Goldenberg, 2013). These individuals realized that the solutions families tried generally resulted in further entrenching the problem. Approaching couples and families with an attitude of experimentation, the therapists were highly active, and they felt free to use any method that was ethical and legal to solve problems or lessen presenting symptoms. Steve de Shazer (1982) and Insoo Kim Berg (1994) (Pichot, 2015), both of whom did postgraduate studies at BFTC, later became two leading figures in the development of *solution-focused family therapy*.

Intrigued by Bateson and inspired by the work of Haley, the early 1970s saw an Italian group, known as the *Milan Group,* become popular (Cazzaniga & Schinco, 2015; Palazzoli, Boscolo, Cecchin, & Prata, 1978). With Watzlawick from BFTC as their consultant, this group borrowed many ideas from Bateson's original work and were also influenced by the work of cognitive and constructivist therapists, who believed that language usage is critical to making meaning and how one comes to make sense of one's family.

With the expansion of behavioral and cognitive approaches to individual therapy in the latter part of the twentieth century, we concomitantly saw these philosophies applied with couples and families. Finally, with what has come to be known as the *postmodern* movement, we have seen the recent rise of what is called *narrative family therapy*. Influenced by Michael White and David Epston (Madigan, 2015; White, 1995; White & Epston, 1990), this approach attempts to understand a couple's or family's narrative, or story, and helps them to *deconstruct* problem-saturated stories and then reconstruct how the couple or family comes to understand itself.

In recent years, the field of couples and family counseling has taken off, with 50 states having licensure for marriage and family counseling, according to the *American Association of Marriage and Family Therapy* (AAMFT, 2002–2013a; 2002–2013b). Today, AAMFT and the *International Association for Marriage and Family Counselors (IAMFC),* a division of the *American Counseling Association (ACA),* are the two main couples and family therapy associations in the country. These associations, along with their respective accreditation bodies that include the *Commission on Accreditation of Marriage and Family Therapy Education (COAMFTE)* and the *Council for the Accreditation of Counseling and Related Educational Programs (CACREP)*, lead the field in setting standards for accreditation, make recommendations to state licensing boards, define best practices and ethical standards, and help to set credentialing requirements in the field of couples and family therapy. Today, some training in couples and family counseling is commonplace in almost all programs that train helpers.

View of Human Nature

Because couples and family counselors can have any of a number of theoretical orientations, their views of human nature can vary dramatically. For instance, a couples or family counselor can be psychodynamically oriented, believing that the unconscious plays an important role in one's life *and* affects the couple or family; behaviorally focused, viewing the individual as conditioned by his or her environment (including a partner and a family); existential–humanistically oriented, seeing the individual and the family as having a growth force that can be actualized; or have leanings toward social constructionism, believing that there is no one reality and that individuals construct their sense of meaning from language used in the social milieu. Despite these differences, most (but not necessarily all!) couples and family counselors share a number of assumptions that are integrated into their theoretical orientations (Barker & Chang, 2013; Turner & West, 2013):

1. The interactional forces between couples and in families are complex and cannot be explained in a simple, causal fashion.
2. Couples and families have overt and covert rules that govern their functioning.
3. How a couple complements each other and the hierarchy in a family (e.g., who's "in charge"; who makes the rules) can help one understand the makeup and communication sequences of couples and of families.
4. Comprehension of the boundaries and subsystems (e.g., spousal, sibling) of couples or families can help one understand the makeup and communication sequences of a couple and of a family.
5. Whether boundaries are rigid, diffuse, or semipermeable impacts how information flows in and out of couples and families and can help one make sense of how communication and change occur in couples and in families.
6. Communication in couples and families is complex, and understanding how couples and family members communicate verbally and nonverbally can give insight into how couples and families maintain their way of functioning.
7. Each couple and family has its own unique homeostasis that describes how its members typically interact. This homeostasis is not "bad" or "good"; it simply is. Change occurs by changing the homeostasis, or the usual patterns in the couple and in the family.
8. Language used by couples, families, one's culture, and in society affect one's sense of self and how individuals, couples, and families come to define themselves.

9. Stress from expected developmental milestones (marriage, birth of a child, etc.) can wreak havoc on an individual, couple, and family, and counselors should be aware of the particular issues involved in developmental crises.

10. All couples will face unexpected stressors in life, and couples and family counselors should have the tools to help couples and families deal with such stressors.

11. In some manner, the past influences personality development and how individuals relate to one another. In solving problems, some couples and family counselors will focus on the past, while others believe that such a focus detracts from dealing with current conflicts and focusing on future goals.

12. Cultural values and beliefs affect every family in conscious and unconscious ways.

Key Concepts

The assumptions listed in the previous section are an outgrowth of a number of ideas that have been generated over the years and will be expanded upon in this section. They include the following concepts: *general systems theory, cybernetics, boundaries and information flow, rules and hierarchy, communication theory, scapegoating and identified patients (IPs), stress, developmental issues,* and *social constructionism.*

General Systems Theory

> *General systems theory is a series of related definitions, assumptions, and postulates about all levels of systems from atomic particles through atoms, molecules, crystals, viruses, cells, organs, individuals, small groups, societies, planets, solar systems, and galaxies.*
>
> (Miller, 1956, p. 120)

Although knowledge of the amoeba and of the universe may seem like a far cry from helping us understand couples and families, in actuality they all have something in common: They obey the rules of a system. The amoeba has a *semipermeable boundary* that allows it to take in nutrition from the environment. This delicate animal could not survive if its boundaries were so rigid that they prevented it from ingesting food, or so diffuse that they would not allow it to retain and digest the food. So long as the amoeba is in balance, it will maintain its existence.

The universe is an exceedingly predictable place, and it has a certain cadence to it. It maintains a persistent structure over a long period of time. However, remove a star, planet, moon, or asteroid, and the system is shaken, momentarily disequilibrated as it moves to reconfigure itself. So long as the universe is in balance, it will maintain its existence. Like the amoeba and the universe, what occurs in couples and families is predictable because they too have boundaries and structure that maintain themselves over long periods of time. So long as the couple and family system is in balance, it will maintain its existence.

General systems theory (von Bertalanffy, 1934, 1968) was developed to explain the complex interactions of all types of systems, including living systems, family systems, community systems, and solar systems. Each system had a boundary that allows it to maintain its structure while the system interacts with other systems around it. As such, the action of the amoeba, one of the smallest of all living systems, affects and is affected by surrounding *suprasystems*, while the universe, the largest of all systems, is made up of *subsystems* that have predictable relationships to one another. Similarly, the action of subsystems in families will affect other subsystems (e.g., the parental subsystem will affect the child subsystem); couples and family units will affect other couples and families; couples and families make up communities that affect society; and so on.

Cybernetics

The study of *cybernetics*, or control mechanisms in systems, has been used to explain the regulatory process of a system (Becvar & Becvar, 2013). The distinctive manner that each system has to maintain its stability is called its *homeostasis*. One type of cybernetic system of which we are all aware is the thermostat. As it becomes colder, the temperature drops, and the thermostat turns on the heating system; as the temperature goes up, the thermostat shuts down the heat. This type of cybernetic system is called a *negative feedback loop* because it keeps the irregularities within the system at a minimum. *Positive feedback loops* are when a change in one component in a system leads to a change in another component within the same system, which leads to a change in the first component, and so forth, eventually leading to a changed system. On the relationship level, cybernetics explains how couples and families maintain their unique ways of regulating themselves (negative feedback loops) or periodically change by employing a positive feedback loop. Negative feedback loops are good if they maintain healthy behaviors in couples and in families (good communication, good feelings, etc.). However, negative feedback loops sometimes will be responsible for the maintenance of dysfunctional behaviors (lack of communication, negative feelings; see Box 6.1).

Because positive feedback loops lead to change, they can be employed by counselors to shake up the system. Typically, what would occur is that a counselor will introduce new information to the couple and family, which will change the way they communicate. Such information can be given verbally, nonverbally, metaphorically, paradoxically, directly, or indirectly. However it is given, the information can be the impetus for shaking up the system and having it move toward healthier ways of communicating. In fact, couples and family counselors will often encourage the *disequilibration* of the "safe" yet unhealthy ways of relating that can be found in some negative feedback loops, such as the one in Box 6.1, so that the couple or family can experiment with new ways of relating. Each couple and family has its unique way of interacting, which includes negative and sometimes positive feedback loop systems. If you examine communication sequences in any couple and family, you can begin to understand the unique boundaries, feedback loops, and homeostatic mechanisms involved.

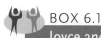

BOX 6.1
Joyce and Antonio: A Positive Feedback Loop

In the dialogue below, Joyce and Antonio are discussing going out to a play. As they realize that their expectations about the evening differ, they begin to get angry at each other. Eventually, there is an altercation, at which point Antonio defuses the situation by leaving. This "typical" pattern of relating is an example of a negative feedback loop and communication pattern that Joyce and Antonio typically take part in. There are many ways in which a counselor might introduce new information to create a positive feedback loop and a new, healthier way of communicating. Can you come up with any?

Joyce: Are you going to the play with me tonight?

Antonio: Well, I was actually thinking I might go out with my friends. You know, I haven't really seen them for a while. Besides, I didn't really think that I committed myself to the play.

Joyce: Well, you did say you thought you would go with me.

Antonio: I don't remember saying that. I was thinking all along that I would go out with my buddies.

Joyce: I remember distinctly you telling me you would go. It's clear as day to me. You're either lying or have early dementia.

Antonio: Look, I don't want to get into a fight. You're always forcing me to get into a fight with you. I don't know why you egg me on like this. You must have a need to fight with me. I bet it has to do with the fact that you never felt loved by your father—you know, we've talked about that before.

Joyce: Not being loved by my father! Who are you kidding? The only one I don't feel loved by is you. At least my father was around. You just take off whenever you damn please! Half of the time you leave me with the kids, as if you have no responsibility around here. You just go out, get blasted and God knows what else.

Antonio: Look, I'm no slacker around here. You don't do a damn thing around this house. Look at it. It's a mess. I do plenty, and you can't even keep this house together. I work hard to fix this place up, and you can't even run a vacuum once in a while. You . . . it's disgusting!

Joyce: Don't call me disgusting!

Antonio: I didn't! I said it's disgusting—the house.

Joyce: No, I heard you, you were going to say I'm disgusting. I hate you! You and your drinking, you and your friends. You and those sluts you hang out with at work. I know what you're doing behind my back!

Antonio: Screw you!

Joyce: Go to hell! (Swings at him.)

Antonio: (Grabs her arm as she swings and throws her on the floor.)

Joyce: You abusive bastard!

Antonio: Screw you. . . . I'm getting out of here. (Leaves the house.)

Joyce: (Sobs as Antonio leaves.)

Boundaries and Information Flow

A healthy system has *semipermeable boundaries* that allow information to come into the system, be processed, and incorporated. When a system has *rigid boundaries*, information is not able to easily flow into or out of the system, and change becomes a difficult process. Alternatively, a system that has *diffuse boundaries* allows information to flow too easily into and out of the system, causing the individual components of the system to have difficulty maintaining a sense of identity and stability (Nichols & Schwartz, 2014; Turner & West, 2013). Rigid boundaries will often lead to disengagement on the part of family members and a heightened sense of autonomy. In extreme cases, such families will have family secrets (e.g., child abuse), with their rigid boundaries maintaining the secret within the family. Diffuse boundaries, on the other hand, often lead to lack of a sense of self, enmeshment, and dependence on one another.

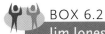

BOX 6.2
Jim Jones and the Death of a Rigid System

During the 1950s and early 1960s, Jim Jones was a respected minister in Indiana. However, over the years, he became increasingly paranoid and grandiose, believing he was Jesus. He moved his family to Brazil and later relocated to California, where approximately 100 of his church followers from Indiana joined him. In California, he headed the "People's Church" and began to set rigid rules for church membership. Slowly, he became more dictatorial and continued to show evidence of paranoid delusions. Insisting that church members prove their love for him, he demanded sex with female church members, had members sign over their possessions, sometimes had members give their children over to him, and had members inform on those who went against his rules. In 1975, a reporter uncovered some of the tactics Jones was using and was about to write a revealing article about the church. Jones learned about this and, just prior to publication of the article, moved to Guyana, taking a few hundred of his followers with him. As concerns about some of the church practices reached the

United States, California congressman Leo Ryan and some of his aides went to Guyana to investigate the situation. Jones and his supporters killed Ryan and the aides, and Jones then ordered his followers to commit suicide. Hundreds killed themselves. Those who did not were murdered.

Jim Jones had developed a church with an extremely rigid set of rules. The writing of a revealing article, as well as the congressman's flying into Guyana, were perceived as threats to the system. As with many rigid systems, attempts at change from the outside were seen as potentially lethal blows to the system. Jones dealt with the reporter's threat to the system by moving his congregation to Guyana. Then, rather than allow new information into the system, Jim Jones killed off the system, first killing the congressman and then ordering the church members to commit suicide. The members had become so mired in the rules of the system that nearly 900 of them ended up committing suicide or being murdered. (Axthelm, 1978)

American culture allows for much variation in the permeability of various systems, but systems that have boundaries that are too diffuse or too rigid tend toward dysfunction. In the United States, it is common to find couples, families, and community groups (e.g., some religious organizations) with a fairly rigid set of rules that maintain their functioning in relatively healthy ways. Alternatively, we may also find couples, families, and community groups that allow for a wide range of behaviors within a fairly diffuse system (e.g., communes). Unfortunately, all too often, we have seen the dysfunction that results from a system whose boundaries are too rigid or too diffuse (see Box 6.2).

Rules and Hierarchy

Families have universal and idiosyncratic rules, which can be overt or covert and are partly responsible for determining the nature of the couple or family. *Universal rules* are those rules that all couples and families tend to follow and are often related to hierarchical structure. For instance, almost all cultures have a hierarchy in which parents, guardians, or an older "wise" person is on a higher level of authority than children. Not following this rule has a consequence, although the kinds of consequences will vary as a function of the culture. *Idiosyncratic rules* are unique to the family. For instance, a family might have a rule that whenever there is tension in the couple's relationship, the youngest child is yelled at for doing something wrong. In a situation such as this, it is likely that the child is being *scapegoated* in an effort to diffuse tension between the couple. There are an infinite number of idiosyncratic rules, and they usually happen in an automatic manner.

Communication Theory

Understanding the complexities of human communication helps counselors recognize the unique characteristics of couples and families and is often the first step toward developing a plan for change. Some of the principles of communication highlighted in the early 1970s by Watzlawick and others at Palo Alto greatly changed the way that couples and family counselors view their clients and are listed below (cf. Watzlawick, Beavin, & Jackson, 1967; Watzlawick, Weakland, & Fisch, 1974):

1. "Normal" or "abnormal" is a contextual phenomenon, not an objective state of being.
2. Behaviors tell a story about communication between people and are often more a sign of what's going on than the actual words that are communicated.
3. One cannot *not* communicate. Not saying anything is a communication about the relationship.
4. A message sent is not necessarily the message received. A person might send one message, but a different message might be heard.
5. Communication has two ways of expression: *digitally*, or the exact meaning of the words; and *analogically*, or the meaning about the meaning, often expressed nonverbally. For example, a person may be angry and say, "I love you" in an angry tone. The digital message "I love you" is at odds with the analogical message.
6. Communication makes a statement about the content of the conversation and about the relationship that one is in. In other words, each statement that a person makes is an expression about the relationship.
7. A series of communications gives important meanings about the relationship (e.g., a husband might always discuss issues with a flat affect to his wife; this continual flat message may be more important than the actual words he says).
8. Any intervention made within the system, be it with one or more of the family members, will reverberate throughout the system.
9. The unconscious is not an important factor in working with individuals; instead, what is important are the current behaviors that people are exhibiting.
10. The *whys* are not as important as *what* is going on between people.

Scapegoating and Identified Patients

All couples bring unfinished business to their relationship. The more serious the issues, the more likely they will affect their relationship and others in the family. For instance, a wife who was sexually molested as a child, and as a result feels mistrust toward men, may choose a man who is emotionally distant (and safe). Perhaps he is a workaholic. Alternatively, a man who has fears of intimacy might choose a wife who allows him to be distant (and safe). Perhaps she was sexually molested and distrusts men. As the relationship unravels, issues that each spouse brings to the marriage are played out on one another or on the children. The emotionally distant workaholic husband may become stressed at work, irritable, and nasty toward his wife, children, or both. The distrustful wife may become discontented with her marriage due to its lack of intimacy and subsequently become depressed and unresponsive toward her husband and children. (Is it surprising that there are so many affairs and divorces?)

When family members are discontented with one another, and when they directly or indirectly take out this unhappiness on a specific family member, that member is said to have been *scapegoated* (Nichols & Schwartz, 2014). Sometimes, when a family member is scapegoated, that person takes on the role of *identified patient* (IP), or the family member who is believed to have the problem. System theorists, however, view the whole family as having the problem. For instance, when a child acts out in the family, in school, or in the community, couples and family counselors will typically view that child as the family member who is carrying the pain for the family. Why is someone in a family scapegoated? Usually, it is because it has become too difficult for the couple to look at some other, more painful issue (Kirst-Ashman & Hull, 2015). Rather than sharing their concerns within the family or seeking marital counseling, the couple scapegoats a member of the family, often a child.

Psychotherapy, particularly marital psychotherapy, threatens to "uncover" the anxious turmoil in the marriage. "If we seek help as a couple," the partners say silently to themselves, "it will all come out." The anger, the bitterness, the hurt, the sense of self-blame that each carries—this will be the harvest of the opening up to each other. "Maybe it will destroy what we have" is their fear. They dread not only losing the stability of the marriage, but damaging their fragile self-images. Rather than risk their painful and tenuous security, they suppress the possibility of working on their marriage together.

(Napier & Whitaker, 1978, p. 148)

Stress

Living is stressful, and at some point in the life of the couple or family, it will be faced with mild to burdensome stress. Families with semipermeable boundaries, clearly defined subsystems and suprasystems, little scapegoating, good communication skills, and a healthy hierarchical structure will have an easier time managing stress (see Box 6.3). On the other hand, families with ill-defined boundaries and poor communication skills will tend to blame others for their problems, fail to take responsibility for their feelings and actions, and have a difficult time dealing with stress. Minuchin (1974) identified four types of stress with which families typically struggle at some point in their development:

➤ *Stressful contact of one member with extrafamilial forces* (e.g., difficulty at work)
➤ *Stressful contact of the whole family with extrafamilial forces* (e.g., a natural disaster such as a hurricane)
➤ *Stress at transitional or developmental points in the family* (e.g., puberty, midlife crises, retirement, aging)
➤ *Idiosyncratic (situational) stress* (e.g., unexpected illness)

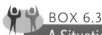

BOX 6.3
A Situational Family Crisis

When I was between the ages of 8 and 13, I had a heart disorder called pericarditis. This was a somewhat debilitating illness that enlarged my heart, caused me much chest pain, and left me periodically bedridden, with a resulting mild depression. Although not considered extremely serious, this illness certainly affected my life in a major way. However, it also affected my parents' lives and the lives of my siblings.

Although my illness potentially could have been a threat to the homeostasis in my family, it became clear that the family was healthy enough to deal effectively with this situation. As my parents' marriage was solid, the added stress did not dramatically affect their relationship. In addition, they were able to maintain the functioning of the family in a relatively normal way. This normalization of family patterns during a period of stress speaks highly of the health in the family.

Developmental Issues

All couples and families face fairly predictable developmental milestones that will result in some amount of stress, as the issues faced within each milestone impact the individual differentially (Becvar & Becvar, 2013; Turner & West, 2013). How couples and families face these developmental issues has a lot to do with their innate ability to handle stress, whether their values are more or less in agreement, and their ability to effectively communicate with one another. For example, review the stages in Table 6.1 and consider how each of the issues listed may be handled by different couples and families. Perhaps you might share how your family of origin seemed to handle these issues. Also consider what stages a childless couple might face.

One function of the couples and family counselor is to be aware of potential *developmental crises* that may affect couples and families and understand how a specific couple or family may tend to respond to stress that results from these normal developmental stages. Helping couples prepare for and respond to stressful situations caused by developmental milestones is an important role of the couples and family counselor.

Social Constructionism

The addition of social construction to systems theory, then, helps address the criticism that systems theory focuses too much on stability, ignores cultural context, and operates as though the research can find objective truth.

(Turner & West, 2013, p. 77)

In recent years, some couples and family counselors have shifted their understanding of how couples and families are formed and make sense of themselves (Tomm, 1998; Turner & West, 2013). Having a *social constructionist* philosophy, these counselors believe that systems theory (and its close cousin, cybernetics) placed too much emphasis on causal factors and did not stress cultural context enough. The social constructionists suggested that earlier couples and family counselors tended to see themselves as experts and objective observers who make interventions to the couple or family. In contrast, the social constructionists focus on the ongoing, changing manner in which

TABLE 6.1

STAGE	ISSUES TO BE CONFRONTED
Coupling with partner	➤ Differences in values ➤ Inclusion of in-laws ➤ Economic concerns related to career paths ➤ Power differentials ➤ Settling into career ➤ Learning how to commit
Having children	➤ Differing parenting styles ➤ Transmission of values ➤ Time commitment ➤ Economic concerns and its impact on playtime for spousal relationship ➤ Infringement on intimacy ➤ Adjustment to new system ➤ Sibling eivalry
Children reaching adolescence	➤ Emotional changes in children ➤ "Holding" children, yet learning how to let them become independent ➤ Mid-life crises as parents grow older ➤ Dealing with extended family issues (boundary issues, health issues) ➤ Settling into career or career-switching
Children leaving home (work/career/college)	➤ Empty nest syndrome can yield depression or anxiety ➤ Learning how to again be intimate with partner ➤ Economic concerns for children and their impact on spousal relationship (i.e., Do we have enough money?) ➤ Existential concerns: What is life about? ➤ Caring for elderly parents ➤ Considering retirement
Late career/retirement	➤ Economic concerns ➤ Reflection on whether life has been fulfilling ➤ Redefining self as one retires ➤ New social network as one leaves the workplace ➤ Health concerns and their impact on the family ➤ Adjusting death of parents , other relatives, and friends

couples and family members come to understand themselves. They believe that couples and families continually co-construct (construct together through ongoing dialogue and nonverbal interactions) their understanding of who they are, and that this construction is a function of the language used by the couple or family, and beliefs from their culture and society. Change occurs, therefore, by the counselor exploring, in a respectful way, how the couple or family co-constructs a sense of meaning for themselves. Then, through the use of thoughtful and respectful questioning, social constructionists believe that they and the couple or family can co-construct a new language that is positive and focuses on solutions. Although many couples and family counselors today integrate this perspective into their existing systems framework

(Becvar & Becvar, 2013), others, such as the narrative and solution-focused purists, question these earlier theories (e.g., systems theory, communication theory) and discard them due to their belief in the importance of how language defines the person, the couple, and the family.

Models of Couples and Family Therapy

The key concepts just discussed drive the various approaches to couples and family counseling. Because some approaches adhere more to certain concepts than others, as you read the theories, reflect on which key concepts tend to drive a particular theory. With many theories of couples and family counseling to choose among, included in this chapter are the most popular ones, as well as those that are most associated with some of the major players in the history of couples and family therapy. The theories that this chapter looks at include the human validation process model, structural family therapy, strategic family therapy, multigenerational approaches, experiential family therapy, psychodynamic family therapy, cognitive–behavioral family counseling, narrative family therapy, and solution-focused family therapy.

Human Validation Process Model

> *All of the ingredients in a family that count are changeable and correctable—individual self-worth, communication, system, and rules—at any point in time.*

> (Satir, 1972a, p. xi)

Considered one of the pioneers of couples and family therapy, Virginia Satir's *human validation process model*, which has also been called a *communication theory* and a *change process model*, integrates many ideas from family systems theory and communication theory, while adding a sense of caring and a focus on self-esteem that is emphasized by the existential–humanistic approaches (Satir, 1972b).

Satir believed that a *primary survival triad* exists that includes parents and the child, with each child's sense of well-being and self-esteem the result of this triad. Individuals with low self-esteem yield one of four unhealthy universal communication patterns: (1) *the placater*, who appeases people so that others won't get angry at him or her; (2) *the blamer*, who accuses others in an effort to diffuse hurt; (3) *the computer*, who acts cool, calm, and collected in an attempt to deal with the world as if nothing could hurt him or her; and (4) *the distracter*, who goes off on tangents in an effort to treat threats as if they do not exist (Satir, 1972a). On the other hand, Satir also believed that children who had healthy parenting would grow into congruent adults who were in sync with their feelings, thoughts, and behaviors and could communicate clearly with others.

Believing that communication and behavioral patterns are a result of complex interactions among family members and the legacy from past generations, Satir felt it was important to obtain graphic information about important past events in one's family. Thus, she would often have families complete

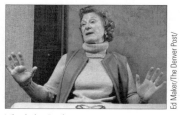

Virginia Satir

Ed Maker/The Denver Post/ Getty Images

a *family life fact chronology*, which is a history of important events within the extended family. Similar to a genogram, the family life fact chronology could be analyzed and reflected upon by all involved in therapy. Additionally, Satir was one of the first therapists to use *family sculpting* in an effort to bring forth blocked and unexpressed emotions (Piercy, Sprenkle, & Wetchler, 1996). This experiential work involves each family member taking a physical position that nonverbally represents how that member interacts with the rest of the family. For instance, a child who is withdrawing might stand near a door as if she were about to leave the room; a mother trying to control her son might stand over him with her finger pointed at him; and a father who is detached through drinking might sit at a table with a make-believe glass of beer in his hand.

Satir believed that a couples and family counselor should be caring and respectful, believe in the ability of the couple or family to heal, actively encourage the couple or family to change, be spontaneous, and act "as a facilitator, a resource person, an observer, a detective, and a model for effective communication" (Becvar & Becvar, 2013, p. 203). By creating a trusting atmosphere that encouraged the letting-down of defenses, Satir hoped to open up communication patterns, look at past hurts, and help clients learn how to be more effective and open communicators. Ultimately, through this process, she hoped that individuals in couples and families could have mature relationships in which each person could:

- ➤ Be responsible for oneself and have a strong sense of self
- ➤ Make decisions based on an accurate perception of self, others, and the social context
- ➤ Be able to make wise choices for which one takes full responsibility
- ➤ Be in touch with one's feelings
- ➤ Be clear in one's communication
- ➤ Be able to accept others for who they are
- ➤ See differences in others as an opportunity to learn, not as a threat (adapted from Satir, 1967, p. 91)

Structural Family Therapy

Although many well-known family therapists see themselves in the *structural school*, certainly the most renowned is Salvador Minuchin (1921–). Minuchin (1974, 1981) states that all families have *interactional* and *transactional rules* that are maintained by the kinds of boundaries in the family, as noted through the structure and hierarchy that exists. He also asserts that all couples and families experience stress, which is handled differently as a function of the existing rules, boundaries, structure, and hierarchy in the couple or family. In order to make change, structural family counselors join with the family, map the family, and provide interventions for restructuring.

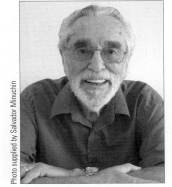

Salvador Minuchin

Joining

Joining is when the counselor is accepted by the family and wins its confidence. Similar to building a working alliance as described in Chapter 1, joining can be done in many ways, such as through empathy, being friendly, or sharing common stories with the family. Joining the family allows the counselor to understand the family's rules, boundaries, structure and hierarchy, and stress. It is only then that the counselor can begin the process of mapping and later restructuring the family.

Mapping

Mapping a family can be done formally or informally, and it involves an examination of how the family communicates, who is in charge, rules used in the family to maintain its homeostasis, and an understanding of the structure and hierarchy of the family. Mapping is the first step toward restructuring, as the counselor cannot facilitate change unless he or she understands the current way in which the family relates.

Restructuring

Restructuring the family occurs after the counselor has joined the family and mapped its structure. It involves creating healthier boundaries and changing structure and hierarchy in order to help the family deal with stress and function in a healthier manner. Restructuring can occur in numerous ways. Box 6.4 shows the restructuring of one family.

Structural family therapy is a deliberate and purposeful approach to working with families; it relies on many of the basic principles discussed in the section "Key Concepts" earlier in this chapter. Many family therapists who are first starting out are trained in this approach, as it helps the therapist view the family from a systemic perspective.

Strategic Family Therapy

The steps involved in *strategic therapy,* whether it be individual therapy or couples and family therapy (i.e., strategic family therapy), are based on an understanding of communication and systems theory. Also, because unconscious motivations play little if any role in this type of therapy, the approach is relatively pragmatic. Relative to the therapeutic process, the strategic approach is not particularly concerned with feelings (although the therapist wants the client to end up having good feelings!). This approach is based on how individuals communicate with one another, how communication sequences can be changed to help people feel better, and how power is dispersed in the family. Power for the strategic therapist is defined in some very nontraditional ways:

> *Power tactics are those maneuvers a person uses to give himself influence and control over his social world and to make that world more predictable. Defined thus broadly, a man has power if he can order someone to behave in a certain way, but he also has power if he can provoke someone to behave that way. One man can order others to lift and carry him while another might achieve the same end by collapsing.*

(Haley, 1986, p. 53)

The therapist most associated with the strategic approach has been Jay Haley (1923–2007), although others, like Cloé Madanes (1945–) and the Milan Group,

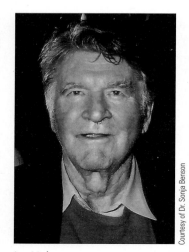

Courtesy of Dr. Sonja Benson

Jay Haley

BOX 6.4
An Example of Family Restructuring

Mom and Dad have three children, aged 15, 12, and 1. Since the birth of their new child, the two oldest children have been fighting constantly and having problems at school. The husband and wife seem depressed. Assessing the situation, you find that the whole family is dealing with transitional and idiosyncratic stress. The baby was not planned, and the family is stretched financially. The therapist notes that the family hierarchy has changed, that the spousal subsystem is showing depression, and that the parental subsystem is not able to maintain control over the two older children. The therapist wants to strengthen the spousal and parental subsystems. The current map of the family is shown below.

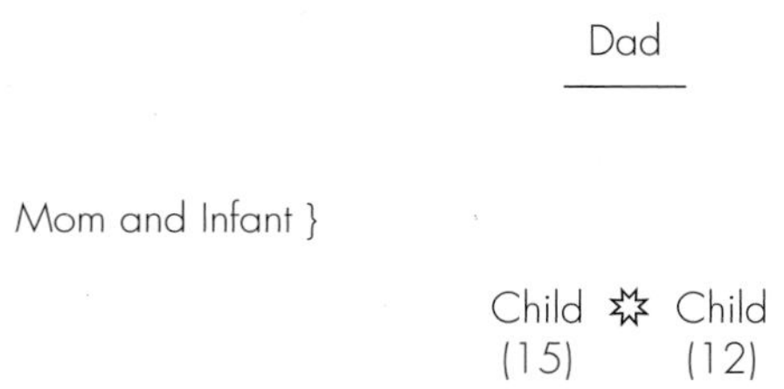
Dad
Mom and Infant }
Child
(15)
Child
(12)

Legend

} = Cutoff

——— = Rigid boundary

✵ = Conflict

- - - - = Permeable boundary

↘ ↕ = Temporarily in other subsystem

The family therapist prescribes the following actions:

- Have the oldest child take a certification course in babysitting to assist with child care.
- Ask the grandmother to assist with child care to relieve some pressure on Mom.
- Have Dad take on some of the responsibilities related to the problems with the oldest children. He must meet with the teachers and school counselors.
- Suggest that Mom, who now has assistance with child care, take on a part-time job to relieve some of the economic stress (she has always worked in the past).
- Establish one evening a week when the grandmother or oldest child will watch the other two children so the parents can go out.

The goal is to reestablish the spousal subsystem while strengthening the parental subsystem. The grandmother and oldest child will periodically take on a position of power in the family, with their power being time-limited. The extra money and reduction of stress for Mom will result in reduced stress in the family. The family map eventually looks like the following diagram:

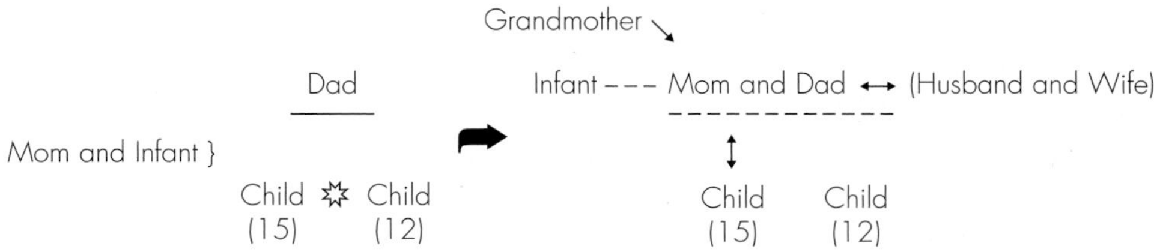
Grandmother
Dad
Mom and Infant }
Child
(15)
Child
(12)
Infant
Mom and Dad
(Husband and Wife)
Child
(15)
Child
(12)

have also become well known. Haley was greatly affected by Milton Erickson (1901-1980), a legend as a therapist because of his uncanny ability to induce change in clients. In Haley's 1976 book, *Problem-Solving Therapy*, he describes four stages of the first interview that lay the groundwork for the change process. Although unique to the way Haley implements strategic therapy, these stages provide a picture of how all strategic family therapists work.

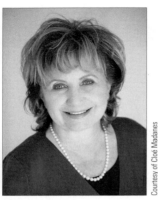

Cloe Madanes

Courtesy of Cloé Madanes

Haley's Stages of the First Interview

1. *The social stage.* This initial stage has the counselor inviting the couple or family to counseling and asking each member to introduce himself or herself. At this point, the counselor can observe where individuals sit, the interactions of couple and family members, and the overall mood of the couple or family. During this stage, the counselor should not share his or her observations with the couple or family, and all formulations about them should be tentative.

2. *The problem stage.* During the problem stage, each couple or family member is asked to describe his or her perceptions of the problem. The therapist should listen carefully, as the problem is often defined differently. Interactions among couple or family members should be carefully observed, and counselor interpretations about the problem should not be shared. Discussion of the problem is important, as the discussion gives the counselor insight into how the couple and family communicates and the hierarchies of the family.

3. *The interaction stage.* The interaction stage is highlighted by the therapist's attempt to get the couple or family to interact during the session in the same manner as would happen at home. This process assists the counselor in viewing how the couple or family is organized around the problem.

4. *Goal-setting stage.* During this stage, the couple or family is asked to clearly define what they would like to change, and, in collaboration with the counselor, they agree upon a problem. However, how the problem gets addressed can vary dramatically (Haley, 1973, 1976). Remember that the focus is on having people change the way they communicate so they will feel better, and sometimes what the couple or family thinks they *should* do will actually make the problem worse. For example, a wife might suggest that a husband does not communicate with her. The husband agrees. However, whenever the couple tries to communicate, they end up in an argument. Thus, instead of suggesting increased communication, the counselor suggests more "date time," which results in both couples having more time together, feeling better about one another, and receiving a very pleasant side benefit: more communication. Thus, the role of the counselor is to help the couple or family change based on the counselor's understanding of the communication problems and how power is used (and abused). The couple or family need not know why the counselor is prescribing certain tasks, but they do need to "buy into" the change process. Haley addresses this change process through the use of *directives*, discussed next.

Directives

It is important to emphasize that directives can be given directly or they can be given in a conversation implicitly by vocal intonation, body movement, and well-timed silence. Everything done in therapy can be seen as a directive.

(Haley, 1976, p. 50)

Directives are the kinds of instructions given to individuals to foster change. If enough progress has been made, directives can be made at the end of the first session, although sometimes it may take two or three sessions. Haley (1976) identifies two types of directives: "(1) telling people what to do when the counselor wants them to do it, and (2) telling them what to do when the therapist does not want them to do it because the therapist wants them to change by rebelling" (p. 52).

In the first case, a counselor can either give good advice or give a directive that changes the structure of the couple or family. Haley admits that individuals rarely follow advice—even good advice. Therefore, he suggests giving directives in which couples or family members want to participate; directives that will address the presenting problem, as well as the broader inherent problems as revealed by the communication sequencing of the couple or family. The counselor generally does not reveal his or her agenda of restructuring the couple or family dynamics, as this is not generally found to expedite change. For instance, parents might identify a problem such as their daughter's use of drugs. However, in therapy, it soon becomes clear that the family isolates and cuts off the daughter from the rest of the family. The counselor could give good advice, such as suggesting to the daughter that she take a drug education class. However, this would most likely be a wasteful suggestion, as the rebellious daughter is unlikely to follow it. Therefore, it would be more useful to offer a directive that deals with the drug use *and* the family organization—a directive in which all would participate. For example, the counselor might ask the family to include the daughter in as many family activities as possible in an effort to ensure that she is not doing drugs. The parents would appreciate this directive, as it is dealing with the problem, and the daughter would appreciate it, as she is finally being included in the family.

The second type of directive, called a *paradoxical directive*, involves subtle challenges to the client, couple, or family to change that often result in the client's doing the opposite of what might seem logical. The expectation is that the directive is likely to fail, and that this failure will lead to success in therapy (Madanes, 2015b). Put simply, "some clients are more invested in the 'cons' of change, not the 'pros' of change" (J. Grimes, personal communication, July 14, 2009). If clients actually do follow the directive, success is also ensured. For instance, a family has a child who is constantly angry and screaming. In this case, the counselor might reframe the situation by stating that this child is actually quite healthy in that he is expressing his feelings. The counselor suggests that listening to the child's feelings is not helpful because the child needs to release his healthy anger. Probably, the counselor remarks, it would be helpful instead to encourage the child to scream more. Parents who rebel against this suggestion end up listening to the child. On the other hand, parents who go with the suggestion are now compliant clients who have reframed the problem into a healthy behavior and are praised at the next session for being good clients.

Another technique to induce change of this kind is through the use of *metaphor*. Look at how Haley (1976) uses metaphor to deal with a couple's uncomfortable feelings about talking directly to their son about his being adopted:

> [The counselor] talked to the boy about "adopting" a dog who had a problem of
> being frightened. . . . When the boy said the family might have to get rid of the
> dog if he became ill and cost doctor bills [the boy had been ill], the therapist

> *insisted that once adopted the family was committed to the dog and would have to keep him and pay his doctor bills no matter what. Various concerns the boy might have had about himself as well as the parents' concerns about him were discussed in metaphoric terms in relation to the proposed adoption of the puppy.* (p. 65)

The use of such metaphors, as noted above, allows couples and families to consider situations abstractly, thereby lessening the likelihood that resistance (which often occurs when counselors give advice) will occur.

Course of Treatment

Strategic therapy tends to be a short-term approach to counseling because it focuses almost exclusively on presenting problems, does not spend time dealing with intrapsychic processes, and uses directives to facilitate the change process (Carlson, 2002). Usually, directives can be made within the first few sessions, with follow-up and revision to the original directives sometimes calling for only a few more sessions.

Being a strategic therapist takes a great deal of training and confidence in one's ability to suggest effective directives. It is interesting to watch some of the more well known strategic therapists work. Criticized as manipulative by some, today's strategic therapists stress collaboration, not manipulation (Carlson, 2002). In fact, for these master therapists, their directives, even ones with hidden agendas, appear to come from a real and caring place.

Multigenerational Family Therapy

Couples and family counselors who take on a *multigenerational approach* focus on how behavioral patterns and personality traits from prior generations have been passed down in families. Therefore, many multigenerational couples and family counselors encourage bringing in parents, grandparents, and perhaps even cousins, uncles, and aunts.

Although multigenerational couples and family counselors focus on intergenerational conflicts, the way they go about this may differ. For instance, Ivan Boszormenyi-Nagy (1920–2007) believed that couples and families are relational systems in which *loyalties*, a sense of *indebtedness*, and *ways of relating* are passed down from generation to generation (Boszormenyi-Nagy, 1973, 1987). Couples enter relationships with a ledger of indebtedness and *entitlements* based on their families of origin and what was passed down to those families. A couple who enters a relationship with an imbalanced ledger will invariably attempt to balance the ledger with each other. This is almost always unsuccessful, as the imbalance is a result of unfinished business from the family of origin, not from the spouse. For instance, one who felt unloved by his mother might attempt to settle his account by trying to have his wife shower him with love. However, because this is unfinished business with the mother, the husband will continue to feel a sense of emptiness, even if the wife fulfills this request. Boszormenyi-Nagy believed that it is crucial for all couples and family members to gain the capacity to hear one another, communicate with one another, and have the ability to understand their interpersonal connectedness to their partner, their current family, and their families of origin (Ducommun-Nagy, 2015).

When each generation is helped to face the nature of the current relationships, exploring the real nature of the commitments and responsibility that flow from such involvements, an increased reciprocal understanding and mutual compassion between the generations results.

(Friedman, 1989, p. 405)

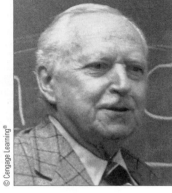

Murray Bowen

Another multigenerational couples and family therapist, Murray Bowen (1913–1990), believed that previous generations could dramatically affect one's ability to develop a healthy ego. He considered the ultimate goal of couples and family therapy to be the *differentiation of self*, which included differentiation of the self from others and the differentiation of one's emotional processes from one's intellectual processes (Bowen, 1976, 1978; McKnight, 2015). He believed that there was a *nuclear family emotional system* made up of all family members (living, dead, absent, and present), which continues to have an emotional impact upon the system. Such an emotional system, said Bowen, is reflective of the level of differentiation in the family and is called the *undifferentiated ego mass*. Thus, previous generations could continue to have an influence on current family dynamics (Klever, 2004; McKnight, 2015). Bowen used the *genogram* to examine details of a family's functioning over a number of generations. Although the basic genogram includes such items as dates of birth and death, names, and major relationships, along with breakups or divorces, the counselor will usually also ask the couple or family to include such things as where various members are from, who might be scapegoated and/or an identified patient (IP), mental illness, physical diseases, affairs, abortions, and stillbirths. Such genograms are excellent tools for examining how families evolve over time and for identifying current issues in families (McGoldrick, Gerson, & Petry, 2008) (see Figure 6.1).

Bowen believed that individuals find others of similar psychological health with whom to form significant relationships. Therefore, an undifferentiated person will find a person with a similar level of undifferentiation, with each hoping that he or she will find completeness in the other. What initially seems like a perfect fit usually ends up as a major disappointment and often ends in divorce. When undifferentiated parents do not deal with their issues, which by their very nature are frequent, a *family projection process* occurs in which parents unconsciously *triangulate* their children or project their own issues onto the children. The purpose of this projection process is to reduce stress within the parental relationship while maintaining each spouse's level of undifferentiation. This allows the couple to continue to avoid their issues. An unhealthy relationship obviously leads to problems with child rearing, and ultimately the child grows into an undifferentiated self, thus continuing the cycle. This process could continue ad infinitum (see Box 6.5).

From a Bowenian perspective, counselors should be detached and take on the role of teachers and consultants, helping their clients to understand family dynamics and systems theory from an intellectual framework. Bowen mostly worked with couples, generally did not include children in the process, and kept emotionality at a minimum during the sessions by having the clients talk to and through the counselor. Bowen's goal was to help couples and family members see themselves as they truly are and to help them move toward differentiation of self.

FIGURE 6.1
Williams-Neukrug Genogram

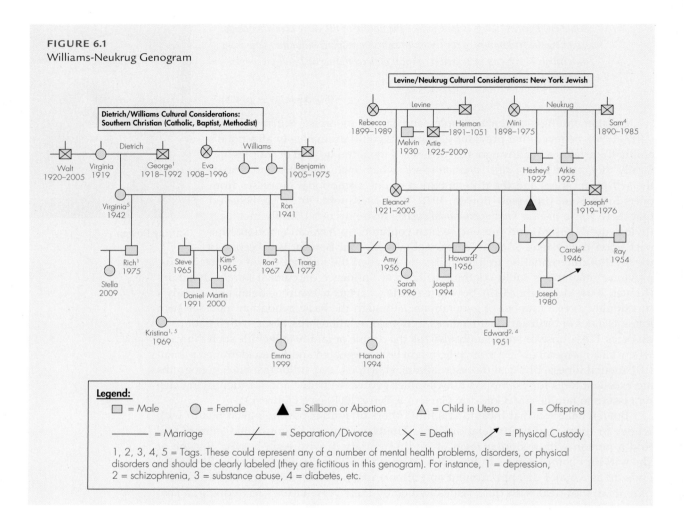

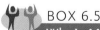 BOX 6.5
Who's More Dysfunctional?

Bowen's belief that individuals generally find others of similar psychological health has always intrigued me. Many times, I have seen clients come for therapy, complaining and even diagnosing their lover or spouse whom they have left. At these times, I've often thought that if the partner were there, that person would likely have a comparable complaint or diagnosis. And it certainly makes some intuitive sense. After all, why would someone who is psychologically healthier than my clients want to be with them? (Or, for that matter, why would someone psychologically healthier than you, or me, want to be with us?) And why would my clients choose to be with someone less healthy than them? (Or, why would we choose to be with those less healthy than us?) Have you ever found yourself diagnosing a person you are with or used to be with? Any thoughts about what they may have been saying about you?

Experiential Family Therapy

As the name implies, experiential family therapy stresses the experience of self, of one another, and of the counselor within the family therapy milieu (Keith, 2015; Napier, 2002). Based mostly on humanistic and existential psychology, this type of therapy has a positive view of human nature, believes that the individual (and the family) has a natural growth tendency, and relies on the relationship between the counselor and the couple or family to induce change. The most well known experiential family therapist is Carl Whitaker (1912-1995), who prided himself on his lack of a theoretical approach: "I have a theory that theories are destructive and I know that intuition is destructive" (Whitaker, 1976, p. 154). Despite this bold statement, it is clear that when working with couples and families, Whitaker conceptualized families from a systems perspective:

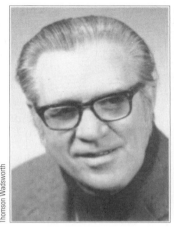

Carl Whitaker

> *The major problem we see in the individual approaches is they fail to take into account the powerful interdependence between family members. . . . The "symptom" is merely a front for the family's larger stress.*

(Napier & Whitaker, 1978, pp. 270–271)

In fact, if you read any of Whitaker's writings, it quickly becomes evident that his approach is strongly influenced by humanistic psychology, with a touch of psychodynamic theory. For instance, Whitaker believes that counselors should:

➤ Respect each member's self-actualizing process.
➤ Respect the couple and family's ability to unravel itself if placed in a trusting environment.
➤ Create an atmosphere of oneness and nondefensiveness in order to make it difficult for the couple or family to flee into defensive patterns.
➤ Assist couples and families in resolving the pain and anger that brings them to therapy.
➤ Assist couples and families in looking at their ghosts from the past.
➤ Be powerful enough to "invade the family" in order to be part of the family and assist in breaking roles that have become solidified over time (Whitaker, 1976, p. 163).
➤ Have an "I–Thou" relationship with co-therapists and the family. This real relationship models openness and the ability to dialogue and to express feeling. "Why should the family expose their tender underbelly if the therapist plays coy and self-protective?" (Whitaker, 1976, p. 164).
➤ Not offer any particular framework or preconceived way in which the couple or family should operate, in an effort to have the family develop their own structure.
➤ Model playfulness, craziness, and genuineness, in an effort to get couple and family members to loosen up and be themselves, and ultimately push them toward individuation.
➤ Assist families in establishing a generation gap, or boundaries between parents and children.

Sometimes sounding strikingly like Carl Rogers, Whitaker suggests that at first, the couple or family is defensive and closed to the counselor. As the counselor joins with the couple or family, they begin to see the counselor as a genuine person and start to open up. This is when past inner hurts and conflicts begin to emerge, and it is at this point that the counselor can facilitate exploration of these hurts and help couple and family members understand how this pain has affected each of them. Each individual can now begin to work on his or her own problems and move toward individuation. In fact, Whitaker and Augustus Napier (Napier & Whitaker, 1978) note that the later stages of couple or family work seem more like individual sessions occurring at the same time:

> *At the end of therapy the family should have resolved their major relationship conflicts, and the individuals should really be individuals in a psychological sense.*

> (Napier & Whitaker, 1978, p. 274)

In family counseling, Whitaker suggested having a co-therapist, as this allows counselors to model the I–Thou relationship. In addition, such a "real" relationship enables counselors to discuss their understanding of the family with each other—usually in front of the family (Napier & Whitaker, 1978). Also, because of the sheer numbers of people involved in family therapy, co-therapy enables counselors to periodically attend to each member of the family. Showing his psychodynamic leanings, Whitaker also suggested that co-therapists will often be perceived as the "parents" of the family, allowing families to make analogies to their families of origin, which can then be discussed. However, co-therapists can also be perceived in other roles, allowing family members to project their issues onto them (Napier & Whitaker, 1972):

> *Carl can be a very big-breasted, tender mother at times and a stern, tough grandfather at others, and I myself don't make a bad rebellious adolescent at times. It's a lot more complicated than the simplistic way in which we often identify personality with biology.*

> (Napier & Whitaker, 1978, p. 92)

If you watch a DVD of Whitaker's work, you see a master therapist who was witty, bright, reflective, real, strong, and willing to take risks. Despite the fact that he insisted he had no theory, you saw consistency in his work, a consistency in the way that he presented himself to the family that allowed the family to grow, learn, deal with painful issues, dialogue, and ultimately change.

Psychodynamic Family Therapy

Psychodynamic couples and family therapy merges concepts from systemic thinking with psychodynamic theory. For instance, when viewing psychoanalysis contextually, couples and family dynamics are seen as a reflection of each member's personality development through the psychosexual stages. The major difference between psychodynamic couples and family counseling and traditional, individual-oriented psychodynamic counseling is that the couples and family counselor places great emphasis on how the client projects his or her internal world onto his or her partner or family and the subsequent interactional processes that take place, whereas the individual-oriented counselor almost exclusively emphasizes the internal world of the client and projections onto the counselor (Becvar & Becvar, 2013).

Nathan Ackerman (1908–1971) (1958, 1966) and Robin Skynner (1922–2000) (1976, 1981) are two well-known psychodynamic family therapists. Like Ackerman and Skynner, most psychodynamically oriented counselors have generally been trained in traditional psychoanalytic methods, and also saw value in taking a systemic view when working with clients. Most converts to the systems approach have found that this combination offers a broader perspective that allows direct involvement with the cast of characters and speeds up the usual slow process of most psychodynamically oriented individual approaches.

For the psychodynamic couples and family counselor, there is generally an emphasis on how effective parents were in assisting their children through the developmental stages (Gerson, 2009; Goldenberg & Goldenberg, 2013). It is also assumed that unresolved issues through the stages are projected onto the other member of the couple or onto the family members in unconscious ways and are reflected in their interactions (Nichols & Schwartz, 2014). Therefore, the major thrust of counseling is to have the couple or family explore their interactions and begin to understand how their behaviors result from these unresolved conflicts. These conflicts may be multigenerational in the sense that the parents pass on their conflicts to their children. It is, therefore, common for psychodynamically oriented couples and family counselors to encourage their clients to bring in grandparents or other extended family members for a session or more and to encourage clients to continue to discuss unresolved issues while at home with their immediate and extended family members.

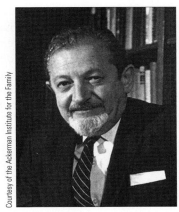

Courtesy of the Ackerman Institute for the Family

Nathan Ackerman

Cognitive–Behavioral Family Counseling

Much like individual approaches to behavior therapy, *cognitive-behavioral family counseling* is oriented toward symptom relief and does not focus on intrapsychic processes, underlying issues, or the unconscious. This approach tends to be highly structured and focuses on specific behaviors and techniques. As in individual behavior therapy, the cognitive-behavioral family counselor has at his or her disposal a wide array of techniques taken directly from *operant conditioning, classical conditioning,* and *social-learning theory* or *modeling.* Also, as in individual behavioral therapy, in recent years there has been a trend toward the inclusion of *cognitive therapy*—thus, the name "cognitive-behavioral family counseling" rather than just "behavioral family counseling" (Becvar & Becvar, 2013). For instance, today's cognitive-behavioral family counselors believe that mediating cognitions can greatly affect couples and family members and therefore should be addressed in treatment. For example, when a parent is continually dismissive of a child, this child begins to make negative self-statements concerning his or her self-worth. Therefore, in addition to behavioral change for the parents, cognitive-behavioral family counselors believe that the child's *negative automatic thoughts* also need to be addressed.

Whereas many traditional behavioral therapists have viewed problem behaviors in a linear, cause-and-effect fashion, today this approach integrates systems theory with cognitive and behavioral theory and views problem behaviors as the result of a number of feedback loops in which the dysfunctional behavior becomes reinforced from a number of different sources, including the couple and family (Barker & Chang, 2013; Goldenberg & Goldenberg, 2013). Because the cognitive-behavioral family counselor is dealing with more than just one individual, it is particularly important to identify symptoms, target behaviors that all members will agree are important to change, and understand how various behaviors are reinforced in the system:

> *The cognitive–behavioral approach is compatible with systems theory and includes the premise that members of a family simultaneously influence and are influenced by each other. Consequently, the behavior of one family member triggers behavior, cognitions, and emotions in other members, which in turn elicit reactive cognitions, behavior, and emotions in the original member. As this process plays out, the volatility of family dynamics escalates, rendering the family vulnerable to negative spirals of conflict.*

(Nichols & Schwartz, 2008, p. 284)

Some common elements that are typically identified in this approach include the following (Gladding, 2011; Goldenberg & Goldenberg, 2013; Nichols & Schwartz, 2014):

1. The importance of building a working relationship
2. Viewing counseling as an active approach that elicits the collaboration of the couple and family
3. Believing that basic learning theory principles can be applied in a systems framework
4. Viewing counseling as brief and time-limited
5. Focusing on specific behaviors or cognitions that will be targeted in treatment
6. Stressing the increase of positive behaviors over the elimination of negative behaviors
7. Teaching and coaching clients about the relationships among events in their lives, behaviors, cognitions, and consequences (e.g., negative or positive feelings)
8. Setting goals that are clear, realistic, concrete, and measurable
9. Actively teaching and supervising the change process within the family
10. Helping couples and families to learn how to self-manage and monitor changes in behaviors and cognitions
11. Evaluating the effects of specific techniques in an effort to measure progress

Whereas some family counselors believe that it is always important to include the whole family in treatment, regardless of the problem (Napier & Whitaker, 1978; Satir, 1967), cognitive–behavioral family counselors take into account what the presenting problem is and tend to include only those members who seem to be directly related to the change process (Nichols & Schwartz, 2014). For instance, if a child is having behavior problems at home and correction of the problem involves only parenting skills training, there may be no need to include the child. Similarly, if a couple is having marital problems, although their problems will be spilling over to the children, the correction of the problem may not directly involve the children, so they may not have to be included. In this process, it is most important for the cognitive–behavioral family counselor to make a thorough assessment of the problem in an effort to determine correct treatment strategies and decide which members of the couple or family should be included in counseling (Becvar & Becvar, 2013; Nichols & Schwartz, 2014).

Narrative Family Therapy

The person or the family is not the problem; the problem is the problem.

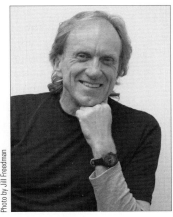

Michael White

This quote from Michael White speaks to one of the newest trends in family therapy—*narrative family therapy*. Based on some of the most recent developments in the counseling field, such as *social constructionism*, *postmodernism*, and *narrative reasoning* (Gladding, 2011), narrative family therapy has at its core the belief that there are no absolute truths and that it is critical to understand the stories that people and families tell in order to help them *deconstruct* how they come to understand their family. Ultimately, the goal of narrative family therapy is to recreate how the family comes to understand itself.

Two of the early founders of narrative family therapy were Michael White (1946–2008) and David Epston (1944–) (White, 1995; White & Epston, 1990), both of whom decided to discard some of the rule-based procedures found in the more traditional family therapy techniques that tended to follow systems and cybernetic theory (Nichols & Schwartz, 2014). This approach has some similarities to solution-focused therapy in that it takes an optimistic, proactive, future-oriented approach to working with people. Counselors who practice this kind of therapy tend to do the following (Fenell, 2012; Nichols & Schwartz, 2014):

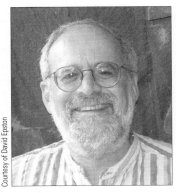

David Epston

1. Show interest and develop a strong, collaborative relationship with the couple or family.
2. Understand the couple's or family's history through the stories they tell and examine how the problem has been dysfunctional for the couple or family.
3. Ask questions in a nonjudgmental manner in order to understand the issues in the couple or family and to begin to help the couple or family redefine the problem.
4. Have individuals, couples, or the family externalize the problem. For instance, instead of defining the problem as "people in the family don't value each other," the problem becomes "time"—there's not enough *time* for everyone to show each other how much they care.
5. Begin to look for exceptions to the problem.
6. Find evidence in the couple's or family's history to show how they have been competent and resourceful and able to combat problems such as this.
7. Help the couple or family reframe the role the problem has played and help them redefine or *re-author* their understanding of themselves by helping them focus on their existing strengths and their possibilities for the future.
8. Help the couple or family reinforce existing strengths and newfound narratives through *ceremonies* and other ways of acknowledging the changes that have been made.

The end goal of narrative family therapy is to help couples and families understand how their narratives (the stories about the family) have defined who they were and how they interacted, and to help them find their own unique, new stories that can re-define them in more positive ways. Ultimately, the couple or family decides what is considered a healthy way of functioning as they deconstruct their past ways of being and find new and better ways of relating.

Solution-Focused Family Therapy

Solution-focused family therapy was originated by Insoo Kim Berg, Steve de Shazer, Bill O'Hanlon, and others (Berg, 1994; de Shazer, 1982; Ratner, George, & Iveson, 2012) and is a pragmatic and future-oriented approach that assumes that clients can change quickly. Because the approach focuses on *solutions*, not problems, discussion of the past is very limited, as such discussion is believed to keep the client mired in the problem. Viewing the client as the expert, this approach asserts that the client has strengths that can be expanded upon. Somewhat based on *social constructionism* and *postmodernism*, the solution-focused counselor helps the client create a new, *problem-free language* associated with new behaviors as he or she finds *exceptions to the problem*, develops solutions, and moves toward creating a new reality.

Like narrative family therapy, but unlike most other forms of family therapy we examined in this chapter, solution-focused family therapy does not rely on the assumptions of general systems theory, cybernetics, boundary or information flow, or many of the other theoretical underpinnings listed at the beginning of this chapter (Nichols & Schwartz, 2014). In fact, solution-focused counselors question the "truth" of those who rely on such theory and do not view problems as being inherently caused by flaws in the couple's or family's structure. Instead, they believe that *language* and *perception of problems* are related to the development of problems. Therefore, solution-focused counselors have clients examine alternative ways of viewing themselves, and they focus solely on helping clients find solutions to their problems based on their existing strengths. Since each member can do this on his or her own, solution-focused counselors do not need to see the couple or whole family together in therapy, but rather only those members who want to work on their own solutions. Underlying assumptions of this type of therapy include:

1. Change is constant and inevitable.
2. The client is the expert on his or her experience.
3. Clients come to us with resources and strengths.
4. If it ain't broke, don't fix it.
5. If it works, do more of it; if it's not working, do something different.
6. Small steps can lead to big changes.
7. There is not necessarily a logical relationship between the solution and the problem.
8. The language for solution development is different from that needed to describe a problem.
9. No problems happen all the time; there are always exceptions that can be used.
10. The future is both created and negotiable.

Solution-focused therapy can be viewed through a series of six stages that include *pre-session change, forming a collaborative relationship, describing the problem, establishing preferred outcomes, problem-to-solution focus, reaching preferred outcomes*, and *ending therapy*. With therapy occurring rapidly, the counselor enters the initial session asking if any pre-session changes were noted, and takes an *ambassador* position with the client in which he or she is *curious, respectful*, and *accepting*. Using *listening* and *empathy* skills and *being tentative* in his or her approach, the solution-focused counselor forms a *collaborative relationship* and slowly moves the client from a description of the problem toward the establishment of *preferred outcomes*. Solutions are eventually determined through the use of a number of questioning techniques that include asking *preferred outcome questions, evaluative questions, coping questions, exception-seeking questions*, and *solution-oriented questions*. In addition, counselors will also *reframe* client responses to view them in a positive light, *amplify exceptions, compliment clients* around solutions that work, and help clients assess progress through the use of *scaling*, where clients subjectively rate their progress on a scale from 0 to 10.

Multicultural/Social Justice Focus
Points to Consider When Working with Minority Families

> *Any comprehensive attempt to understand personal or family functioning must take into account the fundamental influences of gender, culture, and ethnicity in shaping the lives and experiences of men and women.*
>
> (Goldenberg & Goldenberg, 2013, p. 62)

Regardless of theoretical approach, when working with couples and families from diverse cultures and religious orientations, a number of issues should be considered (Goldenberg & Goldenberg, 2013; Ho, Rasheed, & Rasheed, 2004; McGoldrick, Carter, & Petro, 2011; McGoldrick, Giordano, & Garcia-Petro, 2005). The following highlights but a few of the major concerns:

➤ Racism, poverty, and lower-class status are widespread for many clients from nondominant groups and can dramatically affect how couples and families feel about themselves and their relationship to the counselor.

➤ The language used by the dominant culture is often covertly or overtly oppressive of culturally and ethnically diverse couples and families and affects how others see them, how they see themselves, and how they live in society.

➤ Couples and families from nondominant groups will invariably experience some forms of racism and discrimination, and this must be taken into account when working with them.

➤ Many culturally and ethnically diverse couples and families are bicultural and face issues surrounding conflicting value systems between their culture of origin and the larger culture.

➤ Language differences may cause problems of miscommunication (and even mis-diagnosis) for couples and families in counseling.

➤ Clients from culturally and ethnically diverse couples and families are less likely to attend counseling and more likely to end therapy early. Therefore, counselors need to be vigilant about reaching out to such clients and ensuring that they are treating them effectively.

➤ Gender role issues play an increasingly large role in couples and families from all cultures.

➤ Sexual orientation plays an increasingly large role in couples and families from all cultures.

➤ Religion, religious values, and spirituality play significant roles in many cultures, and it behooves the effective counselor to understand the impact that religion and spirituality have on the couple or family.

➤ Couples and families may differ dramatically in terms of a number of key elements, including how the couple and family dress and value appearances, embrace specific beliefs and attitudes, relate to family and significant others, play and use leisure time, learn and use knowledge, communicate and use language, embrace certain values and mores, use time and space, eat and use food in its customs, and work and apply themselves.

The astute cross-cultural couples and family counselor needs to have the knowledge necessary to work with different kinds of families, awareness of his or her cultural biases, and the unique skills needed to work with couples and families from diverse backgrounds.

Why Are the Professional Associations Not Being Inclusive?

You'll notice that the title of this chapter is "Couples and Family Counseling," not "Marriage and Family Counseling." This is because the term *marriage therapy* excludes all of those gay and lesbian couples who still cannot become married in this country, as well as the hundreds of thousands of couples who live together and choose not to get married. Thus, I have used a more inclusive term, "couples counseling." This term is also in sync with the stands of the American Counseling Association (ACA), American Psychological Association (APA), and National Association of Social Workers (NASW) on the normalization of homosexuality. One has to wonder why the American Association of *Marriage* and Family Therapists and the International Association of *Marriage* and Family Counselors have continued to use titles that are exclusive of a substantial portion of our population.

Ethical, Professional, and Legal Issues

Ethical Concerns

There are many unique ethical concerns related to the practice of couples and family counseling, not all of which can be covered in this short section. However, some issues that stand out have to do with withholding treatment, informed consent, confidentiality, and multiple relationships (AAMFT, 2012; IAMFC, 2011; Wilcoxon, Remley, Gladding, & Huber, 2012):

Withholding Treatment

> *Couple and family counselors have an obligation to determine and inform counseling participants who are identified as the primary client. The couple and family counselor should make clear to clients if they have any obligations to an individual, a couple, a family, a third party, or an institution.*

(IAMFC, 2011, Section A.7)

Because some couples and family counselors insist on seeing the whole couple or family rather than one member of the couple or a portion of the family, withholding treatment if one or more members balk at coming into therapy is not unusual. Although most ethical guidelines state that counselors cannot refuse services unless other arrangements are made for the client, a counselor can justify withholding treatment if he or she believes that counseling will succeed only if both members of a couple or the whole family is present. However, if such a position is taken, a couples and family counselor should be able to defend this position from both a pragmatic and theoretical perspective.

Informed Consent

> *Marriage and family therapists obtain appropriate informed consent to therapy or related procedures and use language that is reasonably understandable to clients. The content of informed consent may vary depending upon the client and treatment plan; however, informed consent generally necessitates that the client: (a) has the capacity to consent; (b) has been adequately informed of significant information concerning treatment processes and procedures; (c) has been adequately informed of potential risks and benefits of treatments for which generally recognized standards do not yet exist; (d) has freely and without undue influence expressed consent; and (e) has provided consent that is appropriately documented. When persons, due to age or mental status, are legally incapable of giving informed consent, marriage and family therapists obtain informed permission from a legally authorized person, if such substitute consent is legally permissible.*

(AAMFT, 2012, Section 1.2)

It is the counselor's ethical obligation to ensure that knowledge about the counseling process is given to all clients, and all clients involved in the counseling must willingly understand such informed consent and agree to participate in such a relationship prior to initiating the counseling relationship. Thus, each family member present must understand the nature of counseling, what might be expected of him or her, and any risks that might occur as a result of counseling.

Confidentiality

Couples and family counseling offers some unique challenges to the ethical obligation to maintain confidentiality. For instance, if one member of a couple or family is seen individually and reveals information that he or she does not wish discussed with his or her partner or with the family, and if the counselor thinks this information is critical to the resolution of the problem, should the counselor break confidentiality? Is the client the individual, or the couple or family? Confidentiality also becomes problematic in that one cannot ensure that each member of a couple or all family members will honor it.

> *Couple and family counselors inform clients that statements made by a family member to the counselor during an individual counseling, consultation, or collateral contact are to be treated as confidential. Such statements are not disclosed to other family members without the individual's permission. However, the couple and family counselor should clearly identify the client of counseling, which may be the couple or family system, and inform clients in writing who(m) the identified client is. Couple and family counselors should inform clients that they do not maintain family secrets, collude with some family members against others, or otherwise contribute to dysfunctional family system dynamics. If a client's refusal to share information from individual contacts interferes with the agreed goals of counseling, the counselor may terminate treatment and refer the clients to another counselor. Some couple and family counselors choose to not meet with individuals, preferring to serve family systems.*
>
> (IAMFC, 2011, Section B)

Dealing with such complex issues that don't always have clear-cut answers requires a wise and sensitive counselor. Having clear ground rules before counseling begins can help to avoid these problems.

Multiple (Dual) Relationships

> *Couple and family counselors do not harass, exploit, coerce, or manipulate clients for personal gain. Couple and family counselors avoid, whenever possible, multiple relationships such as business, social, or sexual contacts with any current clients or their family members. Couple and family counselors should refrain generally from nonprofessional relationships with former clients and their family members because termination of counseling is a complex process.*
>
> (IAMFC, 2011, Standard A.9)

Although we are all clear that sexual contacts with current or former clients are forbidden, there may be times when a counselor will unexpectedly run into a client or extended family member outside the counseling relationship. For instance, counselors may see clients at social events that they attend (e.g., a local art festival), contact them at business functions in which they are involved (e.g., a Chamber of Commerce event), see them at recreational facilities (e.g., a road race), and so forth. It is important that counselors are aware of, and are able to keep, appropriate boundaries when they see clients outside the office. Counselors should consider in advance how they should react to clients when they face such situations and remember the importance of keeping their counseling relationship professional and confidential.

Professional Issues

Individual or Family Therapy?

When should a member of a family be referred to individual counseling, as opposed to the whole family being referred for family counseling? Although some therapists have suggested that it is always appropriate to refer the whole family for counseling (Napier & Whitaker, 1978; Satir, 1967), most therapists today agree that it is often a matter of making a wise decision based on a careful assessment of the situation. For instance, a child who comes from an extremely dysfunctional family may be better off seeing a counselor individually because working with the whole family may be seen as an extremely long process, whereas individual counseling may give some immediate relief for the child. Or it may be prudent to refer a spouse for individual counseling to work on her unfinished business while the family undergoes family treatment. This might accelerate the treatment process for everyone.

My own bias for determining individual or family counseling is based on how much the presenting problem seems to reverberate throughout the family. When problems in the family seem to be seriously affecting all family members, I would suggest seeing the whole family. However, if a family member is experiencing a large amount of pain and he or she is attempting not to let this spill into the family (though it always spills over to some degree), then I might opt for individual counseling.

Professional Associations

AAMFT or IAMFC—which professional association should you join? Although there are many more similarities than differences between these two associations, IAMFC (2014) and AAMFT (2002–2013c) suggest different graduate curricula, have different codes of ethics, support slightly different clinical and supervisory experience for licensing, and at times endorse different licensing initiatives. The professional couples and family counselor should investigate both associations to see which seems to be the best fit. But then again, why not join both?

Accreditation and Credentialing

Today, two groups accredit couples and family graduate therapy programs: the *Commission on Accreditation for Marital and Family Therapy Education (COAMFTE)* (AAMFT, 2002–2013d), which is associated with AAMFT; and *the Council on the Accreditation of Counseling and Related Educational Programs* (CACREP), which has a specialty accreditation in marriage and family counseling and is affiliated with ACA (CACREP, 2009; 2014e).

In 1987, the *Association of Marital and Family Therapy Regulatory Boards* (AMFTRB) was established by AAMFT to address licensure and certification issues; today, all 50 states have licensing laws that cover marriage and family counselors (AMFTRB, 2014). Rather than following the guidelines of AMFTRB, some state licensure boards have subsumed the marriage and family credential under the counseling board or other related mental health licensing boards. In addition to licensing, the *International Association of Marriage and Family Counselors* (IAMFC), a division of ACA, developed a certification process through the *National Credentialing Academy* (NCA, n.d.) that enables a marriage or family therapist to become a Certified Family Therapist (CFT).

Legal Concerns

Knowing the Law and Being an Expert

Ethical and effective couples and family counselors know how the knowledge they gain from their sessions could be used in a court of law (Wilcoxon, Remley, Gladding, & Huber, 2012). For instance, information gained relative to child abuse, spousal abuse, family abuse, child custody issues, and separation and divorce of partners can often be accessible to courts. Thus, it is critical that couples and family counselors not assume that information is privileged, know the limits of confidentiality, and know how information gained in sessions could be used in court. It is particularly important that counselors know how such information is likely to be treated in the state where they work, as state laws vary, and that they communicate to their clients the limits of confidentiality.

> *Couple and family counselors inform clients of exceptions to the general principle that information will be kept confidential or released only upon written client authorization. Disclosure of private information may be mandated by state law. For example, states require reporting of suspected abuse of children or other vulnerable populations. Couple and family counselors may have sound legal or ethical justification for disclosing information if someone is in imminent danger. A court may have jurisdiction to order release of confidential information without a client's permission. However, all releases of information not authorized by clients should be minimal or narrow as possible.*

> (IAMFC, 2011, Section B.3)

Insurance Fraud

> *Marriage and family therapists represent facts truthfully to clients, third-party payors, and supervisees regarding services rendered.*

> (AAMFT, 2012, Section 7.4)

With the Affordable Care Act, there will be changes in health care benefits and how clients pay for services. It is important that counselors know how to collect fees for their services and how to report such services to insurance companies. Counselors need to understand that misrepresentation of services (e.g., billing for one client when one sees the whole family) is unethical and may be illegal (Crews, 2005a, 2005b). With insurance fraud being one of the most frequently made complaints against licensed therapists (Neukrug, Milliken, & Walden, 2001), couples and family counselors need to be aware of the idiosyncratic rules of insurance companies, the changing nature of the law with the Affordable Care Act, and specific state laws that might restrict this practice.

The Counselor in Process: Understanding Our Client's Family, Understanding Our Family

Although many counselors will start out individually oriented and slowly develop the skills to work with couples and families, the effective counselor understands the contextual nature of the world in which clients interact whether working individually or with couples and families. This wise counselor understands that the individual has a dramatic impact on the life of his or her family, realizes how the family affects the individual, and sees the interconnectedness between all families and the community and society at large. However, awareness of a client's contextual world is not enough. The effective couples and family counselor has also examined his or her own family of origin, for the counselor who has avoided a family self-examination risks having his or her issues interfere with the effective treatment of clients and families. Although we can never fully know our family as they were, we can continually strive to know ourselves as we become.

Summary

This chapter began with a brief history of the development of couples and family counseling. We started with a discussion of how Charity Organization Societies (COSs) and "friendly visitors" led to a systemic view of problems in families and communities. We noted that Alfred Adler was one of the first to include the family when treating individuals, although family members were usually in separate rooms from the client. We noted that the hold that psychodynamic approaches had on the individual perspective of doing counseling was strong, and that early family therapy approaches tried to adapt this individual approach to working with couples and families. The shift toward couples and family counseling being acceptable was probably related to the impact of those who worked at Palo Alto. The work at Palo Alto, as well as the subsequent research at MRI, influenced the development of a number of family therapy approaches, including strategic family therapy, structural family therapy, and the human validation process model. At around the same time, other approaches to couples and family work evolved, including multigenerational family therapy and experiential family therapy. Later, at MRI, the BFTC at Palo Alto was formed and became the impetus for the development of solution-focused family therapy. Other approaches to family therapy that later took hold included cognitive–behavioral family counseling and narrative family therapy.

As the chapter continued, it examined the view of human nature commonly held by many couples and family counselors and then elucidated a number of key concepts, including general systems theory, cybernetics, boundaries and information flow, rules and hierarchy, communication theory, scapegoating and identified patients, stress in families, developmental issues, and social constructionism.

We examined the more popular approaches to couples and family therapy, including the human validation process model of Virginia Satir; strategic family therapy, used by Jay Haley, Cloé Madanes, and the Milan Group; structural family therapy, popularized by Salvador Minuchin; multigenerational family therapy, as practiced by Murray Bowen and Ivan Boszormenyi-Nagy; the experiential family therapy of Augustus Napier and Carl Whitaker; psychodynamic family therapy, as suggested by Nathan Ackerman and Robin Skynner; cognitive–behavioral family counseling; the narrative family therapy of Michael White and David Epston; and solution-focused family therapy, as popularized by Insoo Kim Berg, Steve de Shazer, and Bill O'Hanlon.

After examining different approaches to couples and family work, we focused on multicultural and social justice issues and pinpointed a number of concerns when working with couples and families from diverse cultures and religious orientations. In addition, we wondered why the professional associations have kept the word *marriage* in their titles, rather than being more inclusive of all couples.

Some ethical concerns discussed in the chapter included withholding treatment of some family members in order to see the whole family, the importance of having all family members give informed consent, the complexities of confidentiality in couples and family counseling, and the intricacies of multiple relationships in couples and family counseling, such as when the counselor sees a client or extended family member at a social or business event. We also highlighted some professional issues, such as when individual counseling may be preferred over family counseling, which professional association to join (e.g., AAMFT or IAMFC), and the status of accreditation, licensing, and certification of couples and family counselors. Some legal concerns noted here included knowing the complexities of legal issues relative to couples and family work (e.g., state laws for reporting abuse) and not becoming involved in insurance fraud by knowing how laws might be changing (e.g., the Affordable Care Act) and by understanding the rules of specific insurance companies with whom the couples and family counselor works. The chapter concluded with a discussion about the importance of examining one's own family of origin, particularly with how it can affect one's work with couples and families.

Further Practice

Visit CengageBrain.com to respond to additional material that highlight the salient aspects of the chapter content. There, you can find ethical, professional, and legal vignettes, a number of experiential exercises, and study tools including a glossary, flashcards, and sample test items. Hopefully, these will enhance your learning and be fun and interesting.

Group Work

I decided I wanted to have a group counseling experience. I had recently finished my master's degree and started a job at a mental health center. I found a counselor whom I trusted who was putting together a group with another counselor. There were eight of us—four men, four women—oh yeah, and the two counselors, that makes ten. But the counselors didn't count as real people!

With the group meeting once a week, it took a while to build trust. However, within a couple of months, it seemed as though things were really taking off. We began to share deeper parts of ourselves. I heard people reveal things about themselves that they had never mentioned to anyone else. I saw transformations take place as members began to work through their unfinished business. I saw the leaders, a man and a woman, model shared group leadership skills and openly work through their own conflicts in front of us.

After we had been meeting for about a year, the leaders suggested having a marathon group session that would last from Friday evening to late Sunday afternoon. I had always heard about such groups and was apprehensive about meeting for such an extensive amount of time. But at the same time, I was excited about what lay ahead for me. The weekend was incredible, as people shared deep parts of themselves.

The group continued for a year longer. It was painful to say goodbye, but necessary. We were finished, at least for now. We had done our work and now were ready to move on in life. We laughed, we cried, we hugged. For a while, some of us continued to maintain contact; others did not. Over time, I lost contact with everyone in the group. I wonder now what those other seven people are doing. Oh yeah, and the two counselors too.

That group experience was crucial for me. It helped me work through unfinished business. It showed me how effective group counseling could be. Watching the counselors taught me how to run groups, and it gave me an appreciation of the group process as the unique unfolding of a group that must be nurtured if it is to blossom.

Since that time, I have participated in other groups and have run a number of them myself. I had a brief flirtation with EST (now Landmark Forum), a very large (250 people) marathon group with a confrontational focus; I joined a leaderless men's support group; I visited some Alcoholics Anonymous (AA) groups; I ran a weight-loss group; I ran groups as part of graduate group counseling classes (which has some ethical complications); I ran a support group for individuals who had been hospitalized for a psychotic disorder; and I ran psychoeducational groups for high school students.

Groups come in all shapes and sizes. They last for different lengths of time. They have different numbers of people in them, and they focus on different things. Groups can seem so different, yet they all share many common elements. This chapter will examine groups—how they are different and how they are the same.

We will begin the chapter by explaining groups from a systemic perspective and then discuss the purpose of group counseling. We will then review how groups evolved during the twentieth century. We will explore the differences among self-help groups, task groups, psychoeducational groups, counseling groups, and therapy groups, and we will look at how theory is applied to group work. We will examine the stages of group development and discuss group leadership skills, particularly as they relate to these stages. Finally, we will take a look at some important multicultural, social justice, ethical, professional, and legal issues related to group work, and then conclude with a brief discussion on the importance of letting groups unravel naturally.

Groups: A Systemic Perspective

In our therapeutic roles with groups, it is important to understand group systems thinking because a systems perspective adds qualities such as boundary conditions; communication inflow, outflow, and between-flow; and group change management to our consideration.

(Connors & Caple, 2005, p. 94)

Groups, like families, can be viewed from a *systemic perspective* in which individuals in the group can be understood by examining the dynamic interaction of its members and how that interaction results in specific *communication patterns*, *power dynamics*, *hierarchies*, and they result in the system's unique *homeostasis* (Agazarian, 2008; Napier & Gershenfeld, 2004). The effective group leader is able to work with the unique issues that the individual brings to the group, and at the same time, understands how system dynamics are a reflection of how these issues play out in the group. Thus, the group leader must be able to both focus with the intensity of a laser beam on each group member and pull back as if he or she is viewing the whole group through a wide-angle lens. In a sense, the effective group leader must see himself or herself as an individual counselor and a systems expert. In addition, an effective group leader not only sees the group as a system, but also understands the place that groups play in larger systems. Thus, at times the group leader may attempt to effect change by working with the larger or *macro* system, such as advocating in communities or for legislative change (Roysircar, 2008).

Many of the same theories discussed in Chapter 6 that illuminate what occurs in families (e.g., *general systems theory*; *cybernetics*) can be applied to an understanding of groups (Agarazian, 2008; Napier & Gershenfeld, 2004). However, one major difference is that in families, our goal is to undo a problematic system and rebuild it so that it's healthier. In groups, there is no prior history to the system, so from the beginning, we are building the system in a manner that will lead the individuals within that system to healthy functioning.

Why Have Groups?

Today, groups are used by all types of counselors and are an important and frequently used intervention method that rivals individual and family counseling (American Mental Health Counselors Association, 2013a; American School Counselor Association, 2013; Barlow, 2014; Perusse, Goodnough, & Lee, 2009). But why should a counselor choose a group over other treatment methods? Table 7.1 summarizes some of the *advantages and disadvantages of group work* (Corey, 2012; Jacobs, Masson, & Harvill, 2012).

Deciding whether individual, family, or group counseling is most beneficial is an important counselor responsibility and should be based on a careful assessment of client needs (Ward, 2004). Based on this assessment, it is sometimes important to offer only individual, group, or family counseling. Other times, group work is an adjunct to individual or family counseling. In addition, if individual or family counseling is not available to the client (e.g., cost of individual counseling is too high; inability to bring family members together), group work can be a viable alternative.

In the history of counseling and therapy, group work is the newest treatment method. Because of this, some consider the training of group counselors to be lagging behind its demand (Corey, Corey, & Corey, 2014; Markus & King, 2003; Ward, 2007). The following section will review how group work has developed, paying special attention to its relatively recent increase in popularity.

TABLE 7.1   Advantages and Disadvantages

ADVANTAGES	DISADVANTAGES
1. *More efficient:* More clients can be seen in a shorter amount of time.	1. *Less focused time:* As compared to individual counseling, each group member has less focused time with the counselor.
2. *Economical:* Group work almost always costs less than individual counseling.	2. *Less intensity with leader:* Groups do not offer the same amount of intense one-on-one time with the group leader as in individual counseling.
3. *Sense of belonging:* Groups offer contact with other people on a deeply personal level.	3. *More intimidation:* Some individuals are intimidated by the group setting.
4. *General support:* Groups can offer foundational support for many clients.	4. *Fear of disclosure:* Some clients will not reveal deeply personal matters in a group setting.
5. *Microcosm of society:* Groups mimic society and offer a "lab" of how others might react to the individual.	5. *Therapeutic effectiveness:* Some problems may be more effectively dealt with in a family or individual setting.
6. *Support for commitment to change:* Groups provide atmosphere where members will support one another as they define goals and follow through on new behaviors.	6. *Increased time commitment:* Generally, clients have to commit more time to group counseling than other forms of counseling—time they may not have.
7. *Vicarious learning:* Through modeling, group members can learn from one another and from the leader.	7. *Lack of flexibility:* One can generally change the meeting times of individual sessions more easily than group sessions.
8. *Feedback:* Groups offer an increased number of people to gain feedback from.	8. *Inability to assure confidentiality:* Leaders cannot assure group members that everyone will keep information confidential.
9. *Practice:* Groups provide a place to practice newly learned behaviors within a trusting environment.	9. *Diversion of focus:* One member could sometimes take up much of group time.
10. *Systemic understanding:* Groups provide information to members about how they react in systems, information that can often be related to family of origin issues.	10. *Psychological harm:* If a leader cannot control one or more destructive members, a member could be harmed psychologically.

The History of Group Work

What occurs in a group has often been described as a microcosm of society (Yalom, 2005); that is, the kinds of values and behaviors exhibited reflect how group members act in society. Perhaps, then, it is not surprising that the ways in which groups have been conducted over the years have reflected the values in society at those times. Let's take a closer look at how some of these groups evolved.

Early History

Gladding (2012) notes that prior to 1900, the purpose of group treatment was to assist individuals in ways that were functional and pragmatic. This often revolved around helping people with daily living skills and arose out of the social group work movement, where individuals like Jane Addams organized group discussions that often had moralistic overtones and centered on such things as personal hygiene, moral behavior, nutrition, and self-determination (Murdach, 2007; Pottick, 1988). Using groups as their vehicle, social reformers like Addams and Mary Richmond were particularly concerned with community organizing as an effort to empower the poor.

At the turn of the last century, a number of parallel movements began to discover the power of groups. For instance, schools began to offer vocational and moral guidance in group settings. Although they were often preachy in nature, and despite the fact that there was little opportunity for group members to discuss personal matters in reflective ways, these group guidance activities acknowledged the importance of groups. At around the same time, Dr. Joseph Henry Pratt became one of the first to practice group treatment with patients. Meeting with about 30 tuberculosis patients weekly, he would start with a lecture, which eventually led to patients revealing their personal stories and offering encouragement to one another. With little if any group theory available at that time, Pratt followed what his predecessors did and practiced a little moral guidance by using persuasion and reeducation (Barlow, Burlingame, & Fuhriman, 2000; Brown, 2015a; Singh & Salazar, 2010a).

At the beginning of the twentieth century, a number of psychoanalytical principles such as primal urges, instincts, and parental influences were used to explain group dynamics (Anthony, 1972; Brown, 2015a; Lonergan, 1994). For instance, some believed that the tendency for group behavior represented a *herd instinct,* where people sought out others for survival purposes. Others believed that a *mob instinct* could emerge from group activities, where the natural aggressiveness of people would come out, and still others believed that one could find in groups a *recapitulation of early family patterns,* and that group members would often blindly give their power over to the group leader (their parent). Although Freud (1922/1975) wrote a book on groups called *Group Psychology and the Analysis of the Ego,* his attachment to individual therapy prevented him from taking his ideas one step further, to develop and practice a broad-reaching theory of group therapy.

In 1914, J. L. Moreno, who was the originator of *psychodrama* and the individual credited with coining the term *group psychotherapy,* wrote one of the first papers on the subject (Barlow et al., 2000; Fox, 1987; Konopik & Cheung, 2013). Although not considered formal group counseling, psychodrama focused on individuals acting out their experiences in front of an audience. This form of therapy emphasized role playing, here-and-now interaction, expression of feeling, and feedback from the audience (the group), and is considered by some the forerunner of group counseling.

The 1920s and 1930s saw the spread of *Adlerian therapy*, with its emphasis on birth order and the importance of belonging and social connectedness. These concepts seemed to fit well in family and group settings, and Alfred Adler was one of the first individuals to practice early forms of family and group work as he and his colleagues worked with prisoners and groups of children in child guidance clinics (Ferguson, 2010; Gladding, 2012). However, their techniques were far from what would be considered group or family counseling today, as they did not fully take into account aspects of group dynamics and group process, so important to present-day group work. At around the same time, the spread of psychotherapeutic theory and sociological concepts concerning group interactions led to some of the first nonpsychoanalytically oriented counseling and therapy groups.

The 1930s saw an increased use of group guidance activities in schools. Mostly performed by homeroom teachers, these guidance activities focused on "helping to establish relationships, determining student needs and abilities, and developing proper attitudes" (Vander Kolk, 1990, p. 5). Continuing into the 1950s, these guidance activities were the forerunner of the psychoeducational groups we see in schools today.

The Emergence of Modern-Day Groups

The 1940s saw the emergence of the modern group movement. In 1947, Kurt Lewin (a founder of modern-day social psychology) and other theorists developed the *National Training Laboratory (NTL)* to examine how group dynamics could help individuals increase self-understanding (NTL, 2014). Still operating today, NTL strives to help individuals become more aware of self and others through group dialogue that focuses on openness and an understanding of group dynamics. NTL has become particularly popular in business and industry in helping individuals understand communication in groups, the group process, and how these relate to organizational goals.

It was also during this decade that Carl Rogers, while working at the Counseling Center at the University of Chicago, was asked by the Veterans Administration to run training sessions for counselors who might be working with returning GIs from World War II. Running the group training using his *person-centered* style, he found that there was increased self-disclosure, deepening expression of feeling, and increased awareness of self. Thus began the *encounter group movement* (Rogers, 1970).

> The key difference between the NTL groups and the Chicago groups was that the former had as their major focus the professional training of leaders, with the personal growth of the participants being a secondary gain; while the latter had the personal growth of the participants as its major focus, with the expectation that this personal growth would enable the individual to become more effective in their helping relationships.

> (Kirschenbaum, 2009, p. 340)

During this period, we also saw the founding of the *American Group Psychotherapy Association (AGPA),* one of the first professional associations to focus on group counseling. However, few then realized the far-reaching effects that groups were about to have on American society.

The Popularity of Groups Surges

The 1960s were tumultuous times: The Vietnam War, the War on Poverty, the civil rights movement, and the assassinations of heroic figures like John F. Kennedy, Robert F. Kennedy, and Martin Luther King, Jr. are but a few of the events that characterized this period of uncertainty. The country was in upheaval, and this chaos was perhaps society's way of saying, "Free us." Free us from racism. Free us from war. Free us from poverty, and let us be free to love. Led by *the encounter group movement*, groups were soon to reflect this need for freedom and love. One outgrowth of this movement was the development of *Esalen* in Big Sur, California, by Michael Murphy. Murphy, who became involved in the encounter group movement, moved to an ashram in India for a year and a half and subsequently came back and established Esalen. A description of Esalen, written in the mid-1970s by Murphy's guru, is still applicable as Esalen continues to offer workshops and related activities today:

> This was a very interesting experimental community, attempting to combine the ideal of self-realization and technology, drawing upon Eastern spirituality and Western thought. The emphasis was on the transformation of your personal life into the divine nature in our language, trying to evoke higher spiritual possibilities out of all your life.

(Gusataitis, as cited in Verny, 1974, p. 10)

It was not unusual to find Carl Rogers, Abraham Maslow, and famous philosophers like Paul Tillich at Esalen. Esalen, as well as other institutes that began to follow its model, were to attract counselors and therapists from around the world, some of whom would eventually become famous in their own right. Fritz Perls, for instance, started doing workshops at Esalen, and his notoriety there, along with his soon-to-be published books, made him a well-known figure (Neukrug, 2011). At Esalen, Perls began to put some of his *Gestalt therapy* ideas into a group framework. Others also applied their theories to the groups at Esalen. Individuals like Bill Schutz, a Harvard faculty member and originally an NTL devotee, developed group physical-contact games and group imagery exercises that had an emphasis on self-awareness:

> Schutz will suggest to one or all members of the group simultaneously that they take a trip through their bodies. They are to enter their bodies by whatever orifice they wish. . . . I recall one lady who entered her body through her vagina and within a few seconds turned into a rat chewing away at herself. Naturally, when she came back from this nightmare it provided us with a lot of material with which to investigate her sexual identity, sexual relations, and related problems.

(Verny, 1974, p. 17)

Esalen and the encounter group movement in general had a particular emphasis on "getting in touch" with one's feelings, and this eventually led to the formation of a number of different types of affect-oriented groups. Some of the more popular types included *marathon groups*, where individuals might spend 48 hours intensely sharing feelings and experiences; *confrontational groups*, like the ones modeled after *Synanon*, a drug and alcohol rehab program where it was common for group members to attack one another verbally in an effort to break down defenses; *Gestalt and sensitivity groups*, which stressed the expression of feelings in order to get to deeper issues; and *nude encounter groups*, which strived to be free of restraints—clothes being one of them. This ever-expanding push to express feelings and get in touch with oneself stretched traditional values and encouraged group members to deal with deep-seated issues. However, the effects of such groups were not always positive. With increasingly larger numbers of groups being run by untrained individuals, and with some people reporting negative results from their experiences, the *American Psychological Association (APA)* in 1973 published *Guidelines for Psychologists Conducting Growth Groups*, which limited what a professional could do in groups (APA, 1973).

The 1960s and 1970s also saw the spread of texts on the theory and practice of group counseling. In addition, professional associations began to establish divisions for members interested in group work. One such association, the *Association for Specialists in Group Work (ASGW)*, was formed in 1973 and is now one of the larger divisions of the *American Counseling Association (ACA)*.

Recent Trends

As groups became more commonplace, helping professionals began to use group counseling as an alternative or additional treatment to individual and family counseling. Group courses became more prevalent in training programs, to the point where it is now unusual for a helping professional to *not* have course work and field experience in group work. As you might expect, group work is one of the content areas required by the Council for the Accreditation of Counseling and Related Educational Programs (CACREP, 2009). Whereas the past 30 years have seen a decline in some of the more outrageous groups of the 1960s and 1970s, there has also been a rise in group counseling and therapy run by well-trained and experienced counselors.

In recent years, the focus of professionally run counseling groups has changed. Whereas the typical counseling group used to be an ongoing, heterogeneous group of individuals who sought increased self-awareness and personality change, today one is more likely to find *common-theme groups* with a specialized focus (e.g., eating disorders); *task groups*, which emphasize conscious behaviors and focus on how group dynamics affect the successful completion of a product; and *time-limited, brief-counseling groups* (usually fewer than 20 sessions) (Gladding, 2012; Southern, Erford, Vernon, & Davis-Gage, 2011). In addition, there has been a steady rise in the popularity of *self-help groups*. These grassroots groups have supported millions of Americans who have struggled with a variety of problems. Whereas the counselor of 30 years ago would rarely refer a client to a self-help group as an adjunct to counseling, the counselor of today who does not refer to a self-help group, in certain instances (e.g., alcoholism, eating disorders), may be acting unethically (Parks-Savage, 2015).

With the continued popularity of group work, ASGW has developed *Best Practice Guidelines,* as well as *Professional Standards for the Training of Group Workers* (ASGW, 2000, 2007). The *Best Practice Guidelines* are "intended to clarify the application of the ACA Code of Ethics to the field of group work" (ASGW, 2007, preamble). The standards define the knowledge, skills, and experiences necessary for the training of group leaders and delineate four specialty areas: *task groups, psychoeducational groups, counseling groups,* and *psychotherapy groups.* The importance of training using these standards has become increasingly recognized in recent years, as more and more counselor education programs adhere to them (Wilson & Newmeyer, 2008).

Today, group counseling is used in most counseling settings. Although the type of group that a counselor conducts will vary as a function of the specialty area and counseling setting, all counselors need to be familiar with the four types of professional groups and be able to conduct such groups or refer to appropriate groups when necessary.

Defining Modern-Day Groups

Today, most groups can be placed into one of five categories: *self-help groups, task groups, psychoeducational groups, counseling groups,* and *therapy groups,* with all but self-help groups being seen as professional groups that counselors may conduct at some point (ASGW, 2000). Although these groups are different in many ways, they all are affected by *group dynamics* and have a unique *group process* (Trotzer, 2013). The term *group dynamics* refers to the ongoing interactions and interrelationships among the group members and between the leader and group members (Gladding, 2006). These interactions are a function of conscious and unconscious forces and are influenced by such things as the structure of the group, the theoretical orientation of the leader, the unique personalities of the leader and the members, and a myriad of other influences such as drives, needs, gender, age, power issues, culture, and other known and unknown factors (Gladding, 2012; Jacobs et al., 2012). Group process refers to the changes that occur in a group as a function of the developmental stages through which the group will pass (AGPA, n.d.; Gladding, 2006). Group process can be affected by the dynamics in the group, but it is ongoing and positive if the group is led effectively. The following are brief descriptions of self-help groups, task groups, psychoeducational groups, counseling groups, and therapy groups, all of which are affected by group dynamics and group process.

Self-Help Groups

Although *self-help groups* have been around for more than 50 years, their growth has been phenomenal over the past 30 years (Southern, Erford, Vernon, & Davis-Gage, 2011). From AA to codependency groups, to eating disorder and diet groups, to men's and women's groups, to groups for the chronically mentally ill, the kinds of self-help groups that have emerged seem endless. Self-help groups tend to espouse a particular philosophy or way of being in the world and generally attract individuals who share a particular diagnosis, symptom, experience, or condition (Lieberman & Keith, 2002). Their purpose is the

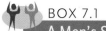

BOX 7.1
A Men's Self-Help Group

For one and a half years, I was a participant in a men's support group established by ten men. The purpose of the group was to have a supportive group of men with whom we could share our feelings, thoughts, and concerns around a wide range of issues, particularly those that were relevant to men. The group was leaderless, although we all periodically would take a leadership role. For all that time, we shared some of our most intimate details about such issues as divorces and marriages, our sexuality, our families of origin, and relationship concerns. But perhaps most important, not having a female present enabled us to share in a way that we probably would not have shared otherwise. Although I did not remain in the group, the group continued for seven years with most of its original members.

education, affirmation, and enhancement of existing strengths of the group members. Generally, there is a nonpaid volunteer leader who focuses the discussion and assists in defining the rules of the group (Humphreys, 2011). However, sometimes there may be no leader at all. Self-help groups are generally free or have a nominal fee and can be facilitated by a trained layperson or mental health professional (see Box 7.1).

Self-help groups are not in-depth psychotherapy groups and generally do not require a vast amount of member self-disclosure. In fact, because self-help groups tend to be open groups, which means that members may come and go as they please, it is sometimes difficult to build group cohesion, a critical element for in-depth work. Usually, individuals in self-help groups are encouraged to share only the amount that feels comfortable. Some self-help groups even discourage intense self-disclosure, as that would be seen as more appropriate for individual or group counseling.

With self-help groups, the number of group members, length of meeting times, and atmosphere of the group setting can vary considerably. Some groups might have 200 members, while others might be limited to just a few people. Some groups might meet in the basement of a church, while others might meet in the comfort of the office of a counselor who has loaned the group space. Some self-help groups may be ongoing, others may be time limited; some might demand confidentiality, while others will not.

Although self-help groups are not generally led by counselors, they have become an increasingly important referral source and are often used as an adjunct to counseling (Parks-Savage, 2015). For these reasons, it has become increasingly important for counselors to be aware of the types of self-help groups available in their communities.

Task Groups

Task groups emphasize conscious behaviors and focus on how group dynamics affect the successful completion of a product (Gladding, 2012; Southern et al., 2011). The formation of NTL was the first systematic effort to understand the dynamics of groups in business and industry, and much of the knowledge learned from NTL is today applied to our understanding of task groups (Hulse-Killacky, Killacky, & Donigian, 2001). Task group specialists utilize

> *principles of normal human development through group based educational, developmental, and systemic strategies applied in the context of here-and-now*

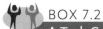

BOX 7.2
A Task Group at a Bank

Ed, a private-practice licensed professional counselor who consults with business and industry, has been approached by the vice president of the local bank because of bickering going on between various bank managers. The conflict seems to have affected their ability to work effectively. Ed decides to meet with the managers for four small-group meetings and analyze some of their interactions. During the first meeting, Ed establishes rapport and asks the managers to define the problem. The next two meetings are spent doing role-play problem-solving activities selected by Ed. He watches the group carefully as they go through the problem-solving process. He is particularly aware of issues of control, hierarchies, and boundaries, especially in relationship to sexism and gender differences, prejudice and cross-cultural style differences, ageism and age style differences, and personal style differences. During the last meeting, he shares what he has seen; and, based on his feedback, he asks the group to develop some problem-solving techniques to work through their interpersonal issues. He tells the group that he will come back in a month to see if they have followed through on their ideas.

interaction that promote efficient and effective accomplishment of group tasks among people who are gathered to accomplish group task goals.

(ASGW, 2000, Section on Specialization Training in Group Work)

Task group specialists enter a system (e.g., agency or organization) and attempt to analyze and diagnose problems. Then they facilitate change in the dynamics of the system, with the goal being the successful completion of tasks (Jacobs et al., 2012). Many times, difficulties within systems are related to problems in differing values and social norms that negatively affect work groups within the system. Such differences among individuals can lead to problems in communication, feelings of dissatisfaction at work, low motivation, low productivity, sexual harassment, cross-cultural problems, and other issues (see Box 7.2).

Psychoeducational Groups

Psychoeducational groups (formerly called *guidance groups*) attempt to increase self-understanding, emphasize education and training, promote personal growth and empowerment, and prevent future problems through the dissemination of mental health education in a group setting (Aasheim, 2010; ASGW, 2000). A few examples of the many topics that psychoeducational groups have focused upon include sex education, bullying, conflict resolution, AIDS awareness, career awareness, communication skills, diversity issues, chemical dependence, and stress management.

Today, the term *psychoeducational groups* is generally used instead of *guidance groups* because the latter term held negative connotations in that it was misconstrued to mean that such groups should be highly advice oriented and have a moral imperative (Gladding, 2012; Kottler, 1994). Although psychoeducational groups had their origins in schools, today such preventive and educational groups can be found in many additional settings, such as business and industry, community centers, and community agencies. Psychoeducational group specialists utilize

the principles of normal human development and functioning through group based educational and developmental strategies applied in the context of

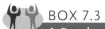

BOX 7.3
A Psychoeducational Group in the Schools (Classroom Guidance)

Jawanda is an elementary school counselor. Her school system requires her to conduct psychoeducational groups four times a year in each class. Each group is followed by four group sessions run by the teacher of the class, who is coached by the school counselor. Some of the classroom guidance activities she does are "How to handle a bully," "Friendship," and "Drug awareness." Jawanda spends approximately one hour in the class, which is split between a presentation, a series of preset questions that she has for the students, and time for discussion and processing at the end of the group. The students seem to particularly enjoy the discussion aspect of the program and become quite active in sharing their experiences and views.

> *here-and-now interaction that promote personal and interpersonal growth and development and the prevention of future difficulties among people who may be at risk for the development of personal or interpersonal problems or who seek enhancement of personal qualities and abilities.*

(ASGW, 2000, Section on Specialization Training in Group Work)

Psychoeducational groups always have a designated, well-trained group leader and focus mostly on *preventive education* and the support of the group members (Brown, 2015b). Leaders will usually offer a didactic presentation, and generally there is limited client self-disclosure, although there is usually an opportunity for discussion and some personal sharing. Such groups may be ongoing or can occur on a one-time basis. Psychoeducational groups can vary dramatically in size and the number of times they meet, although they are generally short term. As with self-help groups, there is little or no charge to participants (see Box 7.3).

Counseling Groups

As with individual counseling and therapy, many people differentiate between *group counseling* and *group therapy* (Capuzzi & Gross, 2010; Gladding, 2012). Usually, group counseling is focused on prevention and wellness, self-enhancement, increased insight, self-actualization, and conscious as opposed to unconscious motivations. Clients in group counseling may be struggling with adjustment problems in life such as the breakup of relationships, deaths, and job transitions. They generally are not dealing with severe pathology or a debilitating psychological problem. Group counseling specialists utilize

> *principles of normal human development and functioning through group based cognitive, affective, behavioral, or systemic intervention strategies applied in the context of here-and-now interaction that address personal and interpersonal problems of living and promote personal and interpersonal growth and development among people who may be experiencing transitory maladjustment, who are at risk for the development of personal or interpersonal problems, or who seek enhancement of personal qualities and abilities.*

(ASGW, 2000, Section on Specialization Training in Group Work)

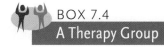

BOX 7.4
A Therapy Group

The group discussed at the beginning of the chapter, in which I participated for two years, I consider to have been a therapy group, although some might call it group counseling (see Figure 7.1). Often, there is a fine line between the two. Although I would not consider any member of the group as having had serious pathology, it was clear that many of us were dealing with major issues in our lives. There was a great push in the group for self-disclosure, insight, and change, and much of the time in the group was spent talking about past issues and uncovering conflicts, as group members attempted to work through unfinished business.

Group counseling tends to be shorter in duration than group therapy but longer than psychoeducational groups. The group leader needs to be well trained in group process and group dynamics. As in group therapy, group counseling is a small-group experience, usually involving four to twelve members. In more recent years, short-term, action-oriented counseling groups that focus on common themes have become increasingly popular (Ivey, Pedersen, & Ivey, 2001).

Group Therapy

In contrast to counseling groups that tend to be preventive in nature and wellness oriented, *group therapy* typically focuses upon deep-seated, long-term issues; remediation of severe pathology; and personality reconstruction (see Box 7.4).

Individuals who participate in therapy groups may suffer from severe emotional conflicts, deep-seated problems, neurotic and deviant behaviors, and severe problems that would need long-term treatment. Group therapy specialists utilize

> *principles of normal and abnormal human development and functioning through group based cognitive, affective, behavioral, or systemic intervention strategies applied in the context of negative emotional arousal that address personal and interpersonal problems of living, remediate perceptual and cognitive distortions or repetitive patterns of dysfunctional behavior, and promote personal and interpersonal growth and development among people who may be experiencing severe and/or chronic maladjustment.*

(ASGW, 2000, Section on Specialization Training in Group Work)

As with group counseling, the therapy group leader needs to be well trained in group dynamics and group process and be able to handle clients who might have extreme emotional responses to a group meeting (Jacobs et al., 2012). In addition, as with group counseling, group therapy has a limited number of members, and continuity of membership is crucial for the development of the group process.

Despite the fact that most authors differentiate counseling groups from therapy groups, there are many similarities. For instance, both counseling and therapy groups have designated highly trained leaders, and generally, there are between four and twelve group members. Also, usually such groups meet for a minimum of eight sessions, although some may continue to meet on an ongoing basis. Most counseling and therapy groups meet at least once a week for one to three hours, and confidentiality of the group is particularly important. Although leadership styles may vary, there is usually some expectation on the part of the leader that members will have the opportunity to freely express their feelings and work on change.

Comparing Psychoeducational, Counseling, and Therapy Groups

Today, counselors can be found running all kinds of groups in a wide range of settings, although master's-level counselors are generally found conducting psychoeducational, counseling, and therapy groups. Figure 7.1 compares the major differences between these kinds of groups.

FIGURE 7.1

Comparison of Psychoeducational, Counseling, and Therapy Groups

Relative Strength of Factors as a Function of Type of Group		Psychoeducational	Counseling	Psychotherapy
	High			
		Wellness Prevention Education	Group process Group dynamics Insight Wellness Self-disclosure Prevention Change	Insight and change Past Group process Group dynamics Pathology Severe distress Unconscious motivation Self-disclosure
	Medium	Insight Group process Group dynamics Self-disclosure Change	Education Past	
			Unconscious motivation Severe distress Pathology	Wellness Prevention Education
		Past Unconscious motivation Severe distress Pathology		
	Low	**Psychoeducational**	**Counseling**	**Psychotherapy**

The Use of Theory in Group Work

Theory is as important in group counseling as it is in individual counseling. As Corey et al. (2014) point out, "A theory can guide you, much as a road map or navigational instrument . . . If you do not have a navigational instrument you may get lost and lose time trying to find your way." (p. 99). As in individual counseling, theory in reference to group counseling (1) gives us a comprehensive system of doing counseling, (2) assists us in understanding our clients, (3) helps us in deciding which techniques to apply, (4) is useful in predicting the course of treatment, and (5) is researchable, thus providing us information about its efficacy. If applied to group work, a counselor's theoretical model should be an extension of that person's personality, for a theory discordant with one's view of human nature will feel awkward and be applied poorly.

Although the vast majority of theories of counseling and psychotherapy were initially developed for individual counseling, most have been applied to group work, with each having advantages and disadvantages when applied to a group setting (Gladding, 2012). The following are brief examples of group counseling as applied by four counseling theories, one from each of the four conceptual orientations examined in Chapter 4: *psychodynamic, existential–humanistic, cognitive–behavioral,* and *postmodern.* More specifically, psychoanalytic group therapy, person-centered group counseling, cognitive–behavioral group therapy, and solution-focused group therapy will be reviewed briefly.

Psychoanalytic Group Therapy

Psychoanalytic group therapy tends to focus upon many of the same elements that are stressed in individual psychoanalysis, such as concentrating on the past, examining unconscious motivations, encouraging insight and self-examination, understanding intrapsychic processes, and learning about one's resistances, defenses, and transferences (Corey, 2012; Wolf, Schwartz, McCarty, & Goldberg, 1972). In group psychoanalytic therapy, it is assumed that group members will unconsciously reenact family-of-origin issues within the group. The group, therefore, offers members a rich opportunity to work on past issues that affect current functioning.

In group psychoanalysis, deep understanding of how past relationships affect current functioning occurs through interpretation of the transference relationship (Godby, Hopper, & Sharpe, 2015). *Transference* is the process of projecting experiences of early relationships onto others, resulting in a distorted view of who they are. Instead of seeing others in the group clearly, they see them through a filter that is symbolic of the early child-rearing practices provided to them. Thus, if parents were consistently abusive and hurtful, the individual unconsciously assumes all adults to be this way and misinterprets the behaviors of others. These projections of early childhood experiences onto others are wonderful fodder for analysis by the leader and the group members and can be examined, interpreted, and studied, and group members can begin to see how early child-rearing practices affect their current relationships. The focus on the past is used by the group leader to help clients understand how defense mechanism and resistances have been developed to protect the client from the trauma that they experienced in early child-rearing from their parents and significant others. Some advantages to group psychoanalytic therapy over individual therapy include:

1. The sheer number of individuals in a group allow more opportunity to recreate past family issues through transference (transferring projections onto the leader and group members).
2. There is ample opportunity for the leader and group members to examine and interpret the projections of any one member onto the leader and other members.
3. There is an increased opportunity for feedback concerning defenses and resistances.
4. There is less chance of extreme dependency on the therapist because some of the authority is dispersed among other group members.
5. Seeing others work through similar issues helps to reduce defensiveness.
6. Observing other members working through resistances can be an encouragement to the client to do the same.

Although the basic techniques used in individual analysis are also used in group analytic therapy, some adjustments are made for the group dynamics. For instance, in a process called *going around*, all group members participate in *free association*, in which they are encouraged to share all their thoughts and feelings willingly and spontaneously with the group (Biancoviso, Bishop-Towle, & Fuertes, 2004). This allows members to move quickly beyond their *defenses* and helps to create group cohesion as members all share deeply personal issues. This sharing can later be interpreted by members, the group leader, or both, as follows:

> It quickly became clear that the encouragement to express associations, thoughts, and feelings freely led to much interaction of a highly charged quality. These interpersonal responses were both appropriate and inappropriate. Patients became increasingly familiar with the characteristic distortions each made and traced these distortions in time to specific familial antecedents. In the course of working through, the patients were encouraged to choose more reasonable alternatives in reality.
>
> (Wolf & Schwartz, 1972, p. 42)

Other psychoanalytic techniques are also easily used in the group setting (Gladding, 2012). For instance, when using *dream analysis*, group members have the opportunity to offer possible interpretations to the dream. Sometimes these meanings may be on target; other times, they are projections of a member's own issues, which also can be worked on. *Transference* can be directed at the leader or the members of the group, and both the leader and the group members can interpret this transference. Finally, *resistance* may occur within a member or with the whole group (e.g., attempting to accuse the leader of poor group skills), and this too can be interpreted by the group leader or by other members.

When psychoanalytic group therapy was originated, groups generally met three times a week for about one and a half hours, and most of the techniques mimicked what occurred in individual counseling (Wolf & Schwartz, 1972). In recent years, however, analysts have tended to meet less frequently with their clients and have adapted new techniques to the group setting. For instance, today some analysts feel comfortable sharing their own inner experience of the client within the group setting and also encourage increased sharing by clients (Levenkron, 2009; Zeisel, 2009).

Although most groups today are not psychoanalytically oriented, many groups borrow some of the tenets and techniques of psychoanalytic group therapy. For instance, the analysis of dreams, discussion of resistances and transference issues, and acknowledgment of the unconscious are commonly discussed in groups of many orientations.

Cognitive–Behavioral Group Therapy

Cognitive–behavioral group therapy combines the best of behavioral therapy and cognitive therapy into one broad counseling approach that relies on learning theory. As discussed in Chapter 4, behavior therapy was developed from three learning paradigms: *classical conditioning*, *operant conditioning*, and *modeling* or *social learning*. Over the years, cognitive approaches were developed that also relied on learning theory and asserted that in addition to behaviors, deeply embedded *cognitive structures*, or *illogical and irrational thinking*, can be conditioned (Neukrug, 2011). Believing that cognitions and behaviors could both be conditioned, counselors began to integrate the two paradigms into what is now called *cognitive–behavioral group therapy*.

Today, many cognitive–behavioral group therapists start by addressing a client's *irrational thoughts* or *cognitive distortions* (I must be perfectly capable in everything that I do!) (Corey, 2012; Neukrug, 2011). As in individual therapy, connections between clients' belief systems and their actions, feelings, and physiological responses are identified. Clients can then take a multipronged approach to dealing with their problems, as they challenge their irrational thinking or cognitive distortions, practice new behaviors, and experiment with new feelings. Because cognitive–behavioral therapy relies on a number of learning theory paradigms, a whole range of techniques can be used (Day, 2007).

Clients of cognitive–behavioral group therapy experience a similar counseling process as do those who participate in individual cognitive–behavioral therapy, with the added benefit of having group members offer assistance through the change process. Initially, the group leader has to ensure that the members experience a sense of group cohesion. This is generally accomplished through the leader's use of foundational skills to build a trusting relationship. Next, the problem has to be clearly defined. Based on problem identification, goals are specified and appropriate techniques are chosen. Evaluating the success of those techniques and working on termination and follow-up issues are the final stages of this process (Corey, 2012; Day, 2007).

There are many advantages to cognitive–behavioral work within a group setting. First, the establishment of group cohesion early in the process allows each group member to receive feedback from other group members concerning problem identification and strategies for change. Second, because relationships are formed, the leader will encourage the group to reinforce the changes made by the members. Third, group members can rehearse new ways of thinking and behaving in the group prior to trying them in the real world. Fourth, group members can act as models for other group members, thereby offering more opportunity to learn from others. Finally, coaching of new behaviors can be offered by the group leader or by group members. In this case, the coach will often sit behind the group member and offer continual feedback concerning a specific behavior being practiced in front of the group.

Leaders of cognitive–behavioral groups are active and directive as they assist clients in working on their cognitive–behavioral goals and assist the group in learning how to respond to one another (Corey, 2012). Such group leaders tend to downplay intrapsychic processes and stress how current cognitions and behaviors are affecting the client. Finally, because cognitive–behavioral therapy does not harp on the past or on intrapsychic and unconscious processes, it is a much shorter process than many other approaches to counseling.

Person-Centered Group Counseling

As with the other approaches we have examined thus far, *person-centered group counseling* uses the basic constructs of its individual approach to counseling and applies them in a group setting (Gladding, 2012). Thus, the person-centered group counselor relies on the qualities of *empathic understanding*, *genuineness*, and *unconditional positive regard* to guide the group process (see Chapter 4).

Person-centered group counselors are not concerned about unconscious motivations, instincts, transference, or spending an inordinate amount of time working on past issues. However, they do believe that increased self-awareness and insight will be achieved by applying the core conditions of empathy, genuineness, and unconditional positive regard. Purists of this approach believe these conditions alone are *necessary and sufficient* to the effectiveness of group counseling. If applied properly, they say, there will be a tendency for the group to move toward health and wholeness.

After leading many groups, Rogers (1970) noted that the same process generally transpired in groups. This process could be described in a series of steps in which clients (1) initially mill around and resist personal expression; (2) begin to share past feelings and negative feelings—feelings that are relatively safe to express; (3) slowly express personally meaningful feelings, deeper parts of self, and feelings about one another in the group; (4) begin to accept all parts of self and find a healing capacity within; (5) are increasingly able to hear feedback about self and let down their facades; (6) become healers themselves and begin to assist others inside and outside of the group; (7) are able to encounter another person fully in an "I–Thou" relationship; and (8) begin to look and act differently inside and outside the group.

The person-centered approach to group counseling is nondirective and worked effectively for Carl Rogers as he traveled the world running groups for peoples in conflict with one another, such as Catholics and Protestants in Northern Ireland (Kirschenbaum 2009). However, the total lack of directiveness, as portrayed by Rogers, is difficult for many counselors. Other existential–humanistic approaches, such as Gestalt therapy and existential therapy, tend to be more directive and have many of the same goals and ideals of the person-centered approach.

Solution-Focused Group Counseling

As detailed in Chapter 4, solution-focused therapy is loosely based on *social constructionism* and *postmodernism*, which assert that reality is a social construction and that problems can be viewed as challenges created by language. Seen from this perspective, how the counselor brings himself or herself into the relationship is critical to helping the individual overcome his or her problems as the counselor attempts to focus on solutions, not harp on problems.

The solution-focused group counselor rejects the notion that individuals have an inherent tendency toward mental health problems or illnesses and focuses almost exclusively on solutions and client strengths, not client deficits or problems (Fernando, 2007). This approach is *pragmatic, optimistic, anti-deterministic,* and *future-oriented* and believes in the ability of clients to change quickly, find *exceptions* to their problems, and build on those exceptions to find new ways of living in the world (O'Hanlon & Weiner-Davis, 2003). Some of the assumptions of solution-focused group counseling that underlie this approach include the following (Colley, 2009; Proudlock & Wellman, 2011):

1. All clients have abilities, resources, and strengths.
2. If what you are doing is working, do more of it.
3. If what you are doing is not working, try something different.
4. Problems are not constant—there are times when they are not affecting the client.
5. Big problems do not necessarily require big solutions.
6. Change in one area will affect other areas.
7. The client is the expert on the problem, not the counselor.
8. Solutions are not necessarily directly related to the problem.
9. Change is inevitable.

Using these assumptions as its basis, solution-focused group counseling can be viewed as going through the following stages (Coe & Zimpfer, 1996; Ratner, George, & Iveson, 2012):

Pregroup Stage.   In this stage, the counselor selects potential group members and prepares them for group counseling. Here, the counselor informs potential clients about the norms of the group, begins to set expectations based on the nine assumptions given above, and sets an expectation that there will be a sense of trust in the group. Also, the counselor will talk with the potential client about the group in a manner that assumes change will occur quickly and that the client has the resources to change. In addition, the counselor might use *presuppositional questions* that offer hope, such as: "What do you think you will do differently between now and the time we first meet?"

Initial Stage.   Here, the counselor takes on a nonexpert role and assumes that the client has the resources and strengths to find solutions to his or her problems. As the counselor listens to the client with curiosity, awe, and interest, trust is built and clients begin to work on setting goals. Counselors use *problem-free talk* as they focus on solutions, not problems, and ask questions focused on helping the client find his or her own solutions. Questions revolve around *preferred futures,* and counselors ask clients what *goals* they would like to pursue, inquiring about when clients have had *exceptions* to problems and successful *coping mechanisms* that clients have used before, asking them to *identify resources and strengths,* and asking them the *miracle question* to help them identify where they want to be:

> *Suppose that one night, while you were asleep, there was a miracle and this problem was solved. How would you know? What would be different?*
>
> (de Shazer, 1988, p. 5)

Working Stage.   In this stage, clients collaborate with the counselor to develop goals and a contract to begin working on them. At this point, clients can practice inside and outside of group, as they work on their solutions while group members encourage and compliment one another. The group leader ensures that a pathology mindset is not reinforced ("I can't change because I'm a major depressive"). Also, members are encouraged to experiment with new behaviors, and they measure their change through a process called *scaling,* in which they identify how close they are to accomplishing their goals by selecting a number on a scale (1 = no progress up to 10 = a great deal of progress).

Termination Stage.   Since clients are encouraged early on to become independent and to change quickly, it is not necessary to spend a great deal of time dealing with issues of closure and termination. Termination occurs when change occurs, and when clients and group members agree that goals are being successfully worked upon. During this stage, clients can be given the option of returning in the future to follow up and amplify any changes that have occurred.

Solution-focused group counseling is a short-term, positive approach to working with clients that assumes that clients can change quickly, that clients have the resources and ability to change, and that change can be long lasting.

Preparing for the Group

Regardless of the type of group that one is conducting, prior to starting, there are a number of practical issues that the effective group leader should consider in order to build the most conducive climate for the group. Some of these include how to recruit members, the composition of the group, whether the group is closed or open, the size of the group, the duration and frequency of meetings, the atmosphere of the meeting place, and the leadership style of the group leader (Corey et al., 2014; Posthuma, 2002; Yalom, 2005).

Getting Members

What if I ran a group and nobody came? Believe me, this is a question that has been asked by many counselors who are considering starting a group. There are a number of ways that members can be obtained, including advertising; seeking referrals from colleagues; seeking referrals from appropriate sources (e.g., teachers, academic advising offices, and physicians); placing signs, if and where appropriate (e.g., a sign in a residence hall); and referring appropriate clients from one's own caseload. Of course, the type of person that the leader wants in the group (group composition) will greatly affect how members are recruited.

Group Composition

The composition of a counseling or therapy group can be a crucial factor in its success. Most significantly, leaders need to decide whether the group will be homogeneous or heterogeneous. In considering this important factor, leaders will reflect on the following factors: age, sex, cultural background, level of functioning, problem focus, and diagnosis of the members. Although research on the effects of group composition on group success is mixed, leaders need to consider all of the potential problems and advantages that might affect the particular group that they will be running (Greenfield, Cummings, Kuper, Wigderson, & Koro-Ljungberg, 2013; Posthuma, 2002; Stark-Rose, Livingston-Sacin, Merchant, & Finley, 2012).

Closed and Open Groups

Groups that do not allow new members to join are called *closed groups*, and cohesion in these groups generally occurs more quickly than in *open groups*. Sometimes group leaders will decide to have a modified closed group, where the leader will replace a member as other members leave. This is particularly useful when running small groups, especially if there is an expectation that members will leave the group at some point. Open groups, such as AA and other self-help groups, generally have members freely joining or leaving.

Size of Group

The size of the group usually depends on the purpose and type of group that one is running. Whereas some self-help groups and psychoeducational groups may have large numbers of individuals (sometimes well over 25), the ideal size for counseling and therapy groups ranges from around 4 to 12 members. Clearly, when the focus of a group is on the sharing of deeply personal issues, a smaller number of clients makes intuitive sense, as small numbers allow the building of trust in an intimate setting. Other factors that should be considered when determining the size of the group include whether there is a co-leader, the length of time that the group meets, the size of the space where the group meets, and the focus of the group.

Duration of Meetings

Groups can generally run from 30 minutes to 3 hours long, with the most common length being 90 minutes to 2 hours (Jacobs et al., 2012). Factors to consider when deciding the length of group sessions include the amount of time available (e.g., school counselors usually have limited time), the focus of the group, the energy level of the leader, the energy level of the participants, and whether there is a co-leader.

Frequency of Meetings

Some groups meet daily, others monthly (Jacobs et al., 2012). Issues to consider in determining frequency include focus of the problem, availability of space, needs of clients, ability to pay, availability of clients, and the availability of the group leader(s).

Securing an Appropriate Space

As in individual counseling, groups should be held in a comfortable, confidential, and safe environment that has few if any distractions (Posthuma, 2002). Because groups often have many members, this is not always an easy task. For instance, some groups, such as psychoeducational groups in schools, are often conducted in a classroom because a separate space would be difficult to find. Classrooms often have uncomfortable hard chairs, may be filled with distractions not related to group content, and may not provide the psychological safety necessary for individuals to open up within the group. In contrast, imagine a private space that is soundproofed, has big puffy chairs, and has artwork that highlights the psyche. This environment seems to call on the group members to share parts of themselves.

Group Leadership Style

Leadership styles will vary based on the leader's personality and theoretical orientation. Prior to starting a group, a good leader should consider the impact that his or her leadership style will have on it (Corey, 2012; Gladding, 2012). For instance, a leader who is more comfortable with a person-centered approach that includes expression of feelings might want to consider whether he or she would be the best person to run a weight loss or bridge phobia group, both of which generally do better with a cognitive–behavioral focus. In addition, good leaders consider the composition of their group and have adjusted their style to the needs of the group members. Finally, research suggests that an effective group leader "will want to be positive, supportive, provide sufficient structure, attend to the developing group cohesion, allow group members to take ownership of their group, and provide a meaningful context for what occurs in the group" (DeLucia-Waack & Nitza, 2014, p. 31). Others have suggested that good leadership also entails being emotionally present, having personal power and self-confidence, being courageous and willing to take risks, being willing to confront oneself, being sincere and authentic, having an identity or strong sense of self, being enthusiastic and believing in the group process, and being inventive and creative (Corey, 2012).

The Stages of Group Development

The development of a group has been shown to occur in predictable stages (Brabender & Fallon, 2009; Yalom, 2005). Although group experts differ on the terms that they use to identify these stages, they tend to describe the characteristics of the stages in fairly consistent ways. One popular series of words, still very much in use today that describes these stages, was developed by Bruce Tuckman (1935–) (1965; Tuckman & Jensen, 1977). Tuckman suggested that the beginning stages have to do with *forming* the group, as members move from being a number of separate individuals to the realization that they are together, in a group. The group then moves into the *storming* stage, when defensiveness and intragroup struggles heighten as members test the waters to see if they can trust one another. Slowly, as trust is built, the group moves into the *norming* stage, where the group becomes a cohesive unit. Soon after, the group members enter the *performing* stage, and they begin to work on their issues. Finally, as members wind down and begin to deal with their feelings about leaving the close-knit relationships that they have built in the group, they move into the last stage, *adjourning*. As you read through the following stages I have identified, take particular note of how Tuckman's stages might apply.

Keep in mind that counseling and therapy groups use continuity of membership to stimulate the development of interpersonal relationships that are necessary for the full development of the group process through all of the stages. On the other hand, the structure of self-help, task, and psychoeducational groups is such that we are unlikely to see passage through all of the stages in every scenario.

The Pregroup Stage (Forming)

> *Counselors screen prospective group counseling/therapy participants. To the extent possible, counselors select members whose needs and goals are compatible with goals of the group, who will not impede the group process, and whose well-being will not be jeopardized by the group experience.*

> (ACA, 2014a, Section A.9.a)

As the ACA ethics code asserts, the group leader needs to find an effective method of pre-screening potential group members. In this process, the group leader assesses the appropriateness of the member for the group. He or she is deciding which potential members will make the best group mix by considering such issues as age, gender, cultural background, group fit, emotional readiness, presenting problem or focus of the group, goals, and educational background (Hines & Fields, 2002). There is no one method of deciding who will be in the group; for instance, sometimes focusing on one attribute (e.g., gender) will increase group cohesion and foster goal attainment, while other times, having a mix of different people (e.g., cross-cultural mix) can be beneficial, such as if the group is working on issues of tolerance.

After deciding who will be in the group, some group leaders will have a pregroup meeting with all potential members, while others will provide potential members with a thorough written or even videotaped summary of the expectations of the group in an effort to have them screen themselves out. However, the most effective and common method is probably the individual interview. Couch (1995) notes that the interview can identify the needs, expectations, and commitment of the potential group member; challenge myths and misconceptions of the potential member; convey and procure information to the potential member; and screen out (or in) potential members. This is also when an *informed consent document* can be given to the member so that he or she is clear about the basic rules and process of the group.

Although deciding on who will be in the group occurs prior to the actual first meeting, it is considered the first stage of the group because of its potential impact on the group process.

The Initial Stage (Forming)

When the group actually does begin, the members are often anxious, apprehensive, and eager to get started—all at the same time. During this stage, group members are adapting to the rules and goals of the group and are wondering whether they can trust the other group members. Because of the initial apprehension and lack of trust, group members will often avoid talking about in-depth feelings during this stage, and discussions are relatively safe. Therefore, it is common for conversations to be superficial, for members to have a focus on others as opposed to a self-focus, and for discussions to revolve around feelings from the past, not "here and now" (Corey et al., 2014). Many behaviors that clients may exhibit reflect their early fears about the group process. Sometimes called *resistance* (although I prefer the word *reticence*), just a few of these behaviors include being silent, laughing or talking excessively, being overly nurturing, monopolizing, intellectualizing, generalizing, being seductive, and so forth.

During this initial stage, group members are often self-conscious, worried about how others might view them, and concerned about whether they will be accepted. Some of the major tasks for the group leader during this stage include defining the ground rules, setting limits, and building a level of trust that will provide members with a sense that they want to continue in the group (Gladding, 2012). If the leader is successful, group cohesion will begin to build by the end of this stage.

In the pursuit of trust and group cohesion, the leader must be able to set limits, ensure that members abide by the ground rules, and simultaneously show empathy and unconditional positive regard. Structure, empathy, and positive regard enable group members to feel psychologically safe, which is the first step toward greater openness. Leaders need to be genuine and only slightly self-disclosing (Corey et al., 2014). This is sometimes a difficult balance, but, ultimately the leader's purpose is to focus on group members, not self.

From a systems perspective, group leaders should be particularly cognizant of *scapegoating*, as this is a convenient way to keep the focus off oneself (Clark, 2002). Thus, the leader should know appropriate strategies for dealing with scapegoating, as such behavior has the potential of limiting self-disclosure and being destructive to group cohesion.

The Transition Stage (Storming and Then Norming)

During the opening phase of the transition stage, group members are beginning to feel comfortable with the technical issues and ground rules of the group. However, anxiety is still felt as trust and safety issues continue. Issues of control, power, and authority become increasingly important in this stage as members position themselves within the system (Corey et al., 2014; Yalom, 2005). What are members trying to accomplish by positioning themselves? Ultimately, they are attempting to be the same person in the group as they are in the rest of their lives:

> Given enough time, group members will begin to be themselves: they will interact with the group members as they interact with others in their social sphere, will create in the group the same interpersonal universe they have always inhabited.

> (Yalom, 2005, pp. 31–32)

As members attempt to find their place in the group, they are likely to experience anxiety, fear, and a myriad of other feelings. At this point in the group process, members may begin projecting onto the group leader and struggle with transference issues (Corey et al., 2014; Yalom, 2005). A dance occurs in the group as members attempt to settle into the group process and simultaneously deal with all the feelings they are having. Attacking and scapegoating are common at this point, as members are fearful of taking ownership of their strong and sometimes confusing feelings and thus blame others for their discomfort. Although empathy and positive regard continue to be important at this stage, it is also vital that the leader actively prevent a member from being scapegoated or attacked as a result of group instability. Failure to do so could prevent the group from progressing further, as members become bogged down with conflict and fail to build cohesion.

If the leader is successful in helping group members pass through the difficult part of this stage, trust will slowly be built, resistance will diminish, and members will begin to settle into their roles and feel safe enough to delve into self and to share personal concerns. Members are now transitioning to a place where they can demonstrate the ability to take ownership of their feelings, have a self- rather than other-focus, talk in the here and now, not blame others for their problems, and have a sense of mutual support and cooperation with the other group members (Yalom, 2005). At this point, the need for the leader to protect members dramatically decreases as members stop blaming others, stop acting out, and increasingly feel a sense of cohesiveness as a group. Near the end of this stage, group members more clearly identify the goals that they would like to achieve. Although goals were probably identified earlier by most group members, defensiveness and lack of clarity of self may have distorted the clients' perceptions of which issues to work on.

From a systems perspective, it is interesting to compare this stage to family counseling. Families come in with a system that has evolved over a number of years. Issues of control, power, and authority have already been decided. Therefore, the purpose of family counseling is to understand the family in order to devise strategies to change the system in a manner that will lead to healthier functioning for all. Groups, on the other hand, are working to build a system (Matthews, 1992), and it is the responsibility of the leader to ensure that strategies are used to develop a healthy, functioning system. Ultimately, the goal for families and groups is the same: to develop a system that has open channels of communications, allows the sharing of feelings, and rebuffs abuses of power that leave people feeling unsafe and victimized. When families and groups arrive at this place, they are ready to work.

The Work Stage (Performing)

As members gain the capacity to take ownership of their feelings and life predicaments, a deepening of trust and a sense of cohesion emerges within the group. Members are now able to give and hear feedback, focus on identified problems, and take an active role in the change process. For instance, they may attempt new ways of communicating, acting, or expressing feelings. During this stage, conflict lessens, but when it does occur, it is handled very differently from the way it was dealt with previously. Members now can talk through conflict and take ownership of their own part in it.

As this stage continues, members will begin to identify and work on behaviors that they would like to change. As members accomplish their goals, they gain in self-esteem as they receive positive feedback from other members and acquire a sense of accomplishment for the work they have done. As members meet their goals, they are near the completion of the group process.

From a systems perspective, during this stage, the group has developed its own unique homeostasis; however, it is important that the group leader prohibit members from becoming too comfortable in their styles of relating, as this can prevent change and growth. Leaders can best facilitate movement during this stage using a variety of advanced counseling skills such as support and confrontation, higher-level empathy, probing questions, and interpretation.

The Closure Stage (Adjourning)

The last stage of the group process is highlighted by an increased sense of accomplishment, high self-esteem, and the beginning awareness that the group process is near completion. Saying good-bye can be a difficult process for many, and it is important that the leader facilitate this process in a direct yet gentle fashion. Often this is done by the leader encouraging members to share what they have learned about themselves, share what they have learned about others in the group, and express their feelings about one another and the upcoming termination of the group. Using empathy, the leader will often summarize the changes that have taken place and focus on the separation process. This important final stage in the group process allows members to feel a sense of completion and wholeness about what they have experienced.

It is important during this stage to ensure that those who need additional counseling, or others who would like additional counseling, be given appropriate referrals. In addition, other members may want to develop a method of ensuring the continuation of changed behaviors. Members might decide to meet periodically on their own in a kind of ongoing support group, or there might be periodic planned meetings with the group leader that focus on reinforcement of changed behaviors. Some members might have periodic check-ins with the group leader on an individual basis.

Finally, to assess if the group has been beneficial, many leaders will complete an evaluation of it. Determining if change has been substantive and continual is often completed during the final group meeting, by distributing a follow-up evaluation at a reasonable amount of time after the group has disbanded, or both.

Multicultural/Social Justice Focus

Principles for Diversity-Competent Group Workers

> *For group counselors to be effective with all populations, it is critical that they are trained to be culturally competent.*
>
> (Bemak & Chung, 2004, p. 31)

In an effort to ensure that individuals who do group work are appropriately knowledgeable about multicultural issues, the ASGW developed and endorsed Multicultural and Social Justice Competence Principles for Group Workers (ASGW, 2012a). These principles include group leaders being aware of self and group members as diverse individuals and being sensitive about differences; having competence as a multicultural group expert and social justice advocate relative to group work; and knowing appropriate group intervention and processing skills while respecting cultural differences. All professionals who practice group work should be knowledgeable about this document.

Social Justice in Group Work: Understanding the Place of Privilege

One of the increasingly important roles of the counselor who does group work is to understand how privilege affects individuals (Holcomb-McCoy, 2008; Singh & Salazar, 2010a, 2010b). It is important that counselors be aware that there is "invisible affirmative action" for a whole range of clients, including males, Whites, and heterosexuals, and that clients who are not bathed in this invisible cloak are often seen as stupid, lazy, or unwilling to put real effort into "making it" (Smith & Shin, 2008). In groups, privilege, or lack thereof, affects each client. One role of the counselor is to help clients see how privilege, or lack thereof, has affected them and to empower them to be advocates for themselves. In addition, counselors can take positive steps in the community and in society to lessen disparities between the haves and have-nots.

Prejudice and the Group as a Microcosm of Society

Because a group is a microcosm of society, prejudices that occur in everyday life are likely to become evident. Therefore, a culturally diverse group offers the potential for clients to work through unconscious, deep-seated feelings of racism and prejudice. Counselors have the opportunity to help heal deeply held prejudices by considering the cultural backgrounds of clients when deciding group membership. By actively seeking out diversity in group membership, counselors are likely to set the stage for group members to work on their prejudices.

Cultural Differences Between a Group Member and the Group Leader

Because misplaced anger is often projected onto the group leader early in the group experience, if a group leader is from a culturally different background from the members, the leader has the opportunity to assist members in understanding their anger, which is sometimes related to deep-seated prejudices but masked as something else. A simple question by a member, like "Why aren't we making quicker progress in the group?" can be related to fears about opening up, as well as prejudices about the ability of a leader who is from a certain cultural group. A skilled group leader can assist members both in examining their anger, which is a natural part of the group process, and in understanding feelings of prejudice.

Ethical, Professional, and Legal Issues

Ethical Issues

Ethical Code and Best Practices Guidelines

The ethical code of ACA (2014a) applies to both group work and individual counseling. However, because the code does not fully address some issues relative to group work, the ASGW developed the *ASGW Best Practice Guidelines* (ASGW, 2007), which helps to clarify the application of the code of ethics "to the planning, implementation, processing, and evaluation in group work practice" (Wilson, Rapin, & Haley-Banez, 2004, p. 20). In addressing ethical and professional concerns, both the code and the *Best Practices Guidelines* should be examined.

Informed Consent and Confidentiality

As with individual counseling, there are a myriad of ethical issues with which the group leader must contend. However, two issues that have particularly stood out over the years include informed consent and confidentiality.

Informed Consent.   Informed consent becomes a particularly important concern in group work because a number of issues not found in other forms of counseling are at play in group work (Corey, 2012; Corey et al., 2014). At the very minimum, when giving informed consent, group members should know (1) the credentials of the group leader; (2) the general therapeutic style of the group leader; (3) the goals of the group; (4) the general ground rules associated with the group; (5) expectations about self-disclosure on the part of the leader and potential members; (6) whether members are free to withdraw from the group at any time and the responsibility they have to the other group members when terminating; (7) the limits of confidentiality; (8) any psychological risks that may arise as a function of the group experience; (9) fees involved; and (10) how the group may or may not be in sync with the values or cultural beliefs of the member.

Confidentiality

> In group work, counselors clearly explain the importance and parameters of confidentiality for the specific group.
>
> (ACA, 2014a, Section B.4.a)

As in all forms of counseling, the group leader must assure group members about the confidential nature of counseling, and also inform them of any limits to confidentiality. Such limits include what the leader might do if he or she suspected foreseeable harm to a client or to others, the fact that the group leader cannot ensure that all members of the group will keep information confidential (see the section "Legal Issue: Confidentiality and the Third-Party Rule," later in this chapter), or any other potential issues that might affect confidentiality (e.g., parents' right to know, subpoenas from the courts).

Professional Issues

Professional Associations

Although a number of professional associations focus on group issues, the major professional association for counselors interested in group work is ASGW, a division of ACA. Its purpose is

> . . . to establish standards for professional and ethical practice; to support research and the dissemination of knowledge; and to provide professional leadership in the field of group work. In addition, the Association shall seek to

extend counseling through the use of group process; to provide a forum for examining innovative and developing concepts in group work; to foster diversity and dignity in our groups; and to be models of effective group practice.

(ASGW, 2012b, para.2)

A few of the many benefits of ASGW include:

- ➤ *Best Practice Guidelines* to augment the ACA ethical guidelines
- ➤ *Professional Standards for the Training of Group Workers*
- ➤ *The Principles for Diversity-Competent Group Workers*
- ➤ A newsletter, as well as the *Journal for Specialists in Group Work*
- ➤ Scholarships for students and group work specialists
- ➤ The sponsoring of workshops and conferences specific to group issues
- ➤ The opportunity to be mentored and learn about supervisory practices relative to group work

Group Versus Individual Counseling

When does one refer a client to group counseling as an alternative or adjunct to individual counseling? With the most current research indicating that group counseling is as effective as individual counseling, some suggest that group work should always be considered as an alternative to individual treatment (Barlow, 2014; Burlingame & Krogel, 2005; Burlingame, MacKenzie, & Strauss, 2004). Although there is no easy method of determining when to use group or individual counseling, a few guidelines might help. For instance, it might be smart to refer to group counseling when, for one or more of the following reasons:

- ➤ A client cannot afford the cost of individual counseling.
- ➤ The benefits for a client of individual counseling have gotten so meager that an alternative treatment might offer a new perspective.
- ➤ A client's issues are related to interpersonal functioning, and a group might facilitate working through these issues in a real-life manner.
- ➤ A client needs the extra social support that a group might offer.
- ➤ A client wants to test new behaviors in a system that will support him or her while simultaneously receiving realistic feedback about the new behavior.
- ➤ The experiences of others who are working through similar issues (e.g., alcoholism or depression) can dramatically improve the client's functioning.

Legal Issue: Confidentiality and the Third-Party Rule

Group workers have the responsibility to inform all group participants of the need for confidentiality, potential consequences of breaching confidentiality and that legal privilege does not apply to group discussions (unless provided by state statute).

(ASGW, 2007, Section A.7.d)

Although group members might justifiably expect that other group members and the leader would respect their right to confidentiality, the legal system generally does not view information revealed to more than one person as confidential. Thus, if a group member were to break confidentiality, such as by revealing information about the group in a court of law, the court might then deem it desirable, and possible, to obtain information from other group members (Wheeler & Bertam, 2012). In addition, if the leader does not hold *privileged communication* status, or the legal right to maintain client confidentiality should the client so choose this privilege (see Chapter 5), the counselor can be compelled by the court to reveal information disclosed in the group. "Privilege" is generally granted to licensed professional counselors through state statutes.

The Counselor in Process: Allowing Groups to Unfold Naturally

Push a group to open up to quickly, and it will push back. The members will resist, protest, confront, and perhaps even leave. A group needs to unfold in its own way as the counselor slowly facilitates the development of the group process. Thus, the counselor's challenge is to facilitate deep knowing on the part of clients as they traverse the stages of group counseling without pressuring them to the point where they will want to leave the group. This delicate balance is not always easily achieved. Perhaps hearing some thoughts shared by Carl Rogers more than 40 years ago can remind us that groups need to move at their own pace:

> . . . *Often there is consternation, anxiety, and irritation. . . . Only gradually does it become evident that the major aim of nearly every member is to find ways of relating to other members of the group and to himself. Then as they gradually, tentatively, and fearfully explore their feelings and attitudes toward one another and toward themselves, it becomes increasingly evident that what they have first presented are facades, masks. Only cautiously do the real feelings and real person emerge. . . . Little by little, a sense of genuine communication builds up. . . .*

> (Rogers, 1970, p. 8)

Summary

This chapter began by noting that groups, like families, are affected by systemic principles, and we then highlighted the fact that group work offers some advantages and disadvantages over other forms of counseling. We discussed how group work has changed over the twentieth century from its early moralistic and preaching orientation, to a rigid psychoanalytic focus, to encounter and training groups that arose in the 1940s. We highlighted some of the well-known individuals who first experimented with different forms of group work, such as Addams, Richmond, Pratt, Freud, Moreno, Adler, Lewin, and Rogers; and discussed the early beginnings of NTL and of encounter groups. In addition, we noted that today, most groups can be classified as one of five types: self-help groups, task groups, psychoeducational groups, counseling groups, and therapy groups. We provided descriptions of each of these types of groups and noted that counselors generally are involved in conducting all but self-help groups.

This chapter discussed the importance of theory in group counseling and noted that a group leader tends to embrace a theory that is an extension of his or her personality. We examined one theory from each of four conceptual orientations, including psychoanalytic group therapy, from the psychodynamic tradition; cognitive–behavioral group counseling, from the cognitive–behavioral tradition; person-centered group counseling, from the existential–humanistic focus; and solution-focused group counseling, from postmodern therapy. We also stated that regardless of the theory chosen, all groups will be affected by group dynamics and reflect group process.

As the chapter continued, we discussed issues to consider when preparing to run a group, including group leadership style, the composition of the group members, whether the group is closed or open, the size of the group, the duration and frequency of meetings, and the atmosphere of the place in which the group meets. We then identified Tuckman's stages of group development (i.e., forming, storming, norming, performing, and adjourning) and showed how they applied to five stages of group development that were discussed: pregroup, initial, transition, work, and closure. We noted that passage through all these stages generally occurs only in counseling and therapy groups and not in self-help groups, task groups, or psychoeducational groups.

In looking at groups from a multicultural/social justice focus, we noted that ASGW has developed *Principles for Diversity-Competent Group Workers*, which can assist in the cross-cultural training of group workers. We next highlighted the part that privilege plays in group counseling and how counselors can address privilege. Next, we noted that because the group is a microcosm of society, prejudice can be sometimes found in groups, and groups can be a place to examine such underlying biases. We also pointed out that if group members are culturally different from the group leader, there is a unique opportunity for group members to safely examine their biases and prejudices as they become projected onto the leader.

The chapter went on to note that most ethical and legal concerns found in individual counseling are also found in group work. However, it highlighted two ethical and legal concerns that are particularly important to group work: informed consent and confidentiality. For instance, we pointed out the increased importance of informed consent in group work due to the many risks involved. In addition, we stated that in group counseling, confidentiality is much less assured, and as reflected in the "third-party rule," cannot be guaranteed through the U.S. legal system.

Near the end of the chapter, we discussed some professional issues related to group work. First, we identified the purpose of ASGW, the group work division of ACA, and highlighted some benefits of joining ASGW, such as the fact that it has developed the *Best Practice Guidelines*, the *Professional Standards for the Training of Group Workers*, and the *Principles for Diversity-Competent Group Workers*. In addition, we noted that they publish a newsletter and a journal, sponsor workshops and conferences, and offer scholarships. Next, we identified some guidelines for choosing group work over individual counseling. Finally, the chapter concluded with a brief discussion of the importance of allowing groups to unfold naturally.

Further Practice

Visit CengageBrain.com to respond to additional material that highlight the salient aspects of the chapter content. There, you can find ethical, professional, and legal vignettes, a number of experiential exercises, and study tools including a glossary, flashcards, and sample test items. Hopefully, these will enhance your learning and be fun and interesting.

CHAPTER 8

Consultation and Supervision

The principal of an elementary school asked me to spend a morning with a third grade class. He wanted to discuss the students' feelings about having had a developmentally delayed young man, who was quadriplegic, mainstreamed into their classroom for six weeks. This was consultation.

Because I was concerned that a client of mine might have an emotional disorder or be learning disabled, I gave him a series of psychological and educational tests. I subsequently met with a colleague of mine to assist me in reviewing the results. This was consultation.

Administrators from a local social service agency asked a colleague of mine to meet with them concerning communication problems at their agency. Following the meeting, they hired him to come to the agency, assess problems, and suggest strategies for change. This was consultation.

Our counseling program invited a counselor educator, who had expertise with the accreditation standards of the Council for the Accreditation of Counseling and Related Programs (CACREP) to review the program's strengths and weaknesses before we applied for CACREP accreditation. This too was consultation.

During my counseling career, I have had numerous supervisors. For instance, when I worked as a counselor at a mental health center, I would meet weekly with my supervisor to discuss my cases. Also, while I was in private practice, we hired a local psychologist to meet weekly, as a group, with me and all my colleagues for supervision. Another time, while in private practice, I contracted with a master therapist for biweekly supervision meetings. This was supervision, a special kind of—you guessed it—consultation.

The preceding examples show that consultation and supervision have become common aspects of every counseling specialty area. As you might surmise, in the CACREP (2009) standards, consultation and supervision are both highlighted as essential skills to master.

In this chapter, we will examine the current status of consultation and supervision. Although supervision may be seen as a type of consultation, there are enough differences between the two to justify discussing them separately. Therefore, the chapter will focus first on consultation and then on supervision.

Consultation

Consultation Defined

. . . me and you talking about him or her with the purpose of some change.

(Fall, 1995, p. 151)

Although I personally like the simple definition offered above, perhaps a more professional one that I might suggest is:

When a professional (the consultant), who has specialized expertise, meets with one or more other professionals to improve their work with current or potential clients.

Although a *consultee* is often referred to as any professional who meets with a *consultant*, the consultee is actually the point person, or the person identifying and inviting the consultant to consult. In fact, in some cases it is not appropriate for the consultee to be included in the consultation. For instance, the administrative head of an agency may hire a consultant to work with all the counselors, but because the administrator is not a counselor, it may be inappropriate for that administrator to be in included in certain types of consultation (e.g., a workshop on a new counseling technique). However, don't be surprised if you see the word *consultee* used rather liberally to mean any person who meets with a consultant.

Although consultants can be hired from outside an agency or institution, the above definition allows for internal consultants. Thus, a person who has specialized expertise within an agency or institution may be able to pass on his or her knowledge to others within that agency or institution (e.g., school counselors often consult with teachers).

As you have probably surmised, consultation involves a *triadic relationship*, in which the work that the consultant does not only affects those who meet with the consultant (e.g., counselors at an agency) but also indirectly affects a third party, which can be an individual (e.g., a client) or a system (e.g., an agency) (Kampwirth & Powers, 2012). Thus, consultation might include the following scenarios:

➤ A principal asking a school counselor to meet with all school staff to help them create a more sensitive multicultural school environment
➤ A mental health agency director hiring an individual to meet with agency personnel to help them better understand changes in the *Diagnostic and Statistical Manual-5 (DSM-5)*
➤ A school system's counseling director hiring an individual to do a workshop for school counselors so they can learn more about how to respond to bullying
➤ A supervisor meeting with a counselor about his or her clients
➤ An administrative director of an agency inviting a consultant to meet with agency personnel to lessen infighting, with the goal being a better-run, friendlier agency
➤ A director of a college counseling center asking one of his counselors to develop a workshop for professors to alert them on how to identify and refer depressed students
➤ A clinical director asking a senior counselor to run a series of workshops for junior counselors on new government regulations concerning confidentiality

Consultation involves some change in the knowledge, skills, or self-understanding of those with whom the consultant meets, and although consultation can affect individuals in important and meaningful ways, it is not therapy. Consultation is *not* a one-to-one, intense counseling experience. However, it does involve a person who has expertise in consultation skills, meeting with others to increase the knowledge and skills of those with whom he or she is consulting.

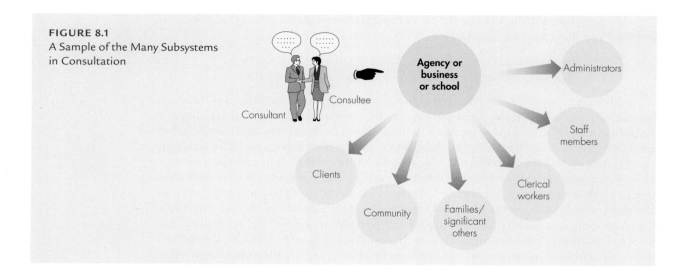

FIGURE 8.1
A Sample of the Many Subsystems in Consultation

Today, consultants can be asked to intervene on one of three levels: *primary*, which is oriented to education and prevention; *secondary*, which is focused on the remediation of nonsevere mental health problems; or *tertiary*, which is concentrated on addressing serious mental health problems (National Public Health Partnership, 2006; Kampwirth & Powers, 2012). In addition, consultation today is *systemic*, in that the effective consultant is able to see the multiple ways that individuals within a system view a problem and realizes that any changes made in the system can affect the lives of many other people (Sears, Rudisill, & Mason-Sears, 2006; Senge, 2006) (see Figure 8.1).

A Brief History of Consultation

The decades of the 1940s and 1950s are considered the beginning of modern consultation methods (Kurpius & Robinson, 1978). At that time, a consultee, who was generally a supervisor or administrator of an organization, would invite a consultant to his or her setting with the expectation that the consultant, "the expert," would solve an existing problem. After coming to the setting, the consultant would have little contact with the consultee, and the consultant was pretty much left to his or her own devices to solve the problem. This became known as the *direct-service approach* to consultation.

> *Example: A principal finds that many parents are complaining about not being able to understand the test scores of their children. The principal asks an expert on assessment to come in and take care of this situation. The consultant decides to run a workshop for parents and designates the counselor to do future workshops for parents. He goes over the test material with the counselor to ensure that she is adequately prepared. The principal remains uninvolved.*

By the end of the 1950s, the consultee would generally be included in the consultation process along with the staff. This would help to ensure that if similar issues were to arise, the consultee would have the training to deal with the problem.

> *Example: After finding a number of insurance forms have been returned for misdiagnosis, and believing that some clients may have been placed on the wrong medication due to similar errors, the clinical director of an agency asks a consultant to come in and teach the staff about the DSM-5. The clinical director sits in on the workshops to also gain knowledge and avoid future problems.*

As consultation models evolved, consultation was increasingly seen as a process in which the consultant would train others or "give away" his or her expertise to staff (Dougherty, 2014; Kurpius & Robinson, 1978).

> *Example: With violence on college campuses increasing in recent years, the director of a college counseling center is concerned that her staff is not adequately trained in crisis counseling and trauma work. Thus, she hires a consultant to come in and train the staff in such counseling. At the end of the weeklong workshop, the staff now feels competent to do such work.*

The latter part of the twentieth century also brought a proliferation of theories about consultation. Many of these theories are similar to the counseling theories examined in Chapter 4, but applied within a consulting framework. The consultant's theoretical perspective represents the prism through which the consultant will come to understand the system, and it affects how he or she will devise strategies for change. Some of these theories will be discussed later in the chapter.

Today, we find an array of models of consultation that speak to how a consultant brings himself or herself into the consulting relationship and are reminiscent of the various models discussed (Cochrane & Salyers, 2006; Dougherty, 2014; Idol, Nevin, & Paolucci-Whitcomb, 2000; Kampwirth & Powers, 2012; Lambert, Hylander, & Sandoval, 2004; Parsons & Kahn, 2005; Schein, 1999, 2013). Often these models are integrated with the particular theoretical orientation of the consultant (to be discussed later in this chapter). What follows are short descriptions of three possible models from a *consultant-centered* perspective, where the consultant imparts knowledge to the system, and three possible models from a *consultee-centered* perspective, where the consultant uses his or her helping skills to elicit knowledge from the system.

Consultant-Centered Consultation

Expert Consultation Model. Here, the consultant is specifically brought into an organization because of his or her expertise in a specific area and asked to use this knowledge to provide solutions to specific problems.

Prescriptive Consultation Model (Doctor-Patient Mode). Here, the consultant collects information, diagnoses the problem, and makes recommendations to the consultee on how to solve the problem.

Trainer/Educator Consultation Model. Often used in what has come to be known as "staff development," this model involves the consultant being hired to come into a system and teach or train staff members.

Consultee-Centered Consultation

Collaborative Consultation Model.   In this type of consultation, a partnership develops in which the consultant offers expertise and also relies on the expertise of individuals in the system to offer input into the problems and solutions. This shared expertise model tends to focus on joint decision making.

Facilitative Consultation Model.   Here, the consultant plays a facilitative role by helping individuals within the system communicate with one another, understand each other, and resolve conflicts among themselves.

Process-Oriented Consultation Model.   This consultant believes either that he or she does not have the answer or withholds expertise, with the confidence that the most effective resolution (resulting in the highest self-esteem and sense of ownership of the problem) would be for the system members to find their own solution. The consultant has faith that system members can change if the consultant is able to develop a trusting environment.

In choosing a model, the consultant needs to know his or her personality style, the people with whom he or she is working, and the problem to be addressed. For instance, one would likely not use an expert model if consulting with master therapists. A consultant whose natural style is directive would have a more difficult time taking on a system-centered style. And a consultant working with counselors who are providing less-than-adequate care on a suicide hotline might start with a consultant-centered style, as it would resolve some issues quickly, which is critical when people's lives are at stake.

Today, CACREP (2009) requires that consultation be taught as part of the curriculum in a counselor education program, and models such as the ones just described are often taught about in classes and may be practiced in practica and internships. Models such as these, along with the theories of consultation described next, are an integral part of the counselor's job.

Theories of Consultation

While models of consultation speak to how the consultant brings himself or herself into the consulting relationship, theories of consultation provide a conceptual framework from which the consultant practices. Sometimes there is overlap between models and theories. For instance, a consultant who bases his or her practice on a person-centered counseling theory would likely use a client-centered consultant style and find it unnatural to take on a consultant-centered style.

Practically any theory of counseling could be applied to consultation. What appears most important in choosing a theory is how it (1) defines itself relative to consultation, (2) is used to conceptualize the consultee's problem, (3) uses intervention strategies to solve problems, (4) deals with problems during the consultation process, and (5) handles termination and follow-up (Brack, Jones, Smith, White, & Brack, 1993). Keep in mind that almost all consultants today integrate their model of consultation with their theoretical orientation while maintaining a systemic and developmental approach.

The following are a few brief examples of theories that have been applied to consultation, but other approaches also exist. Within this section, I took the liberty of matching what

I consider to be the best style (consultee-centered or consultant-centered) with each theory noted. As you read the theories, consider the approach with which you most easily identify.

Person-Centered Consultation

By its very nature, person-centered consultation is consultee-centered because it is the purpose of the person-centered consultant to facilitate the change process in a nondirective fashion (Doughtery, 2014). This consultant would enter a system and attempt to understand each person's perspective on the nature of the system. The use of the basic core conditions of *empathy*, *genuineness*, and *positive regard*, therefore, are crucial for this consultant. Sometimes the person-centered consultant might run groups within the organization in an attempt to have individuals more effectively hear one another's point of view, and with the belief that the natural process of the group will assist the system in healing itself. With the permission of the people in the organization, this consultant might share his or her findings with the whole organization.

Cognitive-Behavioral Consultation

From a cognitive-behavioral perspective, it is crucial that the problem is clearly defined. This requires a careful initial analysis of the system, especially in light of the problem as presented by the consultee (Crothers, Hughes, & Morine, 2008; Doughtery, 2014). Basic counseling skills are crucial to the beginning of this process. Later, as the problem increasingly becomes defined, the cognitive-behavioral consultant uses *behavioral principles, cognitive principles*, and *social learning theory (modeling)* concepts to address identified problem areas and to set identifiable goals. A consultant from this perspective might do well by starting out consultee-centered and ending by being consultant-centered as he or she designs strategies for change.

Gestalt Consultation

As in Gestalt therapy, the Gestalt-oriented consultant's main goal is to increase the awareness of the consultee and others involved in the consultation in an effort to decrease defenses and reduce neurotic behaviors (Barber, 2012). Gestalt consultants believe that by merely bringing the consultant into the system, change will occur. Therefore, this consultant enters the system with a particular way of being that encourages the *expression of feeling* and the *letting down of boundaries* in an effort to promote increased *awareness* and true *encounters with self* and with one another. This approach generally is a combination of consultant-centered and consultee-centered: consultant-centered, because the consultant directs and teaches others how to express feelings and let down defenses; and consultee-centered, because the consultant continues to facilitate such expressions.

Psychoanalytic Approaches to Consultation

A relative newcomer to consultation, psychoanalytic consultation focuses on how unconscious behavior might be affecting the consultee's environment (Kerzner, 2009). The main goal of the consultant, therefore, is to make sense of the *unconscious* forces that are at the root of problems (Czander & Eisold, 2003). Problems are seen as *projections* of the individuals' unconscious processes. *Resistance* is seen as an important defense that protects the individual from examining his or her unconscious processes while at the same time protecting the system from undue stress (e.g., "If I really expressed my anger, things would truly get out of hand"). The consultant works cautiously with members in the system, being careful not to abruptly remove members' resistances and cause chaos and mental decompensation. Eventually, consultants will attempt to explain resistances and assist the members in attempting to understand their part in maintaining systemic problems. The psychoanalytic-oriented consultant would do well to start out consultee-centered as he or she attempts to understand unconscious processes, and then move to a consultant-centered approach as he or she explains the resistances in the organization.

Social Constructionist Consultation

Social constructionist consultation has at its core the belief that *realities are co-constructed through language* (Mortola & Carlson, 2003). Thus, there is no single reality, and it is critical for consultants to understand the different stories or narratives of the individuals with whom the consultant is working. A consultant such as this uses *respectful curiosity* as he or she inquires about and listens to the expression of *dominant narratives*. The narratives of all individuals are accepted as their current realities and those that are problematic are particularly listened to. The consultant can help individuals expand their understanding of problematic narratives by looking at *exceptions* to the problems, seeking other ways of viewing the problems, and creating new *solutions* to the problems. Eventually, the consultant works with individuals toward new solutions that include the co-construction of new, healthier narratives (Carmargo-Borges & Rasera, 2013; Waachter, 2004). This consultant is clearly systems-centered, as he or she is trying to understand clients' narratives and facilitate new ways of understanding for all within the system as they co-create new, healthier narratives.

Chaos Theory Consultation

As opposed to traditional counseling theories that attempt to understand cause and effect in systems, chaos theory assumes that the *world is largely unpredictable* because of the vast number of inputs that can affect the functioning of a system (Peters, 1989). For instance, chaos theory, which has been applied to scientific and social systems, would assume that the dropping of leaves in China would affect the weather across the globe in some unknown ways. Therefore, it would be crucial to discover as many *inputs* as possible that affect the system, in an effort to reduce the unpredictability of the system while keeping in mind that we all must live with a certain amount of chaos. In this approach, consultants first attempt to understand as much of the chaos in the system as possible. Then the consultant takes a proactive role and makes suggestions for change in ways that may be experimental and creative in an attempt to alter the dynamics that have been creating the problematic situation. Although currently far from an exact science, chaos theory offers an interesting perspective to consultation. Chaos theory consultants would probably work best starting with a systems-centered perspective and later moving to a consultant-centered approach as they become more proactive and engage individuals in the change process.

The Consulting Process: Stages of Consultation

A number of authors have defined the process of consultation in similar ways as they explain how a consultant enters a system, facilitates change, and leaves (Crothers, et al., 2008; Dougherty, 2014; Levinson, 2009). These models tend to view the consultation process as consisting of the following stages: pre-entry; entry, goal setting, implementation, evaluation, and disengagement.

Stage 1: Pre-entry

In the initial stage, the consultant conceptualizes and articulates to self and to others what he or she has been asked to do. The consultant, therefore, must have a clear approach to consultation and understand how this approach may be implemented in the particular situation. This pre-entry stage involves an initial contact with the consulting system in which the consultant explains the purpose of consultation and his or her approach. Some ways to do this are through letters to employees, pre-entry meetings, or by having the consultee (e.g., an administrator who initially contacted the consultant) or a designated employee explain the purpose.

Stage 2: Entry

The second stage of consultation is actually a three-pronged process that includes making contact with the consulting system, exploring the problem, and defining the contract between the consultant and the consulting system. Consultants make contact with the consulting system in many ways. For instance, one consultant might call a series of meetings with all the different work groups, while another consultant might decide to meet individually with each person in the consulting system. Yet another third consultant might do both. These stylistic differences are based largely on the particular consultant's conceptual model of consultation.

After contacting the members of the system, the consultant needs to probe the system in such a way that he or she will obtain an initial understanding of the problem. This enables the consultant to discuss the contract with the organization. Such issues as confirming fees; setting up meetings; defining materials needed; deciding purpose, objectives, and ground rules; and setting an approximate termination date are just a few of the items to be determined in the contracting phase of the second stage.

Stage 3: Goal Setting

The third stage, goal setting, involves three phases. The first, information gathering, is essentially a data-retrieval process. Based on the initial assessment of the problem and the contract decided in the second stage, the consultant is well situated to obtain reliable and valid data. This data-collection process ranges from obtaining specific hard numerical data, to sending out questionnaires to employees, to generating data (information) from small group sharing and individual meetings with individuals in the consulting system. In the second phase, these data are analyzed, synthesized, and interpreted. This process allows the consultant to confirm, deny, or revise the initial identification of the problem obtained in the entry stage. Finally, the identification of the problem allows the consultant to set achievable goals for the organization and to begin to examine methods for change.

Stage 4: Implementation

During the fourth stage, the consultant, usually collaboratively with all those involved with the consultation, decides on strategies for change, and the implementation of those strategies begins. Although interventions can vary widely as a function of the consultant's style and theoretical orientation, regardless of style or orientation, the problems addressed should be more or less the same, and the results should focus on solving those problems. Generally, problems are defined contextually and push the system to make deep changes that will prevent future problems.

Stage 5: Evaluation

A good consultant wants feedback. He or she wants to know what worked, what didn't work, and what were his or her strengths and weaknesses. Evaluation includes asking participants for their judgments regarding the interventions that were made and whether the stated goals (change processes) were accomplished. Evaluation can be accomplished verbally or in writing throughout the consultation process (i.e., *formative evaluation*), through a statistical analysis of whether goals were reached near the end of the consulting process (i.e., *summative evaluation*), or through a combination. At times, evaluation may result in the consultant discovering that he or she is off track, and the consultant may decide to recycle the process through the various stages.

Stage 6: Disengagement

Disengagement involves the consultant leaving the consulting relationship, hopefully because goals have been met, and usually at a preset time determined during the contract phase of stage 2, although sometimes this date will be revised based on new information gathered during the consulting process. During this stage, it is important that the consultant processes the results of the consulting relationship, including its successes and any interventions which may have been less successful, with all parties involved. The ending of any relationship involves loss, and the individuals involved should be given the opportunity to share their feelings about ending the consulting relationship.

The Counselor as Consultant

Counselors have long been consultants. In fact, for some, this is their major role. The list of the professionals with whom the counselor may consult is long and includes other counselors and helping professionals, school administrators, parents, teachers, college student service staff and administrators, college professors, administrators of social service agencies, clinical directors, clerical staff, and managers in business and industry. Let's take a brief look at some of the consultation activities of counselors who work at college counseling centers, schools, and community agencies.

Consultation and the College Counselor

Consultation has been an important part of college counseling centers almost since their inception (Stone & Archer, 1990; Westbrook et al., 1993), and continues to be one of the most important activities of college counseling centers, as noted by the *International Association of Counseling Services (IACS)* accreditation standards (IACS, 2010). In fact, consultation is particularly important because it is one of the few activities that make the center visible to everyone in the college environment (Cooper, 2003; Much, Wagener, & Hellenbrand, 2010).

Consultation by college counselors may be defined as any activity where advice and assistance, based on psychological activities, are provided to a group, office, department, club, or others (Stone & Archer, 1990). The kinds of consultation services offered by college counselors are so diverse that their extent could not be covered here. However, some of the major areas in which college counseling centers have used consultation include the following (Cooper, 2003; Love & Maxam, 2011; Much et al., 2010):

1. Faculty, concerning the emotional distress of college students
2. Administration, about diversity issues on campus
3. Directors of residence life, about potential psychological stressors that students might face
4. Students, about their concerns regarding other students
5. Academic advisors, about high-risk students
6. Disability services, in an effort to increase opportunities for the physically challenged
7. Many aspects of the university community, in an effort to increase communication between employees and supervisors
8. Parents, about concerns about their child (e.g., sexual assault on campus)

Consultation at college counseling centers may be consultant-centered or system-centered, depending on the group to which services will be provided. It is, therefore, crucial that the college counselor knows his or her audience and considers the topic to be discussed. Cooper (2003) offers one consultation "cube" model suggesting that consultation by college counselors typically addresses one of four audiences: students, faculty, staff, or administrators; that their interventions can be focused on the individual, a group, or an organization; and that the type of consultation is generally focused on education or training, offering a program, the "doctor–patient" relationship (diagnosing and prescribing), or is process-oriented (see Figure 8.2). (Note the similarities here to the consultant-centered and consultee-centered models discussed earlier in the chapter.)

For instance, where it may be important to come from an education mode if discussing alcohol abuse with students, the same group of students discussing issues of diversity might very well do better with a process orientation. In the same vein, faculty and administrators are likely to be turned off by consultants who take on a doctor-patient role, but more open to obtaining specific education and training on certain topics (e.g., date rape, how to handle violence on campus, etc.). Consultants who work with this population may want to be collaborative, which can be a little less threatening to faculty and administrators.

Consultation at college counseling centers is a wide-ranging service that is becoming increasingly popular. It offers the college counselor one more activity in which he or she can positively affect the lives of others.

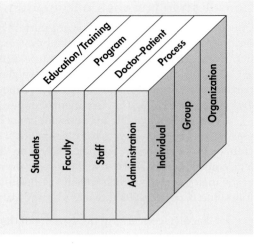

FIGURE 8.2
A Model of College Consultation

SOURCE: Cooper, S. (2003). College counseling centers as internal organizational consultants to universities. *Consulting Psychology Journal: Practice and Research*, 55(4), p. 234.

Consultation and the Agency Counselor

During the 1950s, there were relatively few community mental health agencies in this country. Then, in 1963, Congress passed the *Community Mental Health Centers Act*, and a new era in the delivery of mental health services was upon us (National Council for Behavioral Health, 2014). Providing federal funds for the creation of comprehensive mental health centers across the country, the act provided grants for short-term inpatient care, outpatient care, partial hospitalization, emergency services, and consultation and education services. For the first time, there was an acknowledgment that consultation was an important factor in the prevention of mental health problems. The problem was that consultation in reference to community agencies was not yet firmly defined. However, this was soon to change. Consultation in community agencies went in two directions: outward and inward.

Consulting Outward.   The focus of outward consultation is assisting individuals who have mental health concerns but are not clients directly involved with the agency. For instance, the agency counselor often consults with the parents and teachers of a client (e.g., helping them to cope with a child who has behavioral problems), as well as with other mental health professionals the client might be seeing (e.g., setting up meeting to ensure that future treatment strategies aren't at cross purposes). The community agency counselor may also consult with schools, hospitals, businesses, and other social service agencies in any number of ways. For example, one consultant might assist teachers and counselors from a school system understand mood disorders in children. Another consultant might be asked by a local business to help reduce the general stress level of its employees, and a third consultant might help a social service agency understand some of its employees' internal conflicts.

Consulting Inward.   In 1970, Gerald Caplan published a book called *Theory and Practice of Mental Health Consultation*, which became one of the best-known consultation delivery models. Similar to some of the models of consultation discussed earlier, Caplan's theory defined the role of the consultant in agencies and made suggestions on ways to intervene in organizations (Caplan & Caplan-Moskovich, 2004). His theory, which is still very much in use

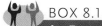

BOX 8.1

An Example of Program-Centered Consultation at a Mental Health Center

A consultant is called in by the administrative director of a local mental health center. The director is concerned about morale at the center, saying that she has heard that people are unhappy and that there is a depressed mood throughout. Not only is she concerned about morale, but also she is worried that the number of billing hours has dropped in the past six months as a result of the mood in the agency. She asks the consultant to evaluate the situation and to make recommendations.

The consultant first writes a letter to all staff and assistants explaining who he is, his consulting style, when he will be coming to the agency, what he will be doing, and approximately how long he will be there. In addition, he discusses the limits of confidentiality, noting that after meeting with everyone at the agency, he will be sharing general feelings, dynamics, and systemic problems that seem to be occurring. He notes that he will keep individual issues confidential, but that his experience as a consultant has shown him that when people begin to discuss personal concerns, things sometimes leak out into the agency. He encourages all agency personnel to avoid this if possible.

Before actually coming to the agency, the consultant develops a hierarchical plan to visit each workgroup. He starts with the administration, meeting separately with the clinical, medical, and administrative directors; next, he meets with the heads of each unit in the center (e.g., outpatient director, day treatment director, and so forth); he then meets with counselors and mental health assistants from each unit, followed by a meeting with the secretarial and clerical staff. He finishes

by meeting with the janitorial staff. Using empathy and basic listening skills, he meets first with each group and then individually with each member. While meeting with the staff, the consultant is also gathering data from the agency on changes in client flow, the economic status of the agency, salaries, types of degrees necessary for varying jobs, information flow (e.g., paper trails), and so forth.

Following the consultant's initial contact with each unit and member of the agency, he gathers all his information and spends two or three weeks determining what he considers to be the major problems in the agency. A report is written with the issues defined, and strategies for change are suggested. This report is sent to the agency director and distributed to the agency personnel. Two weeks later, he meets with the whole agency for a feedback session. Based on the feedback, a revision to the report is written and distributed.

After approval from the agency, the consultant begins to implement the strategies for change. Throughout this process, he is receiving process feedback concerning what is working and what is not. He adjusts his strategies based on this feedback. Finally, after a certain amount of change is completed and directions for continuing the change process in the future are determined, the consultant begins his termination from the agency. Closure is made through a series of agency group sessions where all who want to do so can come and give feedback in person. An anonymous written evaluation form is also made available to all personnel. A follow-up evaluation is completed six months later to see if change was indeed maintained.

today, looks inward at an agency, with the major focus being concern for the clients that the agency serves. He described four roles that a consultant might take on in an agency (Erchul, 2009; Mendoza, 1993): (1) offering specific suggestions to a counselor who has asked for help in working with a client; (2) assisting a counselor in identifying problems the counselor has in working with a client or a number of clients; (3) facilitating communication in the agency and educating agency staff and administrators about identified problems so that the agency runs more smoothly and clients get better service (see Box 8.1); and (4) working solely with administrators to facilitate communication and to educate them about identified problems.

Inward consultation and outward consultation activities are extremely important components of the community agency counselor's job. Such consultation activities clearly assist in providing better services for clients.

The School Counselor as Consultant

Since the 1960s, consultation has consistently been listed as one of the major responsibilities of the school counselor (ASCA, 2012; Baker, Robichaud, Dietrich, Wells, & Schreck, 2009;

Schmidt, 2010). With schools becoming increasingly complex, collaborating with other essential staff in the school is one way that school counselors can help meet the needs of students. For instance, if a school counselor can assist teachers in helping students or assist students in helping other students, then that counselor is expanding the helping relationship from one level to many levels. School counselors act as consultants in many ways, including the following (Baker & Gerler, 2008; Dahir & Stone, 2012; Dougherty, 2014, Kampwirth & Powers, 2012; Schmidt, 2010):

1. Assisting teachers in understanding the psychological, sociological, and learning needs of students
2. Assisting teachers in classroom management techniques
3. Assisting teachers, administrators, and parents in understanding the developmental needs of children and how they might affect learning
4. Meeting with students to help them understand developmental concerns, peer relationship issues, personal concerns, and other issues
5. Meeting with other professionals in the community concerning the needs of a particular student with whom the counselor is working
6. Meeting with parents, teachers, and specialists regarding the individual education plan of a special needs student
7. Assisting students in becoming peer counselors and conflict mediators
8. Assisting school staff in setting up a school environment that is conducive to learning for individuals from all cultures
9. Offering organizational consulting skills to assist administrators and others in the efficient running of the schools
10. Offering administrators, parents, teachers, and students assistance in understanding the purpose of assessment instruments and how to interpret their results

In the role as consultant, the school counselor is in a much more precarious position than the agency or college counselor. A school is a tightly knit organization with clear boundaries between the various professionals. Teachers, administrators, and counselors have very different roles, and they all have responsibilities to students and their parents. Teachers sometimes don't want to be bothered by counselors or administrators, and counselors sometimes don't want to be bothered by teachers. Parents often have views about their children that differ dramatically from those of teachers, counselors, and administrators. The school counselor needs to learn how to balance his or her role as consultant so that each component of the school feels heard and responded to (Kampwirth & Powers, 2012). Ultimately, this balancing act is the most challenging part of a school counselor's job. It is, therefore, essential that the school counselor understands the unique systemic qualities of the school where he or she works if change is to take place. The school counselor's training in interpersonal communication skills, consultation skills, and contextual thinking makes him or her particularly able to do this task. When a school counselor is seen siding with the administration, teachers, students, or parents, his or her consultative techniques have gone awry.

Although schools have their own unique systemic qualities, consultation in the schools can follow many of the same models that have been discussed. Therefore, a school counselor as consultant may be found to be consultant-centered at times (e.g., prescribing a communication skill to a parent or a new behavioral management skill to a teacher), or consultee-centered (e.g., collaborating with the school psychologist, teacher, specialist, and parent on a student's individualized education plan).

Consultation in the schools is one of the main functions of the school counselor and may be the most challenging, invigorating, and creative aspect of the job, as the counselor attempts to find strategies for change that will lead to an increase in self-esteem and learning for all students while satisfying the needs of parents, teachers, and administrators (ASCA, 2012; Dahir & Stone, 2012).

Supervision

Whether one is a counselor at a school, agency, or college, supervision has become an expected and crucial part of a counselor's professional responsibility. This is evidenced by (1) licensing boards requiring clinical supervision as part of the prerequisite to becoming licensed, (2) licensing boards setting more rigid standards for who can conduct clinical supervision and the activities that can count toward licensing, (3) agency and school administrators increasingly supporting the need for supervision, (4) the inclusion of ethical guidelines for supervisors in the ACA code of ethics (ACA, 2014a), and (5) the adoption, by the American Counseling Association (ACA), of the *Standards for Counseling Supervisors* (ACES, 1990). But what exactly is supervision, and how is it related to consultation?

Supervision Defined

> *. . . me and you talking about him or her with the purpose of some change.*

> (Fall, 1995, p. 151)

Remember this simple quote from earlier in the chapter? Although it was previously used to define *consultation*, it also aptly speaks to *supervision*, which involves an ongoing consultative relationship between a supervisor and the counselor that increases the counselor's skills and positively affects clients. A somewhat more involved definition of *supervision* can elucidate this concept further. ACA suggests that supervision is:

> *a process in which one individual, usually a senior member of a given profession designated as the supervisor, engages in a collaborative relationship with another individual or group, usually a junior member(s) of a given profession designated as the supervisee(s) in order to (a) promote the growth and development of the supervisee(s), (b) protect the welfare of the clients seen by the supervisee(s), and (c) evaluate the performance of the supervisee(s).*

> (ACA, 2014a, glossary)

Although it is a type of consultation, supervision differs from most other forms of consultation. For instance, whereas most forms of consultation are time-limited, supervision often involves an ongoing relationship between the supervisor and supervisee. Whereas most forms of consultation do not involve an intense interpersonal relationship that focuses on the consultee, supervision generally does, with the consultee being the supervisee. And whereas in most forms of consultation, the consultant generally does not have a direct evaluative responsibility for the consultee, in supervision, the supervisor is evaluating the supervisee in one fashion or another (Bernard & Goodyear, 2013; Borders & Brown, 2005; Corey, Haynes, Moulton, & Muratori, 2010).

Because supervision is an intense, interpersonal relationship that sometimes delves into some very personal issues of the supervisee and how they may affect the client, it can sometimes be eye-opening, even therapeutic, for the supervisee. However, although supervision can be therapeutic, it is not therapy. When supervision crosses over that imaginary line into therapy, the supervisor must decide if a referral to counseling for the supervisee would be appropriate.

Like consultation, supervision involves a number of systems, the most basic of which is that of supervisor ↔ supervisee/counselor ↔ client. As in all homeostatic mechanisms, if you change one component, the whole system changes. That is the wonderful part of being a supervisor: Impart knowledge to and facilitate growth in your supervisee, and you will see his or her clients change. The system is responding. Take this one step further, and other systems will change. A rebound effect occurs, where the client now affects the systems in which he or she is involved—perhaps his or her family: "Throw a rock into a pond, and the ripples increasingly expand."

The manner in which systems are affected in supervision is complex. First and foremost, the simple act of supervision fine-tunes the counselor's skills and ultimately can positively affect the client and the systems in which he or she is involved. Sometimes a *parallel process* occurs in the supervisory relationship, where the client–counselor relationship is mirrored in the supervisor–supervisee relationship (Bernard & Goodyear, 2013; Corey et al., 2010). This generally occurs when the counselor unconsciously takes on the traits of the client, which are repeated in the supervisory relationship (e.g., taking on the client's anxiety and repeating it in supervision). Parallel process is generally viewed as something that should be addressed in supervision and worked through, with the goal being to help the supervisee work effectively with the client (Pearson, 2001). The scenario in Box 8.2 shows how a parallel process to Juan's work with Suzanne is being created in his supervisory relationship with Carla.

Good supervision will curtail the parallel process seen in Box 8.2, whereby the supervisor acts as an effective model for Juan and offers ideas that Juan can use in his work with Suzanne. However, what would happen if Carla suddenly became anxious, believing that she could not help Juan? You can see why being an effective supervisor is so important to both the supervisee and to the client.

Sometimes it is argued that a reverse parallel process occurs (Borders & Brown, 2005), such as when positive qualities in a supervisor (e.g., good empathic responding) are taken on by the counselor and subsequently passed on to the client. It is hoped that these qualities will ultimately be passed on by the client to others in his or her life.

Whether it is a simple improvement in the knowledge base of the supervisee or the complexity of the parallel process, it is clear that supervision involves a system that can have far-reaching effects.

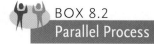

BOX 8.2
Parallel Process

Juan is being supervised by Carla. One of his clients, Suzanne, is having panic attacks. Suzanne has two children, works full time, and is in graduate school. Her marriage is "rocky." Economically, she cannot cut back on work, and her dream is to finish her graduate degree. She comes to Juan pleading for help and noting that throughout the day, she is having panic attacks and at night, she has difficulty sleeping. She is worried about being able to tend to her children and her studies because of her state of mind. A psychiatric consult and subsequent medication has resulted in little relief. She looks at Juan and says, "Please, you've got to help me—what should I do?" Juan is stymied, and at his first opportunity, discusses Suzanne's situation with Carla. Juan notes to Carla, "You know, since I've been working with Suzanne, I am filled with anxiety. I feel inadequate because I can't find a solution for her. I am thinking about her situation all the time, cannot stop obsessing about it, and I am having trouble sleeping because I am worrying about her. It's even affecting my relationship with my partner."

Who Is the Supervisor?

The ACA offers the following brief, but succinct, definition of supervisors:

> . . . counselors who are trained to oversee the professional clinical work of counselors and counselors-in-training.

> (ACA, 2014a, glossary)

Thus, supervisors may be advanced students (e.g., doctoral students) or faculty supervising master's-level students in a counseling skills class, practicum, or internship. Or they may be individuals who are designated to supervise counselors at an agency or a school; or they could be individuals who are hired by counselors (the supervisees) to provide supervision as part of their requirement to become licensed. Whoever the supervisor is, he or she should have obtained knowledge and competency in the following eleven areas, as identified by the *Standards for Counseling Supervisors* (ACES, 1990), with item 12 added by me:

1. Effectiveness as a counselor
2. Healthy personal traits and characteristics
3. Knowledge of ethical, legal, and regulatory issues
4. Knowledge of the nature of the supervisory relationship
5. Knowledge of supervisory methods and techniques
6. Knowledge of counselor development
7. Competency in case conceptualization
8. Competency in the assessment and evaluation of clients
9. Competency in oral and written report writing
10. Ability to evaluate counselors
11. Knowledge of research in counseling and counseling supervision
12. Knowledge of cross-cultural and social justice issues and how they affect the supervisee and the client

The supervisor also has a number of roles and responsibilities, a few of which include ensuring the welfare of the client; informing the supervisors of policies and procedures relative to supervision; meeting regularly with the supervisee and ensuring proper termination; assuring that ethical, legal, and professional standards are being upheld; overseeing the clinical and professional development of the supervisee; and evaluating the supervisee (ACA, 2014a, Section F). Like the effective counselor, the good supervisor is empathic, flexible, genuine, open, concerned, supportive, and able to build a strong supervisory alliance (Borders & Brown, 2005; Corey et al., 2010). In addition, the good supervisor is competent and able to evaluate the supervisee, and knows the appropriate boundaries for supervision. Finally, good supervisors know counseling, have good client conceptualization skills, and are good problem solvers.

Who Is the Supervisee?

The ACA defines the supervisee as follows:

> . . . a professional counselor or counselor-in-training whose counseling work or clinical skill development is being overseen in a formal supervisory relationship by a qualified trained professional.

> (ACA, 2014a, glossary)

One role of the supervisor is to evaluate the supervisee. The supervisee, in contrast, is learning from the evaluative process and building a professional identity (Bernard & Goodyear, 2013). Being subject to the evaluation of the supervisor, the supervisee is in a vulnerable position, and it is inevitable that at some point in the supervisory relationship, supervisee resistance will occur. Of course, the amount and kind of resistance can be the result of a number of factors, including the following (Bernard & Goodyear, 2013; Borders & Brown, 2005):

1. *Attachment and trust:* The ability to build trust and reduce resistance is likely related to the personality traits of both the supervisor and supervisee and their ability to form an effective relationship.
2. *Supervisor style:* Some supervisory styles allow supervisees to feel more in control, less threatened, and result in less supervisee resistance.
3. *Supervisee sensitivity to feedback:* Some supervisees are much more sensitive to evaluation and feedback, increasing resistance.
4. *Countertransference:* Some client issues will elicit defensiveness from the supervisee and result in inadequate responses by the counselor (supervisee). Similarly, supervisees can arouse defensiveness in supervisors, resulting in poor responses by the supervisor. As you can see, there certainly is enough defensiveness to go around. It is clear that unresolved issues on the part of a supervisee or supervisor can lead to problems in supervision (see Figure 8.3).
5. *Developmental level:* Supervisees will tend to become more resistant as they become more autonomous and independent from the supervisor. (A discussion of developmental models of supervision can be found later in this chapter.)
6. *Supervisor characteristics:* A number of characteristics can increase resistance, sometimes in unknown ways. They include age, race, cultural background, gender, power issues, and a wide variety of relationship dynamics.

Individual, Triadic, or Group Supervision?

Supervision can occur one on one, one supervisor with two supervisees (*triadic supervision*), or in small groups (*group supervision*). Each type has its benefits. From

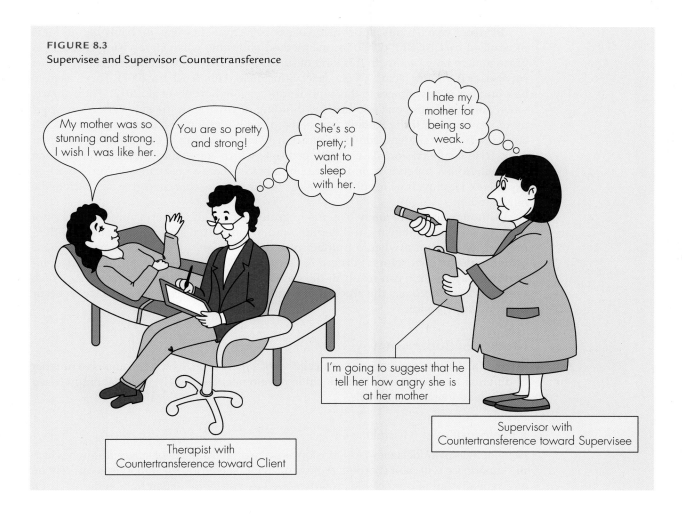

FIGURE 8.3
Supervisee and Supervisor Countertransference

a practical standpoint, group supervision allows a number of people to receive supervision at one time. Therefore, whether taking place in graduate school or at an agency or school, group supervision allows one supervisor to oversee a number of supervisees, usually three to seven. Group supervision has a number of advantages, including being exposed to multiple perspectives about an issue, viewing multiple ways that counselors may respond to clients, hearing about different kinds of interventions and educational opportunities, being able to learn how to do supervision by watching others undergo supervision, obtaining feedback from more than one individual, and normalizing experiences by seeing others that are dealing with similar issues (Bernard & Goodyear, 2013; Borders et al., 2012; Riva & Erickson Cornish, 2008). Another benefit is cost: For those who may be paying for supervision, group supervision is generally much less expensive than the $50 to $150 an hour that a counselor might charge for individual supervision.

In recent years, triadic supervision has become more popular, probably because it is recognized by CACREP (2009) as one method allowable when supervising students in practicum and internship. In this kind of supervision, two students meet together with a supervisor (Lawson, Hein, & Getz, 2009; Stinchfield, Hill, & Kleist, 2007). There seem to be a number of advantages to this type of supervision (Borders et al., 2012). For instance, when students know one another, the building of trust with the supervisor can occur more rapidly than if the student was alone or with a group of students. Also, with triadic supervision, students can learn vicariously from listening to the supervision of their peer. Triadic supervision allows peer feedback, which sometimes is easier to hear than feedback from a supervisor, and this can be a place where a peer can gain his or her first experience learning how to supervise, as he or she gets the chance to give feedback to the other student.

Although there are many benefits to group and triadic supervision, they may not offer the intimacy, intensity, and depth found in individual supervision, and confidentiality is less assured when a number of individuals are involved, even when those individuals are counselors (Bernard & Goodyear, 2013; Borders et al., 2012). Also, individual supervision can result in the development of a mentoring process in which the supervisee becomes the student of a master counselor. This is less likely to occur in group supervision.

Models of Supervision

Corey et al. (2010) suggest three broad classes of supervision, which encompass a number of different models. These classes include developmental models, psychotherapy-based models, and integrative models.

Developmental Models

Developmental models view supervision as occurring in a series of stages through which the supervisee will pass (Borders & Brown, 2005). Therefore, the supervisor can rely on a certain amount of predictable growth as well as resistance, depending on the stage. Of course, individual supervisees may move faster or slower through these stages based on their personality style, their ability, and their fit with their supervisor. Awareness of developmental stages can assist the supervisor in developing strategies for growth based on the supervisee's particular stage (Stoltenberg, 2005). Although there have been a number of developmental models over the years, probably the best known is the *Integrated Developmental Model (IDM)* of Stoltenberg and colleagues (Stoltenberg, 2005; Stoltenberg & McNeil, 2010).

IDM proposes that during the course of supervision, counselors will pass through three levels of development related to awareness of self and of their client, motivation to participate in the counseling process, and developing increasing autonomy in the counseling and supervision process.

In Level 1, counselors are anxious and have difficulty gaining insight into themselves and their clients. New to the field, they are highly motivated but are particularly dependent on their supervisor. As they enter Level 2, counselors are better able to focus on self

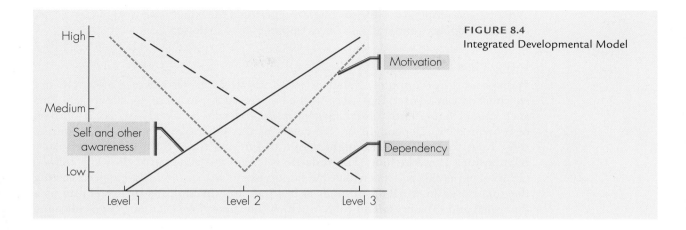

FIGURE 8.4
Integrated Developmental Model

and client and can show greater insight and empathy toward the client. However, realizing the complexity of the counseling relationship, their motivation sometimes decreases as they wonder if they can be effective counselors. They struggle between dependency and autonomy—one moment feeling like they "get it," and the next moment believing that they will never be truly accomplished in this field. Level 3 occurs when the counselor is able to easily understand self and develops deep understanding of the client. Here, counselors again become motivated as they realize their strengths and abilities. This leads to increased independence from their supervisor as they become willing and ready to try new techniques and develop their own sense of professional identity (Stoletenberg, 2005; Stoltenberg & McNeil, 2010) (see Figure 8.4).

Psychotherapy-based Models

Many counselors who practice a particular type of therapy (e.g., Gestalt, person-centered, behavioral, etc.) believe that it is best to receive supervision from a master therapist/supervisor who practices the same approach (Bernard & Goodyear, 2013; Pearson, 2006). This can occur in two ways. The first is when the supervisor structures the supervision so that it models the particular approach that the supervisee is using in counseling. Therefore, a behavioral supervisor would model a behavioral approach by identifying problems in supervision, collaboratively setting goals to work on, and then using techniques to reach those goals. The psychoanalytic supervisor would do analysis with the supervisee, while the person-centered supervisor would use empathy, show unconditional regard, and be genuine with his or her trainee.

In the second psychotherapy-based model, the supervisor uses his or her knowledge base to gently guide and teach the supervisee. For instance, if a trainee were working with a client behaviorally and not making progress, a behavioral supervisor might offer advice on some new behavioral techniques, a psychoanalytic supervisor might suggest a specific psychoanalytic technique and show the supervisee how to use it (e.g., dream analysis), and a person-centered supervisor might suggest that the supervisee work on his or her empathic responses and give specific examples of how to do so.

Integrative Models

Perhaps more appropriately called *meta-theory models, integrative models* are not theory specific and can be used regardless of the theoretical approach of the supervisee. One such model is Bernard's *discrimination model* (Bernard & Goodyear, 2013; Borders & Brown, 2005). Dependent on the needs of the supervisee, this model examines three roles that supervisors might adopt at differing times during the supervisory relationship. These include (1) a didactic role, in which the supervisor is a *teacher*; (2) an experiential role, in which the supervisor is a *time-limited counselor* assisting the supervisee in working through issues that are affecting his or her ability as a therapist; and (3) a *consultant* role, in which the supervisor is an objective colleague assisting the supervisee. As supervisors take on these roles, supervisees can focus on one of three domains: (1) the *interventions* that they are using or would like to use; (2) *conceptualization*, which focuses on how they are understanding client issues; and (3) *personalization*, which examines what personal issues might affect how they conceptualize client problems and the kinds of interventions they make. Referring back to Box 8.2 (with Juan being supervised by Carla), Table 8.1 demonstrates how the supervisor's roles can be applied to each focus of supervision.

TABLE 8.1   Roles and Foci of Discriminant Model

	ROLES OF SUPERVISOR		
FOCUS OF SUPERVISION	*Teacher* ↓	*Counselor* ↓	*Consultant* ↓
Intervention →	Teach the supervisee how to implement relaxation techniques.	Supervisor listens to the supervisee's concerns about her feelings of inadequacy relative to this client.	Supervisee requests specific techniques to use with the client and consultant offers a number of options.
Conceptualization →	Note to the supervisee how the origin of panic attacks may be viewed in a number of ways (e.g., early childhood issues, temperament, situational).	Supervisor connects the supervisee's own childhood issues related to anxiety and wonders if these issues relate to the supervisee's fear of working with the client.	Supervisee asks how temperament can affect anxiety and supervisor responds with research concerning the genetics of temperament and its relationship to anxiety. Possibility of medication to dampen the effects of temperament is discussed.
Personalization →	Define *parallel process* to the supervisee and indicate how that concept might be at play in this case.	Supervisor listens to the supervisee discuss how her own issues raise anxiety and feelings of inadequacy.	Supervisee asks how the parallel process can be halted and supervisor makes a number of suggestions.

Interpersonal process recall (IPR), another integrative model that was developed by Norm Kagan (1980; Kagan & Kagan, 1997), has been particularly popular over the years (Bernard & Goodyear, 2013). In many ways, this model relies on the trainee to uncover his or her own strengths and weaknesses. In this type of supervision, the supervisor and the trainee meet to review an audio or video recording of the trainee with a client. The trainee, supervisor, or both can control the recording, starting and stopping it when it is believed that there is an important moment in the counseling relationship between the supervisee and the client. The supervisor's role is to attend accurately to the feelings and thoughts of the supervisee and, when appropriate, ask leading questions to deepen the session. The following questions have been used in this inquiry session:

1. What do you wish you had said to him or her?
2. How do you think he or she would have reacted if you had said that?
3. What would have been the risk in saying what you wanted to say?
4. If you had the chance now, how might you tell him or her what you are thinking and feeling?
5. Were there any other thoughts going through your mind?
6. How did you want the other person to perceive you?
7. Were those feelings located physically in some part of your body?
8. Were you aware of any feelings? Does that feeling have any special meaning for you?
9. What did you want him or her to tell you?
10. What did you think he or she wanted from you?
11. Did he or she remind you of anyone in your life? (Cashwell, 1994, p. 2)

In the tradition of some of the humanistic therapies, IPR is a model of supervision that gives trainees the ability to explore their feelings and thoughts about a therapeutic relationship within a trusting and safe environment. Trainees, therefore, can get in touch with those aspects of themselves that are preventing clients from moving forward in counseling (Grant, Schofield, & Crawford, 2012).

Each of the above models offers a slightly different take on the supervisory process, and they are not necessarily exclusive of one another. For instance, one can adopt a developmental model and either be orientation-specific or use an integrative approach. In choosing a supervisor, if given the choice, of course a supervisee should pick the supervisor who offers the approach that will best facilitate his or her learning process, as well as the therapeutic experience of the supervisee's clients.

Finally, as with the counseling relationship, there is some evidence that the strength of the working alliance or bond between the supervisor and supervisee, regardless of model, may be the most crucial factor for effective supervision (Grant, et al., 2012; Lyon & Potkar, 2010; Sterner, 2009) Thus, the supervisor who has exceptional knowledge of supervision may be ineffective if he or she cannot build a relationship with the supervisee.

Supervision of Graduate Students

Graduate students in CACREP-approved counseling programs—and, I hope, all counseling programs—will have a number of opportunities to receive supervision. Although the manner in which this occurs will vary from program to program, counseling programs generally offer a course early on that provides supervision of basic counseling skills. Within this course, students usually have the opportunity to record a session with a client or with a fellow student. Supervision of the graduate student is generally given by the professor, an advanced graduate student, peers, or some combination of the three. In addition, students usually have the opportunity to obtain supervision in a practicum and in the culminating graduate school experience, the internship. Supervision in these courses is usually given by an advanced graduate student, a professor, a field supervisor, or a combination.

CACREP requires, and most graduate programs offer, supervision of recorded or live sessions. There are a number of ways this can be accomplished (Bernard & Goodyear, 2013; Borders & Brown, 2005; Champe & Kleist, 2003). First, there is the tried-and-true fashion of video recording a counseling session. Although video recording certainly offers broader feedback to the trainee than audio recording, either can be an invaluable tool for supervisor feedback. In addition to recording a session, most counseling programs today require some kind of live supervision that offers opportunities for immediate feedback that other kinds of supervision cannot provide (though it is anxiety provoking for many). Although live supervision is often face to face, increasingly, we are seeing cybersupervision, where supervisors supervise students or counselors over the Internet. Although there are strengths and drawbacks to such an approach, cybersupervision is undoubtedly here to stay and will increase over the years to come (see the section "Professional Issue: Technology and Supervision," later in this chapter, for more about this topic).

One final method of obtaining feedback about your client is through the time-honored tradition of reviewing written case notes. Well-thought-out and well-written case notes can be invaluable to the counselor-in-training and are one more way for counselors to obtain feedback from their supervisors (Bernard & Goodyear, 2013; Hernández-Wolfe, 2010).

Supervision of Practicing Counselors

Although ongoing supervision has become more popular in recent years, the frequency and kind of supervision varies depending on setting. Today, many counselors receive individual supervision, while a substantial number receive group supervision or peer supervision (Borders & Brown, 2005). Some seek out supervision for professional growth or as a requirement of credentialing, while others receive it as part of their job. Some counselors receive mandated supervision as the result of an ethical violation or professional concern (Cobia & Pipes, 2002).

School counselors have significantly less clinical supervision than agency, college, or private-practice counselors (Dollarhide & Miller, 2006), with one study showing that only 32% are supervised by other mental health professionals (Perera-Diltz & Mason, 2012). In addition, when they do receive supervision, it can often come from many sources and may be less formal than one might hope. For instance, school counselors may receive supervision from their principal (who rarely is trained in counseling and supervision); the director of counseling for the school system, who generally offers only periodic supervision; the head counselor in a school, who often offers sporadic supervision; colleagues for peer supervision, whose supervision can be rather informal; or a private supervisor whom they may hire on their own. Although there has been a call by the counseling profession to develop and implement new, clinical models of supervision in the schools, this kind of systemic change will take time, if it happens at all (Kline, 2006).

Although any style of supervision can be applied to any counseling setting, a number of authors have suggested altering supervisory techniques to fit a particular counseling specialty. Couples and family counselors, addiction counselors, school counselors, mental health counselors, college counselors, and so forth all have unique job functions that might call for changes in the supervisory process (see Chang, 2010; Lee, Nichols, Nichols, & Odom, 2004; Pearson, 2006; Somody, Henderson, Cook, & Zambrano, 2008).

Multicultural/Social Justice Focus

Multicultural Consultation Within a System

> The consultant serves as an agent for change rather than as an agent for maintaining the status quo, and the consultant advocates for both the client and the system rather than advocating for one over the other.
>
> (Hoffman et al., 2006, p. 124)

The consultant is in a unique position when it comes to multicultural issues. Being brought into a system means that one will be dealing with dynamics within the organization and how they may affect the clients who are affected by the system. Cultural differences undoubtedly will affect such dynamics. Thus, when entering a system, the consultant must do his or her best to understand the culture of the system, the culture of subsystems, and the unique background of each individual within the system (Clare, 2009; Homan, 2011).

Because issues of race, ethnicity, gender, and sexual identity, are often difficult to broach, there is generally tension related to cross-cultural issues among individuals within the system. Sometimes this tension may simply be a function of ignorance of differing cultural backgrounds. In other cases, deep feelings of hatred and discriminatory attitudes may prevail. The consultant must assess the degree to which cross-cultural issues play a role in the daily functioning of the system and, based on this assessment, include methods of dealing with these issues in his or her strategies for change. To be successful, the consultant must have an understanding of his or her biases, knowledge of other cultures, and knowledge of the kinds of intervention strategies that can effect positive change in the system. Ultimately, the consultant is in a unique position, as he or she can view the multiple perspectives of the system and advocate for change by empowering those who may be oppressed by the system and by offering new ways to understand the dynamics of the system (Hoffman et al., 2006).

Multicultural Supervision

When conducting supervision, the effective supervisor should be cognizant of the fact that cross-cultural differences (e.g., age, race, ethnicity, gender, sexual orientation, or spirituality) can be a major source of tension between the supervisor and supervisee and between the supervisee and the client (Ancis & Marshall, 2010; Dressel, Consoli, Kim, & Atkinson, 2007; Lassiter, Napolitano, Culbreth, & Ng, 2008; Ober, Granello, & Henfield, 2009). With this in mind, the following is suggested if supervisors are to work effectively on cross-cultural issues with their supervisees:

1. Be up to speed on how multicultural issues affect supervision.
2. Be aware of and address how issues of diversity affect the supervisory relationship.
3. Model cross-cultural sensitivity.
4. Be willing to ask supervisees about their cultural background.
5. Be open to discussing cross-cultural differences with supervisees.
6. Be aware of how power and privilege may affect the supervisory relationship.
7. Help supervisees see how power and privilege may affect their counseling relationships.
8. Assist supervisees in being able to conceptualize clients from a multicultural perspective.
9. Be able to build a strong working alliance with your supervisee.
10. Have and share your knowledge and skills specific to cross-cultural issues.
11. Be a model and provide examples of social advocacy.
12. Be able to use models of cross-cultural supervision.

Ethical, Professional, and Legal Issues

Ethical Issues in the Consulting Relationship

A number of authors, as well as the ACA ethics code, illuminate some key ethical issues specific to the consulting process (ACA, 2014a; Dougherty, 2014; Kampwirth & Powers, 2012). Some of the more salient issues include the following (also, please read Section B.7 and D.2 of the ACA ethics code):

➤ *Agreements:* Counselors should ensure that agreements regarding consultation are obtained from all parties involved, especially with regard to confidentiality.
➤ *Respect for privacy:* Client identities should be protected, and information should be discussed only for professional purposes.
➤ *Growth toward self-direction:* The consultant should have as its primary goals the ability of those involved in consultation to become increasingly independent and able to use the skills that the consultant imparts.
➤ *Disclosure of confidential information:* Information should be kept confidential and discussed only for professional purposes.

➤ *Multiple relationships:* Consultation often involves multiple relationships and consultants should take steps to ensure that all involved are clear about the purpose of the consulting relationships, the limits of the relationships, and its goals.

➤ *Informed consent in consultation:* Counselors should give in writing and verbally to those involved in the consulting relationship information concerning the purpose of the consultation and should jointly decide how goals will be achieved. Those involved in consultation should give consent to the procedures.

➤ *Consultant competency:* Counselors should ensure that they have the competence and the resources to conduct consultation and should refer when they do not.

➤ *Understanding with consultees:* Counselors should develop a "clear understanding" with those involved in the consulting relationship of the problem, goals, and consequences of an intervention.

Ethical Issues in the Supervisory Relationship

Because supervision is technically a kind of consultation, one should be aware of the issues just discussed when supervising. However, some ethical issues that have specifically stood out in supervision include the following (ACA, 2014a; Bernard & Goodyear, 2013; Fall & Sutton, 2004; Glosoff & Matrone, 2010; Scaife, 2008):

➤ *Supervisor preparation:* Supervisors should be trained and competent in supervisory methods.

➤ *Client welfare:* Supervisors have a responsibility to monitor the welfare of the client and take appropriate action if the client is at risk of harming self or another person or if the supervisee cannot effectively work with a client.

➤ *Informed consent:* Supervisors should obtain informed consent from their supervisees and clients should be informed that the supervisee is in supervision with a supervisor and how that might affect confidentiality.

➤ *Multicultural issues:* Supervisors should be aware of and address how issues of diversity affect the supervisory relationship (see the section "Multicultural Supervision" earlier in this chapter).

➤ *Relationship boundaries:* Supervisors should be aware of how power differentials play a role between themselves and their supervisees and thus respect appropriate professional and social boundaries.

➤ *Sexual relationships:* Supervisors do not engage in sexual relationships with supervisees.

➤ *Dual and multiple relationships:* Although dual relationships with some supervisees are inevitable (e.g., a supervisee taking a class from his or her supervisor, having a supervisor serve on a supervisee's dissertation committee), supervisors should be particularly sensitive to the potential for abuse of power in any dual relationship.

➤ *Responsibility to clients:* Supervisors have a responsibility to ensure that adequate counseling is taking place between the supervisee (counselor) and the client.

➤ *Limitations of supervisees:* Supervisors have a responsibility to evaluate supervisees and to find remedial assistance for them if they are not performing adequately. If supervisees are not able to function effectively, supervisors have the responsibility to recommend dismissal from their program or agency, or not recommend them for a specific credential.

➤ *Evaluation and accountability:* Supervisors have a responsibility to evaluate the supervisee's progress in supervision, to ensure ongoing feedback to the supervisee, and to document supervisory sessions.

➤ *Endorsement:* Supervisors do not endorse unqualified supervisees for credentialing, but rather take steps to help them become qualified.

Professional Issue: Professional Association for Counselor Supervision

The Association for Counselor Education and Supervision (ACES), a division of ACA, is specifically focused on issues of counselor training, including supervision. Although admittedly the association has had more involvement with educators as opposed to supervisors, you might want to consider joining it if you are interested in counselor education and in supervision. The association publishes one journal, *Counselor Education and Supervision,* and it offers regional and national workshops, as well as grants in the area of counselor education and supervision.

Professional Issue: Technology and Supervision

Today, almost all counseling programs have rooms equipped with one-way windows, live video streaming, or some other technological advances that allow students to be viewed by supervisors or peers as they are involved in a live counseling session or role-play. Students can receive immediate feedback through a number of methods such as a telephone or a "bug-in-the-ear," which involves an earphone and an electronic transmitting device (e.g., smartphone to smartphone with earphone).

More recently, we have seen an increase in *cybersupervision,* live supervision via the Internet (Chapman, Baker, Nassar-McMillan, & Gerler, 2011; Coursol, 2004; Smith et al., 2007). Advantages to this type of supervision include being flexible about scheduling times, increased number of supervision sites because one is not limited by distance from supervisor, better use of the supervisee's time, and more potential supervisors. Drawbacks include the access and expense of technology, difficulty in building a relationship if a supervisee is not face to face with the supervisor, potential problems with technology, and potential confidentiality issues with technology.

Legal Issue: Liability in Consultation and Supervision

Because consultants and supervisors are directly or indirectly in a position to effect change in clients, they can be held responsible for any potential negative results of their consultation or supervision (Welfel, 2013). This particularly came to light during the Tarasoff decision. In that case (discussed in Chapter 4), after learning that a client was threatening to harm his ex-girlfriend, the client's therapist, a psychologist at a campus counseling center, broke confidentiality and told campus police, who subsequently picked up the client for questioning. The psychologist's supervisor reprimanded the psychologist for breaking confidentiality. The ex-girlfriend was subsequently murdered by the client, and her parents sued everyone involved in the case, including the supervisor. The supervisor, among others, was found liable for not ensuring the safety of the client's ex-girlfriend. Thus, we see how consultants and supervisors can be held responsible for the work they perform.

The Counselor in Process: Committed to Ongoing Consultation and Supervision

Consultation is not just something that you read about in a book. It is your professional responsibility. You are responsible for consulting when you are working with a difficult client, when you are not sure of the best direction in which to move with a client, and when you think you may be working outside your area of competence. Consultation and supervision are living processes. Those who do not seek consultation are not providing the best services they can and are likely harmful to their clients. If we are to be the best at what we do and are committed to the growth of our clients, we must ensure that throughout our professional lives, we are forever seeking out consultation and supervision.

Summary

This chapter examined two important types of helping relationships: consultation and supervision. We began by defining consultation, the consultant, and the consultee, and stated that consultation is a triadic relationship, in that the consultant indirectly affects others with whom the consultant meets. We also noted that consultants can intervene on one of three levels: primary, secondary, or tertiary, but regardless of the level in which they intervene, they are affecting a wider system.

This chapter gave a brief history of consultation, noting that it first became popular during the 1940s and 1950s, when it was known as a direct-service approach. Over the years, however, it became increasingly more process oriented. As the twentieth century progressed, a number of consultation styles or models evolved that could be loosely grouped into one of two categories. Consultant-centered consultation (i.e., expert, prescriptive, and trainer/educator) involves the consultant using his or her body of knowledge to offer suggestions and advice for systemic change. In contrast, consultee-centered consultation (i.e., collaborative, facilitative, and process-oriented) occurs when the consultant assists people in the system to use their own resources in the change process. This same period saw the rise of a number of theoretical approaches to consultation. Sampling some of these theories, the chapter briefly discussed the following approaches as applied to consultation: person-centered, cognitive-behavioral, Gestalt, psychoanalytic, social constructionist, and chaos theory. We noted that consultants generally have a style or model of working related to the theoretical approach to which they adhere.

As the chapter continued, we pointed out that regardless of the approach that a consultant uses, there are a number of fairly predictable stages to the consulting process, including pre-entry; entry, goal setting, implementation, evaluation, and disengagement. Finally, the chapter examined some of the consultation activities of college counselors, agency counselors, and school counselors. Some of the major points noted in this section included Cooper's "cube" model for consultation in colleges; inward and outward consultation, including Gerald Caplan's model of consulting for agencies; and the fact that consultation is one of the more important and complex tasks for school counselors.

This chapter also examined the process of supervision, which was defined as an intense interpersonally focused relationship that involves a number of systems, the most basic being that of the supervisor ↔ supervisee/counselor ↔ client. We described supervision as a special type of consultation and noted similarities and differences between the two. Both consultation and supervision focus on the change process, are systemic, are therapeutic but are not therapy, and involve talking with a third person or persons about another party. Noting the differences, we stated that consultation, unlike supervision, is time-limited and the consultant usually does not have a direct evaluative responsibility to the consultee. In addition, we noted the important role that parallel process can play in supervision.

Next, the discussion offered some definitions of the terms *supervisor* and *supervisee*. It identified twelve competencies of an effective supervisor and noted some of the roles and responsibilities of a supervisor, as well as some of the qualities of good supervisors. Then the chapter went on to discuss the fact that one role of the supervisor is to evaluate the supervisee, and that this can sometimes lead to resistance; and also pinpointed some reasons that resistance can result. In conducting supervision, we have distinguished between individual, triadic, and group supervision and pointed out some of the advantages and disadvantages of each.

This chapter then examined three models of supervision that have evolved over the years. Developmental models, such as Stoltenberg's Integrated Developmental Model (IDM), speaks to predictable stages that a supervisee will go through while in supervision, including three levels of development related to awareness of self and of their client, motivation toward the counseling process, and develop increasing autonomy in the counseling and supervision process.

Psychotherapy-based models approach the supervisory process by using a specific counseling theory as its basis for the supervisory process. These models either model or teach the psychotherapeutic approach. Integrative models are not theory specific and can be integrated within one's theoretical orientation, and the chapter highlighted two integrative models. Bernard's discrimination model looks at the supervisor in the role of teacher, counselor, and consultant and examines domains of supervision that include interventions, conceptualization, and personalization. Interpersonal Process Recall (IPR), developed by Norm Kagan, views the supervisor's role as one in which he or she attends to the feelings and thoughts of the supervisee and, when appropriate, asks leading questions to deepen the session.

Highlighting supervision as a crucial component of graduate school training, we pointed out that supervision is generally provided during skills classes and fieldwork experiences. We noted the various ways that supervisors, today, can view the work of practicing students (e.g., case notes, live observation, electronically), and also stated that a large percentage of practicing counselors continue to seek out supervision after graduate school through individual, group, and peer supervision, and highlighted the difficulty that some school counselors have in obtaining supervision.

As the chapter continued, we detailed the opportunity that the consultant has to effect change in systems based on the dynamics of cultural differences that exist in all systems.

Relative to supervision, we made twelve suggestions for being an effective cross-cultural supervisor. As the chapter neared its conclusion, we identified a number of ethical issues critical to the consulting relationship and others that are critical to the supervisory relationship. In addition, we identified the Association for Counselor Education and Supervision (ACES) as the primary association that addresses supervision. Next, we highlighted some technological advances in the way supervision is conducted, particularly the use of cybersupervision, and then discussed the responsibility that consultants and supervisors have in protecting the welfare of clients. Finally, this chapter concluded by stressing that consultation and supervision should be an ongoing component of the counselor's job. Without consultation and supervision, we are an island unto ourselves, left only to our own resources.

Further Practice

Visit CengageBrain.com to respond to additional material that highlight the salient aspects of the chapter content. There, you can find ethical, professional, and legal vignettes, a number of experiential exercises, and study tools including a glossary, flashcards, and sample test items. Hopefully, these will enhance your learning and be fun and interesting.

THE DEVELOPMENT OF THE PERSON

SECTION

4

Overview

The common theme running through the three chapters in this section is the focus on human development. Although each chapter spotlights a specific area in the development of the person, they all offer a manner of conceptualizing our clients and ourselves as a function of a developmental process. Chapter 9 does this by examining normal development in a number of important domains, including physical, cognitive, and moral development; lifespan development; and the development of faith. Chapter 10 identifies theories about the development of abnormal behavior and presents a way of classifying behavior, and Chapter 11 offers a view of how personality is reflected through one's career development process.

As you read through this section, you might want to consider the developmental aspects of your life. Reflect back on your childhood and the kinds of transitions through which you passed, and then consider the transitions you've experienced in your adult life. Think about the impact that they had upon you and your family. As you continue through this section, reflect on how you developed your sense of self and your state of mental health. Think about how you became you! Finally, think about why you are considering a career in counseling. What kinds of developmental issues have affected this important choice in your life? Clearly, this section offers a framework for working with clients, but it also presents a number of models to help you understand who you are today.

Development Across the Lifespan

With each passage from one stage of human growth to the next, we too must shed a protective structure. We are left exposed and vulnerable—but also yeasty and embryonic again, capable of stretching in ways we hadn't known before. These sheddings may take several years or more. Coming out of each passage, though, we enter a longer and more stable period in which we can expect relative tranquility and a sense of equilibrium regained.

(Sheehy, 1974/2006, p. 29)

I remember going on a trip out west with my parents and my brother. I was 13, and my brother was 8. I was miserable. I sat in the back seat of the car going through the pains of having recently reached puberty. My parents, I think, just thought I was going through a miserable stage. No matter where we went or what we did, I only thought about being in love. Oh yeah, and sex, of course. Somewhere in the middle of this trip, we stopped at a small gift shop. There was a girl who worked there who I had an instant crush on. I was shy but managed to have some small talk with her. No one knew my passion for her; it was my secret. And, in the back of my mind, I also had a curious interest about boys. How was I to make sense of all of this?

My parents took us to national parks. We visited incredible sites where they "oohed" and "aahed," and I just thought about the girl at the gift shop. I even sent her a postcard with a short note and my return address. I hoped so much that I would hear from the girl from the gift shop. I did not. Even today when thinking back on that trip, in my mind I have a hazy picture of the Grand Canyon, Mesa Verde, and Old Faithful, but I have an indelible picture of her. Puberty is a very powerful experience, and it's a part of our normal developmental patterns.

I struggled through puberty. My parents grew up in a time when relationships and sex were not talked about. Well, there could be a few "dirty jokes," but no real conversations. There was no school counselor to go to. And my friends—well, those conversations were certainly limited. I was left to my own devices, struggling with my own needs, desires, and wondering if this was all normal. Like most people, I struggled through this normal phase of development.

This chapter is about normal development across the lifespan. The chapter's goal is to provide you with an understanding of the counselor's role in helping to ease clients through what sometimes can be painful transitions through normal developmental stages. As with my struggle through puberty, we all manage to get through a series of normal and predictable developmental stages in our journey through life. No doubt, I would have struggled through puberty even if I had had Carl Rogers to talk with. However, with Carl by my side, I probably would have felt that what I was going through was normal.

We will start this chapter by briefly reviewing some of the physical and psychological developmental milestones that children, adolescents, and adults face. Next, we will explore the cognitive and moral development of childhood, or how children develop their ways of knowing the world. This discussion will be followed by an examination of adult cognitive development, or how adults develop their ways of understanding and constructing reality. We will then examine lifespan development, or the kinds of tasks and challenges that individuals face as they pass through life stages. Finally, we will explore one model of faith development. Defining faith in a very broad manner, the theory that we will examine reflects elements from all of the theories considered in this chapter. We will conclude by examining multicultural, social justice, ethical, professional, and legal issues related to normal development.

A Little Background

The counseling profession has long prided itself on having a developmental focus. However, despite some attempts at applying developmental models in counseling settings during the 1960s, the concept of development "seemed little more than a catchword" (Blocher, 1988, p. 14). It was not until the 1980s that the application of theory to practice became a reality. The 1980s ushered in the era of true developmental counseling. The establishment of the Council for the Accreditation of Counseling and Related Programs (CACREP) standards in 1981, which included human development as one of its core curriculum content areas, highlighted development as a crucial element in the counseling profession. Then, in 1983, the American Personnel and Guidance Association (APGA) changed its name to the American Association for Counseling and Development (AACD, now ACA). It was becoming increasingly clear that the profession wanted a name that mirrored a developmental perspective in practice.

We have come a long way since the 1980s. Today, we find developmental models being applied to work with clients in all settings, and even to how counselors grow and change over the years. In general, this developmental model challenges us to examine clients from a wellness perspective, in the sense that change and growth is seen as a natural progression that occurs over time, as opposed to a process that is fixed early in life or determined by our temperament.

> *Wellness conceptualized as the paradigm for counseling provides strength-based strategies for assessing clients, conceptualizing issues developmentally, and planning interventions to remediate dysfunction and optimize growth.*
>
> (Myers & Sweeney, 2008, p. 482)

Keeping this wellness notion in mind, this chapter will explore a number of theories of development and discuss how counselors can use them when working with clients.

Understanding Human Development

The development of a person is complex and occurs on many levels. Over the years, a number of models of human development have been described that can assist the counselor when working with clients. Although these models differ tremendously in how they apply developmental theory, they tend to share common elements. For instance, most hold the belief that development is continual, is orderly, implies change, is by its nature painful and growth-producing, can be applied with many differing counseling approaches, and is preventive, optimistic, and wellness-oriented. Let's explore some of these concepts.

Development Is Continual

Whereas earlier theories of development were entrenched in biological determinism, in more recent years development has been viewed as a lifelong journey in which there is *plasticity*; that is, the individual has the ability to stretch and change cognitively, physically, interpersonally, intrapsychically, morally, and spiritually (Santrock, 2013). From this perspective, development begins when we are born and ends when we die. It is nonstop and continuous, and once we step on the ride, we can't get off.

Development Is Orderly and Sequential and Builds Upon Itself

Models that describe human growth have a predictable pattern of development from earlier to later stages, in which the latter stages build on what has already been experienced and integrated into our lives:

> *Development proceeds stage by stage in orderly sequence, and although there are individual variations, these do not basically alter the ground plan that is typical of our species. . . .*

(Di Leo, 1977/2012, p. 1)

This predictable pattern of growth allows the counselor to assess the developmental level of the client and predict the next developmental hurdle the client will face. If an individual does not successfully accomplish a developmental task when it is prime for its ascendancy, then there is greater likelihood of pathological development, or at the very least, it is more likely that the individual will struggle (Crandell, Crandell, & Vander Zanden, 2012; Santrock, 2013).

Development Implies Change, but Our Core Remains More or Less the Same

As we walk down our developmental path, we encounter much that is new to our current understanding of the world. Generally, we *assimilate* this new information, which means that we take it into our existing understanding of the world. Periodically, however, we move into a state of readiness for a dramatic shift in the way that we live in the world, and with support, we *accommodate* or dramatically change the way that we understand the world. Our core remains the same, but as we assimilate and accommodate to the world, we appropriately adapt. Like a piece of clay, we can be molded, sometimes torn apart and then put back together, but the basic material that defines who we are remains the same.

Development Is Painful, Yet Growth-Producing

Developmental theory suggests that there are transition points from one developmental level to another. Such points are generally earmarked by *disequilibrium* as the individual accommodates to a new way of living in the world. Transitions will often be experienced as a state of confusion, anxiety, depression, fear, or exhilaration, and they can occur quickly or last for years.

Transition will be less disequilibrating if the individual has had success in passing through previous developmental milestones and if there is support in the environment to ease the individual through the transition. Support for change comes in many forms; it can be the nurturing needed for the infant to grow physically, the reinforcement given to an adolescent as he or she begins to think in increasingly complex ways, or the psychological support needed by the adult going through a career change. The support can be given by a parent, a friend, or a counselor. However you pass through them, transitions are a signal that you are growing toward something greater than you were previously.

Developmental Models Are Transtheoretical

Developmental theory acknowledges the importance of the interplay among our biology, the environment in which we are brought up, and unique psychological factors of the person in the growth process. Understanding this interplay helps the counselor conceptualize client difficulties in multiple ways and frees the counselor to use strategies from many disciplines and theoretical approaches when working with specific developmental issues (Santrock, 2013, 2014).

Development Is Preventive, Optimistic, and Wellness Oriented

The nature of developmental theory lends itself to prevention and a wellness model of mental health. By knowing expected transitions, counselors can develop workshops and educational seminars to assist individuals in understanding their natural progression from one developmental level to another. It also offers counselors a framework from which to develop strategies when assisting clients who may want to revisit unfinished developmental tasks. Whereas pathological models assume that pathology is an indication of an inborn deficit that is, at best, difficult to fix, developmental models view pathology as either a normal response to a developmental transition or an indication that a past developmental task has remained unfinished (Brown, Johnson, Bender, & Roberts, 2009; Crandell et al., 2012; Santrock, 2014).

In summary, human development is continuous, orderly, sequential, painful yet growth producing, and a natural and potentially positive part of our existence. Developmental counseling offers the counselor a unique perspective when working with clients. The developmentally astute counselor knows (1) a variety of developmental theories, (2) the types of social issues and personal problems often experienced by clients as they pass through specific developmental stages, and (3) the kinds of counseling techniques that might work with clients as they pass through the stages. Clearly, knowledge of human development can go far in assisting the counselor in his or her work with clients.

A Brief Overview of Physical and Psychosocial Development in Childhood

The developing child undergoes major physiological, social, and cognitive changes in the first few years of life (Kail & Cavanaugh, 2013; Santrock, 2013, 2014). Of course, until puberty and usually sometime afterward, there are great gains in height and weight. Gross and fine motor skills change quickly in the first few years of life, and the nervous system is structurally complete but functionally incomplete and will not finish growing until early adolescence. For instance, the myelin sheath that covers the nerves continues to develop until the child is 2 years old, which accounts for the jerky movements of infants, and the cerebral cortex will not be complete until approximately age 12. As the nervous system continues to develop, there are rapid increases in the child's sensory development, speech and language ability, and cognitive and intellectual functioning. Increased physical abilities promote the child's psychosocial development. For example, increased mobility allows the toddler to explore more of his or her environment, and toddlers who are reinforced for their exploratory behavior will develop higher self-esteem than those who are reprimanded.

Because the vast majority of children will develop at fairly predictable rates, a counselor or child specialist who is aware of physiological timetables normed for children can assess whether a child is on target for his or her physiological development. Milestones of normative physical and social development have been described by dozens of authors on a variety of constructs such as intelligence, moral development, memory, motor development, and math and verbal skills (Schneider & Bullock, 2009).

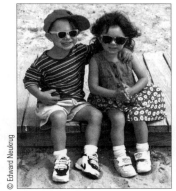

Hannah and Joe

Although the rate of children's physical development is fairly consistent, the scope of a specific child's development is based on the genetic predisposition of the child in interaction with the environment (Brooks-Gunn, 2004; Stearns, Allal, & Mace, 2008). For instance, although most children will be able to do multiplication by the fourth grade, their rate of learning and range of ability will vary based on genetics and environment (see Figure 9.1). Along these lines, a brilliant child is at a major disadvantage if he or she is brought up in a home that has lead paint and lead in the water, or raised by neglectful parents that provide a poor diet and a lack of psychological support, while a child who is less gifted can shine if placed in a stimulating and nurturing environment.

Evidence of the importance of a nurturing environment in a child's development can be seen through the success of the Head Start program. Since the 1970s, Head Start has provided disadvantaged preschool children intellectually stimulating and nurturing environments. On average, these children have done noticeably better academically and socially than children of a similar background who have not received such an opportunity (Puma et al., 2010).

FIGURE 9.1

The Bender Visual Motor Gestalt

The Bender Visual Motor Gestalt is an assessment instrument that is used to determine possible psychological, physiological, and developmental problems in children and adults. In giving the instrument, you ask the individual to reproduce nine figures which are presented to him or her in sequence (the figures are actually much larger than depicted below). For children, difficulties in reproducing some of the figures could be indications of a learning disability, developmental delay, or emotional problems. Below are reproductions of four of the figures of two children who are developmentally on target. When Hannah couldn't reproduce figure 6, she became very frustrated and drew the lines below. Look at how much easier it is for the older child to reproduce the figures.

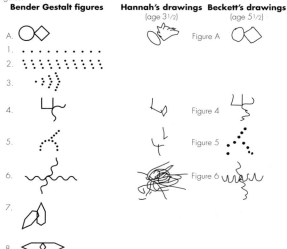

Development in Adolescence and Adulthood

As children grow into adolescence, they face the major task of dealing with the physical and psychological aspects of puberty. Of course, changes in their bodies can greatly affect how they feel about themselves. Adolescence is the time when teenagers will compare themselves to each other as they develop their identity. In adolescence, many teenagers face a myriad of social issues with which they struggle, including drug and alcohol use, crime and violence, dating, sexual identity, and sexually transmitted diseases. Late adolescence marks the time when teenagers will begin to consider their future plans. Older adolescents have to decide whether to go on to college or to work, and consider a career, a college major, or both.

Adolescence and young adulthood bring with them the blossoming of a person's sexuality. Of course, how this issue is dealt with can affect the individual for the rest of his or her life. Body image issues become particularly important now, especially for women who often feel pressure to reflect the image portrayed in the media of what is considered beautiful (Ata, Ludden, & Lally, 2007).

Young adulthood is highlighted by making career choices and, for some, making life-long commitments. Thus, issues of intimacy and how the young adult fits into the world of work are prominent at this time. These issues become increasingly more important as the young adult moves into what is sometimes called *early adulthood*. Success at having a love relationship and committing to a career is often reflected in one's psychological adjustment to the world in this time of life.

As individuals move into middle adulthood, they begin to recognize the slow decline in their physical abilities. When men and women reach their forties most will see slow weight gains and changes in vision, reaction time, strength, and motor ability. The psychological associations to death and dying are likely to increase, especially as parents and grandparents become ill and die. Women will soon face menopause, and for many men and women, midlife physical changes at this time in life coincide with psychological adjustments, and sometimes what's called the "midlife crisis." Adults will begin to assess their worth in the world of work and begin to think about their entrance into late adulthood. Those who have been raising families are likely to reflect on how the family has grown, and those who have not may ponder what it is like not to leave a legacy through their children.

As we move on in life, slow physical changes continue, and in later adulthood, disease and ill health increase and changes in physical abilities occur. These include changes in hearing, taste, smell, visual acuity, and memory, as well as an increasingly fragile skeletal system. As many are now living into their late eighties and nineties, additional health problems become increasingly prevalent. Psychologically, many older adults reflect on their lives and assess whether they are satisfied with their accomplishments.

The Development of Knowing: Cognitive and Moral Changes in Childhood

This section of the chapter will examine cognitive and moral development. Although all of the stages examined next can be reached in adolescence or young adulthood, many individuals do not reach the higher stages at any point in their lives.

Jean Piaget and Cognitive Development

How does a child come to understand the world? This is the question that Jean Piaget (1896–1980) asked when he first began exploring the cognitive development of children (Flavell, 1963). Piaget found that children learn through a process of assimilation and accommodation. *Assimilation* occurs when the child uses his or her existing way of understanding the world to make sense out of new knowledge. *Accommodation,* on the other hand, occurs when the child changes his or her previous ways of knowing to make sense out of this new knowledge (Piaget, 1954).

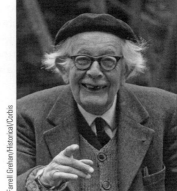

Jean Piaget

Piaget stated that in accommodating to the world, *schemata* (new cognitive structures; e.g., new ways of thinking) are formed that allow an individual to adapt and change his or her ways of thinking and understanding the world. This process of assimilation, forming new schemata, and accommodation occurs throughout the lifespan but is most obvious during childhood. Piaget showed that there were a number of concepts that a child can understand only at the age-appropriate level (see Box 9.1).

BOX 9.1
Hannah's Developmental Readiness

When my daughter, Hannah, was two years old, she loved M&M's®, which we attempted to give to her sparingly. At one point, we discovered small M&Ms (M&M Minis), which are about half the size of the regular ones. Giving her a bunch of these small candies made Hannah ecstatic. After all, now she could have more than she had been given on previous occasions. Hannah had not yet learned the concept that more in number does not necessarily mean more in volume or mass. In a relatively short amount of time, however, she came to understand the concept of differences in size, shape, and mass.

Through his research on child cognitive development, Piaget determined that children pass through predictable stages of development, each highlighted by a particular way of understanding the world (Inhelder & Piaget, 1958; Piaget, 1954). In the *sensorimotor stage* (birth through 2 years), the infant responds almost exclusively to his or her physical and sensory experience. At this stage, the child hasn't acquired full language ability, is not able to maintain mental images, and responds only to the here-and-now of experience. Therefore, not surprisingly, a parent attempting to have a rational conversation with a 1-year-old is pretty much wasting his or her time. However, it may be good practice for the child to hear periodically the tone of rational talk as the child readies him- or herself for the next stage of development.

The *preoperational stage* (2 through 7 years) is marked by the development of language ability and the ability to maintain mental images and to manipulate the meaning of objects (e.g., a doll is a baby, or a block is a car) (Muro & Dinkmeyer, 1977). The child in this stage responds intuitively to the world. Not yet able to think in logical sequences or in complex ways, the child responds to what seems immediately obvious, as opposed to what might be logical. Unless the child is on the verge of entering the next stage of development, trying to explain logical principles would be difficult and usually impossible. Imagine trying to explain to a two-year-old that two kinds of M&Ms had different amounts of mass (see Box 9.1). She just couldn't get it!

From ages 7 through 11 years, the child enters the *concrete-operational stage*, in which he or she can begin to figure things out through a series of logical tasks, can begin to classify objects, and is able to understand a sequence of events. Children can now make mental comparisons and mentally manipulate images. For instance, a child in this stage could create a mental image of a map of how to get to a friend's house. Children in this stage are often adamant about their logical way of viewing the world. For instance, when I was helping a friend's son with a math problem, he became angry when I suggested another way of finding the solution. He did not yet have the cognitive flexibility to examine other ways of knowing.

Children in the concrete-operational stage will have difficulty with metaphors or proverbs because they haven't developed the capacity to think abstractly. However, when children or young adults move into Piaget's final stage, *formal-operational* (11 through 16 years), they are able to apply more complex levels of knowing to their understanding of the world. A child in this stage can understand that objects might have symbolic meaning (e.g., the Liberty Bell is more than just a bell), can test hypotheses, understand proverbs, and consider more than one aspect of a problem at a time.

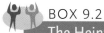

BOX 9.2
The Heinz Dilemma

The following represents one of the more well known of Kohlberg's moral dilemmas. Presenting dilemmas such as these to adolescent boys, he developed his well-known theory of moral development. After reading the dilemma and reviewing the stages and levels, devise responses that a "typical" person might make as a function of the stage he or she is in.

In Europe, a woman was near death from a special kind of cancer. There was one drug that the doctors thought might save her. It was a form of radium that a druggist in the same town had recently discovered. The drug was expensive to make, but the druggist was charging ten times

what the drug cost him to make. He paid $200 for the radium and charged $2,000 for a small dose of the drug. The sick woman's husband, Heinz, went to everyone he knew to borrow the money, but he could only get together about $1,000 which is half of what it cost. He told the druggist that his wife was dying and asked him to sell it cheaper or let him pay later. But the druggist said: "No, I discovered the drug and I'm going to make money from it." So Heinz got desperate and broke into the man's store to steal the drug—for his wife. Should the husband have done that?

(Kohlberg, 1963, p. 19)

Piaget's research on child development has greatly assisted us in understanding how children learn and gives us a healthy respect for age-appropriate developmental limitations. Such knowledge has greatly affected styles of teaching, ways to parent effectively, and methods of counseling children.

Kohlberg's Theory of Moral Development

Like Piaget, Lawrence Kohlberg wondered how children come to understand the world. However, Kohlberg was most interested in how children and adults come to understand and justify their moral behavior. Although Piaget had written about the process of moral development, by having children respond to moral dilemmas (problem situations of a moral nature with no clear-cut answer), Kohlberg greatly extended Piaget's original thoughts (Muro & Dinkmeyer, 1977) (see Box 9.2).

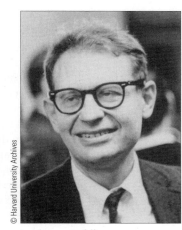

Lawrence Kohlberg

Kohlberg (1981, 1984) discovered that moral reasoning developed in a predictable pattern that spanned three levels of development, each containing two stages. The first level, *preconventional* (roughly ages 2 through 9 years), is based on the notion that children are egocentric and make moral decisions out of a concern of being punished or to be rewarded. In *stage 1* of this level, moral decisions are made to avoid punishment or gain rewards from individuals in authority (*punishment-obedience orientation*), while in *stage 2*, decisions are made with an egocentric/hedonistic desire to satisfy one's own needs (*instrumental-hedonism orientation*). Imagine two 6-year-old children vying for the same toy, both yelling, "I want it!" A parent comes over and asks the children to share, and they comply (wanting to avoid punishment from authority). Suddenly, one of the 6-year-olds gives the other a piece of candy and says, "Here, you have this and give me the toy" ("You scratch my back and I'll scratch yours"). In this situation, the child recognizes the needs of another but is more concerned with having his or her own needs met.

In Kohlberg's *conventional level*, moral decisions are based initially on social conformity and mutualism (*good girl–nice boy orientation*) and later on rule-governed behavior (*law and order orientation*). In *stage 3* of this level, the individual responds in a manner designed

BOX 9.3
Going to Jail for Reasons of Personal Conscience

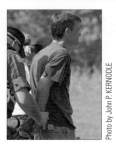

Photo by John P. KERNODLE

My brother-in-law Steve (being hand-cuffed in the photo) was incarcerated for fourteen months because he and others broke into a naval shipyard, sneaked onto an Aegis destroyer, poured their own blood onto the ship, and banged on the ship to protest against nuclear missiles. Some might say that Steve is in Kohlberg's stage 6 because he chose to break the law for the betterment of society and out of his deeply held belief that nuclear arms can only harm people. If Steve had thoroughly reflected upon this, considered all points of view, and come to this decision in a deeply personal and thoughtful manner, he would be in stage 6. If he did this action out of a desire for approval of his social group, or because he adhered strongly to a system of rules, he would be in stage 3 or 4. Often people can do the same actions and be in different stages. You must know the person to determine the stage.

to please others and to avoid the disapproval of significant others. Most children will reach stage 3 by age 13 (Gerrig, 2014). An example of a stage 3 behavior is a 10-year-old who acts appropriately at school to gain the approval of his or her teacher. In *stage 4* of the conventional level, adolescents and adults will emphasize a system of laws and rules as a means of maintaining a sense of order in their lives. Here, there is some recognition that if we violate rules, the social milieu in which we live can be disrupted. If everybody breaks the rules, chaos will result. For example, some 10-year-olds will reason that it is not right to make fun of other kids because it is against the rules at school. Imagine a setting where many, or most people, were violating this rule. What do you think that would look like?

Kohlberg believed that the final level of development, *postconventional morality*, requires formal-operational thinking. He found that most individuals will never reach this level because of the cognitive complexity involved. In *stage 5* of this level, the postconventional thinker believes in the process of democratically devised social contracts (e.g., laws) that can be analyzed, interpreted, and changed, but that ultimately take precedence over individual needs (*social contract orientation*). Here, an individual would likely follow the law because there are governing moral principles that have been used in their development. However, such a person is willing to examine inconsistencies in laws and work on changing laws not seen as good for society.

In *stage 6* of the postconventional level, moral decisions are based on a sense of universal truths, personal conscience, and principles of justice that are seen as being valid beyond current laws and social contracts (*principled conscience orientation*) (Cincotta, 2008). Here an individual would consider moral truths in his or her decision-making process and, after deep reflection, might choose to break a law, deciding that such an action is taken out of respect for the dignity of people and for the betterment of society (see Box 9.3). For instance, during the civil rights movement of the 1960s, some individuals broke laws to advance the cause of civil rights for all people.

Although Kohlberg identified the lowest ages at which some individuals had reached conventional and postconventional thinking, he found that some young adults and adults have not mastered conventional thinking, while most have not reached postconventional thinking. He therefore advised that it would not be unusual to find same-aged adults at different levels of moral development.

Gilligan's Theory of Women's Moral Development

In 1982, Carol Gilligan wrote a book called *In a Different Voice,* which questioned some of Kohlberg's assumptions. Gilligan, who had been a colleague of Kohlberg's, noted that most of his research was based on a small group of boys, and after conducting research with girls and women, she proposed that moral reasoning for females might be based on a different way of knowing or understanding the world. She noted that Kohlberg's theory stressed the notion that high-stage individuals make choices that stress autonomy and individuality, whereas her research seemed to indicate that women at high levels of development value connectedness and interdependence and view the relationship as primary when making moral decisions. In describing the differences between men and women, Gilligan notes the responses of one of Kohlberg's subjects and compares him to a woman she interviewed:

> *Thus, while Kohlberg's subject worries about people interfering with each other's rights, this woman worries about "the possibility of omission, of your not helping others when you could help them."*

(Gilligan, 1982, p. 21)

Gilligan stated that in the development of moral reasoning, especially in stages 3 and above, women will emphasize a *standard of caring* in moral decision making; that is, a concern for the other person will be a core ingredient when making moral decisions. She noted that women are more likely to be concerned about the impact that their choices have on others, whereas men are more concerned about a sense of justice being maintained (Gerrig, 2014). Noting these male and female differences, Gilligan states:

> *Given the differences in women's conceptions of self and morality, women bring to the life cycle a different point of view and order human experience in terms of different priorities.*

(Gilligan, 1982, p. 22)

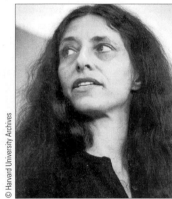

© Harvard University Archives

Carol Gilligan

More specifically, the level 1 preconventional girl is not dissimilar to Kohlberg's level 1 boy, in that her moral reasoning is narcissistic; she reasons from a survival-oriented, self-protective perspective. For Gilligan, the level 2 conventional woman shows a concern for others and feels responsible for others, as opposed to Kohlberg's level 2 person, who is concerned about pleasing others or following the rules. Gilligan's level 3 postconventional woman is a complex thinker who recognizes the interdependent nature of humans and that every action a person takes affects others in deeply personal ways.

Consider how an adolescent or adult woman might respond if her moral reasoning is grounded in a standard of care for others and a sense of responsibility to others, as opposed to the individualistic and rule-following perspective of many men. Gilligan also found that because adolescent girls tend to be more concerned with the feelings of others, they will often lose their "voice" as they defer in decision making. However, as women age and grow, their voice, or strong sense of self, will often return as they realize they can be concerned about others and also have a perspective on the world that they will stand up for (see Gilligan's novel, *Kyra*, published in 2008).

Gilligan has added a unique perspective to the concept of moral development and brings to the forefront major differences in how men and women tend to approach moral reasoning. Understanding such differences is crucial in helping us understand why men and women view moral reasoning in very different ways.

Comparison of Cognitive and Moral Development

There is a logical association between Piaget's stages of cognitive development and Kohlberg's and Gilligan's levels of moral development. The preoperational thinker responds intuitively and cannot think logically or in complex ways. From a perspective of moral development, this person can only be in the preconventional level, responding on a gut level to the rudimentary morality of punishment and reward and acting in a self-centered manner. Although Kohlberg and Gilligan offer different perspectives on their understanding of the conventional person, reflection on self or complex thinking concerning higher moral principles is not possible at this level. Therefore, moral reasoning from the conventional level is likely a function of concrete-operational thinking. Finally, for both Kohlberg and Gilligan, it is clear that the kind of introspection and consciousness necessary for postconventional thinking can be found only by the individual who has conquered formal-operational thought (see Table 9.1).

TABLE 9.1   A Comparison of Piaget to Kohlberg and Gilligan

PIAGET'S STAGES	PIAGET	KOHLBERG'S/ GILLIGAN'S LEVELS	KOHLBERG	GILLIGAN
Sensorimotor	Responds to physical and sensory experience.			
Preoperational	Intuitive responding. Maintenance of mental images. No logical thinking.	Preconventional	1. Punishment/reward. 2. Satisfy needs to gain reward (you get from me, I get from you).	Concern for survival.
Concrete-operational	No complex thinking. Uses logical thinking, sequencing, categorizing to figure things out.	Conventional	1. Social conformity/ approval of others. 2. Rules and laws to maintain order.	Caring for others Sacrifice of self for others; responsible to others.
Formal-operational	Abstract thinking. Complex ways of knowing.	Postconventional	1. Social contract/ democratically arrived at. Rules that can be changed through a logical process. 2. Individual conscience.	Decision making from an interdependent perspective. Every choice we make affects everyone else.

NOTE: Kohlberg's levels are each divided into two stages as shown.

Adult Cognitive Development

For years, tracing the development of knowing in the adult took a back seat to understanding the cognitive development of children. However, a number of recent theories have offered an explanation of how adults make sense of the world. Like their child-development counterparts, which reach upward and attempt to explain pieces of adult development, these theories extend downward and have something to say about child development. However, in practice, these theories tend to be applied to adults. Two of the theories that have gained some prominence in recent years are Kegan's constructive development theory and Perry's theory of epistemological reflection (Kegan, 1982, 1994; Perry, 1970).

Kegan's Constructivist Developmental Model

Robert Kegan believes that our understanding of the world is based on how we construct reality as we pass through the lifespan. His *subject–object* theory states that there are specific developmental stages through which individuals pass that reflect their meaning-making system. Movement from a lower to higher stage necessitates a letting go of the earlier stage. This is not done easily, and Kegan suggests that movement occurs most successfully if there is challenge to one's existing view of the world within a supportive environment (Kegan, 1982).

Kegan (1982) suggests there are six stages of cognitive development (stages 0 to 5), with stages 3, 4, and 5 representing ways in which the adult views the world. Kegan states that the self-absorbed infant, being born into the *incorporative stage,* is all reflexive and has no sense of self as separate from the outside world. However, as the very young child begins to experience the world, reflexes are no longer the primary focus; instead, the young child attempts to have his or her needs met through attainment of objects outside of self. In this *impulsive stage,* the child has limited control over his or her actions and acts spontaneously to have needs met. For instance, a young child might impulsively grab a toy from another child. No wonder the second year of life is often called the "terrible twos":

> In disembedding herself from her reflexes the two-year-old comes to have reflexes rather than be them, and the new self is embedded in that which coordinates the reflexes, namely, the "perceptions" and the "impulses."
>
> (Kegan, 1982, p. 85)

As children gain control over their impulses, they move into the *imperial stage,* where needs, interests, and wishes become primary and impulses can now be controlled (see Box 9.4). Here, the child has a desire for and begins to recognize what he or she wants and has some control over how to obtain it. For instance, in the previous situation, rather than impulsively grabbing for a toy, the child might control his or her impulses and wait until the other child is not looking, or trade a toy for the one that he or she wants.

Although some adults are in the imperial stage of development, most are in the last three stages. During the *interpersonal stage,* the individual is embedded in relationships; that is, relationships are primary, and needs and wishes are met through them.

BOX 9.4
Garrett: Responding from the Imperial Stage

Garrett, a 12-year-old son of a friend, wanted to spend time with a friend of his. However, after being told by his friend that he had already made plans to spend time with another boy, Garrett felt rejected and left out. If Garrett had still been in the impulsive stage, he might have thrown a temper tantrum. Instead, having passed into the imperial stage, he had control over his impulses and devised a way to get his needs met. He manipulated a way to spend time with both of them, disregarding their need to be with one another. You see, in the imperial stage, one can control impulses and therefore develop plans to have one's needs met, and in this stage, there is little empathy for other people's desires. Therefore, Garrett did not yet have the ability to talk over his feelings with his friends. Hopefully, when he's a little older, he'll be able to share his feelings of being left out and understand (have empathy for) his friends' desire to be with one another.

When his father was explaining this situation to me, he said that at first, he was going to try to talk with his son about the other kids' feelings, but then he realized that Garrett just couldn't hear that yet. If you're in the imperial stage and not yet ready to give it up, little can be done to "make" you move to the interpersonal stage.

Symbolically, the interpersonal person lives by the following statements, "I am you, and you are me. I do not exist without you. You make me who I am." As opposed to the narcissistic orientation of the imperial person, the interpersonal person begins to show glimpses of empathy. After all, if your existence is contingent on your relationships with others, you had better periodically show them understanding. However, this stage is mostly symbolized by dependency on others. The interpersonal person's need for relationships can be seen in many of the popular songs of our era, which are often highlighted by dependency messages such as "I will die without you" or "I am no one if you are not in my life."

The individual who moves out of embeddedness with another moves into the *institutional stage*, where a sense of autonomy and self-authorship of life is acquired. Relationships in this stage are still important but no longer seem like the essential ingredient for living. In this stage, the individual's understanding of his or her values and interests become important. Here, the individual may choose a partner because the other person shares similar values; however, the person in this stage does not longingly need the partner as he or she would in the interpersonal stage. The institutional person can sometimes become quite arrogant about his or her point of view. Feeling independent and strong, this person can sometimes angrily stake out his or her position. (Some of my colleagues joke that all New Yorkers are in this stage of development.)

Kegan's final stage, the *interindividual stage*, highlights *mutuality* in relationships; that is, the individual can share with others and learn from others in a nondependent way. Here, there is a sharing of selves, without giving up the self, and difference is tolerated and even encouraged at times. In an effort to be continually self-reflective, this individual encourages feedback about self. Finally, the interindividual person has respect for self and for all others, regardless of their stage. One might say that this person is the epitome of the self-actualized human.

Kegan's *constructivist model* stresses the interpersonal nature of development and the fact that we construct new ways of understanding the world and ourselves as we grow. In his eyes, growth is based on our ability to interact with others and to let go of past, less effective types of relating. Although Kegan gives some general time lines for when movement

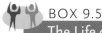

BOX 9.5
The Life of Malcolm X

The life of Malcolm X is a good example of movement through Kegan's stages (see Haley, 2001). As a young adult, Malcolm X found himself involved in a life of crime and drug addiction as he narcissistically tried to have his needs met (imperial stage). Given a ten-year jail sentence for robbery, in prison he was introduced to the Nation of Islam, a Black Muslim religion headed by Elijah Mohammad. Malcolm readily gave up his former lifestyle and became embedded in the values of the Nation of Islam. He lived, slept, and breathed *their* values, and his identity became these values (interpersonal stage). However, as he grew as a person, he realized that he did not agree with some of their ideas, and he moved from embeddedness in their values to a strong sense of his own religious, cultural, and moral values.

Although still an activist, and still somewhat closed to other points of view, he had matured to the point where he was now embracing his own set of values (institutional stage).

Following a pilgrimage to Mecca, he changed his name to Al Hajj Malik al-Shabazz and again modified his views "to encompass the possibility that all white people were not evil and that progress in the black struggle could be made with the help of world organizations, other black groups, and even progressive white groups" (*Encyclopedia of Black America*, 1981, p. 544). Clearly, Al Hajj Malik al-Shabazz had evolved to Kegan's interindividual stage. He could now hear other points of view, be open to feedback, and yet have a clear sense of his own uniqueness in the world.

---

into higher levels could occur, it is common to find older adults who have not moved out of the interpersonal stage, or sometimes even the imperial stage. The life of Malcolm X is an extraordinary example of a person's movement through the stages (see Box 9.5).

Perry's Theory of Intellectual and Ethical Development

William Perry's theory of *epistemological reflection* (Perry, 1970) was developed to examine the cognitive development of adults, particularly college students. The *Perry scheme*, as it is known, describes movement through four stages (King, 1978). In the first stage, *dualism*, students view truth categorically, as right or wrong, and they have little tolerance for ambiguity. Dualists engage in all-or-nothing thinking and believe that experts have answers to almost all questions. Therefore, they believe that they can learn the "truth" from their professor. As individuals develop, they begin to doubt some of their absolutist-type thinking and move into *multiplicity*, or, as reported by some, *transition* (Magolda & Porterfield, 1992), in which a beginning recognition of the limits of authorities occurs.

In the next stage, *relativism*, students are able to think more abstractly and become interested in differing opinions. In relativism, a student comes to understand that there may be many ways of constructing reality and defining truth; that the professor has a body of knowledge, but others have knowledge as well; and that learning can be a joint sharing process between the professor and students. Individuals in this stage are often ambivalent about what values and relative truths to call their own.

Perry's last stage is called *commitment in relativism*. In this final stage, individuals have the capacity to maintain their relativistic outlook while also committing themselves to specific behaviors and values that guide them. Such individuals make a commitment to embracing specific values and beliefs (e.g., pro-life, pro-choice), are open to changing their commitments if given new facts, and can hear different points of view. For example, the committed relativist may make a specific religious or job commitment while at the same time being able to recognize the possibility that new information may modify that choice (Widick, 1977).

Perry's theory has been actively used in college settings to understand how college students think and the cognitive changes they go through while attending college (Magolda & Porterfield, 1992). However, the theory may have broader implications because it may describe a general orientation to how individuals interact in the world, with some people reflecting the rigid, inflexible themes found by the dualists, while other people are capable of the *multiple-perspective-taking* of the relativist. Higher development on the Perry scheme, and related models of cognitive development, appear to be related to the development of many of the counselor qualities discussed in Chapter 1 as critical to effective counseling (Choate & Granello, 2006; Granello, 2002; Granello, Kindsvatter, Granello, Underfer-Babalis, & Moorhead, 2008; Neukrug & McAuliffe, 1993).

Although Perry did not set age limits for individuals who are dualistic, relativistic, or committed in relativism, it would not be too difficult to approximate the lowest ages in which you might find each. The dualist could be as young as the individual in the concrete-operational stage (around 12), while the multiple-perspective-taking of the relativist could take place only somewhat after a person has achieved Piaget's formal-operational stage and Kegan's institutional stage (perhaps a minimum of age 18, but usually much older). The individual who is committed in relativism would also have to be in the formal operational stage, and this person also seems to hold many of the same qualities as Kegan's interindividual person (minimal age of 40).

Comparison of Adult Cognitive Development Theories

Although Kegan's theory is much more broadly based than Perry's, there are many similarities. For instance, both examine how the individual constructs reality and makes meaning in his or her life. Both suggest that as individuals develop, their view of reality becomes increasingly more complex, more open, and seems to embody many of the characteristics of what we might call the *self-actualized person.* Finally, both theories state that adult development is likely to occur if the individual is afforded an environment that is supportive, yet challenging to one's current way of making meaning.

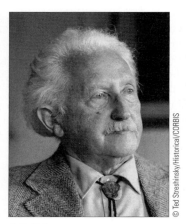

Erik Erikson

Lifespan Development

Some models of understanding the development of the person have taken a lifespan perspective; that is, the individual is seen as continuing to grow over the lifespan, with development not being viewed as suddenly ending in childhood or starting in adulthood. In addition, the previous models examined in this chapter offered stages through which all people *could* pass, although many will not reach the highest stages of development. Lifespan models offer stages through which every person *will* pass.

Erikson's Stages of Psychosocial Development

One of the more recognized models of lifespan development has been Erikson's stages of psychosocial development, which examines how psychosocial forces affect the development of the person. Another model, offered by Daniel Levinson, examines stages of development in a number of arenas (e.g., work, love, and family) experienced by men and women over the lifespan.

Although Erik Erikson started out studying Freud's psychoanalytic approach, he later developed a model that challenged Freud's understanding of the developing ego. Contrary to psychoanalysis, he believed that the influence of instincts and the unconscious were not as great as many had posited and that *psychosocial forces*, in combination with biological and internal psychological factors, were major contributors to the development of a healthy personality. Suggesting that individuals pass through eight life stages, Erikson viewed the individual as changing throughout his or her life and placed considerably more emphasis on the influence of social factors than did any of his predecessors (see Table 9.2). In addition, Erikson's approach was more positive than traditional psychoanalysis, as he believed that when previous stages were not successfully traversed, they could be revisited at a later date (see Erikson, 1963, 1968, 1980, 1982).

TABLE 9.2   Erikson's Psychosocial Stages of Development

STAGE	NAME OF STAGE WITH AGES	VIRTUE OF STAGE	DESCRIPTION OF STAGE
1.	Trust versus Mistrust (birth–1 year)	Hope	In this stage, the infant is building a sense of trust or mistrust, which can be facilitated by the ability of significant others to provide a sense of psychological safety to the infant.
2.	Autonomy versus Shame and Doubt (1–2 years)	Will	Here, the toddler explores the environment and is beginning to gain control over his or her body. Significant others can either promote or inhibit the child's newfound abilities and facilitate the development of autonomy or shame and doubt.
3.	Initiative versus Guilt (3–5 years)	Purpose	As physical and intellectual growth continues and exploration of the environment increases, a sense of initiative or guilt can be developed by significant others who are either encouraging or discouraging the child's physical and intellectual curiosity.
4.	Industry versus Inferiority (6–11 years)	Competence	An increased sense of what the child is good at, especially relative to his or her peers, can either be reinforced or negated by significant others (e.g., parents, teachers, or peers), which leads to feeling worthwhile; or discouraged by others, which leads to feeling inferior.
5.	Identity versus Role Confusion (adolescence)	Fidelity	Positive role models and experiences can lead to increased understanding of temperament, values, interests, and abilities that define one's sense of self. Negative role models and limited experiences will lead to role confusion.
6.	Intimacy versus Isolation (early adulthood)	Love	A good sense of self and self-understanding leads to the ability to form intimate relationships that are highlighted by mutually supporting relationships that encourage individuality with interdependency. Otherwise, the young adult feels isolated.
7.	Generativity versus Stagnation (middle adulthood)	Caring	Healthy development in this stage is highlighted by concern for others and for future generations. This individual is able to maintain a productive and responsible lifestyle and can find meaning through work, volunteerism, parenting, and community activities. Otherwise, the adult feels stagnant.
8.	Ego Integrity versus Despair (later life)	Wisdom	The older adult who examines his or her life either feels a sense of fulfillment or despair. Mastering the developmental tasks from the preceding stages will lead to a sense of integrity for the individual.

Erikson suggested that as individuals pass through the eight stages, they are faced with a *task*, sometimes called a *crisis*. Portrayed as a pair of opposing forces, Erikson described the first opposing task in each stage as *syntonic*, or positive emotional quality, and the second task as *dystonic*, or negative emotional quality. He suggested that individuals needed to experience both syntonic and dystonic qualities. However, in the end, one has to find a balance between the two, with individuals leaning toward the syntonic quality. For instance, trust is a critical factor in all people's lives, as we must generally trust others if we are to get along with one another. However, a certain amount of mistrust is also important. For example, if a person is walking down a dark street and sees an ominous figure, he or she should react with a fair amount of mistrust. More generally, Erikson believed that too much trust would lead to what he called *sensory distortion,* while too much mistrust would lead to *withdrawal* (see Table 9.2). Similarly, too much autonomy would lead to *impulsivity,* whereas too much shame and doubt would lead to *compulsion,* and so forth. Clearly, the role of significant others in the early stages had a greal deal of influence over the ability to find the correct balance between the syntonic and dystonic qualities.

Erikson believed that the development of a healthy ego is contingent on the individual's ability to master these critical periods of development and is highlighted by a particular *virtue* or *strength* that is associated with successful passage through each stage (see Table 9.2). If a positive identity is created and the virtue embraced, the individual can move to the next critical period. On the other hand, the individual who is not able to cope with age-specific developmental tasks will develop a low self-image and a bruised ego and will carry these dysfunctions forward, making it difficult to successfully complete later developmental tasks.

Erikson's eight lifespan stages are often referenced as a means of assisting the helper in understanding typical developmental tasks of the client. Such understanding can aid the helper in developing strategies for clients as they attempt to pass successfully through the stages and can sometimes help normalize problems that may feel quite unbearable in the moment.

Levinson's Seasons of a Man's Life/Seasons of a Woman's Life

Daniel Levinson's book, *The Seasons of a Man's Life* (1978) examined developmental changes of men through the lifespan. His research, which was the basis for Gail Sheehy's bestseller *Passages* (Sheehy, 1976/2006), examined men in a number of occupational groups. He subsequently wrote a book on the lifespan development of women that was finished posthumously by his wife, Judy Levinson (Levinson, 1996).

Levinson expected to find differences between men and women relative to the stages through which they pass in life. However, after intensive biographical interviews with men, and later with women, Levinson identified four comparable *eras* through which men and women pass, including *pre-adulthood, early adulthood, middle adulthood*, and *late adulthood*, but focused on the last three eras (Newton, 1994) (see Table 9.3). (With people living longer, he also hypothesized there might be a fifth era, which he called "late, late adulthood.") Eras are preceded by *transitional periods,* which are followed by *periods* that reflect unique issues or *life structures* that all individuals face in the areas of career, love relationships, marriage and family, relationships with self, uses of solitude, roles in social

TABLE 9.3   Developmental Periods of Levinson

ERA		AGE	DESCRIPTION OF PERIODS
Transition}		17–22	*Transition into Early Adulthood:* Emotional reaction of separating from family and adolescent friends into adult activities such as college, work, intimacy, etc.
	Early Adulthood	22–28	*Entering Adult World:* Considering and sometimes struggling with choices around vocational and occupational goals and commitment to partner.
		28–33	*Transition into the 30s:* Confirmation of choices made versus the need to make new choices relative to work and relationships.
		33–40	*Settling Down:* Settling into choices made and identify one's chief goals as one establishes oneself.
Transition}		40–45	*Transition to Midlife:* "Midlife crisis" and reconsideration of all that one has established. Examination and reassessment of all the choices one has made. Intense psychological turmoil, as people question where they have been and where they are going.
	Middle Adulthood	45–50	*Middle Adulthood:* Examination and reconsideration that occurred in transition to midlife period ends and choices are made that sometimes lead to new relationships, work, and play activities. Wide variation of sense of contentment, depending on the person.
		55–60	*Culmination of Middle Adulthood:* Settling in of new choices that were made during the last period, and sense of fulfillment for some who are settled in.
Transition}		60–65	*Late Adult Transition:* Reflecting on past and resolving issues from past stages when possible. Preparing for later life.
	Late Adulthood	65–80	*Late adulthood:* Reflecting on self, choices made, and whether life has been satisfying and fulfilling. Sense that one has to resolve unresolved issues.
		80+	*Late, late adulthood:* For some, continued psychological development and social changes to adapt to. For others, a sense of movement toward one's ultimate demise.

Adapted from Levinson, D. (1978). *The seasons of a man's life.* New York: Alfred A. Knopf, and Levinson, D. L. (1996). *Seasons of a woman's life.* New York: Alfred A. Knopf.

contexts, and relationships with individuals, groups, and institutions (see Table 9.3). Levinson believed that the eras are universal, cross-cultural, and predetermined by a complex interaction of social forces, biology, and psychological factors.

Although eras and periods were found to be the same for men and women, how they faced the issues and constructed their life structures within the periods varied dramatically. Noting the issue of *gender splitting*, Levinson found that traditional stereotypes were the centerpoint for the struggles of men and women. For instance, in the era of early adulthood, where the individual is dealing with settling into a relationship, career focus, and life goals, women were often struggling with their decision around motherhood and career. The career woman could often be found feeling guilty over her decision to not be a full-time mother, while the stay-at-home mom, having given up a career, often struggled with her sense of identity and with finding meaning and fulfillment in life. In contrast, men's struggles were focused on being a good husband, father, and provider for the family.

Levinson's theory is important because it identifies the ebbs and flows of the developmental process for men and women. Noting that there are periods of great stability and of great fluctuation within each era, he offers an understanding of the normal life tasks that will be faced by most men and women.

Comparison of Lifespan Development Theories

If this developmental sequence does hold to some degree for the species, its origins must be found in the interaction of all these influences as they operate during a particular phase. . . .

(Levinson, 1978, p. 322)

A number of similarities exist between the lifespan theories of Erikson and Levinson. For instance, both state that there are specific developmental stages through which all individuals must pass and that each individual will be dealing with specific developmental tasks within each stage. Both theories are sequential, but not hierarchical; that is, although stages follow one another in an orderly manner, and difficulty in one stage can affect later stages, no stage is considered better than another. Finally, Erikson and Levinson suggest that developmental tasks are a function of biological, psychological, and sociological factors and are probably universal across cultures.

Fowler's Theory of Faith Development

Drawing on the work of Erikson, Piaget, and Kohlberg, James Fowler developed a theory of faith development (Fowler, 1976, 1991, 1995, 2000). Fowler believes that faith is universal and inherent in our nature and relates to how we make meaning. Faith, as defined by Fowler, is much broader than a singular examination of one's religious orientation. It has to do with core values, the images of power that drive the person, and the stories that motivate the individual consciously and unconsciously throughout life (e.g., the stories of Jesus, Martin Luther King, Jr., and Muhammad; the unique stories that drive our families; and so forth):

. . . We shape commitments to causes and centers of value. We form allegiances and alliances with images and realities of power. And we form and shape our lives in relation to master stories. In these ways we join with others in the finding and making of meaning.

(Fowler, 1991, p. 22)

This broad definition of faith means that the atheist, agnostic, fundamentalist, and communist all have some faith experience, for faith does not depend on a belief in God (Fowler, 1991). In fact, it goes deeper than one's belief system because it includes unconscious motivations.

Based on his research, Fowler (1976, 1991, 2000) identified six stages of faith development, with minimum ages at which a person can enter a specific stage. Within this model, one can see pieces of each of the theories examined in this chapter. Thus, as you read through this theory, consider how all of the developmental models examined might explain different aspects of his theory. This can act as a mini-review for this chapter.

Stage 0, Primal Faith (Infancy): Based on Erikson's first psychosocial stage of trust versus mistrust, Fowler believes that infants have a predisposition toward a trusting relationship, which, if developed, will be the basis for the development of faith later in life. (This is not considered one of the actual stages, although it is important to eventual development.)

Stage 1, Intuitive–Projective Faith (Minimum age: 4 years): Based on Piaget's preoperational stage, children in this stage respond mostly to stories, feelings, and imagery. Their world

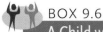

BOX 9.6

A Child with Intuitive–Projective Faith

A friend of mine had twin 5-year-old boys whom she placed in a fundamentalist Christian day-care center. She was of a different faith, but this center was the most convenient for her. One evening, about two weeks after the boys had started at that day-care center, I was having dinner at their house when one of the boys asked me, "Do you believe in God?" I began to respond by saying, "That's a difficult question," and before I could say any more, he yelled out, "You're going to hell!"

My friend's son, in just a few short weeks, had taken in a powerful new belief from a newfound social force in the environment—the day-care center. He projected his newfound belief onto me. If you would want to instill these values in your child, then leaving the child in this school would be important. My friend, however, did not want her malleable children to take on such values, so she removed them from this school.

---

is not logical; it is a symbolic mystery and can be greatly affected by adult views of faith. Symbols and stories are swallowed whole and can be used to expand a child's vision of the world; however, they can also be used to instill fear:

> *My friend told me that the devil will come up out of a hole in the ground and get me if I'm not careful, so now I won't play in the backyard by myself.*

(Fowler, 2000, p. 42)

In this stage, children are quite malleable and will mimic those around them. This stage offers opportunity for faith development, yet it can also restrict a person's ability to develop faith if he or she is placed in a fearful environment (see Box 9.6).

Stage 2, Mythic–Literal Faith (Age 6½–8 years): Having entered Piaget's concrete-operational stage, children in this stage are particularly susceptible to literal interpretations of faith. Symbols, stories, and beliefs from one's traditions are taken one-dimensionally and literally. They are what they are. Children are logical, believe in causation, and rely on the truth held by authorities, such as one's parents, teachers, or ministers. Therefore, others play a particularly powerful role in developing the child's meaning-making system. These ways of making sense out of the world are strikingly similar to what Perry calls "dualistic thinking."

Stage 3, Synthetic–Conventional Faith (12–13 years): As the child moves into adolescence, he or she enters Piaget's formal-operational stage and takes on an increasingly complex and abstract view of the world. The individual is now able to reflect on his or her interactions with others and consider what is important for the development of a value system. Ultimately, the individual in this stage synthesizes many viewpoints from his or her social sphere into a unique meaning-making system. However, because the individual remains embedded within his or her social sphere, this meaning-making system is still naive because it reflects only those values within that sphere. Your faith is therefore unique to your self, yet it is based on those close to you. This may be compared to Kegan's interpersonal stage of development, where the person is embedded in others for the definition of self.

Stage 4, Individuative–Reflective Faith (18–19 years): Like the individual in Kegan's institutional stage, the individual in this stage has the ability to take responsibility for his or her own faith development. This is epitomized by being able to let go of values that are based solely on one's immediate social sphere and being able to develop a new meaning-making system through reflection and introspection. This relativistic individual now recognizes different types of faith experiences and may forcefully move toward a new ideology (e.g., the college student who grew up Baptist and becomes a Buddhist). Certainly, the beginning ability to reflect on self and see different points of view is indicative of postoperational and postconventional thinking. In addition, remnants of Levinson's early adult transition stage can be seen as the individual is symbolically leaving his or her family.

Stage 5, Conjunctive Faith (30–32 years): This relativistic experience of faith happens when the individual is able to honor and affirm others who have different faith commitments while not denying his or her own faith. There is a newfound understanding of symbols and metaphors related to one's own faith tradition, as well as the faith traditions of others. There is openness to other points of view, a commitment to one's own point of view, and a sense of humility regarding all that is known (or not known). This stage has strong leanings toward what Perry called "commitment in relativism."

Stage 6, Universalizing Faith (38–40 years): Few individuals reach this stage of faith, which involves acceptance of others, regardless of stage or faith tradition. Fowler calls this *decentration from self,* or the ability to understand fully the views of others, to be able to see the world through their eyes, a true knowing of others. The individual in this stage experiences faith as universal, beyond particular ideological beliefs, and is therefore able to embrace all others. This individual is able to integrate beliefs from many disparate viewpoints and synthesize them into a faith experience that is unique to himself or herself. This stage shares many similarities with Kegan's interindividual stage, where the person may be described as "self-actualized." This person has compassion for and understands all points of view:

> From primal relationships in the immediate family we gradually widen our circle of awareness and regard to extended family and friends, to those who share our political or religious identifications, and finally beyond those to humankind or being, in an inclusive sense. . . . It means "knowing" the world through the eyes and experiences of persons, classes, nationalities, and faiths quite different from one's own.
>
> (Fowler, 2000, p. 55)

Fowler's model can be used to help counselors and supervisees better understand the nature of their client's faith experience (Parker, 2009; Ripley, Jackson, Tatum, & Davis, 2007). Thus, when counselors understand and advance their own faith development, they in turn will have a deeper comprehension of and appreciation for the values and spiritual orientation of others.

Other Developmental Theories

Many other developmental theories exist. For instance, Loevinger (1976) developed a theory of ego development that examined how individuals develop interpersonally, cognitively, and morally over the lifespan. In studying college students, Chickering developed a theory of college student development that elaborates on Erikson's stages of identity and intimacy (Chickering & Reisser, 1993) and assists counselors and others to understand college student development (see Chapter 18). Similarly, Vaillant (2003) and other researchers have examined adult development over the lifespan and offer stages similar to those of Erikson and Levinson. Other models include Belenky's developmental model of women's ways of understanding the world (Belenky, Clinchy, Goldberger, & Tarule, 1986/1997);

Stoltenberg & McNeil's supervision model (Stoltenberg & McNeil, 2010), which was discussed in Chapter 8; Super's model of career development (Super, Savickas, & Super, 1996), which will be examined in Chapter 11; and various models of cultural and ethnic identity which will be explored in Chapter 14. The theories mentioned in this chapter offer an introduction to some of the more popular developmental theories.

Applying Knowledge of Development

Counselors can assist people of all ages in making smooth psychological transitions as they develop (Santrock, 2013). For instance, a counselor who has knowledge of normative growth in children will be alerted to developmental lags, which can be caused by abuse, poverty, lack of parenting skills, genetics, biology, and other influences. In the areas of cognitive and moral development of children, knowledge of the developmental stages can give the counselor insight into the child's way of understanding the world and help identify stage-appropriate ways to work with children. Similarly, knowing the predictable psychological pitfalls of adolescence can help counselors develop appropriate counseling skills, groups, and workshops to help youth through this often difficult time, making appropriate referrals when necessary.

Adult cognitive development models can offer counselors great insight into understanding how their clients construct reality, thus helping them develop treatment plans that are appropriate to the client's developmental level (Hoare, 2006). Also, such models can be used by school counselors and college student development specialists when trying to help teachers understand their students. These models can then be used to develop new ways of teaching students that are developmentally appropriate. Finally, adult cognitive development models can be used by mental health professionals as a possible alternative to some of the pathological models of development.

Cognitive development models have direct application to counselor training. Research reveals a strong positive relationship between the level of adult cognitive development and the helper's ability to be empathic, nondirective, flexible, cognitively complex, nondogmatic, and problem solving (Basseches, 1984; Benack, 1984, 1988; Eriksen & McAuliffe, 2006; Granello, 2002; Jensen, 2011; Lovell, 1999; Neukrug & McAuliffe, 1993). By assessing their developmental levels, graduate students can examine potential weaknesses and strengths that they may bring with them to the counseling relationship. In addition, counselor educators can adapt their training practices to the developmental level of the student (McAuliffe & Eriksen, 2010).

Through knowledge of lifespan models and the stage-specific developmental issues that clients face, counselors can better comprehend the problems of clients and be less likely to pathologize normal developmental crises. When an issue of adjustment is found to be directly related to a current developmental crisis or unresolved issues from past developmental stages, counselors can devise appropriate strategies to help the client resolve the crisis.

Finally, knowledge of faith development can help counselors understand the values, images, and stories of our clients and help us fully appreciate their uniqueness. The felon and the model citizen, the child and the older person, individuals from diverse cultures and those from mainstream culture—all have been driven by values, images, and stories. Know these, and you know your client. Know your client, and you are much more likely to develop effective treatment strategies.

Comparison of Developmental Models

The varying models of development explored in this chapter offer differing dimensions to the understanding of the person. Some of these models looked at cognitive functioning, others at lifespan development, and still others at moral reasoning and the development of faith. With some of the models, individuals will pass through all the stages; in others, they may never reach the higher stages. Although all the models are sequential (stages build upon stages), only some of the models are hierarchical, which implies that each stage is considered better than the previous stage. Figure 9.2 offers a visual comparison of the varying models looked at in this chapter.

FIGURE 9.2
A Comparison of Developmental Models

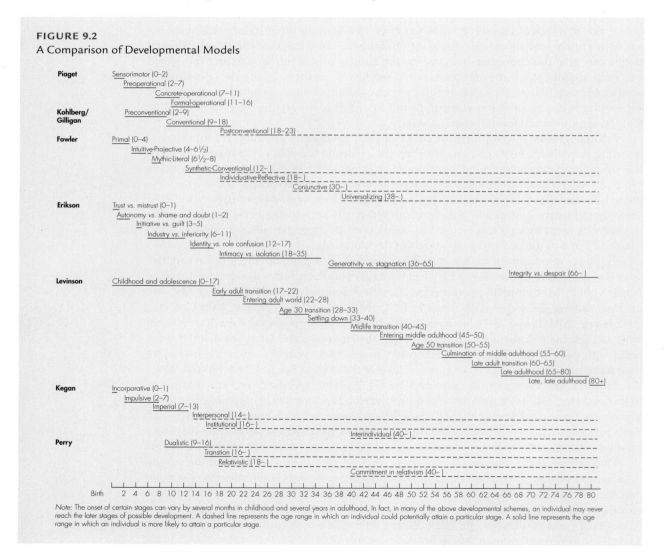

Note: The onset of certain stages can vary by several months in childhood and several years in adulthood, In fact, in many of the above developmental schemes, an individual may never reach the later stages of possible development. A dashed line represents the age range in which an individual could potentially attain a particular stage. A solid line represents the age range in which an individual is more likely to attain a particular stage.

Multicultural/Social Justice Focus

Bias in Developmental Models

Most of the models that you have read about in this chapter were developed by White males, and perhaps even more alarming, most of their research was based on White males who grew up in the mid- to late-1900s. Models that are based on the thinking of White males a good number of years ago does not make them wrong. However, one must pause and consider what the models might look like if they had taken into account differences based on social class, ethnicity, culture, and gender. And might they change if we were to look at them today, as mores and values have changed? There is little doubt that we can gain something from the models in this chapter. But do they apply in the same way to all? As much as they might help us understand one client, perhaps they can hinder our understanding of another client who does not neatly fit into the demographic around which the models were created.

The Development of Cultural Identity

Like many characteristics, how we identify with our cultural or ethnic group can be explained as a developmental process. Thus, we can examine how we have grown and changed as men, as women, as gays, lesbians, or heterosexuals, as Blacks, Whites, or Asians, and so forth (Ponterotto, Casas, Suzuki, & Alexander, 2010). Cultural identity models assume that there is a predictable progression through stages of development of cultural/ethnic consciousness. Chapter 14 will explore some of these models in detail.

In recent years, scholarship has increasingly examined the relationship between cultural identity, cross-cultural training, and perceived and actual counselor competence (Alvarez, & Piper, 2005; Chao & Nath, 2011; Farrell, 2009). And, as you might guess, it has been hypothesized that those who have a better sense of their own cultural identity are better equipped to work with clients who are from different cultures. Thus, it is imperative that as students of counseling, you assess your cultural/ethnic identity. Counseling programs can assist students in examining themselves; but, ultimately, if we are to move toward an identity that embraces and effectively works with all cultures, each of us must be willing to explore our own cultural/ethnic identities.

Ethical, Professional, and Legal Issues

The ACA Code of Ethics: A Developmental Emphasis

The counseling profession today prides itself on having a positive, growth-oriented, and developmental focus. This emphasis is reflected in the preamble of the ACA (2014a) code of ethics, which states, "Counseling is a professional relationship that empowers diverse individuals, families, and groups to accomplish mental health, wellness, education, and career goals," and when it notes that one of its professional values is "enhancing human development throughout the life span."

As counselors, we undoubtedly will come across and work with some clients whom we might consider to be abnormal, mentally ill, or, at the very least, a little out of the mainstream. We may even diagnose and label them, but we must always have respect for our clients' dignity and honor each person's unique developmental journey (Zalaquett, Fuerth, Stein, Ivey, & Ivey, 2008; Zalaquett & Ivey, 2015). Through our caring, our knowledge of development, and our effective use of skills, we can help lift some of the burdens clients feel and assist them in their journey through life.

Professional Associations

One division of ACA particularly focuses on human development and the theories associated with it: the Association for Adult Development and Aging (AADA), which publishes the journal *Adultspan*. However, in general, ACA views development as foundational, and you might want to explore how other divisions tackle this important area also.

Legal Issue: Missing Problems Because We Are Too Positive

Psychiatrists and some clinical psychologists often get a reputation for being too oriented toward psychopathology. They tend to diagnose and label, and this tunnel vision can sometimes prevent client growth. Counselors sometimes have the opposite problem. By seeing only the positive side of human nature, they may sometimes miss serious pathology, suicidal or homicidal thoughts, and deeply troubling feelings. A counselor who misses a serious problem can damage the counseling process and may even have some responsibility for a client's suicide or homicide. Clearly, this is tragic for all involved and can lead to malpractice suits.

Counselors must not be afraid of seeing the dark side of people. One can help a person look at his or her shadow and yet still have an optimistic view of himself or herself. In fact, some would say that only through looking at one's darkest side can healing and growth occur.

The Counselor in Process: Understanding Your Own Development

Recently, a friend of mine was telling me about a theory of development that, unlike Levinson, suggests that we are always in transition, and we never have periods of rest. Hmm, I thought to myself, that certainly feels like my life—it's kind of a roller coaster that sometimes moves fast and smoothly, while other times, it feels like its chugging along an uphill climb. Maybe there are short periods of rest, but they sure do seem to last only a moment or two. I guess I can either go along for the ride or get off. I think I'll keep moving. But maybe while on this roller coaster of life, I can do my best to make sure that the ride is as smooth as possible—oil the wheels, make sure that I'm in the seat snugly, and get to know the person sitting next to me.

Our lives can be unexplored and bumpy, or, as we move along our unique paths, we can check ourselves out, look at the path ahead of us, and make sure that things are as even as possible. This, I believe, means exploring our own development. It means examining the physical, social, and psychological forces that have impinged upon us and continue to affect us. It means looking at the developmental crises in our past that may still be impinging upon us, exploring the developmental phases we are currently experiencing, and thinking about where our future development might take us.

Knowledge of our own development increases our self-knowledge and helps us understand the ways in which we interact with others. But perhaps most important, understanding our own development helps us understand the relationships that we form with our clients.

Summary

This chapter looked at development: child development, adult development, cognitive development, moral development, lifespan development, and the development of faith. We started by noting that development is continual, orderly, and sequential; builds upon itself; and is painful yet growth producing, transtheoretical, preventive, optimistic, and wellness oriented. A developmental framework allows us to understand the common characteristics of people at different ages and stages, the typical problems experienced by people as they pass through the lifespan, the causes of some problems, and therapeutic strategies for change.

The chapter began by presenting an overview of development through the lifespan and particularly focused on some of the physical and associated psychosocial changes that occur in childhood, adolescence, and adulthood. It was noted that development occurs at fairly predictable rates, and a counselor or developmental specialist who is aware of physiological and psychological timetables can assess whether a person is on target in his or her development.

The chapter examined a number of developmental models. We started by looking at cognitive and moral development, and then noted that Piaget examined how cognitive development unravels and identified a number of stages that he called sensorimotor, preoperational, concrete-operational, and formal-operational. He found that as children move through these stages, there is an orderly progression that begins with the child's ability to maintain mental images and language skills, leads to the child's ability to think in a logical and orderly manner, and culminates in adolescence with the child's ability to think abstractly and in complex ways.

Next, the text examined Kohlberg's theory of moral development, in which he identifies three levels of development called preconventional, conventional, and postconventional thinking. These stages reflect Kohlberg's belief that moral reasoning goes through a series of stages that move from extreme narcissism toward concern for democratic principles and personal conscience. We also mentioned Gilligan's argument that unlike men's moral development, which tends to be individualistically oriented, women's development includes a standard of care whereby women are concerned with how their choices affect others. Gilligan also found that adolescent girls will often lose their voice, but as grown women find it again.

Looking at adult cognitive development, the chapter examined two theories: Kegan's theory of constructive development and Perry's theory of epistemological reflection. Both Kegan and Perry believe that humans continually construct reality and that this occurs in stages, with many individuals never having the opportunity to reach the higher stages of development. Although Kegan's stages span the life cycle, his theory is mostly applied to adult development. His stages are called incorporative, impulsive, imperial, interpersonal, institutional, and interindividual. Kegan believes that in adulthood, individuals move from a narcissistic position to a position of mutuality, to a place where the individual develops a strong sense of self, and then to the final position, where the person is a complex thinker who can perceive situations from many perspectives, have a strong sense of self, and be able to hear feedback. Perry's theory, which focuses mostly on college students, mapped the potential changes of young adults as they move from being dualistic, black-and-white thinkers to becoming relativistic people who can see differing perspectives. The highest stage for Perry is being committed in relativism, epitomized by the person who can see varying perspectives yet has a strong commitment to specific values.

Lifespan development was another frame from which the chapter examined the development of the person. Reviewing the theories of Erikson and Levinson, we noted that both offer age-specific stages through which all people must pass. Erikson's stages include trust versus mistrust, autonomy versus shame and doubt, initiative versus guilt, industry versus inferiority, identity versus role confusion, intimacy versus isolation, generativity versus stagnation, and integrity versus despair. Erikson suggested that through all these stages, individuals are faced with a task (sometimes called a crisis), and that each task can be syntonic (positive emotionally) or dystonic (negative emotionally). Balance between the two is critical. Levinson's theory identified four eras in the lives of men and women that include childhood and adolescence, early adulthood, middle adulthood, and late adulthood. He also proposed a probable late late adulthood era. Levinson believed that each era is marked by transition and periods of stability and has its own unique tasks to master. Although men and women pass through the same eras and periods, the tasks they address within each of them will vary dramatically as a function of gender issues.

The final theory examined in this text was Fowler's model of faith development. Defining faith as a person's core values, the images of power that drive that person, and the stories that motivate the individual consciously and unconsciously, we stressed that Fowler's model is much broader than a religious focus on faith. Presenting six stages of faith development, Fowler suggests that the development of faith parallels many other developmental theories and moves from a rigid adherence to a point of view, toward a relativistic understanding of varying points of view, to an acceptance of and love for many different perspectives while simultaneously having one's own faith experience.

As the chapter zeroed in on multicultural and social justice issues, we noted that most of the theories were developed by White males in the 1900s and their research samples tended to be White males. Thus, one must consider the efficacy of these theories with this in mind. In addition, like many characteristics examined here, we noted that our identity with our cultural or ethnic group can be explained as a developmental process. We stressed the fact that if we are to work effectively with all clients, we must risk looking inward and gain an understanding of our own cultural/ethnic identity.

As the chapter neared its conclusion, we highlighted the notion that the foundation of our profession is development. We pointed out that ACA has stressed the importance of having a developmental lens, and we particularly noted one division of ACA dedicated to this focus, AADA. This developmental focus stresses the dignity and growth of the client while discouraging labeling and diagnosing. While on the one hand this is a strength, on the other hand, this positive, future-oriented focus may make some counselors become too lax at times and miss a serious client problem. This could have devastating effects and lead to ethical complaints and lawsuits against the counselor.

Finally, we stressed that knowledge of our own development can greatly assist us in understanding ourselves, the ways in which we interact with others, and the ways in which we form relationships with our clients.

Further Practice

Visit CengageBrain.com to respond to additional material that highlight the salient aspects of the chapter content. There, you can find ethical, professional, and legal vignettes, a number of experiential exercises, and study tools including a glossary, flashcards, and sample test items. Hopefully, these will enhance your learning and be fun and interesting.

CHAPTER 10

Abnormal Development, Diagnosis, and Psychopharmacology

Not too long after obtaining my master's degree, I was as an outpatient therapist at a community mental health center. Suddenly, I was working closely with clinical psychologists and psychiatrists. I had a caseload that included a number of clients with serious emotional disorders, and every time I conducted an intake interview, I was required to follow up with a consultation with the psychiatrist. Invariably, the psychiatrist wanted me to talk diagnosis and clinical terms that I had never considered or learned about in school or in past jobs. I had to catch up quickly. However, part of me didn't want to do that because I really didn't believe in making a diagnosis. I had to use this book called the *Diagnostic and Statistical Manual-II* (DSM-II) that had descriptions of the various emotional disorders. It soon became my bible.

I learned rather quickly about making diagnoses, and I didn't find it half bad. It helped me categorize clients, which seemed to help organize my thinking about them. It made me understand which medications might be appropriate for specific disorders. And it sometimes gave me guidance in treatment planning. However, I was still doubtful. A part of me thought, "Is this real, or are we making up these categories? And maybe diagnosing these people increases the likelihood that they'll remain ill, like a self-fulfilling prophecy. We see them that way, we label them that way, and they become that way." Most of all, it bothered me when some of the other clinicians would smugly say things like, "Oh, he's borderline, he can't act any other way."

It's quite a few years later now, and I hope I've become a little more sophisticated about psychopathology and diagnosis. However, whenever I listen to someone diagnosing a client, there's still a part of me that asks, "Is this real?" This response, I believe, is a healthy part of me and is reflective of the history of our profession—a profession that has, in the past, balked at the use of diagnosis and the concept of "abnormal behavior" or psychopathology. On the other hand, maybe there is something to categorizing behavior and using diagnosis. I would hope that I could understand psychopathology, reap the possible benefits of using diagnosis, and continue to have a healthy, questioning attitude.

In this chapter, I will explore abnormal development, diagnosis, and psychopharmacology. I will start by examining reasons that each of them may be important and take a look at the close relationships among them. I will then describe the development of abnormal behavior (interchangeably called *psychopathology* in this chapter) from genetic and biological, psychodynamic, learning theory, humanistic and postmodern perspectives. This discussion will be followed by an overview of the *Diagnostic and Statistical Manual-5*

(DSM-5), the current diagnostic system used in the United States and throughout much of the world. In addition, the chapter will offer a brief overview of many of the psychotropic medications currently used in the treatment of various disorders. As usual, the text will offer some perspectives from a multicultural/social justice focus, discuss some relevant points related to ethical, professional, and legal issues, and conclude with a comment about the "counselor in process."

Why Study Abnormal Development, Diagnosis, and Medication?

John is in fifth grade and has been assessed as having a conduct disorder and attention deficit hyperactivity disorder (ADHD). John's mother has a panic disorder and is taking antianxiety medication, and his father is bipolar and taking lithium. Jill is John's school counselor. It is written into John's individualized educational plan (IEP) that he should see Jill for individual counseling and group counseling. Jill must also periodically consult with John's mother and father.

Tenesha is a sophomore in college. She has just broken up with her boyfriend, is severely depressed, and cannot concentrate on her schoolwork; her grades have dropped from A's to C's. She comes to the counseling center and sobs during most of her first session with her counselor. She admits having always struggled with depression but states that, "This is worse than ever; I need to get better if I am going to stay in school. Can you give me any medication to help me so I won't have to drop out?"

Eduard goes daily to the day treatment center at the local mental health center. He seems fairly coherent and generally in good spirits. He has been hospitalized for schizophrenia on numerous occasions and now takes Abilify to relieve his symptoms. He admits to Jordana, one of his counselors, that when he doesn't take his medication, he believes that computers have consciousness and are conspiring through the Internet to take over the world. His insurance company pays for his treatment. He will not receive reimbursement from his insurance company unless Jordana specifies a diagnosis on the insurance form.

With evidence that over one-fourth of Americans have a diagnosable mental disorder within any year (Bagalman & Napili, 2014), regardless of where you are employed, you will be working with clients who (1) have serious emotional problems that are sometimes labeled as abnormal behavior or as an emotional disorder; (2) have been given or are in need of a diagnosis for treatment purposes, for legal reasons, or both; and (3) are taking or in need of medication. Although controversy exists about defining abnormality, developing a diagnosis, and using psychotropic medications (Frances, 2013; Kapur, Phillips, & Insel, 2012; Madesen & Leech, 2007; Shorter, 2013), all counselors today deal with these issues. This has not always been the case.

Counselor educators and counselors have historically had a disdain for diagnosing and labeling and have at times opposed the use of psychotropic medication (Eriksen & Kress, 2005, 2006, 2008; Hansen, 2003). In fact, within counseling programs, learning about psychopathology (the development of mental disorders) was practically unheard of until recently. There were many reasons for this. First, the early history of the counseling profession was largely influenced by the humanistic approaches to counseling, which downplayed the notion of abnormal development, the role of diagnosis, and the use of medication. This influence also led to counseling professionals believing that training in psychopathology and diagnosis would lead counselors to stigmatize individuals unduly. In addition, many counselors and counselor educators believed that counselors should be working with "normal" individuals and in a preventive and wellness role. They felt that the role of the counselor should be to focus on normal developmental issues and the positive side of human nature, not on psychopathology. Recently, however, many counseling programs have included in their curriculum a focus on psychopathology, diagnosis, and psychopharmacology (CACREP, 2009). There are many reasons for this change:

➤ Counselors in all specialty areas are increasingly working with clients who are severely disturbed.
➤ In contrast to past years, when most graduates from counseling programs obtained jobs in schools where they less frequently encountered individuals with serious emotional disorders, a large portion of graduates now work in community agencies, often with individuals with mental illness.
➤ Federal and state laws (e.g., PL94-142, IDEA) now require that students with severe emotional disorders be serviced in the schools. Thus, today's school counselor is more likely to be dealing with students with severe emotional problems.
➤ Many licensing boards require knowledge of diagnosis and psychopathology for counselors to obtain a license.
➤ Today, many counselors need to know diagnostic procedures if they are to receive reimbursement from insurance companies.
➤ Society has become more tolerant of individuals with emotional problems and mental disorders, and there is less stigmatizing of individuals with diagnoses.
➤ A diagnostic system offers clinicians a common language with which to discuss client issues.
➤ There has been a retreat by some from the rigid adherence to a philosophy that all mental illness is a social construction.
➤ Diagnosis can sometimes be helpful in the development of treatment plans, and treatment plans sometimes may include the use of medication.
➤ There is a growing body of evidence that our biology contributes to, and in some cases may even determine, some forms of mental illness.
➤ Some people get better with medication, and we now understand that we had best not throw out the baby with the bathwater (the concepts of abnormal behavior and diagnosis are inextricably tied to the use of medications).

You Can't Have One Without the Other: Abnormal Behavior, Diagnosis, and Medication

What comes to your mind when you ponder the word "abnormal"? Most people probably think of something unnatural or out of the norm, as the word itself suggests. When applied to a clinical situation, abnormality entails an infrequent and unusual emotional, cognitive, or behavioral response:

> *Patterns of emotion, thought, and action deemed pathological for one or more of the following reasons: infrequent occurrence, violation of norms, personal distress, disability or dysfunction, and unexpectedness.*

(Kring, Davison, Neale, & Johnson, 2007, Glossary, p. 1)

No doubt, at moments in our lives we have all seen or experienced what might be considered abnormal behaviors, thoughts, or feelings. If one experiences these on an ongoing basis, then they become the norm for the individual, but are deviations from what is considered usual or normal in society. As a species, when we observe deviations from the norm, we tend to want to understand them and classify them. This is what diagnosis does. It is a classification of thoughts, feelings, or behaviors that deviate from the norm. Classification systems, such as those found in the *Diagnostic and Statistical Manual* published by the American Psychiatric Association (APA, 2013a). Offer clinicians a mechanism for understanding how some individuals deviate from more typical behavior. In addition, if you can classify individuals into different categories, you can research which treatment strategies, including the use of medications, will best apply to each diagnostic category. For instance, research has shown that psychoanalytic therapy is probably not the best type of therapy for a person who has an obsessive–compulsive disorder, whereas this used to be the treatment of choice.

Today, there is less controversy about the concept of abnormality, with most clinicians believing that the development of mental disorders is the result of a complex interaction of genetic, biological, sociological, and psychological factors. We may and probably should argue about the term *abnormal*, but no matter what you call it, there are individuals who exhibit some types of behavior that deviate from the norm. We may and probably should argue that diagnosis is stigmatizing, but there are individuals who are helped because of adequate diagnoses and subsequent treatment plans. And we probably should argue about the overuse of medication, but it is now clear that some people are helped, and even miraculously changed, by taking medication.

Personality Development and Abnormal Behavior

A number of models of personality development offer us an understanding of "abnormal behavior," sometimes simply referred to as *the development of mental disorders (psychopathology).* This section will examine five such models, including the genetic and biological model, which assumes that there are inherited factors that, when expressed, will show certain personality traits; the psychoanalytic model, which proposes a relationship between psychosexual stages of development and abnormal behavior; the learning perspective, which views abnormal behavior as the result of learned dysfunctional behaviors and faulty cognitions; the humanistic approach, which stresses the importance of the relationship with significant others in the development of personality variables; and the postmodern and social constructionist approach, which views reality as a function of language used in a person's social milieu and questions the whole assumption of abnormality.

Genetic and Biological Explanations of Development

It is not about nature versus nurture, as that old cliché would have it. It is about nature-on-nurture-on-nature-on-nurture, round and round and round.

(Baker, 2004, p. 28)

Genetics, which is the science of hereditary characteristics, is a subset of *biology*, which is the science of life. Biology, therefore, includes genetic factors, but genetics does not include all biological factors. For instance, if we say that biological factors can affect the development of intelligence in children, we are referring to such things as prenatal care, nutrition, exposure to toxins, hormonal changes, genetics, and so forth. However, when we assert that genetics can affect the development of intelligence in children, we are referring to how the expression of genes, not other factors, can affect cognitive ability.

The *nature-versus-nurture* debate as it relates to personality formation has a long and turbulent history and continues today. However, the schisms among genetic determinists, environmental advocates, and intrapsychic zealots are clearly much less than ever before. This is partially because the concept of *heritability* has changed, with genes no longer being seen as deterministically causing behavior. Today's views of genetics assume that in most cases, there are *complex environmental influences* on the action of genes (Duncan, 2005; Griffiths & Stotz, 2013). For instance, after an extensive review of the literature, Clark and Watson (2008) note that genetics and the individual's unique experiences both play an essential role in the expression of personality traits. They go on to remark that "it is largely through gene–environment interactions that each individual's unique personality develops" (p. 277).

The linking of biology, including genetics, with environmental factors in the development of personality moves the counseling profession toward an approach that is truly holistic. Understanding the intricate interaction among these variables can be very powerful in the effective use of counseling. Clinicians in today's world should no longer be shy about consulting experts familiar with genetics and biology, as these efforts can help provide the most broadly based treatment for their clients.

Which emotional disorders are most likely to be biologically based? Conduct a literature review, and you'll find research that suggests that most mental disorders have some genetic basis. However, the actual expression of those disorders is complex, and for any individual a disorder only gets expressed if a number of genes are turned on by environmental influences at specific times (Clark & Watson, 2008; Griffiths & Stotz, 2013). Thus, the old idea that one gene determines a specific mental disorder is no longer believed to be true:

> *The vast majority of mental disorders are believed to be polygenic: health problems occur when disease-related alleles are inherited for many different genes. Most mental disorders also are multifactorial, which means that multiple environmental and genetic factors are operating in an intricate, epigenetic fashion to upset the stable development and functioning of cells.*

(Baker, 2004, p. 63)

Finally, it would seem to make intuitive sense that if a disorder has a genetic or biological basis, one might consider using biological interventions in addition to psychotherapy. Biological interventions can be defined broadly to include such things as stress reduction, exercise, how we eat, how we sleep, the amount of light we receive, psychopharmacology, and so forth. All of these factors, in some manner, affect one or more major biological systems and can affect our mood positively or negatively. Although the use of medication to alleviate symptoms has shown efficacy across a wide range of mental disorders (Leucht, Hierl, Kissling, Dold, & Davis, 2012), some still consider their use controversial, noting that most medications have side effects, some potentially devastating ones, and the relative effectiveness of some medications are still questioned (Murray, 2006; Whitaker, 2010).

Freud's Model of Psychosexual Development

As we remember from Chapter 4, Freud believed that we are born with sexual and aggressive instincts that unconsciously affect our behaviors throughout life (Bishop, 2015). He identified a *structure of personality* that includes the *id*, the depository of all of our instincts; the *ego*, the development of the rational part of our mind; and the *superego*, which constitutes the moral part of our mind. Freud believed that infantile sexuality is an expression of instinctual body urges associated with different pleasurable bodily functions. Based on these *erogenous zones*, Freud identified stages of development through which each individual will pass. How the erogenous zones are satisfied is related to ego and superego development and the mental health of the individual (Neukrug, 2011).

Born all id, the infant is immediately thrust into the first stage of psychosexual development, the *oral stage*, in which pleasure is received through feeding. The hungry infant wants to be fed, and his or her main goals are to obtain pleasure through feeding and to reduce stress caused by hunger and lack of tactile stimulation received through the mouth. The major developmental task of this stage, which occurs between birth and 1½, is how the child becomes attached to the mother (or the major caretaker) as a function of feeding. Poor parenting at this early stage can lead to mistrust of others, difficulty in forming close relationships, dependency needs, aggression, greediness, acquisitiveness, and sarcasm (Corey, 2013; Neukrug, 2011). From this perspective, one can see how abusive or neglectful parenting can lead to pathological behavior.

During the *anal stage*, the child receives pleasure from bowel movements, and the child's instinctual urges become focused on the anal erogenous zone. This stage, which occurs between ages 1½ and 3, is distinguished by a child's physiological readiness to be toilet trained. The main function of this stage is for the child to develop his or her capacity to retain or evacuate, which becomes a metaphor for the child's ability to master his or her impulses. The parents' attempts at introducing the idea that there are socially appropriate behaviors (the prototype being using the potty) are significant in the development of the child's ego and superego. However, defecating is pleasurable, and the child resists learning how to control this pleasurable experience. Consequently, the child becomes embroiled in a battle of control, independence, power, and doing the socially correct thing (Hall, 1954/1999). Ultimately, the child has to learn how to control his or her feelings of aggression, housed in the id, and does so by the development of the ego, which learns to deal rationally with the world, and through the use of *defense mechanisms* (see Chapter 4), which are now being spawned in an effort to have the child restrain his or her impulses and channel them into acceptable behaviors.

Parental attitudes about defecation, cleanliness, control, and responsibility have a major effect on personality development. For instance, strict parents may have children who retaliate and aggress against them and grow into adults who have little respect for authority, and are irresponsible, messy, disorderly, extreme, and controlling of others. On the other hand, some children with punitive and strict parents may assume their parents were right and become adults who are extremely neat, fastidious, compulsive about orderliness, disgusted by and fearful of dirt, and generally exhibit overcontrolled behavior (Hall, 1954/1999). You might say that these individuals are constipated in their relationship to the world.

In contrast, parents who extensively praise children for their ability to go to the potty can lead them to have an exaggerated sense of self. As adults, these individuals may make things to please others or may be generous, philanthropic, charitable—and maybe even gravitate toward the helping professions. On the other hand, too much emphasis on toilet training may leave the child feeling he or she has lost something when defecating, ultimately leading toward a sense of depression and anxiety of future losses. These individuals become *fixated* upon the erotic pleasure of defecating and may become adults who have a strong desire to collect and possess things (e.g., hoarders), or, in a defensive posture, these individuals may respond in the opposite way by becoming reckless, gambling, and giving away possessions.

In the third stage of development, the *phallic stage*, which occurs from ages 3 to 5, the erogenous zone again shifts, this time to the child's genitals. Here, the child becomes aware of pleasurable feelings associated with touching his or her genitals and receives pleasure from self-stimulation. The types of permission that parents give the child in this stage can greatly affect the child's attitudes and values and are crucial in the development of the individual's superego.

During this stage, an *Oedipus* or an *Electra complex* is awakened as instinctual urges emerge related to the child's wish to possess the opposite-sex parent and eliminate the same-sex parent. However, the child soon realizes that this is not achievable, and the subsequent guilt as a result of the child's attempts to possess the opposite-sex parent is resolved by the child developing a sense that everything in life is not attainable, identification with the same-sex parent, and an understanding that we must live responsibly in the world. Thus, this stage is crucial for the development of the nature of attachments to significant men and women in one's life, the identification with masculinity or femininity, and the development of the superego. The values learned in this stage are stored in the superego, which is reflected in who we are as parents and shapes the morality of our social system. Imagine the kinds of behaviors an adult might exhibit if his or her parents were extremely permissive or strict during this stage!

The *latency stage* (ages 5 through puberty) is a period of relative relaxation for the child, where he or she replaces earlier sexual feelings with a focus on socialization. Here, the child becomes more aware of peers and there is increased attention placed on peer-related activities. Freud's final stage of development, the *genital stage*, begins at puberty and continues through the lifespan. Sexual energy, in this stage, is focused on social activities with peers and on love relationships. During this stage, we discover whether earlier stages of development were resolved adequately, as the adult's behavior will reflect unresolved issues from the earlier stages. These issues will often be cloaked by defense mechanisms but can generally be deduced through analysis.

As reflected in the above discussion, parenting behaviors through the developmental stages affect the formation of the ego and superego and establish the precarious balance among the id, ego, and superego:

> *Thus the ego—driven along by the id, held back by the superego, repulsed by reality—struggles to master its economic task of creating harmony among the forces and influences acting within it and upon it: and we understand why we are so often unable to stop ourselves from crying out: "Life is so difficult!"*

> (Freud, 1940/2003, pp. 71–72)

Ultimately, how the id, ego, and superego impinge on our lives, unconsciously and to a lesser degree consciously, determine the individual's level of health or dysfunction. Our defense mechanisms, created to ward off anxiety resulting from tension among the id, ego, and superego, give us a peek into our early development and the kinds of parenting that we received.

Conclusion

Freud was quite specific in his description of disorders and their roots, with the oral, anal, and phallic psychosexual stages holding the potential for the later development of dysfunctional behavior. However, some of these assertions have not held up under research. Despite this fact, the basic core of his theory remains tenable. For instance, the concept that development occurs as we pass through a series of erogenous zones and that early parenting can affect personality formation is considered, at the very least, to be an important factor in understanding emotional disorders. Also, the role of unconscious impulses has remained an important concept for most therapists in their understanding of behavior. Finally, the idea that we can explore our early development and examine how it has affected our personality style is important in many counseling approaches. Whether or not one agrees with most of what Freud conceptualized, it is clear that the lens through which counselors and others view the developing person has been greatly affected by the psychoanalytic view of development.

Learning Theory and the Development of the Person

> *The child is born empty of psychological content into a world of coherently organized content. Like a mirror, however, the child comes to reflect his environment; like an empty slate he is written upon by external stimuli; like a wax table he stores the impressions left by these stimuli; and like a machine he may be made to react in response to stimulating agents.*

> (Langer, 1969, p. 51)

This radical quote, reflecting early behavioral thought, shows the rigid views that many learning theorists held about the development of the person. Drastically differing from

Freud's notion on instincts, B. F. Skinner and other early learning theorists believed that "the most important causes of behavior are environmental and [that] it only confuses the matter to talk about inner drives" (Nye, 2000, p. 80). However, the vast majority of learning theorists today have a much broader view of development, with many now believing that genetic factors, cognitive structures, and even intrapsychic forces play a role in personality development (Neukrug, 2011). However, the basic core of this nonstage theory is still learning theory.

As we learned in Chapter 4, learning theorists believe that individuals learn behaviors through *operant conditioning*, *classical conditioning*, or *modeling* (*social learning*) and therefore place emphasis on how *positive or negative reinforcement*, *models*, and the pairing of an *unconditioned stimulus* with a *conditioned stimulus* affect our personality development (Bandura, Ross, & Ross; 1963; Jozefowiez & Staddon, 2015; Maia & Jozefowiez, 2015; Skinner, 1971; Wolpe, 1969). Operant conditioning is generally considered to be the most common type of conditioning and occurs when behavior is reinforced, thus increasing the probability of that response occurring again, or punished. Over the years, through rigorous research, Skinner and others delineated many principles of operant conditioning, each of which is crucial to the shaping of behaviors and the development of personality. A small portion of these include:

➤ *Positive reinforcement:* Any stimulus that, when presented following a response, increases the likelihood of that response.
➤ *Negative reinforcement:* Any stimulus that, when removed following a response, increases the likelihood of that response.
➤ *Punishment:* Applying an aversive stimulus to decrease a specific behavior. Punishment is often an ineffective method of changing behavior, as it may lead to undesirable side effects (e.g., counteraggression).
➤ *Schedules of reinforcement:* The numerous ways in which a stimulus can be arranged to reinforce behavior; based on elapsed time and frequency of responses.
➤ *Discrimination:* The ability of a person to respond selectively to one stimulus but not respond to a similar stimulus.
➤ *Generalization:* The tendency for stimuli that are similar to a conditioned stimulus to take on the power of the conditioned stimulus.
➤ *Extinction:* The ceasing of a behavior because it is not reinforced.
➤ *Spontaneous recovery:* The tendency for responses to recur after a brief period of time after they have been extinguished.

Skinner and other learning theorists maintain that reinforcements often occur very subtly and in ways that we may not immediately recognize (Nye, 2000; Skinner, 1971; Wolpe, 1969). Therefore, things like changes in voice intonation, subtle glances, TV shows that appeal to us, or body language could subliminally affect our personality development. They note that by examining a situation closely enough, one could attain an understanding of the types of reinforcement contingencies that were instrumental in shaping an individual's behavior.

Over the years, many learning theorists have included a cognitive framework within their conceptualization of development. Such cognitive therapists as Albert Ellis (Ellis & Harper, 1997), Michael Meichenbaum (1977), and Aaron Beck (J. Beck, 1995; 2005) believe that not only do behaviors of individuals become reinforced, but so do the ways in which people think. Therefore, thinking can dramatically affect behavior, and behavior can dramatically affect thinking in a complex interaction. Cognitive-behaviorists have challenged the beliefs of the original behavioral purists and have changed the manner in which most learning theorists conceptualize the development of the individual.

Because abnormal development is seen as a result of *reinforcement contingencies*, learning theorists believe that change can occur at any point in the life cycle. Therefore, one can identify dysfunctional behaviors and irrational thinking, determine which reinforcers continue dysfunctional ways of living in the world, and devise methods of reinforcing new behaviors and different cognitions.

Summarizing some of the major factors that can lead to healthy or abnormal development, modern-day learning theorists believe the following:

➤ The individual is born capable of developing a multitude of personality characteristics.

➤ Behaviors and cognitions are continually reinforced by significant others and by cultural influences in our environment.

➤ Reinforcement of behaviors and cognitions is generally very complex and can occur in very subtle ways.

➤ Abnormal development is largely the result of the kinds of behaviors and cognitions that have been reinforced (other factors such as genetics may also affect development). By carefully analyzing how behaviors and cognitions are reinforced, one can understand why an individual exhibits his or her current behavioral and cognitive repertoire.

➤ Through the application of principles of learning, old dysfunctional behaviors can be extinguished and new healthy behaviors can be learned.

Conclusion

Learning theory offers a unique, objective, straightforward method of understanding personality development. Maladaptive behavior is believed to be the result of dysfunctional behaviors and faulty cognitions that are conditioned, sometimes in very subtle ways. Because maladaptive behavior is believed to be at least partly learned, it can be unlearned and new functional behaviors can be adopted. Thus, modern-day learning theorists generally have an optimistic view of the person in that they believe people can change their way of living in the world. Today's behaviorists, therefore, have an anti-deterministic view of human nature, in that they believe people can use reinforcement contingencies and biological interventions (e.g., medication) to become better human beings.

The Humanistic Understanding of Personality Development

The humanistic approaches that have probably had the most impact on our understanding of the development of the individual have been the *person-centered approach* of Carl Rogers (1951) and Abraham Maslow's *hierarchy of needs* (1943, 1968, 1970), among others. As highlighted by the following quote of Maslow's, humanistic ideas are in stark contrast to the views of psychoanalysts and the learning theorists:

> *I think it is now possible to be able to delineate this view of human nature as*
> *a total, single, comprehensive system of psychology even though much of it has*

arisen as a reaction against the limitations (as philosophies of human nature)
of the two most comprehensive psychologies now available: behaviorism (or
associationism) and classical, Freudian psychoanalysis. . . . In the past I have
called it the "holistic-dynamic."

(Maslow, 1968, p. 189)

Maslow stated that people have what he called a "hierarchy of needs," with lower-order needs having to be satisfied before the next need on the hierarchy can be assimilated (see Figure 10.1). This has great implications for understanding the motivations of individuals. For instance, by examining Figure 10.1, we can see that an individual who is hungry or in need of shelter probably has little ability to focus on the needs of love and belonging; the individual who feels unloved and does not have some sense of a social support will necessarily have lowered self-esteem; and so forth. The highest need to be satisfied, stated Maslow, was *self-actualization*, in which one has the desire to become self-fulfilled and to live out the person one actually is. Individuals who are self-actualized are in touch with their feelings, have high self-worth, are alive and spontaneous, and have developed a sense of their spirituality. Although Rogers's theory is not hierarchical, on many occasions, he stated his support for the ideas of Maslow and implied that an individual who is given a nurturing environment would develop according to Maslow's hierarchy (Kirschenbaum, 2009).

FIGURE 10.1
Maslow's Hierarchy of Needs

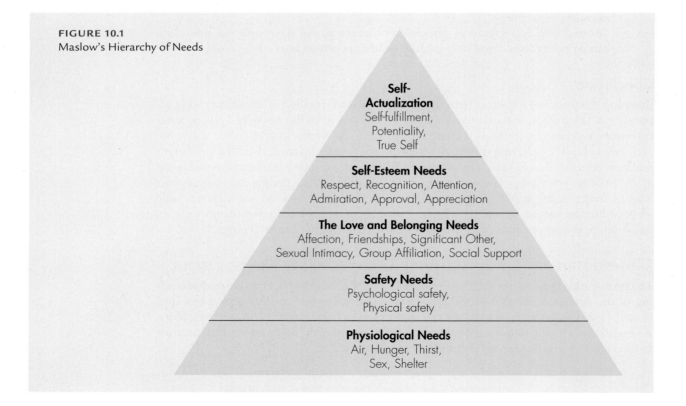

BOX 10.1
The Story of Ellen West

As described by Rogers (1961/1989), Ellen West was a client who underwent psychotherapy by a number of well-known nonhumanistically oriented therapists (a client Rogers knew about but never saw himself). Rogers noted that Ellen felt that she had to follow her father's wishes (conditions of worth) and not marry the man whom she loved. Consequently, she disengaged herself from her feelings by overeating and becoming quite obese. A few years later, she again fell in love but instead married a distant cousin due to pressure from her parents. Following this marriage, she became anorectic, taking 60 laxative pills a day, again as an apparent attempt to divorce herself from her feelings. She saw numerous doctors, who gave her differing diagnoses, treated her dispassionately, and generally denied her humanness. Eventually, disenchanted with her life, Ellen committed suicide.

This story, Rogers noted, gives a poignant view of what it's like to lose touch with self—to be incongruent. As Ellen West felt she needed to gain the conditional love of her parents, she gave up the most valuable part of self—her "real" self. This led to a life filled with self-hate and a sense of being "out of touch." Eventually, she was viewed by therapists as mentally ill, which Rogers implied might have added to her feelings of estrangement and her eventual suicide.

Rogers believed that individuals are born good and have a natural tendency to actualize and obtain fulfillment if placed in a nurturing environment that includes *empathy*, *congruence*, and *unconditional positive regard* (Neukrug, 2015). Unlike Freud, Rogers did not emphasize the importance of instincts, the unconscious, or developmental stages in the formation of personality development. Unlike Skinner, Rogers did not place much value on reinforcement contingencies in creating the personality of the individual. In fact, during 1960s, Rogers and Skinner did a series of debates that highlighted their differences. One such difference was Rogers's strong belief that the quality of the relationship between the child and his or her major caretakers is one of the most significant factors in personality development (Rogers, 1951, 1957, 1959, 1980).

Rogers believed that we all have a need to be loved. He stated that significant people in our lives often place upon us *conditions of worth* or expectations about the ways we should act if we are to receive their love. Therefore, as children, we will sometimes act in ways to please others in an effort to obtain a sense of acceptance, even if the pleasing self is not our real self. In essence, the child has learned that by acting in an *incongruent* or *nongenuine* fashion, he or she will receive acceptance. This nongenuine way of living then becomes the way of relating to the world and prevents the person from becoming self-actualized, becoming one's true self. This is when our self-actualizing tendency is thwarted.

Rogers would not have used the term *abnormal*. He felt strongly that this term and others like it are stigmatizing and not accurate. He believed that all dysfunctional behaviors were the result of individuals having conditions of worth placed upon them that would eventually result in disengagement from self. In fact, he believed this response to conditions of worth was a natural reaction to an unhealthy environment. The story of Ellen West epitomizes this kind of response to an untenable situation, with unfortunate results (see Box 10.1).

Conclusion

The humanistic approach downplays, and in many cases challenges, the concept of abnormality. Instead, so-called abnormal behavior is seen as an attempt by reductionist and dispassionate clinicians to objectify and isolate the client. If we call the individual "abnormal," we take away his or her humanness and no longer need to deal with the person. In fact, humanists would say that abnormal behavior is a healthy response to an unhealthy situation. In other words, abnormal behavior is the individual's attempt to survive in a world that places conditions of worth on the person. What is abnormal, say the humanists, is the attempt to call something abnormal that is actually natural.

Postmodernism's and Social Constructionism's View of Development

Postmodernism has sometimes been defined as the questioning of *modernism*, which states that truth could ultimately be uncovered and that underlying structures are responsible for shaping how one comes to understand the world. Postmodern therapists, such as Michael White and David Epston, suggest that much of what has been handed to us as "truth" by the modernists is only the modernist's particular "take" on reality (Rice, 2015) Therefore, counselors who act in an "objective" manner and assume there are certain inherent mechanisms that lead a person down a path toward a particular personality style have become entrenched in believing that particular truth. *Social constructionism* views knowledge and truth as something that is constructed through conversations (Gergen, 1985, 2009; Rudes & Guterman, 2007). Fitting comfortably alongside postmodernism, this philosophy suggests that language used and the discourses that we have with others are key factors in the development of reality. In other words, nothing is fixed. Freedman and Combs (1996) suggest four premises that summarize postmodernism and social constructionism: *realities are socially constructed, realities are constituted through language, realities are organized and maintained through narrative*, and *there are no essential truths*.

Because language creates reality through discourse, the major responsibility of a counselor would be to recognize that the language he or she uses will likely affect the client (as will the client's language likely affect the counselor) (Rice, 2015). Therefore, the counselor must carefully choose his or her words knowing the influence of language on the person. In fact, *not* saying certain things will reinforce existing ways of being for the client. Also, because reality is constantly changing and a function of language, it is assumed that one can never fully know the inner world of another, "all one can know is the verbal expressions of another's experiences" (Rudes & Guterman, 2007, p. 388). For postmodernists and social constructionists, even the idea of an "inner world" is seen as a cultural by-product, not something that necessarily exists. From this perspective, it would make sense to question any counselor who states he or she knows the client's inner world as a result of understanding the functioning of some hypothesized inner structures (e.g., id, ego, superego; incongruent vs. congruent self, self-actualization, etc.). Hypothetically, what I say is the color blue may be someone else's red, and what I say is depression may be experienced differently by another, and what I say is happiness also may be experienced differently by another (see Box 10.2).

Conclusion

You can see that the postmodern and social constructionist approaches turn the concept of abnormality on its head. From their perspective, abnormal behavior is simply a social construction—a construct that has been developed by certain individuals within the

BOX 10.2
Color Therapy

Imagine there was a counseling approach that stated color preference was an indication of mental health, and the closer a person's favorite color was to "red," the healthier he or she was. Those that liked red most were very healthy, those that liked orange were pretty healthy, those that liked yellow were somewhat healthy, and so forth down the spectrum to green, then blue, and then those who liked violet, who were really unhealthy. Now imagine that this approach became so popular that it was accepted throughout the land and most people "know" that color preference is related to mental health.

Now, imagine a client sees a counselor who is a "Color Counselor." Naturally, one of his first questions is to ask the client what her favorite color is. She says "blue." Well, immediately, the counselor assumes the client is not mentally healthy. After all, blue is way down the list toward violet. So, the counselor begins to treat her and tries to change her favorite color. He even has a systematic way of having her work up the hierarchy toward red. If she practices the system every day, she will eventually get closer to red, says the counselor. After a few months, she has worked her way up to green, and the counselor says he thinks that she might want to consider taking some medication, for medication will help her experience the red more often. And, the counselor tells her that after a few years of experiencing more red, she can

try to reduce her medication because maybe she can begin to like red on her own.

Frustrated that she is not making progress fast enough, the client decides to see a new counselor. The new counselor is clearly unconventional and does not even believe in color therapy. She asks the client to tell her what her problem is. The client states "Well, everyone says that liking blue is bad, and so I must be mentally ill. What do you think?" This counselor replies by saying, "How about we don't focus on the color right now. Instead, let me ask you: What do you want your life to look like? Where do you want to take therapy? What do you want as your end goal? And, what would make you happier?"

With counselor number one, there is an external reality based on preconceived notions about colors. And this reality has been bought into by many. In fact, a whole system of working with clients has been developed. And, almost everyone "knows" and believes in this approach. The second counselor, however, does not have these preconceived ideas, and indeed even questions the moral authority that asserts that this reality exists. This counselor does not believe there are any internal structures that mediate mental health based on color. This counselor is the postmodern, social constructionist counselor!

helping professions who have tended to be in power (e.g., psychiatrists) and have subtly, but forcefully, pushed their viewpoint onto the rest of the mental health field. They also believe that through dialogue and new knowledge, people can build new constructions of their sense of self.

> One might wonder how the field of counseling could have been enhanced if, in the early 1950s when the DSM was first published, the American Counseling Association (then the American Personnel and Guidance association) had published a complementary diagnostic framework, perhaps a "Manual of Client Core Issues" (MCCI). This diagnostic guide would not have focused on symptoms of pathology but rather on psychosocial and relational formulations of client struggles that tend to be problematic....

> (Halstead, 2007, pp. 6–7)

Comparison of Models

Table 10.1 shows a comparison of the five models we examined. Each approach offers a unique perspective on the development of the person. Today, attempts have been made to

TABLE 10.1   Comparison of How Different Models View Psychopathology

	BIOLOGICAL	PSYCHOANALYTICAL	LEARNING THEORY	HUMANISTIC	POSTMODERN/ SOCIAL CONSTRUCTIONIST
Developmental Focus	Traits exhibited at varying times based on our biological timetable; other traits we are born with.	Psychosexual stages of development are oral, anal, phallic, latency, and genital.	Learning occurs from birth and people can continue to learn throughout the lifespan.	Maslow's hierarchy may loosely be considered developmental with no age parameters. People are capable of moving toward self-actualization.	Not a developmental focus, although there is a belief that people can change over time
Developmental Stages/Major Themes	Traits are a function of multiple genes as the person interacts with the environment over one's lifespan.	Psychosexual stages. Structure of personality: id, ego, superego. Unconscious. Instincts. Defenses.	Reinforcement contingencies. Schedules of reinforcement. Learning/relearning. Generalization. Discrimination. Recently: Intervening cognitions.	People are born with an actualizing tendency optimized by empathy, unconditional positive regard (UPR), and genuineness. Conditions of worth are sometimes placed on people. The need to be regarded can lead to an inability to actualize self.	Reality is socially constructed through language and organized and maintained through narratives. There are no essential truths.
Development of Healthy Self	Traits may be a function of the draw of the cards (genes). Environment can affect biology and ultimately development of healthy self (e.g., prenatal care).	Early healthy parenting is crucial, as is ability to master psychosexual stages and suitable development of id, ego, and superego.	Reinforcement of specific behaviors and/ or thoughts will lead to a healthy sense of self.	Conditions in environment need to be conducive for the individual to expose his or her true self. Conditions include empathy, UPR, genuineness. The true self is always healthy.	The concept of a "healthy self" is a construction, as there is no "one" healthy self. Individuals define what is healthy or unhealthy for themselves.
Treatment	Genetic engineering, healthy environment, care of body, and medication.	Psychodynamic therapy, long-term treatment, and resolution of unresolved conflicts.	Identifying problem behaviors, setting goals, and using behavioral and cognitive change strategies.	Exposure to environment that will be conducive to development of one's true self (can be through therapy).	Help people see how they have constructed their reality and invite them to construct a new reality that works more effectively for them.

integrate many of these approaches. To view a more in-depth description of these models (with the exception of the biological model), see Chapter 4.

Diagnosis and Mental Disorders: What Is DSM-5?

Derived from the Greek words *dia* (apart) and *gnosis* (to learn), the term diagnosis refers to the process of making an assessment of an individual from an outside, or objective, viewpoint (Harper, 2014). Although attempts have been made to classify mental disorders since the turn of the century, it was not until 1952 that the American Psychiatric Association (APA) published the first comprehensive diagnosis system, called the *Diagnostic and Statistical Manual (DSM-I)*. Although DSM-I had many critics, and was indeed a crude effort at a diagnostic system, it did represent the first -modern-day attempt at the classification of mental disorders.

The DSM has been revised multiple times over the years. In 1994, DSM-IV was released, and in 2000, an additional text revision of DSM-IV became available (DSM-IV-TR) and contained 365 diagnoses (American Psychiatric Association, 1994, 2000). Although there were many critics of the DSM-IV-TR (Beutler & Malik, 2002; Thyer, 2006; Zalaquett, Fuerth, Stein, Ivey, & Ivey, 2008), it became the most widely utilized diagnostic classification system for mental health disorders of its time (Seligman, 1999, 2004). A DSM-IV diagnosis consisted of five axes that included clinical disorders, personality disorders and mental retardation (now called *intellectual disabilities*), medical conditions, psychosocial and environmental factors, and a global assessment of functioning (GAF) scale, which gave specific ratings for the severity of an mental disorder that ranged from 1 through 100 (see Table 10.2).

The practice of utilizing the multiaxial diagnostic system allowed mental health professionals to present a thorough description of clients and communicate their concerns and symptoms to other professionals (Neukrug & Schwitzer, 2006). However, there was much criticism to a multiaxial approach and to the notion of diagnosis in general (Eriksen & Kress, 2005, 2006, 2008; Halstead, 2007; Kress, Eriksen, Rayle, & Ford, 2005; Madesen & Leech, 2007; Seligman, 2004) (see Table 10.3). Although the DSM-5 certainly has its

TABLE 10.2   Former Five-Axis Diagnostic System

AXIS	CATEGORY	EXAMPLES
Axis I	Clinical disorders	Depression, anxiety, bipolar, schizophrenia, etc.
Axis II	Personality disorders and mental retardation	Borderline personality disorder, antisocial personality disorder, etc.
Axis III	General medical conditions	High blood pressure, diabetes, sprained ankle, etc.
Axis IV	Psychosocial and environmental factors	Recent loss of job, recent divorce, homelessness, etc.
Axis V	Global assessment of functioning	A single score from 1 to 100 summarizing one's functioning and symptoms

TABLE 10.3 Advantages and Disadvantages of DSM

DISADVANTAGES	ADVANTAGES
1. Does not predict outcomes of counseling	1. Can help with case conceptualization
2. Does not examine etiology	2. Proper diagnosis can lead to good treatment planning including proper use of medication
3. Use can reinforce the counselor's tendency to use a medical model of treatment	3. Facilitates communication among professionals
4. Does not fully account for contextual and social factors	4. Fosters research on diagnostic categories
5. Can lead to labeling and stigmatization of client	5. Helps client understand their emotional problems
6. Can be dehumanizing to client	6. Offers a model to test hypotheses concerning treatment outcomes
7. Fosters an objective view of client and minimizes the counseling relationship	7. Provides a sense of what is "normal" for most people
8. Problems with the "scientific" evidence supporting diagnostic categories	8. Provides a forum for professionals to discuss nomenclature and treatment

critics (Jackson, 2012; Miller, 2012), the most recent edition of the manual, published in 2013, has attempted to update its diagnostic categories and has moved toward a one-axis approach.

The DSM-5[1]

The newest diagnostic manual, DSM-5 (APA, 2013a), was under development from 1999 to 2013 and first published in May of 2013. Subsequent editions, like computer software, will follow with editions 5.1, 5.2, 5.3, and so on. In addition to the print version of DSM-5, an online component (www.psychiatry.org/dsm5) is available for supplemental materials. Diagnosis codes for mental disorders in DSM-5 are the same as those in the *International Classification of Disease (ICD) Manual,* 10th edition (ICD-10). This serves to unify the diagnostic and billing process between psychological and medical professions.

Single-Axis vs. Multiaxial Diagnosis: Perhaps the most significant change in the DSM-5 was the return to a single-axis diagnosis (APA, 2013a; Wakefield, 2013). Whereas mental retardation (now called *intellectual disabilities*) and personality disorders were listed under a separate axis (Axis II), collapsing them into a single axis with the other disorders reduces their stigma and removes the misguided belief that personality disorders were largely untreatable (Good, 2012; Krueger & Eaton, 2010). In DSM-5, medical conditions, which had been listed on Axis II in DSM-IV, will likely take a more significant role in mental health diagnosis as they can be listed side by side with the mental disorder (Wakefield, 2013). Also, psychosocial and environmental stressors, previously listed on Axis IV of DSM-IV, will be listed alongside mental disorders and physical health issues. In fact, DSM-5 has increased the number of "V codes" ("Z codes" in ICD-10), which are considered nondisordered conditions that sometimes are the focus of treatment and often are reflective of a host of psychosocial and environmental issues (e.g., homelessness, divorce, etc.). Finally,

[1] Much of this section is paraphrased from DSM-5 (American Psychiatric Association, 2013a).

the APA decided to do away with the GAF scale (Axis V) due to its unreliablity and is now looking for a possible replacement (APA, 2013a).

Making and Reporting Diagnosis.   In the diagnostic process, a specific ordering process is used. In addition, subtypes, specifiers, and severity codes help distinguish diagnoses, and sometimes a specific form of provisional diagnosis will be used.

Ordering diagnoses. Individuals often have more than one diagnosis, with the first diagnosis being called the *principal diagnosis*, which is usually the most salient factor that resulted in the person seeking treatment (APA, 2013a). The secondary and tertiary diagnosis should be listed in order of need for clinical attention.

Subtypes, Specifiers, and Severity. Subtypes for a diagnosis can be used to help communicate greater clarity. They can be identified in the DSM-5 by the instruction "Specify whether" and represent mutually exclusive groupings of symptoms (i.e., the clinician can only pick one). For example, the ADHD has three different subtypes to choose from: predominantly inattentive, predominantly hyperactive/impulsive, or a combined presentation. *Specifiers*, on the other hand, are not mutually exclusive, so more than one can be used. The clinician chooses which specifiers, if any, apply. The ADHD diagnosis offers only one specifier that is "in partial remission" (APA, 2013a, p. 60). Some diagnoses offer an opportunity to rate the *severity* of the symptoms. Referencing the ADHD diagnosis, there are three options of severity: mild, moderate, or severe. Severity can also be identified through *dimensional diagnosis.* For instance, the Autism Spectrum Disorder has "Table 2 Severity levels of autism spectrum disorder" (APA, 2013a, p. 52), which classifies autism on three levels of severity "requiring support," "requiring substantial support," and "requiring very substantial support." Similarly, schizophrenia has the user go to a "Clinician-Rated Dimensions of Psychosis Symptom Severity" chart (pp. 743–744) to rate symptoms on a five-point Likert scale.

Provisional Diagnosis. When a clinician has a strong inclination that a client will meet the criteria for a diagnosis, but does not yet have enough information to make the diagnosis he or she may use a *provisional* diagnosis. Once the criteria are later confirmed, the provisional label can be removed. These situations often occur when a client is not able to give an adequate history or further collateral information is required. They include the following:

➤ *Rule-out*—the client meets many of the symptoms, but not enough to make a diagnosis at this time; it should be considered further (e.g., rule out major depressive disorder).

➤ *Traits*—this person does not meet the necessary criteria; however, he or she presents with many of the features of the diagnosis (e.g., borderline traits or cluster B traits).

➤ *By history*—previous records (another provider or hospital) indicate this diagnosis; records can be inaccurate or outdated (e.g., alcohol dependence by history).

➤ *By self-report*—the client claims this as a diagnosis; it is currently unsubstantiated; these can be inaccurate (e.g., bipolar by self-report).

Specific Diagnostic Categories.   The DSM-5 offers an in-depth discussion of twenty-two broad diagnostic categories and their subtypes. The following offers a brief description of these diagnostic categories and is summarized from DSM-5 (APA, 2013a). Please refer to the DSM-5 for an in-depth review of each disorder:

➤ *Neurodevelopmental Disorders.* This group of disorders typically refers to those that manifest during early development, although diagnoses are sometimes not assigned until adulthood. Examples of neurodevelopmental disorders include intellectual disabilities, communication disorders, autism spectrum disorders (incorporating the former categories of autistic disorder, Asperger's disorder, childhood disintegrative disorder, and pervasive developmental disorder), ADHD, specific learning disorders, motor disorders, and other neurodevelopmental disorders.

➤ *Schizophrenia Spectrum and Other Psychotic Disorders.* The disorders that belong to this section all have one feature in common: psychotic symptoms; that is, delusions, hallucinations, grossly disorganized or abnormal motor behavior, and/ or negative symptoms. The disorders include schizotypal personality disorder (which is listed again, and explained more comprehensively, in the personality disorders category in the DSM-5), delusional disorder, brief psychotic disorder, schizophreniform disorder, schizophrenia, schizoaffective disorder, substance/ medication-induced psychotic disorders, psychotic disorders due to another medical condition, and catatonic disorders.

➤ *Bipolar and Related Disorders.* The disorders in this category refer to disturbances in mood in which the client cycles through stages of mania or mania and depression. Both children and adults can be diagnosed with bipolar disorder, and the clinician can work to identify the pattern of mood presentation, such as rapid-cycling, which is more often observed in children. These disorders include bipolar I, bipolar II, cyclothymic disorder, substance/medication-induced, bipolar and related disorder due to another medical condition, and other specified or unspecified bipolar and related disorders.

➤ *Depressive Disorders.* Previously grouped into the broader category of "mood disorders" in the DSM-IV-TR, these disorders describe conditions where depressed mood is the overarching concern. They include disruptive mood dysregulation disorder, major depressive disorder, persistent depressive disorder (also known as dysthymia), and premenstrual dysphoric disorder.

➤ *Anxiety Disorders.* There are a wide range of anxiety disorders, which can be diagnosed by identifying a general or specific cause of unease or fear. This anxiety or fear is considered clinically significant when it is excessive and persistent over time. Examples of anxiety disorders that typically manifest earlier in development include separation anxiety and selective mutism. Other examples of anxiety disorders are specific phobia, social anxiety disorder (also known as *social phobia*), panic disorder, and generalized anxiety disorder.

➤ *Obsessive-Compulsive and Related Disorders.* Disorders in this category all involve obsessive thoughts and compulsive behaviors that are uncontrollable and the client feels compelled to perform them. Diagnoses in this category include obsessive-compulsive disorder, body dysmorphic disorder, hoarding disorder, trichotillomania (or hair-pulling disorder), and excoriation (or skin-picking) disorder.

➤ *Trauma- and Stressor-Related Disorders.* A new category for DSM-5, trauma and stress disorders emphasize the pervasive impact that life events can have on an individual's emotional and physical well-being. Diagnoses include reactive attachment disorder, disinhibited social engagement disorder, posttraumatic stress disorder (PTSD), acute stress disorder, and adjustment disorders.

➤ *Dissociative Disorders.* These disorders indicate a temporary or prolonged disruption to consciousness that can cause an individual to misinterpret identity, surroundings, and memories. Diagnoses include dissociative identity disorder (formerly known as *multiple personality disorder*), dissociative amnesia, depersonalization/derealization disorder, and other specified and unspecified dissociative disorders.

➤ *Somatic Symptom and Related Disorders.* Somatic symptom disorders were previously referred to as "somatoform disorders" and are characterized by the experiencing of a physical symptom without evidence of a physical cause, thus suggesting a psychological cause. Somatic symptom disorders include somatic symptom disorder, illness anxiety disorder (formerly *hypochondriasis*), conversion (or functional neurological symptom) disorder, psychological factors affecting other medical conditions, and factitious disorder.

➤ *Feeding and Eating Disorders.* This group of disorders describes clients who have severe concerns about the amount or type of food they eat to the point that serious health problems, or even death, can result from their eating behaviors. Examples include avoidant/restrictive food intake disorder, anorexia nervosa, bulimia nervosa, binge eating disorder, pica, and rumination disorder.

➤ *Elimination Disorders.* These disorders can manifest at any point in a person's life, although they are typically diagnosed in early childhood or adolescence. They include enuresis, which is the inappropriate elimination of urine, and encopresis, which is the inappropriate elimination of feces. These behaviors may or may not be intentional.

➤ *Sleep-Wake Disorders.* This category refers to disorders where one's sleep patterns are severely affected, and they often co-occur with other disorders (e.g., depression or anxiety). Some examples include insomnia disorder, hypersomnolence disorder, restless legs syndrome, narcolepsy, and nightmare disorder. A number of sleep-wake disorders involve variations in breathing, such as sleep-related hypoventilation, obstructive sleep apnea hypopnea, or central sleep apnea. See *DSM-5* for the full listing and descriptions of these disorders.

➤ *Sexual Dysfunctions.* These disorders are related to problems that disrupt sexual functioning or one's ability to experience sexual pleasure. They occur across sexes and include delayed ejaculation, erectile disorder, female orgasmic disorder, and premature (or early) ejaculation disorder, among others.

➤ *Gender Dysphoria.* Formerly termed *gender identity disorder,* this category includes those individuals who experience significant distress with the sex they were born and with associated gender roles. This diagnosis has been separated from the category of sexual disorders, as it is now accepted that gender dysphoria does not relate to a person's sexual attractions.

➤ *Disruptive, Impulse Control, and Conduct Disorders.* These disorders are characterized by socially unacceptable or otherwise disruptive and harmful behaviors that are outside of the individual's control. Generally, more common in males than in females, and often first seen in childhood, they include oppositional defiant disorder, conduct disorder, intermittent explosive disorder, antisocial personality disorder (which is also coded in the category of personality disorders), kleptomania, and pyromania.

➤ *Substance-Related and Addictive Disorders.* Substance use disorders include disruptions in functioning as the result of a craving or strong urge. Often caused by prescribed and illicit drugs or the exposure to toxins, with these disorders the brain's reward system pathways are activated when the substance is taken (or in the case of gambling disorder, when the behavior is being performed). Some common substances include alcohol, caffeine, nicotine, cannabis, opioids, inhalants, amphetamine, phencyclidine (PCP), sedatives, hypnotics or anxiolytics. Substance use disorders are further designated with the following terms: intoxication, withdrawal, induced, or unspecified.

➤ *Neurocognitive Disorders.* These disorders are diagnosed when one's decline in cognitive functioning is significantly different from the past and is usually the result of a medical condition (e.g., Parkinson's or Alzheimer's disease), the use of a substance/medication, or traumatic brain injury, among other phenomena. Examples of neurocognitive disorders (NCDs) include delirium and several types of major and mild NCDs, such as frontotemporal NCD, NCD due to Parkinson's disease, NCD due to HIV infection, NCD due to Alzheimer's disease, substance- or medication-induced NCD, and vascular NCD, among others.

➤ *Personality Disorders.* The 10 personality disorders in DSM-5 all involve a pattern of experiences and behaviors that are persistent, inflexible, and deviate from one's cultural expectations. Usually, this pattern emerges in adolescence or early adulthood and causes severe distress in one's interpersonal relationships. The personality disorders are grouped into the three following clusters, which are based on similar behaviors:

  ➤ *Cluster A: Paranoid, schizoid, and schizotypal.* These individuals seem bizarre or unusual in their behaviors and interpersonal relations.

  ➤ *Cluster B: Antisocial, borderline, histrionic, and narcissistic.* These individuals seem overly emotional, are melodramatic, or unpredictable in their behaviors and interpersonal relations.

  ➤ *Cluster C: Avoidant, dependent, and obsessive-compulsive* (not to be confused with *obsessive-compulsive disorder*). These individuals tend to appear anxious, worried, or fretful in their behaviors.

➤ *Paraphilic Disorders.* These disorders are diagnosed when the client is sexually aroused to circumstances that deviate from traditional sexual stimuli *and* when such behaviors result in harm or significant emotional distress. The disorders include exhibitionistic disorder, voyeuristic disorder, frotteurisitc disorder, sexual sadism and sexual masochism disorders, fetishistic disorder, transvestic disorder, pedophilic disorder, and other specified and unspecified paraphilic disorders.

➤ *Other Mental Disorders.* This diagnostic category includes mental disorders that did not fall within one of the previously mentioned groups and do not have unifying characteristics. Examples include other specified mental disorder due to another medical condition, unspecified mental disorders due to another medical condition, other specified mental disorder, and unspecified mental disorder.

➤ *Medication-Induced Movement Disorders and Other Adverse Effects of Medications.* These disorders are the result of adverse and severe side effects to medications, although a causal link cannot always be shown. Some of these disorders include neuroleptic-induced parkinsonism, neuroleptic malignant syndrome, medication-induced dystonia, medication-induced acute akathisia, tardive dyskinesia, tardive akathisia, medication-induced postural tremor, other medication-induced movement disorder, antidepressant discontiunation syndrome, and other adverse effect of medication.

➤ *Other Conditions That May Be a Focus of Clinical Assessment.* Reminiscent of Axis IV of the previous edition of the DSM, this last part of Section II ends with a description of concerns that could be clinically significant, such as abuse/neglect, relational problems, psychosocial, personal, and environmental concerns, educational/occupational problems, housing and economic problems, and problems related to the legal system. These conditions, which are not considered mental disorders, are generally listed as V codes, which correspond to ICD-9, or Z codes, which correspond to ICD-10.

In addition to the above categories, the DSM offers *other specified* and u*nspecified disorders* that can be used when a provider believes an individual's impairment to functioning or distress is clinically significant; however, it does not meet the specific diagnostic criteria in that category. The "other specified" should be used when the clinician wants to communicate specifically why the criteria do not fit. The "unspecified disorder" should be used when he or she does not wish, or is unable to, communicate specifics. For example, if someone appeared to have significant panic attacks but only had three of the four required criteria, the diagnosis could be "Other specified panic disorder—due to insufficient symptoms." Otherwise, the clinician would report "unspecified panic disorder."

A diagnosis can be critical to the determination of whether one is to recommend the use of psychotropic medication. Let's look at this sometimes important adjunct to counseling.

Psychopharmacology

Whether medication should be used as an adjunct to counseling and how one broaches this possibly delicate topic with clients are increasingly important issues for the counselor and other mental health professionals (Ingersoll, 2000; Preston, O'Neal, & Talaga, 2013). If counselors are to make informed decisions about a referral for medication, they should know the pros and cons of their usage (see Table 10.4) and should have some basic knowledge about psychotropic medications (Preston, et al., 2013). With a host of possible medications available (see Schatzberg & Nemeroff, 2009), the following represents a brief overview of some of the more commonly used psychotropic drugs. Although classification systems of psychotropic drugs vary, almost all systems describe medications in most or all of the following five groups: *antipsychotics, mood-stabilizing drugs, antidepressants, antianxiety agents,* and *stimulants* (National Institute of Mental Health, 2010; Preston, et al., 2013; Videbeck, 2014). Let's look at each of these.

TABLE 10.4   Advantages and Disadvantages of Psychotropic Medications

ADVANTAGES OF MEDICATION	DISADVANTAGES OF MEDICATION
➤ The efficacy of medication use is easily studied. ➤ If they work, medications can help quickly. ➤ The quick response of medications can instill hope. ➤ The quick response of medication can lead to more effective work in therapy. ➤ The quick response of medication can reduce the likelihood of a serious mental illness (e.g., schizophrenia) occurring again. ➤ Medication may help some people that psychotherapy won't help. ➤ Sometimes medications are more cost effective than psychotherapy. ➤ Due to their biological basis, some mental disorders can only be treated by medication.	➤ Only counseling can address the complexity of the human condition. ➤ Counseling leads to autonomy, drugs lead to dependence. ➤ The quick effects of medications lessen the desire for clients to work on their problems. ➤ Most psychotropic medications have some side effects. ➤ The effects of some psychotropic medications are serious and long-lasting. ➤ Research on the effects of some psychotropic medications are mixed and confusing. ➤ Psychotropic medications do not solve life's problems, only the individual can do this.

Antipsychotics

During the early 1950s, the first wave of antipsychotic drugs was discovered (Nasrallah & Tandon, 2009). These were soon to change the field of mental health dramatically. For the first time, individuals with severe psychotic symptoms could be treated with some success; this became one reason for the release of hundreds of thousands of individuals from mental institutions around the country.

Antipsychotic drugs, sometimes called *neuroleptics*, are generally used for the treatment of schizophrenia, as well as schizoaffective disorders, and the manic phase of bipolar disorder (Videbeck, 2014). Less frequently, these drugs are used in the treatment of Alzheimer's disease, aggressive behavior, and anxiety and insomnia. There are three broad classes of antipsychotic drugs that include the *conventional antipsychotics*, the *atypical antipsychotics*, and the new, *second-generation antipsychotics* (Patterson, Albala, McCahill, & Edwards, 2010; Videbeck, 2014). Some of the classic antipsychotic and second-generation drugs used in these disorders are listed in Table 10.5.

TABLE 10.5   Antipsychotic Medications

CONVENTIONAL ANTIPSYCHOTICS		SECOND-GENERATION ANTIPSYCHOTICS	
GENERIC NAME	*TRADE NAME*	*GENERIC NAME*	*TRADE NAME*
Chlorpromazine	Thorazine	Clozapine	Clozaril
Haloperidol	Haldol	Risperidone	Risperdal
Thioridazine	Mellaril	Olanzapine	Zyprexa
Trifluoperazine	Stelazine	Quetiapine	Seroquel
Fluphenazine	Prolixin	Ziprasidone	Geodon
Perphenazine	Trilafon	Aripiprazole	Abilify
Thiothixene	Navane		
Loxapine	Loxitane		
Molindone	Moban		

Antipsychotics can dramatically alter the course of an individual's life who is having an acute psychotic episode. This is important because the quicker an individual can recover from a psychotic episode, the greater the likelihood of eliminating (or at least decreasing) the intensity of future psychotic episodes. Although antipsychotic medications can help an individual who has a long history of psychotic behavior live a more normal life, they are often not a cure. For these individuals, normal cognitive functioning is often not restored, and they are frequently left seeming somewhat stilted in their thinking and ability to respond.

Depending on the type and dosage of medication, a number of side effects may occur. For instance, some individuals may have one or more of the following side effects (Goldberg & Ernst, 2012):

➤ *Anticholinergic side effects* include dry mouth, blurred vision, constipation, urinary retention, decreased memory, and a decreased libido.

➤ *Extrapyramidal side effects (EPS)* include muscle spasms, Parkinson-type symptoms, and motor restlessness.

➤ *Tardive dyskinesia,* which includes involuntary movements of the tongue, lips, and facial muscles, can occur in some individuals who have taken high dosages of antipsychotic medications over a long period of time, although it has occasionally been seen when the medications are taken for short periods in lower doses.

➤ *Blood disorders,* which can lead to death if not treated, have been found with some of the newer antipsychotic medications.

➤ *Other effects,* such as a fast heartbeat, rigidness, agitation, sedation, weight gain, and skin pigmentation.

Mood-Stabilizing Drugs

During the 1800s, an element called *lithium* was discovered that was found to have positive effects for the treatment of a number of bodily afflictions (Freeman, Wiegand, & Gelenberg, 2009). In the early 1950s, lithium was rediscovered as an effective treatment for bipolar disorder (then called *manic-depression*). Lithium seems to act particularly well in lessening the effects of manic symptoms in an individual with bipolar disorder. Because it does not have the same dramatic effects with the depressive end of the illness, antidepressants are often also prescribed. For individuals who take lithium, the level of drug in the system has to be assessed through a blood test because too much lithium can cause severe side effects and too little will be ineffective in treatment. Like antipsychotics, lithium can produce a number of side effects, including gastrointestinal problems, excessive thirst, excessive urination, hand tremors, a metallic taste, fatigue, lethargy, and mild nausea; however, the side effects are generally viewed as less serious than those with the antipsychotic medications. Although lithium has been used in the treatment of other disorders (Freeman, et al., 2009), it is often an early treatment of choice for bipolar disorder.

Lithium has been shown to be a very effective drug for the treatment of bipolar disorder, often restoring an individual to a normal lifestyle. However, some individuals do not respond to treatment with lithium. For those individuals, a number of other drugs have shown some success, including *anticonvulsant medications,* such as Depakote and Tegretol (Freeman, et al., 2009; Patterson et al., 2010). In addition, some *benzodiazepines* (antianxiety drugs) may also be helpful in treating manic episodes (McElroy & Keck, 2009).

Antidepressants

The use of *amphetamines* during the 1930s was one of the first attempts to treat depression psychopharmacologically (Pirodsky & Cohn, 1992). Known as "speed," this medication did little except to stimulate a person's central nervous system temporarily, which often would eventually lead to a "crash" and more serious depression. In addition, consistent use of amphetamines can lead to paranoia and health problems.

The 1950s saw a dramatic shift in the treatment of depression with the identification of two classes of antidepressants called *monoamine oxidase inhibitors* (MAOIs) and *tricyclics* (Krishnan, 2009; Nelson, 2009). Until recently, these classes of drugs were the medications of choice in the treatment of depression, with the tricyclics being used more frequently because they tended to have fewer side effects. However, the last twenty years have seen the widespread use of a new class of antidepressants called *selective serotonin reuptake inhibitors* (*SSRIs*) (Videbeck, 2014). *SSRIs* have been called "miracle drugs" by some due to their limited side effects and often dramatic results. In fact, these drugs have been so effective that there is some evidence that they can help make an individual who already feels relatively well feel even better. For these reasons, such drugs as Prozac, Luvox, Paxil, Lexapro, Celexa, and Zoloft have very quickly become commonplace in American society. However, in recent years, research has suggested that these drugs increase the risk for suicide, especially in children (Bridge et al., 2007). As a result, warnings have been given to individuals taking these medications. In addition to the treatment of depression, SSRIs also show promise in treating other disorders, including obsessive–compulsive disorder, panic disorder, some forms of schizophrenia, eating disorders, alcoholism, obesity, and some sleep disorders.

Besides SSRIs, there are a number of what have been called *atypical anti-depressants* that also have fewer side effects than the tricyclics or the MAOIs and seem to be promising in the treatment of depression. Some of these include Serzone, Effexor, Wellbutrin, and Desyrel.

Antianxiety Medications

The use of modern-day antianxiety agents started with the discovery of Librium, which came on the market in 1960 and was soon followed by Valium. These medications and other *benzodiazepines* were better tolerated and less addictive than barbiturates (e.g., *phenobarbitol*), the previous treatment of choice (Sheehan & Raj, 2009). However, tolerance of and dependence on benzodiazepines can be developed, and there is a potential for overdose on these medications.

Today, benzodiazepines, such as Valium, Librium, Tranxene, Xanax, and others, are frequently used for generalized anxiety disorders as they have a calming effect on the individual (Videbeck, 2014). In conjunction with psychotherapy, these medications can be an effective agent in treating such disorders. Benzodiazepines have also been shown to be helpful in reducing stress, relieving insomnia, and managing alcohol withdrawal (Nishino, Mishima, Mignot, & Dement, 2009). In addition, they have been used in conjunction with some antidepressants for the treatment of obsessive–compulsive disorder (OCD) and in treating social phobias and posttraumatic stress disorder (PTSD) (Sheehan & Raj, 2009). Two other *nonbenzodiazepines*, *Buspar* and *Gepirone*, have been found to be effective for use in generalized anxiety disorders and can be an alternative to the the more popular benzodiazepines.

In addition, these drugs show some efficacy in the treatment of depression, especially with those who are exhibiting anxiety disorders (Robinson, Rickels, & Yocca, 2009).

Stimulants

Probably the first modern-day stimulant used to treat emotional disorders was *cocaine*, which was first discovered in the mid-1800s. However, due to its addictive qualities, cocaine has never become a treatment of choice in this country. In 1887, *amphetamines*, which had many of the same stimulant qualities as cocaine but were less addictive, were synthesized (Ballas, Evans, & Dinges, 2009; Fawcett & Busch, 1998). Over the years, amphetamines were used, mostly unsuccessfully, as diet aids, as antidepressants, and to relieve the symptoms of sleepiness. However, during the 1950s, amphetamines were found to have a *paradoxical effect* in many children diagnosed with ADHD—they seemed to calm them down and help them focus. Today, the use of stimulants in the treatment of ADHD is widespread, with the three most common drugs being Ritalin, Cylert, and Dexedrine. In addition to treating ADHD, stimulants have been found to be successful in the treatment of *narcolepsy* and are somewhat successful in treating residual attention deficit disorder in adults.

Psychopharmacology has come a long way since the 1950s, when the first modern-day psychotropic medications were introduced. Increasingly, the medications used for a wide array of disorders are more effective and have fewer side effects than in the past. As the mechanism for psychological disorders becomes increasingly understood, new and even more effective medications can be developed to target the underlying physiological mechanism causing the disorder.

Multicultural/Social Justice Focus

DSM-5 and Cultural Sensitivity

Because people from diverse cultures may express themselves in different ways, symptomatology may differ as a function of culture (Mezzich & Caracci, 2008). Thus, some have argued that although diagnosis can be helpful in treatment planning, it can lead to the misdiagnosis of culturally oppressed groups (Caetano, 2011). Others have noted that the DSM tends to diagnose from an individual perspective and does not account for the effects of the broader system on the individual (Gallagher & Streeter, 2012).

The APA has attempted to combat some of these problems by asking clinicians to understand and acknowledge "culturally patterned differences in symptoms" (APA, 2013a, p. 758). For example, Latin American culture acknowledges that *ataque de nervios* ("attack of nerves") is a common disorder related to difficult and burdensome life experiences and may exhibit itself through "headaches and 'brain aches' (occipital neck tension), irritability, stomach disturbances, sleep difficulties, nervousness, easy tearfulness, inability to concentrate, trembling, tingling sensations, and mareos (dizziness with occasional vertigo-like exacerbations)" (p. 835). A clinician who ignores the client's culture could easily misdiagnose a client who presents with symptoms like this and begin to treat the client with inappropriate strategies. Best practices for multicultural counseling suggest that the clinician have some understanding of differences in the cross-cultural expression of symptoms and that the clinician explore the client's culture with him or her when deciding on appropriate treatment strategies (APA, 2013c). Finally, DSM-5 offers a section entitled "Cultural Formulation Interview (CFI)," which helps clinicians understand the kinds of values, experiences, and influences that have come to shape the client's worldview and provides an outline for how to interview clients from diverse backgrounds appropriately. In addition, DSM-5 offers definitions of some cross-cultural symptoms and identifies how cross-cultural issues impact a wide range of diagnoses.

Ethical, Professional, and Legal Issues

Ethical Issues

Noting the potential misuse and abuse of diagnosis, the code of ethics of the American Counseling Association (ACA) addresses a number of important issues when making a diagnosis (ACA, 2014a, Standard E.5: Diagnosis of Mental Disorders), including the importance of making a proper diagnosis, being culturally sensitive, knowing the historical and social prejudices related to diagnosis, and the right to refrain from making a diagnosis.

Proper Diagnosis

"Counselors take special care to provide proper diagnosis of mental disorders. Assessment techniques (including personal interview) used to determine client care (e.g., locus of treatment, type of treatment, or recommended follow-up) are carefully selected and appropriately used." (Section E.5.a)

Cultural Sensitivity

"Counselors recognize that culture affects the manner in which clients' problems are defined and experienced. Clients' socioeconomic and cultural experiences are considered when diagnosing mental disorders." (Section E.5.b)

Historical and Social Prejudices in the Diagnosis of Pathology

"Counselors recognize historical and social prejudices in the misdiagnosis and pathologizing of certain individuals and groups and strive to become aware of and address such biases in themselves or others." (Section E.5.c)

Refraining from Diagnosis

"Counselors may refrain from making and/or reporting a diagnosis if they believe it would cause harm to the client or others. Counselors carefully consider both the positive and negative implications of a diagnosis." (Section E.5.d)

Professional Issues

Challenging Abnormality and Diagnosing

For years, authors have argued about the causes of emotional problems and whether using a diagnostic classification system is worthwhile (Gallagher & Streeter, 2012; Glasser,

1961; Ivey & Ivey, 1998; Laing, 1967; Madsen & Leech, 2007; Rogers, 1961; Szasz, 1961, 1970, 1990, 1995). For instance, both R. D. Laing and Thomas Szasz viewed mental illness as a normal response to a stressful situation. In fact, Laing even encouraged people to get in touch with their own psychoses as a means of letting go of their stressors, and he would periodically allow himself to "go insane" in his own hospitals. Szasz believed psychopathology is the client's way of communicating about social and cultural forces that impinge on him or her. In a similar vein, William Glasser believed that psychopathology is a client's clumsy attempt at meeting his or her needs. If you help clients understand their needs and wants, you can help them find more effective behaviors toward those ends.

Ivey and Ivey (1998) suggest that rather than assuming there is something inherently wrong with a person, we should view problems as a "logical response to developmental history" (p. 334) and natural responses to issues in the family, community, and broader culture. This approach does not suggest discontinuing the use of diagnosis; rather, it offers a humanistic and antideterministic alternative to understanding the person (see Table 10.6).

Finally, Corey and associates (2015) summarize some reasons that clinicians might want to be tentative when making a diagnosis:

➤ Diagnosis is an objective process in which the person making the diagnosis is really "not in the shoes" of the person being diagnosed.
➤ Diagnosis tends to rob people of their uniqueness.
➤ Diagnosis can lead to a self-fulfilling prophecy for both the client and clinician (I think, therefore I am).
➤ Diagnosis leads to tunnel vision, where the clinician attempts to fit all problems into the specific diagnostic category.
➤ Diagnosis tends to view individuals from an individual perspective and not a contextual one, thus minimizing the effect of family and social systems.
➤ Diagnoses are sometimes cross-culturally biased.
➤ Diagnoses tend to look at pathology at the expense of the strengths of the client.

T A B L E   10.6   Positive Reframe of Personality Disorders

PERSONALITY STYLE	PARANOID	SCHIZOID	SCHIZOTYPAL	ANTISOCIAL	BORDERLINE	HISTRIONIC
Positive frame	It is important to watch out for injustice.	It is useful to be a loner or independent of others at times.	Ability to see things differently than others see them.	It is sometimes necessary to be impulsive and take care of our own needs.	Intensity in relationships is desirable at all times.	All could benefit at times with open access to emotions.
PERSONALITY STYLE	NARCISSISTIC	AVOIDANT	DEPENDENT	OBSESSIVE-COMPULSIVE	PASSIVE-AGGRESSIVE	
Positive frame	A strong belief in ourselves is necessary for good mental health.	It is useful to deny or avoid some things.	We all need to depend on others.	Maintaining order and a system is necessary for job success.	All of us are entitled to procrastinate at times.	

SOURCE: Ivey & Ivey (1998, p. 338).

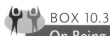

On Being Sane in Insane Places (Rosenhan, 1973)

A group of eight pseudopatients presented themselves to mental hospitals. One was a psychology graduate student, three were psychologists, one a pediatrician, one a psychiatrist, one a painter, and one a housewife. These subjects presented themselves to 12 mental hospitals in five states. The only symptoms they displayed in the admissions offices were saying that they felt their lives were empty and hollow and that they heard voices saying "empty, hollow, thud." The researchers chose these symptoms because they could not find one case of "existential psychosis" in the literature. Once admitted, the pseudopatients ceased showing any symptoms at all. Mental health professionals diagnosed all but one of these people as schizophrenic, and the length of hospitalizations ranged from 7 to 52 days. The professional staffs of the hospitals never detected the fraud, although many actual patients were suspicious and questioned the fake patients. (Swenson, 1997, p. 449)

Today, the controversy over the use of diagnosis still exists, although it has calmed down a bit. When you are called to diagnose a client (and you will be), you may want to reflect on the above issues and carefully consider how your diagnosis will be used.

To Diagnose or Not Diagnose

Wheeler and Bertram (2012) suggest that there are two polar opposites relative to the use of diagnosis. On one side are those who reject diagnosis outright, suggesting that cross-cultural problems with diagnosis and the complexity of being human make it almost impossible to diagnose. And there is certainly evidence to suggest that this is true (Alarcon, 2009; Kapur, et al., 2012) (see Box 10.3). On the other side are those who adhere to the medical model. They suggest that the scientific nature of diagnosis makes it reasonable and efficacious to use—that diagnosis is helpful and useful in treatment planning (APA, 2014a). And there is evidence to suggest that most diagnoses are reasonable. So, where does that leave us? Wheeler and Bertram suggest that most counselors probably are in the middle between these two perspectives. However, for those who are at one extreme or the other, they warn that it is best to not become hopelessly bound to one position or the other, and to work carefully with clients in the best and most reasonable way that you can—regardless of the "side" you find yourself on.

Legal Issues

Confinement Against One's Will

One controversial role that diagnosis has played over the years has been its importance in having a person hospitalized against his or her will. Prior to the mid-1970s, if a client was given certain diagnoses (e.g., acute schizophrenia), he or she would almost assuredly be placed involuntarily in a psychiatric hospital. However, as a result of the *Donaldson v. O'Connor* (1975) decision (see Chapter 2), individuals can no longer be involuntarily held in mental institutions for extended periods of time if they are not in danger of harming themselves or others. In most states, severely impaired clients can be hospitalized for short periods of time, perhaps two to three days. At that point, a certification by two or more experts or a court hearing is generally needed to continue short-term hospitalization of two or three weeks. Long-term confinement against the patient's will would necessitate a court hearing and is very unusual today.

Insurance Fraud

Today, certain diagnoses are often not reimbursed by insurance companies. Although there may be a tendency by some to alter a client's diagnosis so that he or she would obtain reimbursement, this act is unethical and constitutes insurance fraud. With this practice being one of the more commonly cited complaints made against Licensed Professional Counselors (LPCs) (Braun & Cox, 2005; Neukrug, Milliken, &Walden, 2001), counselors must learn to inform clients of what will and will not likely be re-imbursed, work with clients when faced with certain diagnoses that are not reimburs-able (ACA, 2014a, Section H.2.a), and be honest with insurance companies and other third parties:

> Counselors are accurate, honest, and objective in reporting their profes-
> sional activities and judgments to appropriate third parties, including
> courts, health insurance companies, those who are the recipients of evalua-
> tion reports, and others.

(ACA, 2014a, Section C.6.b)

The Counselor in Process: Dismissing Impaired Graduate Students

I have, at times, sat in a faculty meeting when a faculty member brought up the name of a student and suggested that the student be approached because it seemed appar-ent that he or she had severe emotional problems. Sometimes I have agreed with the faculty member's assessment; other times I have not. For me, this issue is similar to the old debate concerning the use of the term *abnormal behavior.* In terms of students, it first challenges me to define what a "severe emotional problem" is, and then asks me to ponder whether I believe such students can be assisted to the point that they can be effective counselors (see Foster & McAdams 2009). The ACA ethical code suggests the following:

> Counselor educators, through ongoing evaluation, are aware of and address
> the inability of some students to achieve counseling competencies. Counselor
> educators do the following:
>
> 1. assist students in securing remedial assistance when needed,
> 2. seek professional consultation and document their decision to dismiss or
>   refer students for assistance, and
> 3. ensure that students have recourse in a timely manner to address decisions
>   requiring them to seek assistance or to dismiss them and provide students
>   with due process according to institutional policies and procedures.

(ACA, 2014a, Section F.9.b)

If I were conceptualizing a "problem student" from a developmental and wellness perspective, as presented in Chapter 9, I would assume that he or she could change. However, if I were to look at this student from an abnormal development perspective, I might think that there is something inherently wrong with him or her, and that change would be particularly difficult, if possible at all. In this latter example, I might ask the student to drop out of the program. Perhaps there is a middle point between these two extremes; however, the issue remains: Do we believe that any student can eventually overcome his or her personal limitations and be effective as a counselor, or do we think that some individuals are simply too impaired? What do you think?

Summary

This chapter introduced the concepts of abnormal behavior, diagnosis, and psychopharmacology, noting that the three are inextricably connected. Whereas it used to be unusual for counseling programs to examine these concepts, changes in the field have made it increasingly common and important.

In attempting to explain abnormal behavior, this chapter looked at five models. The genetic and biological model posits that there are inherited factors that, when expressed, will produce certain personality traits. It also asserts that some genetic factors are expressed only when a person is exposed to certain environmental factors. In addition, the biological model states that environmental factors can greatly affect the development of certain traits, regardless of one's genetics. The psychoanalytic model, on the other hand, assumes that abnormal development is a function of the ability to master the psychosexual stages. Individuals who are parented poorly as they pass through the first five years of life will develop a precarious balance among their id, ego, and superego, which ultimately will lead to dysfunctional ways of being. This model is particularly deterministic, stating that personality development occurs very early in life and is difficult to change. In contrast, the learning perspective assumes that what was learned can be unlearned, and new behaviors and ways of thinking can be learned. Learning theorists believe that through operant conditioning, classical conditioning, and modeling, we learn either healthy or dysfunctional ways of living. In recent times, most learning theorists have included a cognitive perspective that stated that our cognitions are also reinforced and can lead to healthy functioning or to irrational ways of thinking. The humanistic perspective suggests there is a natural growth force in people, and, if a person is placed in a nurturing environment (e.g., empathy, genuineness, positive regard), the individual will develop a healthy personality and high self-esteem. However, if conditions of worth are continually placed upon the person, growth will be thwarted and there will be a tendency toward dysfunctional ways of living in the world. Humanists believe that the individual can change at any point in his or her life if placed in a supportive environment. Finally, postmodernists and social constructionists view reality as being socially constructed through language and organized and maintained through narratives. Therefore, they believe abnormal behavior to be socially constructed such that there are no essential truths and that individuals can change through dialogue with others.

If one believes that there are deviant behaviors, then it is natural to want to classify them. This is what diagnosis achieves. The chapter offered a brief history of DSM and then described DSM-5, the major diagnostic classification system for emotional disorders, as well as some of the advantages and disadvantages of DSM. We noted that the DSM-5 has moved away from the multiaxial system used to describe and communicate mental disorders of DSM-IV-TR and now uses a single-axis system. However, we noted that medical conditions and psychosocial and environmental stressors can be listed alongside mental disorders, and mentioned that the DSM-5 has increased the number of "V codes" ("Z codes" in the ICD-10), which are often reflective of psychosocial and environmental issues, and that the DSM-5 has done away with the GAF scale found in DSM-IV-TR. In addition, the chapter pointed out that mental retardation (now called *intellectual disabilities*) and personality disorders were collapsed into the same axis as all other disorders with the hope that this will reduce the stigma they received by being on a separate axis and remove the misguided belief that personality disorders were largely untreatable.

As we continued to discuss DSM-5, we pointed out that in the diagnostic process, a specific ordering system is used that lists the major disorder first, that subtypes, specifiers, and severity codes help distinguish diagnoses, and that sometimes a specific form of provisional diagnosis will be used (e.g., rule-out, traits, by history, and by self-report). We then went on to offer very brief descriptions of the twenty-two broad diagnostic categories and their subtypes.

If an accurate diagnosis is made, then treatment planning becomes easier, one aspect of which may be the use of psychotropic medication. Thus, the chapter examined five classes of drugs often used in the treatment of a wide range of emotional disorders. They included the antipsychotics, mood-stabilizing drugs, antidepressants, antianxiety agents, and stimulants. A brief history of the use of various psychopharmacological agents was provided, along with descriptions of some of the major psychotropic medications currently in use.

Near the end of the chapter, we explored how DSM-5 addresses cultural sensitivity and noted that some have argued that although diagnosis can be helpful in treatment planning, it can lead to the misdiagnosis of culturally oppressed groups. The APA has attempted to combat some of these problems by asking clinicians to understand and acknowledge "culturally patterned differences in symptoms" and that it offers a section entitled "Cultural Formulation Interview (CFI)," which helps clinicians understand the kinds of values, experiences, and influences that have come to shape the client's worldview and provides an outline for how to appropriately interview clients from diverse backgrounds.

As the chapter continued, it highlighted a number of ethical issues addressed in ACA's ethical code that spoke to the potential misuse and abuse of diagnosis, including the importance of making a proper diagnosis, being culturally sensitive relative to diagnosis, knowing the historical and social prejudices related to diagnosis, and the right to refrain from making a diagnosis.

Moving on to professional issues, we noted how diagnosis is viewed by some as a way to legitimize the oppression of minorities and those who are labeled mentally ill. The text reviewed the ideas of Thomas Szasz, William Glasser, Carl Rogers, and R. D. Laing and noted that they all refused to use the term *mental illness*, stating that it tends to depersonalize and oppress the individual. We also highlighted Ivey and Ivey's work on trying to understand diagnosis from a developmental perspective and Corey's points concerning why we all should be careful when making diagnoses. Next, the discussion raised a final professional issue to ponder—to diagnose or not diagnose. We noted that there are two polar opposites relative to diagnosis—the belief in the medical model and the efficacy of diagnosis or the belief that cross-cultural problems and the complexity of human beings makes it very difficult to diagnosis. We pointed out that most counselors are probably in the middle and warned counselors to not get locked into one extreme position

This chapter also discussed two legal issues. First, it noted that it is no longer easy to confine a person in a mental institution against his or her will. Today, evidence that a person is in danger of harming self or others, or is gravely ill, must be presented if a person is to be committed for a short period of time. We also discussed the importance of making an accurate diagnosis, of being honest with clients and insurance companies about diagnoses, and of being careful not to commit insurance fraud by changing a diagnosis in order to be reimbursed. Finally, the chapter ended with a brief consideration of the impaired graduate student and whether counseling programs should view students such as this as incapable of change and therefore problematic for continuation in a program.

Further Practice

Visit CengageBrain.com to respond to additional material that highlight the salient aspects of the chapter content. There, you can find ethical, professional, and legal vignettes, a number of experiential exercises, and study tools including a glossary, flashcards, and sample test items. Hopefully, these will enhance your learning and be fun and interesting.

Career Development: The Counselor and the World of Work

My father was a building contractor. When I was young, he used to take me to various construction sites, and I would watch buildings slowly being built. As a teenager, during the summers, I assisted a carpenter or laborer at the sites. I remember getting picked up at five-thirty in the morning, sitting cramped and half-asleep in the cab of a well-seasoned truck, to be taken on a bumpy ride to work. I would think to myself, "Is this what I want to do for the rest of my life?" However, because I did well in school, I knew I'd be going on to college; but to do what?

Majoring in biology and thinking that I would not be accepted to medical school, I chose dentistry as my eventual occupational choice. My mind was made up, I thought. But something did not feel right. Although a part of me said, "Go to dental school," another distant voice said, "This is not for you—you have other things to do in your life, other things that involve helping people in other ways." These divergent feelings and thoughts were certainly an outgrowth of many things, including my family values, placement in my family, my interests, my own emerging values, and my abilities.

Although it was a tough decision, I eventually chose to listen to my inner voice, and I switched my major to psychology. Eventually, through trial and (occasional) error, I ended up in the field of counseling. No doubt my life would have been made somewhat easier if I had had the benefit of a career counselor who could have helped me assess my likes and dislikes, my values, and my abilities; helped me understand my personality; facilitated self-knowledge and self-reflection; and assisted me in applying all of this knowledge to my career development journey.

As I proceeded in my career, I continued to face a number of choices. Should I go on for a doctoral degree? Should I go toward clinical work or academia? Should I change career paths totally? Again, my choices often seemed to be a product of trial and error. I would try something out to see if I liked it and if I was good at it, and would then make a decision about my future career direction. However, as I gained more awareness and began more fully to understand the career development process, I saw that I could choose my own direction in life if I had adequate knowledge of myself and knowledge of the world of work. No longer would my career decision making be an accident. I began to choose my future!

Despite the fact that I have been pretty satisfied with my chosen occupation, there were times when my life did not feel complete. Therefore, other activities began to fill in some of the empty spaces. In my mid-twenties, I began to jog. As the years continued, running and other workout routines became a focal point in my life. They offered an outlet for my stress, a place for me to meet other people, and an activity that took me away from my work. In my early forties, I married, and soon after, I became a father. As new life roles emerged, I found that I had to balance my roles of professor, clinician, exerciser, and writer with those of husband and father. Now, as my children grow and leave the home, and as I near the twilight of my career,

I wonder—did I do all right? Was I a good father and husband? Was I productive in my job, and what, if any, positive impact have I had on others?

My story, with its twists and turns, is fairly common. People tend to haphazardly go through life without the benefit of guidance, sometimes intuitively moving in the direction that serves them best. However, many times, people are unhappy with their jobs and other life roles. If afforded the opportunity for career counseling, many would have an easier time in their journey through life. They would be able to make smart occupational and life choices. That is why this chapter is so important. It explains the career development process, its importance to life satisfaction, and the role of the counselor in facilitating career development.

This chapter will survey the career development process and specifically examine how individuals make career choices, the meaning of work in people's lives, the major theories of career development, and some of the career information systems available. It concludes by examining multicultural and social justice issues related to career development, and ethical, professional, and legal issues in the realm of career development.

Some Definitions

The career development process is perhaps the most misunderstood counseling-related subject. Therefore, it is particularly important to start out with some basic definitions. The following definitions, synthesized from several prominent authors, are terms related to the career development process (Brown, 2012; Greenhaus & Callanan, 2006; Herr, Cramer, & Niles, 2004; Sharf, 2013). Keep in mind that some of these definitions may not be the same as the common, lay definitions of these terms:

➤ *Avocation.* A chosen activity that is pursued by an individual because it gives satisfaction and fulfills an important aspect of the person's life. It may or may not be income-generating.
➤ *Career.* The totality of work and life roles through which an individual expresses himself or herself. It may include work, leisure, and avocational activities.
➤ *Career awareness.* One's consciousness about career-related decisions, which can be facilitated through self-examination of one's values, abilities, preferences, knowledge of occupations and life roles, and interests.
➤ *Career development.* All of the psychological, sociological, educational, physical, economic, and other factors that are at play in shaping one's career over the life span.
➤ *Career counseling.* Individual or group counseling with a focus on increasing career awareness and fostering decision making relative to career goals.
➤ *Career guidance.* A program, designed by counselors, that offers information concerning career development and facilitates career awareness for individuals.
➤ *Career path.* The sequence of positions and jobs that typically signifies potential advancement.
➤ *Job.* Specific work tasks that one is responsible for accomplishing.
➤ *Leisure.* Time taken from required effort (e.g., job or occupation) in order to pursue self-chosen activities that express one's abilities and interests.

➤ *Occupations.* Jobs of a similar nature that can be found within several work environments and connote the kinds of work a person is pursuing.
➤ *Work.* Effort expended at a job, occupation, or avocation in order to produce or accomplish something.

Is Career Development Developmental?

You might be wondering why a chapter on career development is included in a section on human development. In fact, career development can be considered developmental because it examines the career decision-making process of an individual as it unfolds through distinct stages. Unfortunately, I find that when most people think about career development, they often think that it is just a process of finding a job. In actuality, it is much more than that. In fact, career development includes all of the following:

➤ The 3-year-old who plays house or hammers a peg into a hole
➤ The 5-year-old who joins a T-ball league
➤ The 10-year-old inner-city youth who has few positive role models
➤ The 12-year-old who begins to examine his or her abilities, likes, and dislikes
➤ The 14-year-old who suddenly discovers that her parents are getting divorced
➤ The 17-year-old who considers what college to go to, and the 17-year-old who ponders what job to take after high school
➤ The 25-year-old who takes a new job and also leads an aerobics class
➤ The 30-year-old who gives up a full-time job to do child care
➤ The 37-year-old who is promoted and is vice president of the local PTA
➤ The 45-year-old who hates her job but continues to work at it to make money while maintaining an exciting hobby on the side
➤ The 50-year-old who wonders, "Is this all there is?"
➤ The 60-year-old who ponders whether she should retire in a couple of years
➤ The 70-year-old who never worked, has raised a family, and has become a fairly good tournament bridge player
➤ The 85-year-old who reflects back on his various life roles

Our career development is expressed through the jobs, occupations, leisure activities, and avocations we have chosen throughout our lifespan (Ethridge, Burnhill, & Dong, 2009; NCDA, 2008). Most important, it is how we experience ourselves in all of our life roles. It is affected by the kinds of messages we received from our parents, from our community, from our religious affiliation, and from society. It is ongoing, ever-transforming, and doesn't end until we die.

Why Career Development and Career Counseling?

I hope that by now, you see that career development is not just the process of finding a job, but the development of all of our various life roles and the factors that go into shaping them. It is reflected in how we express our identity through the roles we choose. Career counseling helps an individual navigate the career development process. Thus, career counseling is helping the 3-year-old develop a sense of self, assisting the 12-year-old in understanding what she is good at and what she likes, helping the 17-year-old choose a college or a job, helping a client weigh the relative importance of being a parent and working at a job, assisting a person through a midlife crisis, helping an individual as she readies for retirement, and reminiscing with an older person about his life. Career counseling helps to raise a person's awareness about the choices he or she is making in life.

Adequate career counseling can assist us in making smart choices around our work and other life roles. The work we choose is a large part of the career development process and serves interpersonal needs, psychological needs, family needs, and societal needs (Herr et al., 2004) (see Figure 11.1). Numerous studies show that career planning and career counseling are related to job satisfaction and positive mental health (Duffy, Bott, Allan, Torrey, & Dik, 2012; Lent & Brown, 2013a; Rehfuss, Gambrell, & Meyer, 2012; Verbruggen & Sels, 2010).

It is not a big leap to realize that adequate career planning and career counseling can help us feel better about our lives. This is why career counseling is so vital to facilitating a client's career development.

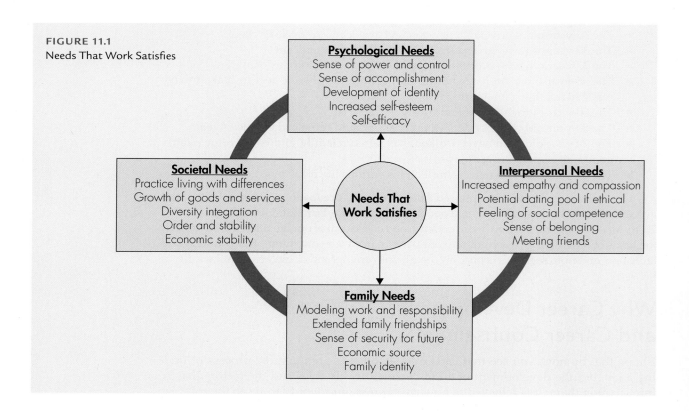

FIGURE 11.1
Needs That Work Satisfies

Psychological Needs
Sense of power and control
Sense of accomplishment
Development of identity
Increased self-esteem
Self-efficacy

Societal Needs
Practice living with differences
Growth of goods and services
Diversity integration
Order and stability
Economic stability

Needs That Work Satisfies

Interpersonal Needs
Increased empathy and compassion
Potential dating pool if ethical
Feeling of social competence
Sense of belonging
Meeting friends

Family Needs
Modeling work and responsibility
Extended family friendships
Sense of security for future
Economic source
Family identity

A Little Bit of History

The counseling profession owes its existence to *vocational guidance*. At the turn of the twentieth century, on the heels of the Industrial Revolution, there came many demographic changes throughout the United States. Almost overnight, there was a large influx of people who moved from rural areas to the cities, an increased number of immigrants who settled mostly in urban areas, and, with this, a large increase in the number of children in city schools. Shifts in the types of available jobs were evident, as was the need to assist these new city dwellers and students in their vocational development.

One of the first persons credited with developing a systematic approach to vocational guidance was Frank Parsons (Briddick, 2009a; McDaniels & Watts, 1994). As noted in Chapter 2, Parsons envisioned systematic vocational guidance in the schools, a national vocational guidance movement, and the importance of counseling to assist individuals in their vocational development (Briddick, 2009b; Jones, 1994). Parsons, a humanitarian and social justice advocate, later became known as the founder of vocational guidance, and he suggested that vocational guidance involved a three-step process that included knowing oneself, knowing job characteristics, and making a match between the two through *true reasoning* (Parsons, 1909/2009; Pope & Sveinsdottir, 2005). Realizing the importance of vocational guidance, others jumped on the bandwagon. Individuals like Jesse Davis in Grand Rapids, Michigan, Eli Weaver in New York City, and Anna Reed in Seattle established guidance services in their respective school systems (Aubrey, 1977).

In 1932, during the midst of the Depression, the *Wagner O'Day Act* was passed. It established the U.S. Employment Service, which provided vocational guidance for the unemployed. Also around this time, the testing movement began to spread. The merging of vocational guidance with testing formed a natural partnership because assessment offered a relatively quick and reliable means of determining individual traits. It was also during this time frame that the U.S. Department of Labor published the *Dictionary of Occupational Titles (DOT)*, which represented one of the first attempts at organizing career information. Now, individuals could assess their traits and match them to existing jobs.

The 1950s was the beginning of an explosion of career development theories. For instance, it was at this time that Ann Roe developed her classification system of career counseling, which promoted the idea that early childhood experiences were responsible for later career choices. Other theories began to broaden the concept of career to include such things as leisure activities, avocations, occupations, and postvocational patterns related to retiring. One theory, proposed by a team composed of an economist, a sociologist, a psychiatrist, and a psychologist (Ginzberg, Ginsburg, Axelrad, & Herma, 1951; Ginzberg, 1972), and a second theory, developed by Donald Super (Super, 1953, 1957), were instrumental in transforming the static vocational guidance model, which viewed career choice as a moment in time decision, into a model that viewed career development as a lifelong process (Hershenson, 2009).

With the emergence of humanistic approaches to counseling as well as government initiatives such as the *National Defense Education Act (NDEA)*, which stressed career guidance in the schools, new comprehensive models of career guidance were developed in the 1960s and 1970s. These models viewed career guidance broadly and included (1) focusing on lifelong patterns of career development; (2) assisting individuals in making choices that reflected their sense of self; (3) examining leisure and avocational activities when working with clients; (4) viewing career development as a flexible and changeable process as compared to the rigid, irreversible process of earlier times; and (5) emphasizing the individual, not the counselor, as the career decision maker (Herr et al., 2004). During the 1970s, we also saw the emergence of John Holland's personality theory of career counseling, which examined the importance of how an individual's personality "fit" into differing work environments.

The 1980s and 1990s expanded the notion that career development was a lifelong process in which counselors could assist individuals in defining their life roles. As the 1990s unfolded, the computer age took firm hold, delivering a wealth of accessible information that allowed quick exploration of the world of work. The evolution of career development models in conjunction with this new technology made career exploration an exciting and in-depth process. In recent years, we saw the expansion of some of the earlier models of career development, as well as the addition of some newer models, including *social cognitive career theory* and *constructivist theory*, which increasingly looked at how an individual develops a sense of self relative to his or her career. Recently, we have seen authors attempt to integrate many of these various career development models.

Today, career guidance and career counseling are important components of what all counselors do. This is one of the reasons that career and lifespan development has been selected by CACREP as one of the eight content areas that all counseling students must learn in graduate school.

Theories of Career Development

Before Phrenology [the study of the shape and size of the cranium] was known, there was no means of determining, with any degree of certainty, what might be the character, disposition, and talents of any stranger who should be presented.

(Sizer, 1872, pp. 382–383)

Although career counseling theories likely can be traced to the phrenologists of the nineteenth century (Hershenson, 2008), I doubt that today, one can find a career counselor who relied on the shape and size of the bumps of the cranium when doing career counseling! However, there are many theories of career development today that do help counselors understand how the client has come to approach the world of work and provide a framework for devising strategies to assist clients in their career search (see Sharf, 2013). Although this text cannot go into all of the theories, we will explore some of those that have been highlighted in the literature, including modern-day *trait-and-factor theory*, Roe's *psychodynamic theory*, Holland's *personality theory of occupational choice*, Super's *lifespan development theory*, *social cognitive career theory*, and *constructivist career counseling*. The section, "Integatrating Models of Career Development," later in this chapter, will demonstrate how these theories can be combined when conducting career counseling.

Trait-and-Factor Approach

The *trait-and-factor approach*, which grew out of the early work of Frank Parsons, was the major career development theory for many years, maintaining its popularity until the 1950s (Blustein, 2006; Gysbers et al., 2009). Originally, this approach was a straight-forward process that involved the counselor assisting the client in assessing his or her strengths, examining the availability of jobs, and using a rational process to make career decisions. Largely focusing on assessment of ability and interests, this approach tended to be didactic and directive.

Although trait-and-factor theory has maintained its emphasis on the importance of a fit between the individual and the environment, the application of current-day trait-and-factor theory looks very different than it did years ago. The following summarizes some of the important principles held by current-day trait-and-factor theorists (Herr et al., 2004; Niles & Bowlsbey, 2013; Sharf, 2013):

1. Individuals have unique traits that can be measured, discussed, and examined. Some of these include aptitudes, needs and interests, values, stereotypes and expectations, psychological adjustment, the propensity to take risks, and aspirations.
2. Occupations require individuals to have certain traits if they are to be successful.
3. The better the ability of the individual to match his or her traits to occupations, the greater the likelihood that the individual will succeed and feel satisfied.
4. The interaction between client and therapist is a dynamic process that includes both affective and cognitive components.
5. The ability of an individual to match his or her traits with occupations is a conscious process that can occur in a deliberate fashion. However, such matching can be effective only if a person has insight into self and knowledge of his or her unique traits and the sociological factors that may affect potential decisions.
6. Cultural values are important when conducting career counseling (e.g., interaction between client and counselor) and affect the success of the individual on the job (how the person sees self and is viewed by others at work).

Today's trait-and-factor counselor does not simply match abilities and interests with jobs, but uses a variety of techniques to examine how the vast array of the client's skills, interests, and personality variables might affect eventual career choices. This is done in a dynamic manner in which the counselor, through the use of modern-day counseling techniques, facilitates client understanding of self and assists the client in making decisive career choices.

Ann Roe's Psychodynamic Theory

In 1956, Ann Roe developed a rather elaborate theory that based career choice on the kinds of early parenting received (Roe, 1956). Roe hypothesized that parents can be classified as either *warm* or *cold,* and that these two styles result in one of three types of *emotional climates: emotional concentration on the child, acceptance of the child,* or *avoidance of the child* (see Figure 11.2). The type of emotional climate in the home will result in one of six types of parent–child relationships, which, often unconsciously, influences the kinds of occupational choices the child will eventually make (Roe & Siegelman, 1964). Parenting style, said Roe, ultimately results in the individual having one of the following eight orientations toward the world of work: *service* (I), *business* (II), *organization* (III), *technology* (IV), *outdoor* (V), *science* (VI), *general culture* (VII), and *arts and entertainment* (VIII) (see Figure 11.2).

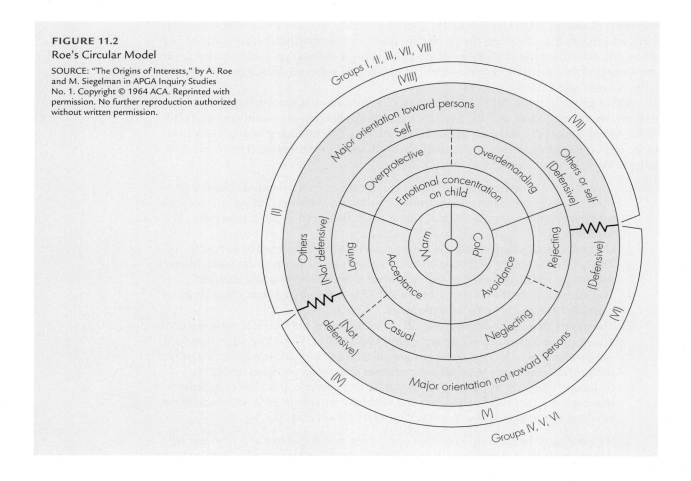

Although research has not borne this out, Roe suggested that parenting styles lead to the different orientations noted in Figure 11.2. The following briefly describes them (Sharf, 2013):

1. *Protective.* Parents are indulgent and restrict exploring and curiosity, and children are dependent. Occupational areas: service (I), arts or entertainment (VIII) fields.
2. *Demanding.* Parents expect excellence and high expectations. Occupations: general culture, such as lawyers, teachers, scholars, and librarians (VII) or to the arts and entertainment fields (VIII).
3. *Rejecting.* Nonaccepting parents who withhold love from and criticize their children. Occupation: science-related fields (VI).
4. *Neglecting.* Parents ignore their children and give little positive or negative attention. Occupations: outdoor interests (V) and science (VI).
5. *Casual.* Low-key parents who give minimal attention to their children after their needs are attended to. Occupations: technological occupations (engineers,

aviators, applied scientists) (IV) or organizational occupations (bankers, accountants, clerks) (III).

6. *Loving.* Warm, caring, helpful, and affectionate parents who are not intrusive. Occupations: service (I) or business-contact occupations (promoters, salespersons) (II).

Although Roe's approach is rarely talked about these days as an important career counseling theory, her focus on such factors as parenting styles, the unconscious, gender issues, and societal factors such as the economy (Brown, Lum, & Voyle, 1997; Herr et al., 2004; Sharf, 2013) set a tone that counselors should be doing more than simply matching one's traits with available jobs. Today, when a counselor conducts career counseling, all of these factors should be considered in helping the individual understand his or her orientation to the world of work.

John Holland's Personality Theory of Occupational Choice

John Holland's (1919–2008) theory of occupational choice proposes that people express their personality through their career choices (Holland, 1973; Holland & Gottfredson, 1976). Considered both a personality theory and a trait-and-factor theory (Spokane, Luchetta, & Richwine, 2002; Swanson & Schneider, 2013), Holland's theory suggests that genetic and environmental influences lead people to develop "a hierarchy of habitual or preferred methods for dealing with social and environmental tasks" (Herr et al., 2004, p. 211). In essence, Holland suggested that if individuals could identify their unique personality styles, they could find a job that best fits their personality and ultimately find satisfaction in their careers. Identifying six personality types, Holland stated that each type represents a way that a person relates to the world and assigned each type a name that reflected its general personality style, including *realistic, investigative, artistic, social, enterprising,* and *conventional* (RIASEC) (see Box 11.1). Holland believed there were numerous occupations that could fit each individual's personality type and ability level.

Although one can be a pure type (i.e., their personality is almost exclusively one type), it is more usual for an individual to have two or more types that dominate. By listing an individual's top three types in order of preference, we can find what is called one's *occupational code,* often referred to as one's *Holland Code.* Holland conducted research that supported the notion that the six personality types could be viewed on a hexagon, with adjacent types sharing more common elements than nonadjacent ones (see Figure 11.3). Generally, an individual's predominant type and secondary types are close to one another on the hexagon. For instance, if an individual was highest in the social type, then it would not be surprising if the artistic and enterprising types were also high because they are next to the social type on the hexagon.

Holland also asserted that jobs could be classified by type. Thus, he hypothesized that if you accurately matched an individual's code to a job that has the same code, you increase your chances of having a person who is satisfied at the job and ultimately in his or her career. For instance, the individual with the SAE code could be matched with the occupation "counselor," which has the same corresponding code. Research on the Holland Codes, which has been plentiful, has shown that accurate matches indeed increase the chances for job satisfaction (Ohler & Levinson, 2012). Keep in mind, however, that there are many other SAE choices besides counselor.

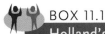

BOX 11.1

Holland's Personality and Work Types

Realistic: Realistic persons like to work with equipment, machines, or tools, often prefer to work outdoors, and are good at manipulating concrete physical objects. These individuals prefer to avoid social situations, artistic endeavors, or intellectual tasks. Some settings in which you might find realistic individuals include filling stations, farms, machine shops, construction sites, and power plants.

Investigative: Investigative persons like to think abstractly, solve problems, and investigate. These individuals feel comfortable pursuing knowledge and manipulating ideas and symbols. Investigative individuals prefer to avoid social situations and see themselves as introverted. Some settings in which you might find investigative individuals include research laboratories, hospitals, universities, and government-sponsored research agencies.

Artistic: Artistic individuals like to express themselves creatively, usually through artistic forms such as drama, art, music, and writing. They prefer unstructured activities in which they can use their imagination and creative side. Some settings in which you might find artistic individuals include theaters, concert halls, libraries, art or music studios, dance studios, orchestras, photography studios, newspapers, and restaurants.

Social: Social people are nurturers, helpers, and caregivers and have great concern for others. They are introspective

and insightful and prefer work environments in which they can use their intuitive and caregiving skills. Some settings in which you might find social people are government social service agencies, counseling offices, churches, schools, mental hospitals, recreation centers, personnel offices, and hospitals.

Enterprising: Enterprising individuals are self-confident, adventurous, bold, and sociable. They have good persuasive skills and prefer positions of leadership. They tend to dominate conversations and enjoy work environments in which they can satisfy their need for recognition, power, and expression. Some settings in which you might find enterprising individuals include life insurance agencies, advertising agencies, political offices, real estate offices, new and used car lots, sales offices, and management positions.

Conventional: Individuals of the conventional orientation are stable, controlled, conservative, and sociable. They prefer working on concrete tasks and like to follow instructions. They value the business world and clerical tasks and tend to be good at computational skills. Some settings in which you might find conventional people include banks, business offices, accounting firms, and medical records offices.

FIGURE 11.3
Holland's Hexagon Model

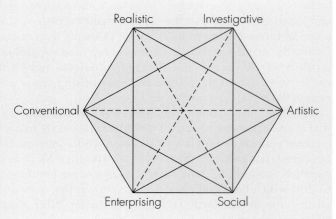

Holland and others have worked hard to identify the codes that best represent various jobs. For instance, Gottfredson and Holland (1996) identified the occupational codes for more than 12,000 jobs and published these codes in the *Dictionary of Holland Occupational Codes*. By taking one or more of a number of assessment instruments such as the *Strong Interest Inventory* (CPP, 2004, 2009a) or the *Self-Directed Search* (PAR, 2013), an individual can determine his or her Holland Code and then match it with occupational codes. If you want to get a sense of what your Holland Code is, review Box 11.1 and pick your top three codes. Then put them in order based on your subjective ranking (for me, it would be "SIA"). This would be your code. Through the use of the *Dictionary of Holland Occupational Codes*, the O*NET website (discussed later in this chapter), and other related tools, your code can be cross-referenced with the various kinds of jobs that match that code.

Holland's theory has been used extensively by career counselors, and it is to his credit that numerous assessment instruments to determine one's code have been developed. In addition, research has consistently shown the importance of the Holland theory when working with clients to achieve job satisfaction. John Holland has certainly added much to career counseling.

Super's Lifespan Development Approach to Career Counseling

During the 1950s, Donald Super drew from a number of developmental models to come up with his lifespan approach to career choice. This approach, which quickly gained in popularity, involves an individual passing through a series of sequential and predictable stages. Initially known as a *developmental self-concept theory*, Super's theory (1953, 1957, 1976, 1990; Super & Hall, 1978; Super, Savickas, & Super, 1996) contended the following:

1. Career development is an ongoing, continuous, and orderly process starting in early childhood and ending with death.
2. People's abilities, personality traits, and self-concepts differ, and individuals are qualified for a number of different types of occupations based on their characteristics.
3. Occupations tend to be specifically appropriate for people with certain kinds of qualities, although there is enough variability in occupations to allow for some differences in the kinds of people who will be drawn to them.
4. Self-concept is both a function and result of one's career development process and can change as one passes through developmental stages.
5. Movement from one occupational level to another is influenced by a number of factors, including parental socioeconomic level, status needs, values, interests, skill in interpersonal relationships, economic conditions, and intelligence.
6. Starting in early childhood and continuing into late adulthood, career development can be assisted by helping individuals understand and develop their abilities and interests and by assisting them in understanding their strengths and weaknesses.
7. By understanding the developmental level of the individual, counselors can make appropriate interventions that can assist individuals in learning about themselves

and their career development process, thus making occupational choices more likely to lead to satisfaction at work and a high self-concept.

8. Career development is generally irreversible, although some people who face important developmental crises may recycle through the stages at any point in their career.

Super (1990; Super, et al., 1996) saw career development as a five-stage process, with each stage having substages distinguished by unique developmental tasks (see Figure 11.4). During the *growth stage* (ages birth through 14 years), children identify with others, gain an awareness of interests and abilities, and begin to develop a career self-concept. Included in this stage is the very young child becoming aware of the world of work and the middle school youth comparing his or her abilities and interests to those of peers. In the *exploration stage* (ages 14–25), adolescents and young adults begin to tentatively test their occupational fantasies through work, school, and leisure activities. Later in this stage, individuals begin to *crystallize* their vocational preferences by choosing an

FIGURE 11.4
Super's Stages and Substages

SOURCE: Donald E. Super, *New Dimension in Adult Vocational and Career Counseling* (Columbus, Ohio: The Center on Education and Training for Employment [formerly NCRVE], The Ohio State University). Copyright 1985. Used with permission.

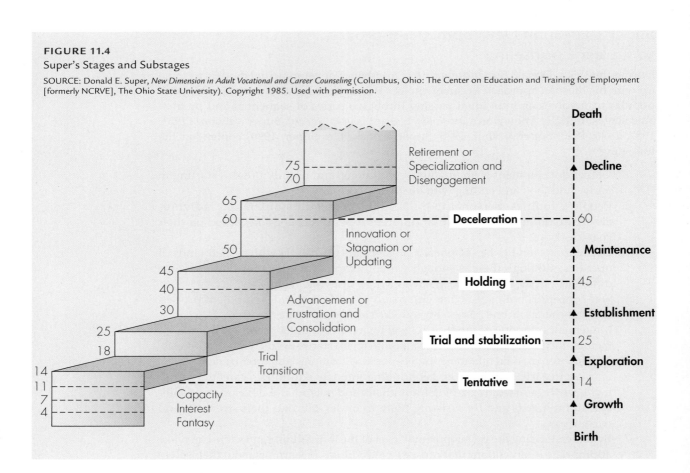

occupation or further professional training. The *establishment stage* (ages 25–45) involves stabilizing career choices and advancing in chosen fields, while the *maintenance stage* (ages 45–60) encompasses the preservation of one's current status in the choices made and avoidance of stagnation. During the *decline stage* (ages 60 and over—sometimes called the *disengagement stage*), people begin to disengage from their chosen fields and increasingly focus on retirement, leisure, and avocational activities.

If counselors are going to design effective strategies that will work with clients, they should be familiar with each stage and substage so that they can tailor their techniques to the particular tasks unique to that developmental milestone. For instance, an elementary school counselor would be foolish to assist a child in making specific career choices, and a college counselor would be remiss to encourage a college student to become established quickly in a career.

Super's developmental approach has added an important dimension to the understanding of the career development process by making us aware of the universal developmental tasks that people face throughout their lifetimes.

Social Cognitive Career Theory

> . . . SCCT highlights people's capacity to direct their own vocational behavior (human agency)—to assemble their own puzzle, so to speak—yet it also acknowledges the many personal and environmental influences (e.g., sociostructural barriers and supports, culture, disability status) that serve to strengthen, weaken, or in some cases, even override human agency in career development.
>
> (Lent, 2005, p. 102)

In recent years, *Social Cognitive Career Theory (SCCT)* has become one of the more popular theories of career development (Lent, 2013; Patton & McIlveen, 2009). SCCT pulls together ideas from a number of career development concepts. Anchored in self-efficacy theory (Sharf, 2013), SCCT states that the types of choices we make are based on our current beliefs about whether we can perform certain behaviors (Albert & Luzzo, 1999; Bandura, 1997). However, SCCT suggests that self-efficacy is related to our family experiences (e.g., what we're told we're good at), sociological influences (e.g., discrimination, mobility, sexism, and the economy), our abilities and aptitudes, our interests, our sense of our personality style (e.g., the kinds of work environments we seem to fit into most comfortably), and the goals we have in life.

SCCT suggests that individuals are affected by *objective factors* and *perceived environmental factors* (Johnson, 2013; Lent, Brown, & Hackett, 2002). For instance, economic hardship, educational experiences, and societal factors (e.g., societal values around gender, culture, disability status, etc.) can all affect the kinds of choices available to a person. However, an individual's perceptions of environmental factors can also affect career decisions. For instance, discrimination may legitimately affect the ability of an individual to obtain a certain job. However, perceived discrimination (as opposed to discrimination that actually exists) may prevent one person from obtaining a job, but it may not affect another person from the same minority group from acquiring the same job. SCCT therefore examines how objective and perceived factors shape an individual's self-efficacy. The example of very different responses by two individuals faced with the same objective factors suggests the important role a phenomenological perspective (understanding the unique worldview of the client) plays in SCCT (Lent et al., 2002).

SCCT has particular implications for the counselor's role in working with clients by affecting their environment while simultaneously working on their belief system. For instance, high school counselors can work with teachers to help them understand that their beliefs about their students, and how those beliefs become translated behaviorally (whom they pick to respond in class, nonverbal messages sent to students, and so on), can affect how students view themselves. Embedded, often unconscious racist beliefs about the inability of some minority groups to achieve can be counteracted by counselors doing workshops for teachers and helping them see how they have held such beliefs and the importance of believing and behaving in ways that give all students the message that they can achieve. Simultaneously, counselors can work with students to effect change in their beliefs about themselves. Students who have not been supported by significant others in their academic pursuits often need such direct support. Girls and boys who have been reinforced for gender and social stereotypes that might negatively affect their career choices can have their horizons broadened.

Like school counselors, counselors working in agencies or college settings can influence the ways in which young adults and adults view themselves and direct them toward a broader understanding of the world of work. In addition, they can advocate for social change by working to break down societal barriers that some clients might face (e.g., discrimination). SCCT theory has wide implications for the greater society, as it potentially can break many of the stereotypes and beliefs that individuals hold about themselves and the beliefs we all hold about one another relative to the world of work.

Constructivist Career Counseling: A Postmodern Approach

Career construction theory, through the power of narrative, addresses what, how, and why people construct their careers as they translate their storied identity into work roles.

(Del Corso & Rehfuss, 2011, p. 335)

Another relatively recent addition to career development theory has been promulgated by *constructivist theorists*, who believe that career decision making is related to how clients "construct" or make meaning of their career process (Gysbers et al., 2009; Hutchison & Niles, 2009; Schultheiss, 2007). In the *postmodern* tradition, these theorists do not believe that reality is fixed or that there is one "correct" path for any individual (Sharf, 2013). Instead, they believe that knowing about self in relationship to career is an ongoing, active process that can change as the individual interacts with others and sees new aspects of self. They believe that reality shifts based on conversations that people have with others. They also suggest that narratives in society, disseminated by people in positions of power (usually the "majority"), become part of the reality of society and often result in the oppression of minorities and women.

One method that constructivists often rely on in an effort to unravel the client's meaning-making system is the narrative, or life story (Bujold, 2002; Del Corso & Rehfuss, 2011). By hearing the client's narrative, one can obtain a sense of where the client has come from, where he or she is now, and how the client is thinking about the future. *Dominant narratives* often drive how a person acts in the world and can sometimes be destructive. "I can't do statistics because I could never do it and because girls are not good at statistics" can be related to narratives in the client's life, stories in society about women doing math, and may have nothing to do with the "reality" of an individual's ability at statistics. Such narratives can be deconstructed, and new stories can be constructed through dialogue with the counselor and others.

Constructivists argue that most career development theories do not explain changes in an individual's cognitive functioning over the lifespan. They suggest that an individual's unique meaning-making—or ways in which an individual comes to "know" the world—changes as he or she experiences the world. By meeting with clients and hearing their narratives, counselors can both understand clients' unique meaning-making systems and develop conversations with them to foster new possibilities for the decisions that a person makes relative to his or her career. When meeting with clients, counselors will often ask questions and show respectful curiosity in trying to understand the narratives that drive a person and the other narratives in a person's life that they may not have been particularly aware of.

Some of the basic goals of the counselor when applying this approach include:

1. Trying to understand the client's sense of his or her career self by listening to the client's narratives, or life stories
2. Helping clients, through conversation, understand the dominant narratives that drive their lives and push them to certain career-related decisions
3. Helping clients identify career-related dominant narratives that are detrimental to their lives
4. Helping clients deconstruct negative career-related dominant narratives and develop new, positive narratives that can offer better career choices
5. Understanding that there are barriers in society, created through language, that affect a large number of people, particularly oppressed groups, and influence how these individuals come to understand the world and the choices they have in the world of work
6. Focusing on changing dominant societal language and the resulting barriers that they create, which differentially affect minorities and women

Constructivist career development theory is an exciting new approach in which client growth is possible if the counselor is able to understand the unique ways that clients view the world, identify their dominant narratives, and help them develop new narratives that can expand client choices.

Integrating Models of Career Development

After examining the theories of career development in this chapter, you can see how varied they are in their approach to working with clients. In an attempt to pull positive components from all the approaches, many counselors integrate the various theories. Look at Angela (Box 11.2), and then let's examine how each theory discussed could offer a different and important perspective on her situation.

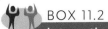

BOX 11.2
Integrating Career Development Theories: Angela

Angela is a 24-year-old African American in her first year of graduate school in counseling. Her mother, who is a school counselor, and her father, who is a head nurse, have both encouraged her to go into the counseling profession. Angela has a brother, John, who is two years older and going to medical school. She describes her relationship with her parents as loving, but sometimes a little overwhelming and claustrophobic. Angela lives at home and is beginning to feel frustrated because her parents continue to want to know where she is most of the time. Angela has done particularly well in school, especially in the sciences and math. In fact, while working toward her bachelor's degree, she switched majors her junior year from psychology to chemistry with the distant thought that, like her brother, maybe she too would go to medical school. Although Angela is doing well in her courses, she continues to have a "funny feeling" about being a counselor. Deep inside, she thinks that maybe she should be doing something else.

Trait-and-Factor Theory and Holland's Personality Theory

By using a modern day trait-and-factor approach, a counselor can have Angela take some interest inventories, personality measures, and ability tests that will help her to explore her traits, including her interests, aptitudes, values, and personality qualities. In addition, by using the trait-and-factor approach, the counselor can help Angela explore the stereotypes she holds about specific occupations, as well as her beliefs about the kinds of occupations she thinks she can do (e.g., self-efficacy). This approach can also help Angela examine the world of work and give her a better understanding of all the occupations that might fit her personality type (e.g., Holland), as well as the sociological factors that could affect her choices.

Developmental Theory

Angela is in the exploration stage of her career development process. A person in this stage usually wonders about the choices he or she has made and considers other options. Knowing this, when a counselor uses this approach, he or she might want to assure Angela that it is usual for young adults to be questioning their decisions. At the same time, it would be important for the counselor to understand the nature of Angela's doubts about her decision to be a counselor and help her explore these doubts. Ultimately, the goal of the career counselor who uses developmental theory would be to help Angela move toward a more stable position relative to whatever career-related decisions she makes.

Psychodynamic Theory (e.g., Roe)

The career counselor who employs a psychodynamic approach would assume that, in unconscious ways, Angela's parents have strongly influenced the kinds of career choices she has made. Having had loving parents who were somewhat overprotective and who are both in service occupations could push Angela toward a service occupation such as counseling (see Figure 11.2). However, one would not want to rule out many other service occupations. In addition, examining the kinds of early modeling and messages that she received from her parents and their general parenting style, as well as how that may have affected her personality development (e.g., dependency needs), can offer the counselor a wealth of information about Angela. Also, the counselor would want to examine Angela's position in her family and understand what it was like being the youngest in the family, the only daughter in the family, and the younger sister of a successful older brother.

Social Cognitive Career Theory

The career counselor who uses a social cognitive career approach is concerned about objective factors and perceived factors in building Angela's self-efficacy. This is especially important in that Angela seems to be interested in the sciences, and yet she is pursuing a field that she has a "funny feeling" about. In particular, the counselor might want to examine the kinds of messages that Angela has received from her parents and from society relative to her career choices. Sometimes, despite the fact that one does well in school, reinforcement for certain jobs may not occur due to stereotypes that teachers and others hold of African American students. For Angela, these stereotypes might have affected her perceived notions of what she can (and cannot) do in the world of work. The counselor might also want to look at blocks that have been put in Angela's way toward achieving in the medical field. For instance, have there been opportunities that have been missed because of her cultural background (e.g., not being chosen in class for special projects, not being told about certain "paths" to medical school, etc.)? Both perceived and objective factors have built Angela's self-efficacy, or belief in what she can and should do, all of which affect the choices she makes about her future.

Constructive Development Theory

From the constructivist perspective, the counselor wants to understand how Angela makes meaning out of her career decisions. Ultimately, the counselor wants to listen to the narratives, or stories, Angela tells herself relative to her career path. What dominant stories are driving her current decision to be a counselor, and are there other, nondominant stories, that present a different scenario for Angela? Whether these others stories can and should take on a more dominant role in Angela's life might be something for her to consider. Being respectfully curious, the counselor might ask such questions as:

- ➤ Tell me how you ended up pursuing a counseling degree.
- ➤ What factors affected your choices to go into counseling?
- ➤ What stories do you tell yourself about being a counselor?
- ➤ Are there specific memories you have about being a counselor? What are those?
- ➤ Are there other careers that you have fantasized about?
- ➤ Are there memories you have about pursuing a career in the medical field? What are those?
- ➤ What prevented you from pursuing these other careers?
- ➤ Do you think the stories you have about other careers would be important for you to explore?
- ➤ What do you think about focusing on the "other" stories rather than the dominant story of being a counselor?

Ultimately, Angela will want to look at her narratives and make a decision about which stories have dominated her life and which stories she wants to have dominating her life.

Bringing It All Together

As you can see, each theory offers a unique perspective about Angela; when used together, they can provide Angela the best opportunity to understand herself and make choices that would work best for her. As you can imagine, fully assisting Angela would take some time and would involve understanding that Angela is working through expected developmental struggles, exploring her past and the influences that it has had on her, assessing her lifespan developmental level, taking time to understand her present ways of making sense out of the world, assessing her traits, helping her examine opportunities that are available to her, understanding her self-efficacy, exploring stereotypes that may have influenced her, exploring her dominant and nondominant narratives, and assisting her in making a transition to a new way of perceiving the world. Indeed, we are not simply talking about finding Angela a job or changing her major, but helping Angela gain deep knowledge about herself so that she can make the wisest decisions for her life.

The Use of Career-Related Information

An extensive amount of occupational information is available in the field of career counseling and career development, which can assist clients in understanding the nature of work, increase client self-understanding, and help counselors understand their clients. This section will examine some of the more prevalent informational resources available. Keep in mind that these represent just a few of the many ways of obtaining information about the world of work.

Occupational Classification Systems

O*NET OnLine and O*NET Dictionary of Occupational Titles

The *Occupational Information Network (O*NET,* www.onetcenter.org) is an online database developed by the Department of Labor that provides a large array of worker attributes and job characteristics for approximately 1,000 occupations. A related, hardcopy resource called the *O*NET Dictionary of Occupational Titles* is also available (Farr & Shatkin, 2013).

O*NET OnLine replaces the *Dictionary of Occupational Titles (DOT),* which for years was the major occupational classification system of the Department of Labor and gave descriptions of approximately 13,000 occupations. Although far fewer occupations are listed in O*NET OnLine, the ones that are listed make up a large percentage of occupations in which you find Americans.

O*NET OnLine offers a much richer and more elaborate amount of occupational information than previous tools, such as the DOT. In addition, much of the information can be cross-referenced and examined from different perspectives, making the site a valuable resource for individuals involved with occupational exploration. Figure 11.5 is the content model from which O*NET is based. Each of the occupations listed in O*NET describes the different kinds of information listed in this model (for a detailed discussion, see http://www.onetcenter.org/content.html).

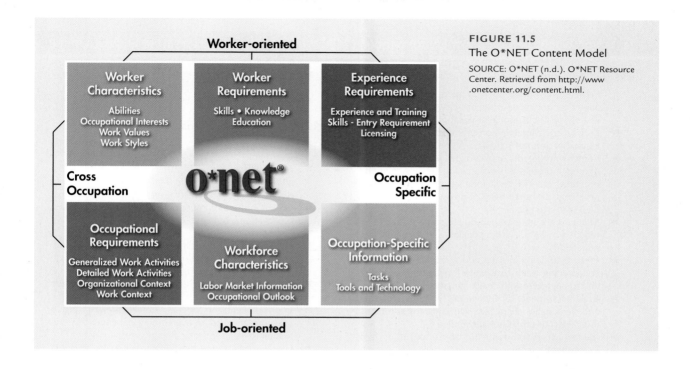

FIGURE 11.5
The O*NET Content Model

SOURCE: O*NET (n.d.). O*NET Resource Center. Retrieved from http://www.onetcenter.org/content.html.

Box 11.3 shows two items from the content model for school counselors and mental health counselors: "Job Tasks" and "Wages and Employment" (Labor Market Information) and offers a glimpse of the extensive information that O*Net offers.

The Guide for Occupational Exploration (GOE)

Originally published in 1979 as a companion volume to the DOT, the *Guide for Occupational Exploration (GOE)* recently underwent a major revision and now includes 16 *interest areas* (see Box 11.4) (Farr & Shatkin, 2006). The GOE lists approximately 900 occupations that are cross-referenced with the interest areas and work groups. Based on the O*NET system, the GOE includes such information as job descriptions, projected growth rate, education and training needed, values, skills, and working conditions. In addition, the GOE provides a mechanism to cross-reference interests, skills, values, and other elements to potential occupations.

The Occupational Outlook Handbook (OOH)

The Occupational Outlook Handbook (OOH) (U.S. Department of Labor, 2014, 2015) is an online and hard-copy "handbook," developed by the Department of Labor, that includes information on such items as the following for a few hundred popular occupations:

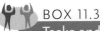

BOX 11.3
Tasks and Wages and Employment for School and Mental Health Counselors from O*NET Online

Tasks (School Counselor*)

➤ Counsel individuals to help them understand and overcome personal, social, or behavioral problems affecting their educational or vocational situations.

➤ Provide crisis intervention to students when difficult situations occur at schools.

➤ Confer with parents or guardians, teachers, administrators, and other professionals to discuss children's progress, resolve behavioral, academic, and other problems, and determine priorities for students and their resource needs.

➤ Maintain accurate and complete student records as required by laws, district policies, and administrative regulations.

➤ Prepare students for later educational experiences by encouraging them to explore learning opportunities and to persevere with challenging tasks.

➤ Evaluate students' or individuals' abilities, interests, and personality characteristics using tests, records, interviews, or professional sources.

➤ Identify cases of domestic abuse or other family problems and encourage students or parents to seek additional assistance from mental health professionals.

➤ Counsel students regarding educational issues, such as course and program selection, class scheduling and registration, school adjustment, truancy, study habits, and career planning.

➤ Provide special services, such as alcohol and drug prevention programs and classes that teach students to handle conflicts without resorting to violence.

➤ Conduct follow-up interviews with counselees to determine if their needs have been met.

Wages and Employment Trends (School Counselor)

➤ Median wages (2013): $25.77 hourly, $53,600 annual

➤ Employment (2012): 262,000 employees

➤ Projected growth (2012–2022): Faster than average (8–14%)

➤ Projected job openings (2012–2022): 87,000

Tasks (Mental Health Counselor)

➤ Maintain confidentiality of records relating to clients' treatment.

➤ Encourage clients to express their feelings and discuss what is happening in their lives, helping them to develop insight into themselves or their relationships.

➤ Collect information about clients through interviews, observations, or tests.

➤ Assess patients for risk of suicide attempts.

➤ Fill out and maintain client-related paperwork, including federal- and state-mandated forms, client diagnostic records, and progress notes.

➤ Prepare and maintain all required treatment records and reports.

➤ Counsel clients or patients, individually or in group sessions, to assist in overcoming dependencies, adjusting to life, or making changes.

➤ Guide clients in the development of skills or strategies for dealing with their problems.

➤ Perform crisis interventions with clients.

➤ Develop and implement treatment plans based on clinical experience and knowledge.

Wages and Employment Trends (Mental Health Counselor)

➤ Median wages (2013): 19.51 hourly, $40,580 annual

➤ Employment (2012): 128,000 employees

➤ Projected growth (2012–2022): Much faster than average (22% or higher)

➤ Projected job openings (2012–2022): 64,000

SOURCE: Retrieved June 2, 2014, from O*NET Online from "School Counselors" and "Mental Health Counselors."

* "School Counselor" can be found under Educational, Guidance, School, and Vocational Counselors.

median pay, entry-level education, work experience needed, if there is additional training needed to obtain the job, what is typically done by those in the occupation, the type of work setting, and other jobs similar to the job being described. If you want to find out some quick information on the occupation of "counselor," go to http://www.bls.gov /ooh/home.htm and enter "counselor" into the search engine. You might find some interesting facts!

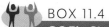

BOX 11.4
GOE's Sixteen Interest Areas

1. Agriculture and Natural Resources
2. Architecture and Construction
3. Arts and Communication
4. Business and Administration
5. Education and Training
6. Finance and Insurance
7. Government and Public Administration
8. Health Science
9. Hospitality, Tourism, and Recreation
10. Human Service
11. Information Technology
12. Law and Public Safety
13. Manufacturing
14. Retail and Wholesale Sales and Service
15. Scientific Research, Engineering, and Mathematics
16. Transportation, Distribution, and Logistics

Assessment Instruments

Interest Inventories

Over the years, a number of assessment instruments have been developed to assist individuals in their career exploration process. Probably the most important of these have been the *interest inventories*, such as the *Strong Interest Inventory* (CPP, 2004, 2009a), the *Career Decision-Making System (CDM)* (PsychCorp, 2014a), and the *Career Assessment Inventory (CAI)* (PsychCorp, 2014b). Interest inventories examine a client's interests in such areas as school subjects, types of people, types of occupations, amusements, and/or personal characteristics. Some interest inventories, like the *Self-Directed Search* (PAR, 2013), and the *Strong* (again) use the Holland codes to examine an individual's personality orientation toward the world of work and usually provide occupations in which the client might find a good fit.

Assessment of Aptitude

Aptitude testing allows individuals to examine whether occupational preferences match their ability. For instance, an individual who is interested in becoming a researcher but has little math ability may have a difficult time achieving his or her occupational goals, and a person who is found to have high mechanical ability might consider various jobs that relate to this aptitude. Two of the popular aptitude tests include *the Differential Aptitude Test (DAT)* (Pearson, 2014), and the *Armed Services Vocational Aptitude Battery (ASVAB)* (ASVAB, n.d.), which was developed for the military and is sometimes given in high schools for free.

Personality Assessment

Numerous personality tests have been used in conjunction with career counseling. Tests such as the *Myers-Briggs Type Indicator* (CPP, 2009b) and the *California Psychological Inventory (CPI)* (CPP, 2009c). Can help a client focus on basic personality dimensions and examine whether or not his or her personality profile might fit certain jobs (see Box 11.5).

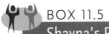

Shayna had definitely decided that she was interested in an occupation that would provide her with an opportunity to help people. A personality inventory indicated that she was very reserved and nonassertive and deferred to others. She agreed with the results of the personality inventory and further agreed that these characteristics would make it difficult for her to accomplish her occupational goal. Shayna became convinced that she would have to modify these personality characteristics through a variety of programs, including self-discovery groups and assertiveness training. (Zunker, 2012, pp. 163)

Computer-Assisted Career Guidance

The expansion in the use of personal computers has made career information systems available to a vast number of individuals. Today, there are numerous software programs that allow individuals to assess abilities, interests, values, and skills and other related information. For instance, self-directed, comprehensive, computer-based career guidance programs that help individuals explore their interests, personality, and skills can now be found on the Web or purchased as stand-alone software programs. Two common programs include *Discover* (ACT, 2014) and the *System of Interactive Guidance and Information-Plus (SIGI-Plus)* (Valpar, 2014), which can often be accessed at college career counseling centers and other settings where career guidance is offered. Of course, today, a host of interest inventories and personality tests related to career choice can be accessed directly on the Web. In addition, other career information is available from sites like O*NET, OOH, and other government and nongovernment sources, as discussed earlier.

Other Sources of Occupational Information

The amount of occupational information available is enormous, and much of it is free! For instance, printed and web-based materials can be obtained from a number of government agencies, commercial publishers, professional associations, and educational institutions. In addition, many colleges and trade schools have career centers available for use by their students, and even sometimes for the general public as well. In addition to free materials, numerous books offer career information. Today, there are even best-selling paperbacks that can assist in career development, such as *What Color Is Your Parachute?* (Bolles, 2014). Finding information about occupations is relatively easy; it just takes a little bit of time.

The Clinical Interview: The Lost Child in Career Development

The field of career counseling is so replete with theories, career information, and career assessment instruments that sometimes it seems like our most precious counseling tool, the clinical interview, is forgotten. A good clinical interview can help the counselor gain an enormous amount of information about a client, information that can be effectively used in helping the client make career choices. The clinical interview is a good way of operationalizing career development theories. It can be used to assess family-of-origin issues that have had an impact on the client's career development, the meaning-making system of the client, client desires and wants, how the client tends to present himself or herself, and emotional problems that might interfere with seeking out or maintaining certain jobs.

The clinical interview is a major part of the total assessment process for the client, and the counseling skills learned in a graduate program are the vehicle for that assessment. If career counseling meant only assessing traits and matching those traits with jobs, we would be operating out of a turn-of-the-last-century paradigm and would hardly need an advanced degree to work with clients.

Integrating Theory, Career Information, and Career Assessment

Between the numerous theories of career counseling and the enormous amount of occupational information available to counselors, you may be asking, "Where do I start when doing career counseling?" The following offers general guidelines for what you might want to cover when doing comprehensive career counseling:

1. Conduct a thorough clinical interview. Assess factors crucial to the client's career development process, including the following:
   - ➤ How early childhood issues may have affected the client's propensity toward certain careers (e.g., placement in family, parenting styles, traumatic events, etc.)
   - ➤ How socioeconomic status of the family of origin may affect the client's aspirations (affordability of continuing one's education)
   - ➤ How parents' career development may affect the client's aspirations (e.g., stories we are told about our parents' work lives and how that translates into stories about our career path)
   - ➤ How emotional problems may interfere with career decision making (e.g., depression, anxiety disorder, etc.)
   - ➤ How sociological issues may affect career decision making (stereotyping, discrimination, economic issues, and so forth)
   - ➤ How certain dominant stories drive the client's career decision-making process
   - ➤ An assessment of the tasks to be completed based on the client's career development level (e.g., using Super's model or a related model to assess career development)
   - ➤ How perceived factors and client's self-efficacy affect the choices that the client makes
   - ➤ How past, current, and future barriers might deleteriously affect the client's career decision-making process
2. Assess the client's abilities, interests, and personality characteristics through the use of appropriate assessment instruments (e.g., the Holland Code, the CPI, the Strong).

3. Devise treatment strategies in collaboration with your client that are congruent with his or her developmental readiness and the information gathered about your client.

4. Make available appropriate informational resources that can be used in conjunction with your treatment plan.

5. Assist the client in understanding the world of work and factors that may potentially affect career choices (such as economic conditions or market saturation).

6. Help the client examine issues related to self-efficacy, dominant narratives, and perceived factors that prevent the client from taking his or her best career path.

7. Examine barriers to career choices and what can be done to eliminate them (e.g., racism, economic hardship, lack of educational opportunities, etc.).

8. Have the client make tentative career decisions.

9. Explore the practicality of the career decisions chosen and begin to narrow down the choices.

10. Have the client take preliminary steps toward choosing a career path by doing such things as informational interviews with individuals who have taken a similar path, shadowing people at a job, and reading literature about the career path.

11. Follow up with the client to ensure satisfaction and closure of the career development process.

12. Recycle if necessary. If the client is unsatisfied with his or her progress, start the process over and reexamine all the issues.

As you can imagine from the above, a thorough career assessment can be a rather lengthy process. However, the use of such a process creates career choice, not career happenstance.

Multicultural/Social Justice Focus

Multicultural Theory of Career Development

Although no one method of conducting career counseling for individuals from diverse backgrounds has been developed, a number of unique issues have been highlighted for counselors to consider when working with culturally diverse clients. Some of these include the following (Arthur & Collins, 2011; Arthur & McMahon, 2005; Byars-Winston & Fouad, 2006; Gysbers et al., 2009; Leong & Flores, 2013):

1. Cultural values and practices may make full access to the workplace more difficult for some people (e.g., certain religious practices, such as praying every day and taking time off for certain holidays, may be frowned upon at the workplace).

2. Whereas mainstream America has lived a life of upward mobility, some cultures and classes have not lived this dream and approach career development with different goals and aspirations.

3. Acknowledgment that there is a wide range of influences on a person (e.g., geography, family, media, workplace, etc.) and that they differentially affect people of color.

4. The expression of self and the development of self-concept are central to the career development process, regardless of cultural background.
5. The person environment (personality workplace) fit, regardless of cultural background, is crucial for satisfaction at work.
6. The better the client understands his or her cultural identity development (see Chapter 14), the easier it will be for the client to find a fit between self and environment.
7. Discrimination in attaining jobs and at the workplace is a reality and needs to be addressed and acknowledged by career counselors.
8. Discrimination and racism have resulted in some people having serious doubts about their ability to obtain jobs and be upwardly mobile.
9. There are probably more differences within a cultural group than between cultural groups. Avoid uniformity of assumptions or thinking that all clients from one culture are the same.
10. Career counseling theories and assessment procedures, so prevalent in career counseling, may have inherent biases and may need to be adapted, or not used, for some culturally diverse groups and women.
11. Knowing one's own biases and stereotypes and how to address them while counseling clients from nondominant groups is critical.
12. Have the knowledge and skills necessary to be able to work effectively with a wide range of clients (see the discussion of multicultural career counseling and development competencies in the next section).

Multicultural Career Counseling and Development Competencies

In 2009, the *National Career Development Association (NCDA)* developed a set of *Minimium Competencies for Multicultural Career Counseling and Development*. These competencies speak to the ability of the career counseling professional to "promote the career development and functioning of individuals of all backgrounds" (NCDA, 2009a, para. 1). The competencies touch on multicultural competence in a wide variety of areas, including career development theory, counseling skills, assessment, information technology, program development, coaching and consultation, supervision, ethical and legal issues, and research and evaluation.

Social Justice Focus: Reshaping Clients' Stories

> *Yet is it possible to prepare students [and clients] for the vagaries of an uncertain world without ensuring that they have a critical understanding of how social, political and economic discourses impact on constructions of "career," "opportunity," "self," and "justice"?*

> (Irving, 2010, p. 51)

Recent approaches to the understanding of career counseling and career education have increasingly focused on how a client's sense of their "career" is affected by the kinds of relationships and discourse that he or she has with others. This relational cultural constructivist approach assumes that in interaction with the world around us, there are forces that shape one's view of how people make sense of who they are relative to their occupational choices and career path (Schultheiss, 2007). This approach assumes that change does not reside "within" the person, but is a function of interactions with people, and that individuals can understand these interactional forces and see how biases, racism, discrimination, and so forth have affected their development and meaning-making system. Taking this perspective, counselors are increasingly charged to have a new discourse with clients and help them see how their stories or narratives have been shaped by those around them. In the case of career counseling, this means helping clients understand how relationships have embedded certain belief systems within their understanding of their world of work (I am not capable, people will prevent me from making it, I cannot achieve in _____ , etc.). Today, the dual role for the career counselor includes listening to clients' stories and helping them hear how they have developed their stories and being an advocate for oppressed groups to lessen the negative impact that social factors have on them (Del Corso, 2011; Marchand, 2010; McMahon, Arthur, & Collins, 2008).

Ethical, Professional, and Legal Issues

Ethical Issues

Ethical Standards for Career Counseling and Consultation

NCDA has its own code of ethics (see NCDA, 2007) which is designed to be used in conjunction with ACAs (2014a) code. The following represents its major headings, but you are encouraged to view the code in its entirety. The code is now undergoing a revision process.

> Section A: The Professional Relationship
> Section B: Confidentiality, Privileged Communication, and Privacy
> Section C: Professional Responsibility
> Section D: Relationships with Other Professionals
> Section E: Evaluation, Assessment, and Interpretation
> Section F: Use of the Internet in Career Services
> Section G: Supervision, Training, and Teaching
> Section H: Research and Publication
> Section I: Resolving Ethical Issues

Competency Guidelines for Career Development

In addition to the *Multicultural Career Counseling and Development Competencies* already mentioned, NCDA offers a broad-based description of competencies needed for all counselors who practice vocational and career counseling (NCDA, 2009b). These competencies include a focus on eleven areas that an effective career counselor should master: Career Development Theory, Individual and Group Counseling Skills, Individual/Group Assessment, Information/Resources, Program Management and Implementation, Consultation, Diverse Populations, Supervision, Ethical/Legal Issues, Research/Evaluation, and Technology.

Professional Issues

Professional Associations

The NCDA and the *National Employment Counselors Association (NECA)*, both divisions of ACA, are two associations oriented toward career development. (You can reach these divisions through the ACA website: www.counseling.org.) The *Career Development Quarterly*, published by NCDA, and the *Journal of Employment Counseling*, published by NECA, are circulated quarterly and are two of the many benefits to those who join the associations.

Optimizing Career Development

Recently, when teaching a class, I asked my students to share why they had decided to enter the helping professions. An African American student told me about her school counselor, who had treated most African American students in her high school in a manner that would discourage them from pursuing jobs in professional fields. She said, "This is why I have decided to become a school counselor—so I could assist African Americans in reaching their potential." Unfortunately, this is not the first time I have heard a story such as this.

Career counselors should be optimizing choices for clients, whether they are school counselors working with disadvantaged youths, college counselors assisting college students in job choices, agency counselors working with middle-aged adults who are seeking a job change, vocational rehabilitation counselors working with individuals who recently became paraplegic, or graduate students considering their options concerning doctoral work. Counselors should never say, "I don't think you can make it," "You don't have the ability," "You don't have the skills," or "You won't be able to take the pressure." Instead, they should be encouraging clients, increasing options, and helping clients reach their potential. Be realistic, but don't be discouraging. At best, discouraging clients in the pursuit of career dreams is incompetent; at worst, it is racist, sexist, ageist, and discriminatory toward individuals with disabilities.

Legal Issues: Important Laws

Carl Perkins Career and Technical Education Act

Originally passed in 1984, and updated since that time, this act seeks to support academic, career, and technical skills of secondary and postsecondary students who are enrolled in career and technical education, formerly called *vocational education* (U.S. Department of Education, 2007).

Americans with Disabilities Act

This law, passed in 1992, ensures that qualified individuals with disabilities cannot be discriminated against in job application procedures, hiring, firing, advancement, compensation, fringe benefits, job training, and other terms, conditions, and privileges (U.S. Department of Justice, n.d.).

PL94-142 (The Education of All Handicapped Children Act)

Concerning career guidance, this law, along with the *Carl Perkins Act*, requires that students in occupational education programs must be given vocational assessment to assist them in their career development.

Rehabilitation Act of 1973

The *Rehabilitation Act of 1973* ensures access to vocational rehabilitation services for adults if they are severely physically or mentally disabled, if they have a disability that interferes with their ability to obtain or maintain a job, and if assessment has shown that employment with their disability is feasible.

School-to-Work Opportunities Act

Passed in 1994 by Congress, this act provides incentives to help schools and community colleges develop programs that integrate academic learning with on-the-job experiences.

Title VII and Title IX

Title VII of the *1964 Civil Rights Act* and Title IX of the *Education Amendments of 1972* prohibit discrimination against women and minorities in all aspects of employment. In addition, Title VII and subsequent amendments set standards for the use of tests to ensure that they do not discriminate against culturally diverse populations.

The Counselor in Process: Career Development as a Lifelong Process

Career development is a lifelong process. It starts at birth and continues until we die. It is not just the process of finding a job, but how we actualize all our life roles. An astute counselor understands this process. He or she views it much like navigating a flowing river—a river that has twists and turns; parts that seem shallow, dangerous, and scary; and parts that are deep, still, and stable. This counselor understands that the river starts to flow in infancy, when the child first begins to imitate adult behaviors, and continues into young childhood, when the youngster wonders about the world of work. Such a counselor sees this river pick up speed in adolescence, with the teenager who begins to explore his or her interests, values, and abilities, and watches it move more rapidly and dangerously in young adulthood, when the individual tentatively chooses a career. This river soon deepens and slows in mid-adulthood with the person who feels established, or suddenly takes sharp twists and turns with the middle-aged person who decides to take a fresh look at his or her career choices. The river begins to slow in later life, with the individual who moves out of work and into leisure activities, or the person who decreases the amount of work that he or she is doing. The committed and wise career counselor is willing to flow, for a short while, along this river with his or her client; and, perhaps, if the helper is a good navigator, he or she can assist in guiding the client down the river along the most direct and stable route.

Summary

This chapter examined the counselor and the world of work. It began by defining a number of terms relevant to understanding career development, and then went on to examine a number of psychological, interpersonal, family, and societal needs that work serves.

Presenting a brief history of career counseling, we noted that career development, formerly called *vocational guidance,* is the origin of the counseling profession and can be traced back to the early 1900s with the work of Frank Parsons and his concept of true reasoning. We pointed out that vocational guidance started out as a concrete and somewhat directive trait-and-factor approach, and then listed a number of events that highlighted the expansion of career counseling, such as the development of vocational guidance in the schools, the *Wagner O'Day Act,* the and the publishing of the *Dictionary of Occupational Titles.* With the advent of new theories by Donald Super and others during the 1950s, career counseling became a more humanistically oriented, developmental approach. The National Defense Education Act expanded career guidance in the schools during the late 1950s and 1960s and soon, we saw a general expansion of career counseling and career development and the emergence of new theories.

We next went on to describe some of the more popular and researched theories on career development, although we noted that a number of other theories are used as well. Starting with trait-and-factor theory, we talked about how it has expanded over the years, and today, users of this approach assess how a wide range of client skills, interests, and personality variables might affect eventual career choices. Next, the chapter examined the psychodynamic theory of Ann Roe, who advanced the idea that early parenting styles were instrumental in shaping occupational choice. We looked at John Holland's theory, which states that people express their personality through the types of career choices they make ("RIASEC"), and examined Super's developmental theory, which suggests a person's self-concept is both a function and result of one's career development process. Moving on to a more recent approach, we highlighted Social Cognitive Career Theory (SCCT) and noted that this theory suggests that objective factors, such as environmental factors (e.g., social influences) and perceived factors, both affect the kinds of decisions that one makes about career choices. Finally, the chapter reviewed constructive developmental theory, which stresses the importance of understanding how the client makes meaning of his or her career development process. We noted that narratives are often used to assess meaning and to help identify a client's meaning-making system. We concluded by noting that most career counselors today attempt to integrate many of these approaches when doing career counseling.

The next part of this chapter examined some of the prevalent kinds of career-related information that is available. We first presented an overview of occupational classification systems, beginning with the Occupational Information Network (O*NET), which is an online database developed by the Department of Labor that provides a large array of worker attributes and job characteristics for about 1,000 occupations. In addition, there is a related, hard-copy resource called the *Dictionary of Occupational Titles (DOT).* Next, we discussed the *Guide for Occupational Exploration (GOE),* which lists approximately 900 occupations that are cross-referenced with 16 interest areas. The last system examined in the chapter was the *Occupational Outlook Handbook (OOH),* which includes a wide range of information on the nature of work for a select group of a few hundred occupations. We then discussed how the assessment of interest inventories, aptitudes, and personality is important in career counseling and highlighted a few of the more popular instruments. Next, the text went on to cover the growing use of computers in career guidance and noted that comprehensive, computer-based programs, computer-assisted assessment, and career resources on the Internet are becoming increasingly popular.

Having discussed theories, occupational information, and assessment techniques, we pointed out that the clinical interview is one of the most important tools the counselor has when working with clients. Next, we presented an outline for the integration of career development theories, occupational information, assessment techniques, and the clinical interview when doing career counseling.

Although there is no theory of multicultural career development, there are some general guidelines that should be considered when working with diverse clients. For instance, in 2009, NCDA developed Minimum Competencies for Multicultural Career Counseling and Development that promotes the career development of all individuals. We then suggested that counselors should take stock in developing a relationship with clients that challenges embedded beliefs that they cannot achieve in certain areas—embedded due to oppressive social factors that have stressed these beliefs.

Near the end of the chapter, we mentioned the two major associations in the field of career development: the NCDA and the NECA. The chapter then highlighted the NCDA code of ethics and noted that it is to be used in conjunction with ACA's code of ethics. We also noted that NCDA offers a broad-based description of competencies needed for all counselors who practice vocational and career counseling. We then suggested that counselors should be optimizing choices for clients, not limiting them, and went on to highlight some important laws whose purpose is to assist individuals in their career counseling process. Finally, we emphasized that career counseling is a lifelong process that has twists and turns, and that an effective career counselor helps the client make this ride a little more satisfying.

Further Practice

Visit CengageBrain.com to respond to additional material that highlight the salient aspects of the chapter content. There, you can find ethical, professional, and legal vignettes, a number of experiential exercises, and study tools including a glossary, flashcards, and sample test items. Hopefully, these will enhance your learning and be fun and interesting.

RESEARCH, PROGRAM EVALUATION, AND ASSESSMENT

Overview

Research, program evaluation, and assessment have much in common, and therefore, it is natural to find them together in Section V of this text. For instance, some form of quantification is involved with the application of research, program evaluation, and assessment. Program evaluation can be loosely seen as a kind of research, in that you are researching the value and worth of a program. Research often will use assessment techniques to examine the question at hand. Finally, research, program evaluation, and assessment all involve close scrutiny of people. In research, you are examining people in reference to a hypothesis or research question; in program evaluation, you are examining how people respond to a program being offered; and in assessment, you are trying to determine a person's typical or habitual ways of responding. As you read through these chapters, consider the common factors that you find in these important content areas and think about ways in which you might apply research, program evaluation, and assessment in your role as a counselor.

Testing and Assessment

One day while living in Cincinnati and working on my doctorate, I was walking on a downtown street when a person came up to me and said, "Do you want to take a personality test?" I said, "Sure!" I was led into a storefront and proceeded to spend about 30 minutes completing an inventory. When I finished, I was asked to wait a few minutes while they scored it. Then, a person came into the room and said, "Well, you have a pretty good personality, and you're fairly bright, but if you complete Ron Hubbard's book on *Dianetics* (the basis of "Scientology") you will have a better personality and be even brighter."

Ten years later, I was walking down a street in Minneapolis when I passed a store that was again selling books by Ron Hubbard. I walked in. Someone approached me and said, "Would you like to take a test?" I responded by noting that a number of years back I had taken such a test and was not convinced it was well made. We bantered back and forth, and finally the Scientology devotee and I came to an agreement. The deal was that I would purchase the book, *Dianetics*, and after the devotee sent me information on the reliability and validity of the test he wanted me to take (thus showing me if it was a well-made test), I would read the book. I gave him my home address. I never heard from him again.

You will be tested on this chapter! Just kidding; well, at least *I* won't be testing you on it. Tests create anxiety! *Tests*! Some of the most interesting, feared, misused, disliked, and potentially valuable tools that we have as counselors are tests. What are they all about? This chapter will examine tests, as well as other assessment techniques.

We will begin this chapter by defining testing and assessment and then exploring why assessment is important. Then we will give a brief overview of the history of tests and assessment. We will survey some of the many different kinds of tests and review the use of basic test statistics in the development and the interpretation of assessment instruments. We will discuss the concepts of reliability, validity, cross-cultural fairness, and practicality and relate these concepts to how worthwhile a test is. Also, we will suggest ways of finding good tests, discuss the importance of writing assessment reports, and review how the use of computers has affected the administration, scoring, and interpretation of tests. Finally, we will discuss multicultural/social justice, ethical, professional, and legal issues related to testing.

Defining Testing and Assessment

There is much ignorance about very basic measurement, evaluation, and research topics among the practitioners . . . and among those who are ignorant, there is, on occasion, a fair amount of hostility toward some useful data.

(Mehrens, 1992, p. 439)

Unfortunately, although written over twenty years ago, the above quote continues to be true today. In fact, after teaching testing and assessment for close to thirty years, I find that students initially know little about this CACREP content area. Perhaps worse, they often don't think it's an important part of what a counselor does. So, let's start with some basic definitions, and let's see if by the end of the chapter, I can convince you of the worth of testing and assessment (if you're not already a believer).

Today, the word *assessment* includes a broad array of evaluative procedures that yield information about a person. Assessment includes a number of techniques, such as conducting a clinical interview to establish the overall functioning of a person; using personality tests to assess temperament, affect, and habits; administering ability tests to assess learning and cognitive functioning; and utilizing informal assessment techniques to assess a wide range of a person's behaviors (Figure 12.1).

Tests are considered a subset of a broad pool of assessment techniques and yield scores based on the gathering of collective data (e.g., adding a number of correct answers on a multiple-choice exam). Tests and other assessment procedures can be formal, where the procedure is scientifically shown to be sound (or valid and reliable); or informal, which implies that such rigor has not been demonstrated, although the procedure might still yield valuable information. But why assess a person at all?

Why Testing and Assessment?

As a counselor, you will be involved with testing and assessment (Neukrug, Peterson, Bonner, & Lomas, 2013; Peterson, Lomas, Neukrug, & Bonner, 2014). You may be administering assessment instruments. You are likely to interpret assessment instruments. You may be a consultant to others on the proper use of assessment techniques or supervise others who interpret tests and assess clients. You may use assessment procedures in research and evaluation, and you will read about assessment techniques in the professional literature. Assessment techniques have permeated many aspects of our society, but there are only a handful of professionals who know them well enough to use them properly. As a counselor, you will be one of those few.

In many schools, counselors are the only individuals who have expertise in testing and assessment (Baker & Gerler, 2008). Although school psychologists are highly trained in assessment (Agresta, 2004; Merrell, Ervin, & Peacock, 2012), they generally float from school to school. Meanwhile, school administrators and teachers, although trained in how to create and administer teacher-made tests, are generally grossly undertrained in the understanding of other kinds of assessment (Behuniak, 2003; Elmore & Elkstrom, 2003). Also, although special education teachers and learning disability specialists generally

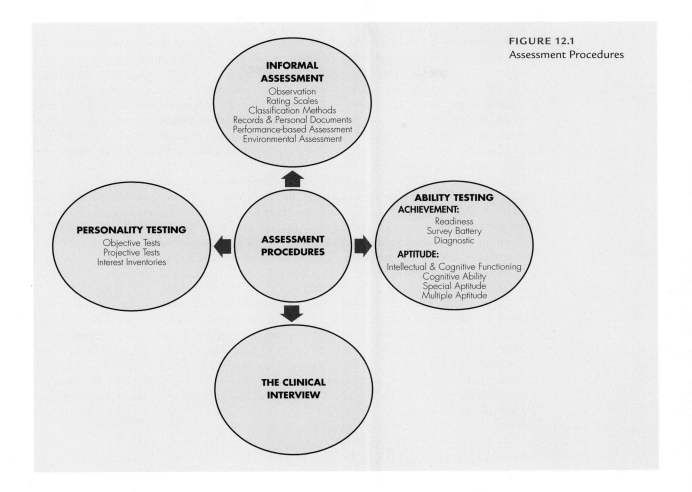

FIGURE 12.1
Assessment Procedures

have strong backgrounds in diagnostic testing, they have limited focus and are generally not trained in a wide birth of assessment instruments (Neukrug & Fawcett, 2015). School counselors, on the other hand, report that assessment is a broad and critical part of their job (Neukrug et al., 2013; Peterson et al., 2014).

The role of school counselors in assessment varies and may include communicating test results to students and parents, assisting teachers and administrators in understanding assessment results, using assessment techniques in program evaluation and research, providing workshops and individual consultation for teachers on test use and test interpretation, and using test results and other assessment techniques to assist in the development of educational plans for children with learning disabilities, and more (Neukrug & Fawcett, 2015; Peterson et al., 2014). In addition, school counselors will periodically receive and need to understand test reports from agency counselors who are working with students.

Although in agencies and higher education, there is a greater likelihood that related mental health professionals (e.g., psychologists) will be well versed in testing and assessment, there is still the possibility that the counselor will be the only individual with such expertise. But whether or not the counselor is the expert, in most settings, counselors will find themselves periodically administering and interpreting educational and psychological tests for their clients (Naugle, 2010; Peterson et al., 2014). In addition, counselors in almost all settings are asked to understand assessment reports completed by other clinicians, and many counselors will be reviewing the test records of the children with whom they work. Finally, in these days of accountability, counselors are often asked to evaluate the efficacy of clinical programs, and assessment instruments are crucial for this process. It is clear that in agency and higher education settings, testing has become a core component of the counselor's work.

Although tests have been criticized over the years for being poorly made or having bias, with advances in statistical analysis and improvement of test quality, tests today can offer an additional way of exploring the inner world of clients (Neukrug, 2015). Today, the professional counselor should be engaged in a cycle of formulating a hypothesis about a client, gathering information from the client, and reformulating the hypothesis. In addition, to increase the accuracy of one's hypothesis, it is often suggested to increase the number of procedures used, as this will more likely yield a clearer snapshot of the client (JCTP, 2004; Neukrug & Fawcett, 2015).

Why testing? Why *not* testing? Tests offer an additional venue for helping us understand the ability and personality of our clients. They can be useful in diagnosis. They can help in goal setting and treatment planning, and assessment procedures are often critical aspects of research and evaluation. Because of past experiences with tests or personal biases about tests, some have made assumptions that testing is not useful. However, such assumptions should not and cannot lead one to dismiss a potentially powerful aspect of the counseling process. Let's see how testing and assessment can be an important part of what the counselor does.

A Little Background

Broadly speaking, assessment takes place whenever a person is asked to show the existence or amount of a particular trait or ability. In this sense, Abraham's faith was assessed when he was asked by God to kill his first-born son, Isaac. And early Olympians were assessed as they compared their performances to one another. One of the earliest assessment techniques, used for purposes with which we're more familiar, was developed in 2200 B.C. by the Chinese, who gave an essay-type test for the selection of what today would be called "civil service employees" (DuBois, 1970; Higgins & Sun, 2002). However, it was not until the 1800s that psychological and educational assessment turned into a more formal process.

Modern-day assessment was formed out of two distinct processes occurring in the late 1800s. On the one hand, this period saw increased acceptance of Charles Darwin's theory that differences within a species and between species held the key to natural selection. Soon psychologists picked up the call to examine individual differences in people (Juve, 2008; Kerr, 2008). Individuals like Wilhem Wundt and Gustav Fechner become particularly interested in *experimental psychology* and developed some of the first *psychology labs*. It was this impetus that led to an understanding that rigorous experimental control was crucial to scientific inquiry regarding individual differences and that tests were often critical to this process (Kaplan & Saccuzzo, 2013).

One of the first tests was developed by Alfred Binet at the end of the nineteenth century. Hired by the Ministry of Public Education in Paris, Binet was asked to develop an instrument that could differentiate those who could function in a classroom from those who could not (Kerr, 2008; Ryan, 2008; Watson, 1968). This scale, which was later revised by Lewis Terman at Stanford University, became known as the *Stanford-Binet* intelligence test, a revised version of which is still used today.

A number of developments at the beginning of the twentieth century saw the spread of assessment instruments in other realms. For instance, the popularity of psychoanalysis and its emphasis on personality development influenced the beginning of objective and projective personality assessment. In addition, on the heels of the Industrial Revolution, there was an influx of people to large cities, which resulted in a need for objective tests of achievement and of vocational aptitudes in the schools. Finally, World War I saw a sudden need for the widespread use of personality and ability tests to help in the placement of recruits in the military. The assessment movement had taken hold in the United States.

With advancements in statistical knowledge and its application to test construction, assessment instruments began to take on a modern look in the 1940s and 1950s. As the 1960s and the 1970s progressed, the advent of the computer made it easier to examine the statistical properties of tests and improve their quality. The 1980s saw the proliferation of personal computers, which increased the ability of researchers to examine the quality of tests even more (Sampson, 1995), and the 1990s saw a revolution in the ways that many tests were administered, scored, and interpreted. This revolution has continued into the twenty-first century.

Today, assessment instruments are pervasive throughout society. There are long tests, short tests, extremely long tests, and very short tests; instruments to measure knowledge and instruments to measure passion; procedures to properly diagnose, and others that can tell if you're self-actualized; tests for admission into graduate school and assessment procedures to finish graduate school. Tests are everywhere. Let's look at some of the different kinds of assessment instruments in existence today.

Types of Assessment Techniques

Although assessment techniques today are appreciably better than their ancestors from the turn of the twentieth century, the basic assessment categories have pretty much stayed the same. The following discussion offers an overview of ability tests, personality tests, informal assessment techniques, and the clinical interview (see Figures 12.1 and 12.2–12.4).

Assessment of Ability

Ability tests measure a range of cognitive abilities and include *achievement tests*, or tests that measure all of what one has learned; and *aptitude tests*, or tests that measure all that one is capable of learning. Achievement tests include *survey battery, diagnostic,* and *readiness tests*. Aptitude tests include *cognitive ability tests, individual intelligence tests, neuropsychological testing, special aptitude tests,* and *multiple aptitude tests* (see Figure 12.2).

FIGURE 12.2
Tests in the Cognitive
Domain

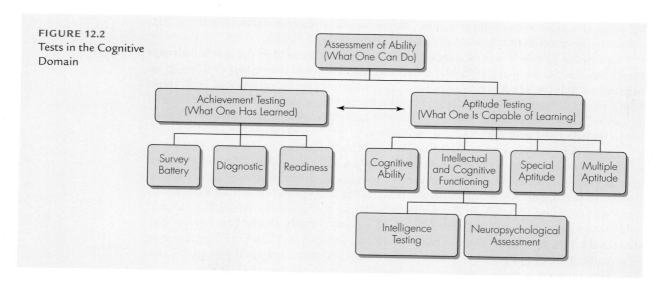

FIGURE 12.3
Assessment in the
Affective Domain

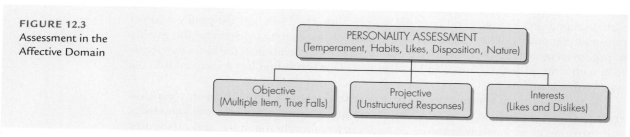

FIGURE 12.4
Informal Assessment
Procedures

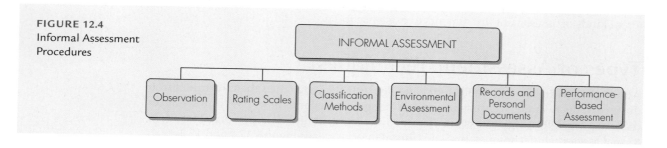

Achievement Tests (Survey Battery, Diagnostic, and Readiness)

Achievement tests include survey battery tests, diagnostic tests, and readiness tests (see Figure 12.2). Usually given in the schools to assess progress, *survey battery tests* measure content areas (e.g., fifth grade math) and are generally administered to large groups of students. Probably you are familiar with these types of tests through your own education. The *Iowa Test of Basic Skills* and the *Stanford Achievement Test* are two examples of survey

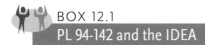

BOX 12.1
PL 94-142 and the IDEA

With the passage of *Public Law 94-142* (PL94-142) in 1975, as well as the more recent *Individuals with Disabilities Education Act (IDEA)*, millions of children and young adults between the ages of 3 and 21 who were found to have a learning disability were assured the right to an education in the least restrictive environment (U.S. Department of Education, 2010). These laws also asserted that any individual who was suspected of having one of a number of disabilities that interfere with learning has the right to be tested, at the school system's expense, for the disability. Thus, diagnostic testing, usually administered by the school psychologist or learning disability specialist, became one of the main ways of determining who might be learning disabled. These laws also stated that a school team would review the testing, and other assessment information obtained, and that the learning-disabled student would be given an individual education plan (IEP) that states which services would be offered to assist the student with his or her learning problem.

battery achievement tests. The many uses of survey battery achievement tests include assessment of a student's ability level, determination of teaching effectiveness, and examination of the general level of students' ability throughout a school or school system.

Diagnostic achievement tests, which are used to delve more deeply into areas where there are suspected learning problems, are often given one on one by an experienced examiner, usually a school psychologist or learning disabilities specialist. Often these tests are recommended following the results of a survey battery achievement test and when, in consultation with parents and teachers, it seems probable that a student may have a learning disability. This means that it is suspected that the student's ability is much lower in one or more specified areas than his or her average ability in other areas. Today, if an individual is found to have a learning disability, laws protect the child's right to an education (see Box 12.1).

Readiness tests are used to assess an individual's ability to move to the next educational level. These days, readiness tests are mostly used to determine if a child is developmentally ready to move to first grade. However, it should be emphasized that any differences found at these young ages may not be found at later ages, as children's ability at very young ages is much more variable and more affected by environment than at later ages (Hoekstra, Bartels, & Boomsma, 2007).

Aptitude Tests

The five major kinds of aptitude tests include cognitive ability tests, individual intelligence tests, neuropsychological assessments, special aptitude tests, and multiple aptitude tests (see Figure 12.2). *Cognitive ability tests* generally require true/false or multiple choice responses in an effort to measure the cognitive skills necessary to be successful in school. Often given in groups, these tests are frequently used to determine a student's overall potential in school. These tests can also aid in identifying those who are learning disabled and gifted. For instance, it is common for students who have a learning disability to score significantly higher on a cognitive ability test, which measures capability, as compared to a survey battery achievement test, which measures what one has learned in specific -content areas. Other cognitive ability tests are used for placement and as predictors of ability in college (e.g., ACTs, SATs), graduate school (e.g., MATs, GREs), and professional schools (Mattern & Patterson, 2012; Richardson, Abraham, & Bond, 2012).

Individual intelligence tests, which are given one on one to measure general intellectual ability, are administered by highly trained examiners, most often psychologists. These tests have a broad range of uses, such as helping to identify individuals who are learning disabled, developmentally delayed, intellectually disabled (formerly called "mentally retarded"), or gifted, and can even be used as an indicator of personality characteristics. Usually, when a comprehensive assessment of an individual is requested, an individual intelligence test is included.

Neuropsychological assessment measures a broad range of behaviors related to brain functioning. It is used to identify brain damage, to measure change in one's overall cognitive functioning, to compare changes in cognitive functioning to one's norm group, to provide rehabilitation treatment and planning guidelines, and to provide specific guidelines for educational planning in the schools (Kolb & Whishaw, 2009; Lezak, Howieson, & Bigler, & Tranel, 2012).

Special aptitude tests focus on measuring specific segments of ability (e.g., spatial ability, eye-hand coordination, mechanical ability) and are often used to predict the potential for success at specific jobs or training programs. For instance, one's aptitude on an eye-hand coordination test may be used to predict success at operating complex machinery in a factory, or a drawing test may be used to predict success in art school.

Multiple aptitude tests, which measure a series of specific segments of ability, are used to understand an individual's aptitude on a broad range of abilities. Results of these tests can be used in occupational decision making. Some examples of multiple aptitude tests include the *Differential Aptitude Test (DAT)*, which is frequently used by high school counselors, and the *Armed Services Vocational Aptitude Battery (ASVAB)*, which was developed by the military and generally administered for free in the schools.

Although achievement testing measures what a person has learned and aptitude testing measures one's potential for learning, in fact there is often much overlap between the two. This is why there is a two-headed arrow connecting these categories in Figure 12.2. For instance, one would be naive to assume that the SAT or the GRE does not measure what one has learned. However, because they are both used to predict future performance, they are considered aptitude tests.

Personality Assessment

The assessment of personality includes measuring one's temperament, attitudes, values, likes and dislikes, emotions, motivation, interpersonal skills, and/or level of adjustment (Neukrug & Fawcett, 2015). The three types of personality assessment that are most commonly used today are *objective tests*, *projective techniques*, and *interest inventories* (see Figure 12.3).

Objective Personality Tests

Objective personality tests are questionnaires or inventories that require true/false, yes/no, multiple-choice, or related responses in an effort to measure some aspect of personality. Thus, we might find tests measuring anxiety, depression, psychosis, suicidal tendencies, eating disorders, extroversion-introversion tendencies, marital satisfaction, and so on. Some of these tests, like the *Minnesota Multiphasic Personality Inventory-2 (MMPI-2),* measure psychopathology and assess some aspects of one's temperament, or deeply embedded personality style, while others, like the *Myers-Briggs Type Indicator (MBTI),* measure common personality styles that are likely not to be related to temperament. A few functions of objective personality tests are to deepen client insight, to help in the determination of clinical diagnosis, to make predictions about future behaviors, to determine personality characteristics for the court (e.g., child custody or child molestation accusations), and to screen applicants for sensitive jobs (e.g., working with children or nuclear arms).

Projective Techniques

Projective techniques attempt to assess personality characteristics by having an individual respond to *unstructured stimuli* (e.g., an inkblot). Stimuli presented allow for a broad range of responses that are representative of conscious and unconscious needs, desires, likes, drives, and personal struggles. For instance, the *Rorschach,* one of the most widely used projective tests, uses inkblots as stimuli to which the individual responds. After all the responses are collected, the examiner interprets their meaning. Other types of projective techniques include *sentence completion tests,* where a client completes a stem of a sentence with the first thing that comes to mind; *drawings,* where the client is asked to make a specific drawing that is later interpreted (e.g., a drawing of the client's family all doing something together); and techniques in which the individual is asked to develop stories from pictures that are presented.

Interest Inventories

Although strictly speaking, they are a type of objective personality test, *interest inventories* are generally classified separately because of their popularity and very specific focus. Used to determine the likes and dislikes of a person, as well as an individual's personality orientation toward the world of work, interest inventories are almost exclusively used in the career counseling process. These instruments can moderately predict job satisfaction based on occupational fit. For instance, if a person chooses a job that seems to match his or her personality type based on the results of an interest inventory, then that person is more likely to be satisfied in that occupation than a person who does not have an occupational fit (Duffy, Bott, Allan, Torrey, & Dik, 2012; Lent & Brown, 2013; Rehfuss, Gambrell, & Meyer, 2012). With a variety of interest inventories having been developed, and with millions of individuals taking one or more each year, these assessment instruments have become big business in career counseling. Two of the more popular include the *Strong Interest Inventory* and the *Self-Directed Search.*

Informal Assessment Procedures

Informal assessment instruments are generally developed by the individual giving the procedure (e.g., the counselor or teacher) (Neukrug & Fawcett, 2015). Although they are often less valid than other kinds of instruments, they offer an important and relatively easy method of examining a slice of behavior of an individual. There are many kinds of informal assessment instruments, with some of the more common ones being *observation, rating scales, classification methods, environmental assessment, records and personal documents,* and *performance-based assessment* (see Figure 12.4).

Observation

Conducted by the professional who wishes to observe the individual (e.g., school counselors observing students in the classroom), by significant others who have the opportunity to observe the individual in natural settings (e.g., parents observing a child at home), and even by the client, who when in counseling is asked to observe specific targeted behaviors he or she is working on changing (e.g., eating habits), *observation* can be an easy and important tool for understanding the individual. When observing, observers often conduct an *event sample*, which is when a specific event is observed without regard for time (e.g., observing empathic responses on a video recording), or a *time sample*, when observation occurs over a specific amount of time without zeroing in on an event (e.g., observing two five-minute segments of all counseling responses on a video recording). Sometimes time and event sampling are combined, such as when one might only listen for empathic responses on two five-minute segments of recordings.

Rating Scales

Rating scales allow an individual to give a subjective rating of a behavior on a scale to obtain a quantity of an attitude or characteristic. Rating scales come in many different forms, with a few of the more popular kinds of rating scales being *Likert-type scales, semantic differential scales, rank order scales,* and *numerical scales* (see Box 12.2).

Classification Methods

In contrast to rating scales that tend to assess a quantity of specific attributes or characteristics, *classification methods* provide information about whether an individual has or does not have certain attributes or characteristics. Some of the more common classification methods include *behavior checklists* (see Box 12.3) or *feeling word checklists*. The kinds of classification methods that one can create are innumerable and are limited only by one's imagination. For instance, classification methods can be developed that ask clients to examine and choose items that represent their "irrational thoughts"; or an older person might be asked to pick from a long list of physical barriers to living fully (difficulty getting out of the bath, problems seeing, etc.).

Environmental Assessment

Environmental assessment includes collecting information from a client's home, school, or workplace, usually through observation or self-reports. This form of appraisal is more systems oriented and naturalistic and can be eye-opening because even when clients do not intentionally mislead their therapists, they will often present a distorted view based on their own inaccurate perceptions or because they are embarrassed about revealing

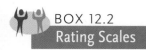

BOX 12.2
Rating Scales

Below are examples of four rating scales. Consider how you might use them as a counselor.

Numerical Scale:
With "0" being equal to the worst depression you ever had and a 10 being equal to the best you could possibly feel, can you tell me where on a scale of 0–10 your depression is today?

| 2   3   4   5   6   7   8   9   10

Worst Depression   Best I Could Feel

Semantic Differential Scale
Place an "X" on the line to represent how much of each quality you possess:

sadness_____happiness
| 2   3   4   5   6   7   8

introverted_____extroverted
| 2   3   4   5   6   7   8

anxious_____calm
| 2   3   4   5   6   7   8

Rank Order Scale
Please rank order your preferred method of doing counseling. Place a 1 next to the item that you most prefer, a 2 next to the item you second most prefer, and so on down to a 5 next to the item you prefer least.

_____ I prefer listening to clients and then reflecting back what I hear from them in order to facilitate client self-growth.
_____ I prefer advising clients and suggesting mechanisms for change.
_____ I prefer interpreting client behaviors in the hope that they will gain insight into themselves.
_____ I prefer helping clients identify which behaviors they would like to change.
_____ I prefer helping clients identify which thoughts are causing problematic behaviors and helping them to develop new ways of thinking about the world.

Likert-Type Scale
Please indicate how strongly you agree or disagree with each of the following statements:

	Strongly disagree	Somewhat disagree	Neither Agree nor disagree	Somewhat agree	Strongly agree
It is fine to view a client's personal Web page (e.g., MySpace, Facebook) without informing the client.	1	2	3	4	5
It is okay to tell your client you are attracted to him or her.	1	2	3	4	5
There is no problem in counseling a terminally ill client about end-of-life decisions including suicide.	1	2	3	4	5

BOX 12.3
Checklist of Abusive Behaviors

Check those behaviors that you have exhibited toward your partner and your partner has exhibited toward you.

	Exhibited by You to Your Partner	Exhibited by Partner to You
1. Hitting	———	———
2. Pulling hair	———	———
3. Throwing objects	———	———
4. Burning	———	———
5. Pinching	———	———
6. Choking	———	———
7. Slapping	———	———
8. Biting	———	———
9. Tying up	———	———
10. Hitting walls or other inanimate objects	———	———
11. Throwing objects with intent to break them	———	———
12. Restraining or preventing from leaving	———	———

some aspect of their lives (e.g., a person living in poverty might not want to reveal an unpleasant home situation). Some of the more common environmental assessments include using *direct observation* by the counselor; applying *sociometric procedures* to identify the relative position of an individual within a group (e.g., asking preschool children which students in class they like best and mapping all their responses), conducting a *situational assessment* where a person's responses to a contrived but natural situation is assessed (e.g., when, as part of a doctoral admissions process, a potential doctoral student counsels a role-play client and his or her responses are assessed), and completing an *environmental assessment instrument* that uses rating scales and checklists to assess a client's environment.

Records and Personal Documents

A number of common forms of *records and personal documents* are used to inquire about the client, including asking the client to write an *autobiography*, collecting *anecdotal information* (e.g., typical or atypical work behaviors in a personnel file), completing a *biographical inventory* (a detailed picture of the client from birth created by conducting an involved interview or by having the client answer a series of questions on a checklist), examining *cumulative records* (e.g., school records), completing a *genogram* (see Figure 6.1 in Chapter 6), or having the client keep *diaries* or write *journals* (e.g., a sleep journal, where one writes down his or her dreams and explores patterns among the dreams).

Performance-based Assessment

This kind of assessment evaluates an individual using a variety of informal assessment procedures based on real-world responsibilities that are not highly loaded for cognitive skills. *Performance-based assessment* is seen as an alternative to traditional standardized testing and is often used when individuals from nondominant groups have performed lower on traditional tests and when other procedures can be shown to predict as well as traditional tests. Thus, rather than giving a highly loaded cognitive test that may predict well for Whites who want to become firefighters, but not predict well for some minority groups, individuals can be given a series of alternative procedures, such as assessing how quickly they can respond to realistic yet contrived situations that they might actually face on the job as firefighters.

The Clinical Interview

Another assessment technique, the *clinical interview*, allows the counselor to obtain an in-depth understanding of the client through an unstructured or structured interview process. The *structured interview* allows the examinee to respond to a set of preestablished items verbally or in writing. This kind of interview generally allows for a broad assessment of client issues but sometimes does not allow for in-depth follow-up in one area. The *unstructured interview*, on the other hand, does not have a preestablished list of items or questions, and client responses to examiner inquiries establish the direction for follow-up questioning. Some counselors prefer using a *semi-structured interview*, which is a cross between the two kinds of interviewing techniques. The clinical interview serves a number of purposes (Neukrug & Fawcett, 2015). For instance, the interview:

1. Sets a tone for the types of information that will be covered during the assessment process
2. Allows the client to become desensitized to information that can be very intimate and personal
3. Allows the examiner to assess the nonverbal signals of the client while he or she is talking about sensitive information, thus giving the examiner a sense of what might be important to focus on
4. Allows the examiner to learn firsthand the problem areas of the client and place them in perspective
5. Gives the client and examiner the opportunity to study each other's personality style to ensure that they can work together

Norm-Referenced, Criterion-Referenced, Standardized, and -Non-Standardized Assessment

Generally, assessment techniques are either *norm-referenced* or *criterion-referenced*. In norm-referenced assessment, the individual can compare his or her score to the conglomerate scores of a peer or norm group. Usually, norm groups consist of a national representative sample of individuals. Many tests that are sold by national publishing companies are norm-referenced. In contrast, criterion-referenced assessment techniques are designed to assess specific learning goals of an individual. Attainment of these goals, as measured

TABLE 12.1   Comparison of Standardized, Nonstandardized, Norm-Referenced, and Criterion-Referenced Assessment

	STANDARDIZED	NONSTANDARDIZED
Norm-Referenced	These assessment instruments must be given in the same manner and under the same conditions each time they're given. Often, they are highly researched objective instruments that are developed by publishing companies. Usually, large norm groups are available, with which the individual can compare his or her results.	These assessment instruments may vary in how they are administered and generally are not as rigidly researched as the standardized tests. However, because of their informal nature, they may be more practical for the purpose for which they are being used. Scores that are later compared to a norm group should be viewed more tentatively than standardized tests.
Criterion-Referenced	These instruments are given in a standard manner and have preset learning goals that are based on an individual's personal educational objectives. Often created by large publishing companies, individuals who take these tests generally have the ability to tackle their individualized learning goals and have their results compared to national norm groups.	These instruments are informally made, often by teachers, and are based on the teacher's knowledge of his or her students and the content area being tested. The teacher can develop an individualized test that has preset learning goals for each student. The informal nature of these instruments means that norm groups are rarely available for comparisons.

by a criterion-referenced procedure, shows mastery of the subject matter at hand. Often, criterion-referenced procedures are used with individuals who are learning disabled because goals can be individualized for the student based on his or her specific learning problem.

Standardized assessment procedures are administered in the same manner and under the same conditions each time they are given. In contrast, *nonstandardized assessment procedures* are not necessarily given under the same conditions and in the same manner at each administration. Often, informal assessment procedures are nonstandardized. However, this is not a hard-and-fast rule (see Table 12.1).

An example of a standardized, norm-referenced test is an individual intelligence test. This kind of appraisal instrument is given the exact same way across the country, and an individual's score is then compared to national norm group scores (e.g., the individual's age group scores). A second example of a standardized test is the *Counselor Preparation Comprehensive Exam (CPCE)* administered by the *Center for Credentialing and Education (CCE)* (see http://www.cce-global.org/Org/CPCE). In this case, all schools that use this exam have the choice of comparing their school's scores to a national sample (the norm group) or deciding on a criterion cutoff (e.g., number of correct responses needed to obtain a "passing" score).

Examples of standardized, criterion-referenced assessment procedures include nationally made individual achievement tests, which are often given to students with learning disabilities. These tests are administered the same way each time, but a student takes only those parts of the test relevant to his or her individual learning goals as defined by a special education teacher. This test could additionally be norm-referenced if a comparison to a national norm group is desired and available.

Using a checklist to measure self-concept while observing a child in a class and then comparing the child's scores to those of a local norm group (e.g., students in the school) might be an example of a nonstandardized and norm-referenced test. In a case like this, specific test items can be developed to assess for the attribute that is being measured (e.g., "self-concept") and an individual's placement relative to his or her norm group (e.g., "students in the school") can be assessed.

Finally, a counselor-made assessment procedure that has targeted learning goals for students might be an example of a nonstandardized, criterion-referenced assessment procedure. For instance, a counselor who is working with children with behavioral problems might develop a set of nonstandardized procedures (e.g., counting child-specific behaviors related to the problem behaviors of each child). After counting the behaviors, the counselor would determine whether they have reached their targeted goals (the criterion).

Basic Test Statistics

Relativity and Meaningfulness of Test Scores

If Joshua receives a score of 47 on a test, and Mariana receives a score of 95 on a different test, how well have they done? If Joshua's score was 47 out of 52, one might assume he has done fairly well. But if 1,000 people had taken this test and all others received a higher score than Joshua, we might view his score somewhat differently. And to make things even more complicated, what if a high score represents an undesirable trait (e.g., cynicism, depression, or schizophrenia)? Then clearly the lower his score compared with his norm group, the comparatively better he has done, and vice versa.

What about Mariana's score? Is a score of 95 good? What if it is out of a possible score of 200, or 550, or 992? If 1,000 people take the test and Mariana's score is the highest, and if a higher score is desirable, we might say that she did well compared with her norm group. But if her score is on the lower end of the group of scores or a high score is not the goal, then comparatively, she did not do well.

By comparing Joshua and Mariana's scores to the scores of their peers or norm group, we can assign meanings to their scores. This is because *norm group comparisons*:

1. Allow individuals to compare themselves with their peer group. For instance, Joshua and Mariana can compare their scores with those of people who took the same test and are like them in some important way (e.g., similar age, same grade).
2. Allow test takers who took the same test but are in different norm groups to compare their results. For instance, a parent with two children who are two grades apart could determine which one is doing better in reading (e.g., one might score at the 50th percentile and the other at the 76th relative to the peer groups); or a school counselor might be interested in the self-esteem scores of all fifth graders compared to all third graders.
3. Allow an individual to compare his or her results on two different tests. For instance, as noted earlier, it is sometimes valuable to know an individual's score on an achievement test and on a scholastic aptitude test because a discrepancy

between the two tests might indicate a learning disability. Alternatively, when doing personality assessment, it is not unusual to give a number of different tests with an effort made to finding similar themes (e.g., high indications of anxiety on a number of different tests).

Finally, let's not forget that Joshua and Mariana will have their own opinions about how they think they should do on a test. Thus, a high score to one person would be a low score to another. The individual who consistently scores at the highest percentiles on a math test may feel upset about a score in the average range, while an individual who consistently scores low may feel good about that same score. Similarly, an individual who has struggled with lifelong depression may feel good about a moderate depression score on the *Beck Depression Inventory*, while another person might be concerned about such a score.

Measures of Central Tendency

Measures of central tendency tell us what is occurring in the midrange of a group of scores. Thus, if you know a person's score, you can compare that score to one of three scores that represent the midrange of the group. Three measures of central tendency include the *mode*, or the most frequent score; the *median*, or the middle score (50% of the scores fall below and above that score); and the *mean*, or the average of all of the scores. Although measures of central tendency do not tell a lot about general trends in the whole group, they do give a sense of whether a known score is higher or lower than the mean, median, or mode.

Measures of Variability

Measures of variability tell us how much scores vary in a distribution. Three measures of variability include the *range*, or the number of scores between the highest and lowest scores on a distribution; the *interquartile range*, which measures how 50% of the scores vary from the median; and the *standard deviation*, or the manner in which scores deviate around the mean in a standard fashion. Although all three measures of variability are important for the interpretation of test scores, in normally distributed curves, the standard deviation takes on a particular importance.

To better illustrate the concept of standard deviation, let me tell a quick story. A number of years ago while visiting the Museum of Science in Boston, I saw a device called a *quincunx* (also known as *Galton's Board,* named for Sir Francis Galton), through which hundreds of balls would be dropped onto a series of protruding points (see Figure 12.5 and www.odu.edu/~eneukrug/galton.htm). Each ball had a 50/50 chance of falling left or right every time it would hit one of the protruding objects. After all the balls were dropped, they would be collected and automatically dropped again. This machine would drop those balls over and over again, all day long. Now, this in and of itself was not so amazing. However, what did seem extraordinary was the fact that each and every time those balls were dropped, they would distribute themselves in the shape of a *normal curve* (also called the *bell-shaped curve*). Mind you, they were not distributing themselves in that manner because they were being sent in that direction. In fact, the resulting bell-shaped

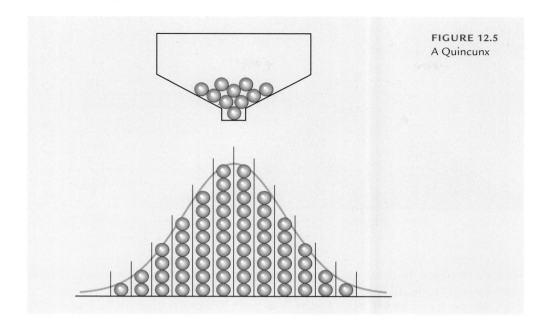

FIGURE 12.5
A Quincunx

curve is a product of the natural laws of the universe and is explained through the laws of probability. So perfect are these natural laws that minds as great as Einstein have given religious connotations to them (Isaacson, 2007). However, no matter what label is used to describe it, it is amazing that such a predictable pattern occurs over and over again. What does this have to with testing? Like the balls dropping in this device, when we measure most traits and abilities of people, the scores often approximate a bell-shaped distribution. This is very convenient, for the symmetry of this curve allows us to understand the most important measure of variability: *standard deviation.*

Let's take a look at one trait, depression, to help us understand how standard deviation works. If we examine scores of American adults on a test to measure depression, we might find something like the hypothetical curve in Figure 12.6. In this case, as in all normally distributed curves, the mean or average score always represents the 50th percentile and splits the distribution in half. In addition, the standard deviation distributes itself in a consistent manner. For instance, in all normally distributed curves, approximately 34% of the scores will fall between the mean and what is called "+1 standard deviation," and another 34% between the mean and "−1 standard deviation." Similarly, 14% will fall between +1 and +2 standard deviations and 14% will fall between −1 and −2 standard deviations. Finally, about 2% will fall between +2 and +3 standard deviations, and another 2% between −2 and −3 standard deviations.

Furthermore, in the normally distributed curve in Figure 12.6, as in all scores that have a distribution that approximates a bell-shaped curve, certain assumptions can be made about how scores deviate around the mean. For instance, if an individual scores above the mean, we immediately know that he or she has scored better than at least 50% of the population who took the test. If the individual scores at about the point of one

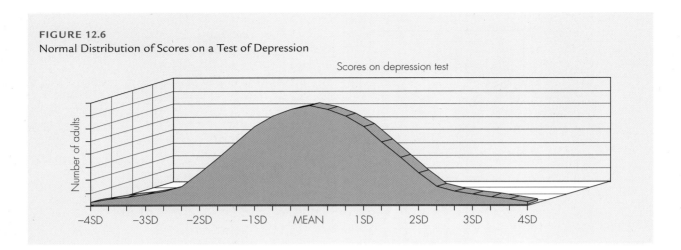

FIGURE 12.6
Normal Distribution of Scores on a Test of Depression

standard deviation, he or she has scored at approximately the 84th percentile, and so forth (see Figures 12.6 and 12.7).

Consider for a moment that a test has a mean of 52 and the standard deviation of 20. For this test, most of the scores (about 68%) would range between 32 and 72 (plus and minus 1 standard deviation; see Test 1, Figure 12.7). On the other hand, a second test that had a mean of 52 and a standard deviation of 5 would include 68% of its scores between 47 and 57 (again, plus and minus 1 standard deviation; see Test 2, Figure 12.7). Clearly,

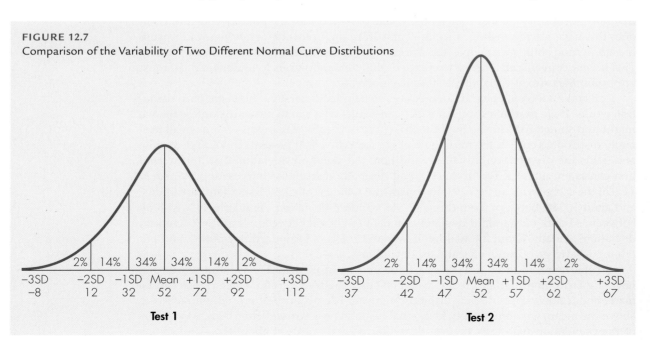

FIGURE 12.7
Comparison of the Variability of Two Different Normal Curve Distributions

even though the two tests have the same mean, the range of scores around the mean varies considerably. An individual's score of 40 would be in the average range on the first test, but well below average on the second test. This example shows why measures of central tendency and measures of variability are both important to understanding test scores.

Derived Scores

Usually, when a large group of individuals takes an assessment instrument, each person's reported score is not the actual raw score obtained by that person. Similarly, the mean is generally not the actual mean of all the raw scores. Instead, to make scores easier to interpret, the raw scores are converted by publishing companies to what are called *derived scores*. You are probably already aware of a number of derived scores such as *percentiles, stanines, SAT-type scores,* and *ACT-type scores*. If scores were not converted in this fashion, every individual who wanted to interpret his or her score would need knowledge of standard deviation and how it varies from test to test. In addition, converting scores to derived scores makes it easier to compare scores on different tests because their units of measurement are made comparable (e.g., percentiles on one test can be compared to percentiles on another).

Although the means and standard deviations of tests can vary dramatically, normal (bell-shaped) curves will always have the same percentage of scores distributing between the mean and one standard deviation above the mean (approximately 34%) or below the mean (another 34%). Similarly, all normally distributed curves will have the same percentage of scores between the mean and 2 standard deviations above the mean (approximately 48%) or below the mean (another 48%) and, of course, between the mean and 3 standard deviations above the mean (approximately 50%) or below the mean (another 50%). This property allows us to convert scores from any test that is normally distributed to a derived score of our choice. For instance, imagine two persons taking the same test. One obtains a raw score of 32 and the other a raw score of 92. When we discover that the mean is 52 and the standard deviation is 20 points, we immediately know that the first person scored at about the 16th percentile (1 standard deviation below the mean, or 52 minus 20) while the second person scored at about the 98th percentile (2 standard deviations above the mean, or 52 plus 20, and plus 20 again) (see Figure 12.7, Test 1). Now we know that on this test, one person scored at the 16th percentile while another scored at the 98th percentile; these scores are derived from the original raw scores. However, there are also other types of derived scores. For instance, if this was a test to measure depression, we might use a derived score called a *Transformed-score* (*T-score*). Having a mean of 50 and standard deviation of 10, T-scores are often used with personality assessment. Therefore, for the two individuals noted above, the first would have obtained a T-score of 40 (1 standard deviation below the mean), while the second would have obtained a T-score of 70 (2 standard deviations above the mean).

In addition to comparing two individuals on the same test, derived scores allow us to compare the same individual on different tests or on different subtests of the same test. For instance, a person might receive a T-score of 56 on a test of depression and a T-score of 32 on a test that measures trait anxiety. Thus, on the first test, that person scored above the mean (mean of T-scores is 50), and the same person obtained a score quite a bit below the mean (almost 2 standard deviations; e.g., 50 minus 10 and minus

10 again would be a derived score of 30). Below are some of the more typical derived scores that are used:

> *Percentile rank.* A derived score that describes the percentage of scores that fall at or below a given score. Percentiles are used with many different types of tests.
> *T-scores.* A derived score having a mean of 50 and a standard deviation of 10 and generally used with personality tests.
> *Deviation IQ.* A derived score having a mean of 100 and a standard deviation of 15 and generally used with intelligence tests.
> *SAT type scores.* A derived score having a mean of 500 and a standard deviation of 100; used mostly to report SAT scores.
> *ACT scores.* A derived score having a mean of 21 and standard deviation of 5; used with the ACT. Along with the SAT's, one of the most widely used college entrance exam.
> *Normal Curve Equivalents (NCE) scores.* A derived score having a mean of 50 and standard deviation of 21.06; often used with educational testing; ranges from 1 to 99.
> *Stanines.* A derived score having a mean of 5 and standard deviation of 2; generally used with achievement tests; ranges from 1 to 9.
> *Sten scores.* A derived score having a mean of 5.5 and standard deviation of 2; generally used with personality inventories and questionnaires; ranges from 1 to 10.
> *Grade equivalent scores.* A derived score generally used with achievement tests to determine an individual's position relative to his or her grade level. The grade level of the student represents the mean of the grade equivalent. Probably the most misunderstood of derived scores, grade equivalents above the current grade level do not mean that the individual can thrive at that grade level. Instead, it means that the student is doing much better than most students within his or her own grade level.
> *Idiosyncratic publisher-derived scores (scaled scores).* On some tests, particularly survey battery achievement tests, publishers create a derived score, sometimes called a *scaled score,* unique for that test. Therefore, a specific achievement test might have a mean of 150 and a standard deviation of 20, or a mean of 200 and a standard deviation of 25, and so forth—whatever specific mean and standard deviation that publisher decides to use. Usually, test publishers pick numbers that allow test takers to interpret their scores relatively easily.

Correlation Coefficient

A basic statistic that is not directly related to the interpretation of tests but is crucial in test construction is the *correlation coefficient.* Correlation coefficients show the relationship between two sets of scores, range from $+1$ to -1, and generally are reported in decimals of one-hundredths (see Figure 12.8). A *positive correlation* shows a tendency for two sets of scores to be related in the same direction. For instance, if a group of individuals took two tests, a positive correlation would show a tendency for those who obtained high scores on the first test to obtain high scores on the second test and for those who obtained low scores on the first test to obtain low scores on the second test.

FIGURE 12.8
The Range and Strength of Correlation Coefficients

−1, −.99,... −.80............ −.51.... −.25... −.10... −.02, −.01,0, +.01, +.02... +.10... +.25.... +.51,........... +.80... +.99, +1

| strong | moderate | low | none | low | moderate | strong |

A *negative correlation* shows an inverse relationship between two sets of scores; for instance, individuals who obtain high scores on the first test would be likely to obtain low scores on the second test. A correlation that approaches −1 or +1 shows a particularly strong relationship, while a correlation that approaches 0 shows little or no relationship between the two factors. For instance, if I wanted to show that the GREs predict performance in graduate school, I would have to show that the correlation coefficient does not approach zero and is significant enough to warrant its use (Burton & Wang, 2005).

Similarly, if I wanted to show that my newly made test of depression was worthwhile, I could correlate scores on my new test with an established test of depression. In this case, I would hope to find a relatively high correlation coefficient, as evidenced by the fact that individuals who scored high on my test would have a tendency to score high on the established test and individuals who scored low on my test would have a tendency to score low on the established test. Knowledge of the correlation coefficient concept is particularly important in assessing some aspects of the worthiness of a test.

Test Worthiness

> *The challenge to specialists in test theory is to continually broaden their methodology, to extend the toolkit of data-gathering and interpretation methods available to deal with increasingly richer sources of evidence, and more complex arguments for making sense of that evidence.*
>
> (Mislevy, 2004, p. 243)

Good tests are well-researched tests that can show evidence for the establishment of four qualities that are particularly important to *test worthiness*: (1) *validity*, whether a test measures what it is supposed to measure; (2) *reliability*, the ability of a test to measure a trait or ability accurately; (3) *cross-cultural fairness*, whether the test measures what it is supposed to measure in a consistent manner for all subgroups to whom the test is given; and (4) *practicality*, the ease of administration and interpretation of the test. Let's take a closer look at these qualities.

Validity

How well does a test measure what it's supposed to measure? That is the primary question that *validity* attempts to answer. Over the years, a number of methods have been developed to determine the validity of a test. Logically, it makes sense that the more methods that one can use to provide evidence of a test's validity, the stronger the case that one can make that the interpretation of test scores is accurate for its purposes (JCTP, 2004). Various types of validity that help to provide the evidence needed to demonstrate the worthiness of a test include *content validity; criterion-related validity*, which includes *concurrent validity* and *predictive validity*; and *construct validity*, which includes methods of *experimental design, factor analysis, discriminant validity*, and *convergent validity*. But first, let's describe a type of validity that is really not validity—*face validity*.

Face Validity

Often said not to be a real type of validity, a test can have *face validity* yet not be valid, or not have face validity and be valid. Face validity has to do with how the test superficially looks. If you were examining the test, would it appear to be measuring what it is supposed to measure? Although most tests should have face validity, some tests could be valid and yet not have it. For instance, there might be some items on a personality test that, on the surface, do not seem to be measuring the quality that the test is attempting to assess. Look, for example, at the hypothetical item below, which is assessing whether an individual may have a panic disorder:

1. In the past week, check the following symptoms that you have experienced:

_____ a. sweaty   _____ c. racing heart   _____ e. distracted myself
_____ b. numbness   _____ d. trouble breathing _____ f. avoided events

Even though the symptoms listed above might not seem obvious to a person unfamiliar with panic disorder, they are often associated with the disorder, as noted in the *Diagnostic and Statistical Manual-5* (APA, 2013a). On the surface, this item might not seem to be measuring the construct, but individuals with panic disorder often have some or all of these symptoms, and thus such a question might be an important indicator for test validity.

Content Validity

Content validity has to do with whether test items are constructed in a manner showing that they represent the defined body of knowledge being tested. Content validity is most important in ability testing, especially achievement testing, in which items picked to be included in the instrument need to be representative of the content area being tested. Content validity is generally achieved by surveying well-known texts, the professional literature, and experts in the test content area and then developing items based on the knowledge gained.

Criterion-Related Validity

Criterion-related validity exists when an assessment instrument is shown to be related to some external criterion or reference. Two types of criterion-related validity are concurrent validity and predictive validity. *Concurrent validity* occurs when a test shows sizable correlation to a criterion in the present. For instance, using a correlation coefficient, a newly made test of depression can be correlated with experts' clinical judgments of clients' depression. A high correlation would show criterion-related validity. A low correlation would mean the test's validity is questionable. *Predictive validity* takes place when a test is shown to be predictive of a future criterion. For instance, again using a correlation coefficient, ACT or SAT scores can be correlated with students' GPAs in college. A high correlation would show that the ACT or SAT can predict college grades to some degree. However, a low correlation would leave us questioning the ability of the test to predict college grades and the usefulness of the test for college admissions.

Construct Validity

Construct validity is used to support a theoretical assumption that the construct being measured by a test exists (Goodwin, 2002; Neukrug & Fawcett, 2015). Construct validity is much more important for more ambiguous constructs such as depression, empathy, or intelligence and less important for something like geometry or botany. As an example, let's say that I created a new test of depression. I would certainly expect that my test would be able to support my hypothesis that those who are depressed (e.g., psychiatric admissions for depression) would score higher on my test compared to those who are not depressed (e.g., a group of identified nondepressed individuals). If my test can distinguish these two groups, I have shown *experimental validity*, a type of construct validity that uses validation of a research hypothesis to support the construct. A second type of construct validity, *convergent validity*, examines if my test is related to an already existing, valid test (e.g., correlating my test with the existing Beck Depression Inventory). *Discriminant validity*, a third way to show construct validity, demonstrates that a test is not related to another test (e.g., there would be no relationship between scores on my depression tests and scores on an established test that measures anxiety). Finally, if my test had subscales that were supposed to be unique (e.g., hopelessness, suicidal ideation, and sadness), then when correlating the subscales with one another, we should find only a negligible relationship among them (*factor analysis validity*). This type of construct validity supports the notion that subscales on a test are separate and unique, although they all might be related to the larger construct (in this case, depression).

Reliability

The second quality examined in determining the adequacy of an assessment instrument is *reliability*. Whereas validity is used to show that a test is measuring what it's supposed to measure, reliability examines the accuracy of test scores. Put another way, reliability measures the amount of *error* in a test—the less error, the better the test. As with validity, reliability measures the adequacy of the test and is not making a statement about the people taking the test. There are a number of ways of examining such accuracy, including *test–retest, alternate forms, split-half,* and *internal consistency reliability.*

Test–Retest Reliability

One common type of reliability, *test–retest reliability* examines the relationship between scores on one administration of a test with scores on a second administration of the same test to the same group of people. For instance, if I wished to show that my test was accurate, I might administer the instrument to a large group of individuals and, after a short time (perhaps one week) has passed, administer it a second time. I would then correlate the scores from the first administration with the scores from the second administration of the test. A test that is poorly made (has a fair amount of error) will result in many individuals having large deviations between the first and second administrations of the test. One problem with this kind of reliability is in sorting whether deviations between the first and second administration of a test are the result of changes in individuals or because of error in the test (remember, we are measuring error in the test, not changes in the person). For instance, if individuals are given a test to measure depression, then seek out therapy, and one month later are given the same test, it would be difficult to determine if changes in test scores are a result of therapy or reflective of a poorly made test. This is why other types of reliability that do not rely on a second administration of the test are often used in addition to or in lieu of test–retest reliability.

Alternative Forms Reliability

Also called *parallel forms or equivalent forms reliability, alternative forms reliability* measures the accuracy of a test by correlating one form of a test with a second form that is considered to be a close mirror of the first form. Because the two forms are generally given at the same time, the possibility that the correlation is a result of changes in the individual between the first and second administrations of the test is eliminated. One problem with this kind of reliability is the difficulty of making a second form that is a true mirror of the first. Also, for many tests, it is not practical to devise a second, equivalent form of the test.

Split-Half Reliability

Sometimes called *odd-even reliability, split-half reliability* eliminates the problem of having to create a second form of the test. In this kind of reliability, the instrument is split in half in some rational manner that assumes that scores on the first half of the test should be equivalent to scores on the second half. The two halves are then correlated to show the accuracy of the test. A major problem with this kind of reliability revolves around the fact that two halves of a test are generally not perfectly equivalent to one another, and therefore this does not assess as accurately for error within the test.

Internal Consistency

Like split-half reliability, *internal consistency reliability* gives an estimate of consistency based on a single administration of a test. The reliability estimate found reflects the average of all split-half reliabilities. With the advent of computers, this kind of reliability has become quite popular. Two popular types of internal consistency reliabilities include *Cronbach's Coefficient Alpha* and *Kuder-Richardson* (see Table 12.2 for a summary of validity and reliability).

Cross-Cultural Fairness of Tests

> . . . *Information gained and decisions made about the client or student are valid only to the degree that the test accurately and fairly assesses the client's or student's characteristics. Test selection and interpretation are done with an*

TABLE 12.2   Summary of Types of Validity and Reliability

VALIDITY	RELIABILITY
Content: Content analysis; experts contribute test questions and are consulted, and items are created from well-known sources.	*Test–retest:* The ability of a test to show consistency in scores from one testing to a second testing.
Concurrent: A kind of criterion-related validity that evaluates the relationship between the test and a criterion in the present (e.g., another test, expert judges' ratings).	*Alternate forms:* The correlation of one form of a test with a second equivalent form of the test. Also called *equivalent* or *parallel form reliability.*
Predictive: A kind of criterion-related validity that evaluates the relationship between the test and a future criterion.	*Split-half:* The relationship between items on one half of a test with items on the second half of the test. Also called *odd-even reliability.*
Construct: The ability of a test to show that a certain construct exists and can support a theoretical assumption of the test. There are four types: experimental design, factor analysis, discriminant validity, and convergent validity.	*Internal consistency:* The average of all possible split-half reliabilities. Two types are Cronbach's Coefficient Alpha and Kuder-Richardson.

> *awareness of the degree to which items may be culturally biased or the norming*
> *sample not reflective or inclusive of the client's or student's diversity . . .*
>
> (ACA, 2003, Standard 6)

Cross-cultural fairness is critical in determining whether an assessment instrument is fair for all individuals who may be taking a test or assessment instrument. Although it is impossible to eliminate all bias from tests and other assessment instruments, one should expect that the bias is small enough to allow for justifiable interpretations of any individual's responses. When examining cultural bias, test publishers should have exhaustively reviewed the extent to which the content of a test has cultural bias. For instruments used to predict future behavior, the test should be shown to be predictive for minority groups. This does not mean that it will predict in the same manner for all groups, but that the predictive validity of each subgroup was examined and the test was shown to predict accurately for each subgroup (Aiken & Groth-Marnta, 2006). In fact, the U.S. Supreme Court case of *Griggs v. Duke Power Company* (1971) asserted that tests used for hiring and advancement at work must show that they can predict job performance for all groups.

Cross-cultural bias in testing is an important issue when assessment instruments are used with individuals from diverse cultures. Examiners need to be aware of bias in testing, ethical issues related to assessment and multiculturalism, and state and national laws concerning the use of tests with minorities. Some related issues will be discussed later in this chapter.

Practicality

Suppose that I have a test that can accurately assess mental health problems, but each administration costs $1,000. This test may be good at what it does, but the cost may be prohibitive for most people. Or suppose that we have an instrument than can accurately measure learning disabilities but takes a school psychologist two days to administer. These are some of the questions with which we must struggle when deciding whether or not a test is practical.

Practicality examines whether the test is realistic to give. It includes issues related to the cost of testing, the time it takes to administer the test, the ease of administration, the format of the test, the readability of the test, and the ease of interpretation. A test can have good validity and good reliability and be cross-culturally fair, and yet not be practical to give.

Where to Find Tests and Assessment Techniques

Today, there are thousands of tests available for a wide variety of assessment procedures (Buros Center for Testing, 2014). Because there are so many options, finding a test or assessment technique that meets one's specific needs is not always easy. However, a number of sources are available to assist in the proper selection of tests for use with a desired population:

1. *Publisher resource catalogs.* Publishing companies freely distribute catalogs that describe the tests and assessment procedures they sell.
2. *Journals in the field.* Professional journals, especially those associated with measurement, will often describe assessment procedures that they have used in research or give reviews of new instruments in the field.
3. *Source books and online source information on testing and assessment procedures.* There are a few comprehensive books that provide the names of the test author(s), the publication date, the purpose of the test, critical reviews, bibliographical information, information on test construction, the name and address of the test publishing company, the costs of the test, and other basic information. Two of the most important source books are the *Buros Mental Measurement Yearbook,* which can now be accessed online, and its companion volume, *Tests in Print.*
4. *Books on testing and assessment.* Textbooks that present an overview of testing and assessment techniques are usually fairly good at highlighting a number of the better-known procedures that are used today.
5. *Experts.* School psychologists, learning disability specialists, experts at a school system's central testing office, psychologists at agencies, and professors are some of the people who can be called on for assistance with information on assessment procedures.
6. *The Internet.* Today, publishing companies have home pages that offer information about assessment procedures they sell. In addition, the Internet has become an increasingly important place to search for information about a variety of assessment procedures. Of course, one needs to be careful to ensure that any information from the Internet is accurate.

Writing Assessment Reports

In-depth information on the writing of assessment reports is not within the purview of this text. However, because some counselors will write such reports, and all counselors will read the assessment reports of others, it is crucial that they understand the basics of report writing. Although the content of a report will vary based on the purpose of the assessment, a report will generally include the following categories: demographic information, reason for referral, family background, other relevant information (e.g., legal, medical, vocational), behavioral observations of the client, a mental status, test results, a diagnosis, recommendations, and summary (Neukrug & Fawcett, 2015).

As with clinical case reports, assessment reports should not be longer than a few pages, and the examiner should use language that most professionals can understand—even ones who have little or no background in testing and assessment. Some common problems that have been identified in the writing of assessment reports include the overuse of jargon, focusing on the assessment procedures and downplaying the person, focusing on the person and deemphasizing the assessment results, poor organization, poor writing skills, and failing to take a position about the person who was assessed (e.g., not making specific recommendations) (Goldfinger, & Pomerantz, 2014; Neukrug & Fawcett, 2015). Ideally, as you proceed through your training program, you will obtain many opportunities to practice writing assessment and case reports.

Multicultural/Social Justice Focus

Caution in Using Assessment Procedures

As noted earlier, so important are cross-cultural issues in testing today that they are included as one of the four aspects in determining the worthiness of an assessment instrument (Neukrug & Fawcett, 2015). Because bias in testing has been a problem since the beginning of assessment procedures, a number of standards have been developed to address this important issue. For instance, the *Association for Assessment and Research in Counseling (AARC)*, a division of ACA, has developed *Standards for Multicultural Assessment* that provides 68 standards in the areas of advocacy, selection of assessment procedures, administration and scoring, interpretation and application of results, and training in the use of assessments, (AARC, 2012). In addition to the standards, the ACA *Code of Ethics* speaks to the importance of the careful use of testing with minorities:

> Counselors select and use with caution assessment techniques normed on populations other than that of the client. Counselors recognize the effects of age, color, culture, disability, ethnic group, gender, race, language preference, religion, spirituality, sexual orientation, and socioeconomic status on test administration and interpretation, and place test results in proper perspective with other relevant factors.

(ACA, 2014a, Standard E.8)

Also, the *Code of Fair Testing Practices in Education* has been developed, with its intent being to ensure that testing is "fair to all test takers regardless of age, gender, disability, race, ethnicity, national origin, religion, sexual orientation, linguistic background, or other personal characteristics" (JCTP, 2004, p. 1). Finally, there are many other standards and guidelines for the proper use of tests, and all address this important issue in some manner (see the section "Guidelines for the Use of Assessment Procedures," later in this chapter).

Take a Stand—Do Something!

All too often, I have seen counselors idly stand by and do nothing when they know that:

➤ Tests have been administered improperly

➤ A learning-disabled student should have been removed from testing because he or she was not at his or her optimum [e.g., a child with attention deficit hyperactivity disorder (ADHD) did not take medication, was hyper, and could not focus on the test questions]

➤ Tests were used that were culturally biased

➤ Tests were used that had limited validity or reliability

➤ Cheating has taken place

It is our duty, our moral responsibility, and our ethical obligation to speak out. When you do nothing for fear of losing your job, when you do nothing for fear of being a rebel, when you do nothing for fear of reprisal, and when you do nothing because you simply do not care, you are part of the problem, not the solution. Do not make excuses for not responding—speak out.

Ethical, Professional, and Legal Issues

Ethical Issues

Guidelines for the Use of Assessment Procedures

To guide practitioners and the public, a number of codes and standards address a myriad of assessment issues. If you are interested in becoming more involved in assessment, you may want to take the time to examine some of the following standards:

a. *The ACA ethical code* (ACA, 2014a)
b. *The Code of Fair Testing Practices in Education* (JCTP, 2004)
c. *Standards for Multicultural Assessment* (AARC, 2014a)
d. *Standards for the Qualifications of Test Users* (ACA, 2003)
e. *Responsibilities of Users of Standardized Tests* (RUST) (AARC, 2003)
f. *Rights and Responsibilities of Test Takers: Guidelines and Expectations* (JCTP, 2000)
g. *Standards for Educational and Psychological Testing* (American Educational Research Association, 1999)
h. *Competencies for testing in School Counseling; Mental Health Counseling, Marriage, Couples, and Family Counseling; Career Counseling, and Substance Abuse Counseling* (see AARC, 2014a)

Nature and Purpose of Assessment

Similar to informed consent, prior to being assessed, clients should be explained the nature and purpose of assessment, as noted in the ACA (2014a) code of ethics:

> Prior to assessment, counselors explain the nature and purposes of assessment
> and the specific use of results by potential recipients. The explanation will be

> *given in terms and language that the client (or other legally authorized person*
> *on behalf of the client) can understand.*

> (Section E.3.a)

Although individuals have the right to refuse testing or other assessment procedures; in some cases, such as court-ordered testing to assess fitness of a parent in a child custody case, a client may not have such a right or refusal to be tested could have negative implications.

Invasion of Privacy and Confidentiality

Assessments invade one's privacy. However, concerns about invasion of privacy are lessened if the client has given informed consent, has some real choice in whether he or she can refuse an assessment, and knows the limits of confidentiality, such as when testing is court ordered (Wheeler & Bertram, 2012).

Competence in the Use of Tests

To properly administer, score, and interpret test results, test givers must have adequate knowledge about testing and familiarity with any test they may use. To establish who is qualified to give specific tests, during the 1950s the American Psychological Association (APA) adopted a three-tier system for test user qualifications. Although APA reevaluated this system and currently provides rather extensive guidelines for test user qualifications (see Turner, Demers, Fox, & Reed, 2001), many test publishers continue to use the original three-tier system:

> *Level A tests are those that can be administered, scored, and interpreted by*
> *responsible nonpsychologists who have carefully read the test manual and are*
> *familiar with the overall purpose of testing. Educational achievement tests fall*
> *into this category.*
>
> *Level B tests require technical knowledge of test construction and use and*
> *appropriate advanced coursework in psychology and related courses (e.g.,*
> *statistics, individual differences, and counseling).*
>
> *Level C tests require an advanced degree in psychology or licensure as a*
> *psychologist and advanced training/supervised experience in the particular test.*

> (APA, 1954, pp. 146–148)

To highlight some examples based on the above categories: teachers can administer most Level A survey battery achievement tests, while master's-level counselors can administer Level B tests (e.g., interest inventories and many objective personality tests). Level C tests are reserved for those who have at least a master's degree, a basic testing course, and advanced training in the specialized tests they may be giving (e.g., school psychologists, learning disabilities specialists, clinical and counseling psychologists, and master's-level therapists who have gained additional training).

Technology and Assessment

The expansion of the use of technology has brought some challenges to counseling and to the use of tests in this medium. The most recent ACA (2014a) code of ethics expanded its coverage of technology, and a number of items apply to testing and assessment. Some of these include knowing one's limitations relative to technology and assessment, being competent on the use of technology and assessment, ensuring security of tests results; ensuring confidentiality and privacy, and maintaining results electronically in ways that ensure compliance to the law.

The next decade will undoubtedly bring with it an ever-increasing reliance on technology in the assessment realm, and counselors will need to be ever vigilant about the proper use of assessment instruments as new technological advances are made.

Other Ethical Issues

In addition to the issues already noted, other ethical issues should be considered when administering and interpreting test results, and you are encouraged to read the ACA (2014a) ethical standards carefully to familiarize yourself with them. Briefly, a few of these include knowing how to (1) properly release test results; (2) select tests; (3) administer, score, and interpret tests; (4) keep tests secure; (5) pick tests that are current and up to date; and (6) assess whether tests are properly constructed.

Professional Issues

Computer-Driven Assessment Reports

Today, there are computer programs that can assist in the assessment process. One such program has the interviewer or the client complete 120 items that requests information about a wide range of personal issues, and the user receives a computer-generated report that describes the client's presenting problems, legal issues, current living situation, tentative diagnosis, emotional state, treatment recommendations, mental status, health and habits, disposition, and behavioral/physical descriptions (see Schinka, 2012). After obtaining the information, computers can generate sophisticated test reports, and often, pieces of these reports can be moved directly into the examiner's written assessment report (Berger, 2006; Michaels, 2006). However, whether it is a computer-generated report that resulted from a client interview or a report that includes aspects of computer-generated test reports, it is still up to the examiner to make sure that the correct questions are being asked of the client, the correct assessment procedures are being used, and that the material used in the development of the examiner's assessment report is chosen wisely by the examiner:

> While the computer may administer these [tests] and even prepare a report, what the test looks like, how it responds, what it achieves, and any reports generated are predetermined by the author, and it is a person who puts it all together to make the interpretation.
>
> (Berger, 2006, p. 70)

Professional Association

The AARC is the one division of ACA that has one of its major focuses on assessment. In fact, its vision is to advance "the counseling profession by promoting best practices in assessment, research, and evaluation in counseling" (AARC, 2014b, para. 1). Consider joining AARC if you are interested in testing, assessment, diagnosis, and the training and supervision of those who do assessment, if you are interested in developing and validating assessment products and procedures, or both. AARC publishes the journals *Measurement and Evaluation in Counseling and Development* and *Counseling Outcome Research and Evaluation.*

Legal Issues: Laws That Have Had an Impact on Testing

A number of laws have been passed that impinge on the use of tests. Some of the more important ones include:

- ➤ *Americans with Disabilities Act.* This law states that accommodations must be made for individuals who are taking tests for employment and that testing must be shown to be relevant to the job in question (U.S. Equal Employment Commission, n.d.).
- ➤ *Family Education Rights and Privacy Act (FERPA).* This law affirms the right of all individuals to their school records, including test records (U.S. Department of Education, 2014b).
- ➤ *Carl Perkins Act (PL 98-524).* This law ensures that individuals with disabilities, or who are disadvantaged, have access to vocational assessment, counseling, and placement (U.S. Department of Education, 2007).
- ➤ *Civil Rights Acts (1964 and amendments).* This series of laws asserts that any test used for employment or promotion must be shown to be suitable and valid for the job in question. If not, alternative means of assessment must be provided. Differential test cutoffs are not allowed.
- ➤ *Freedom of Information Act.* This law ensures the right of individuals to access their federal records, including test records (U.S. Department of Justice, 2013). Most states have expanded this law so that it also applies to state records.
- ➤ *PL 94-142 and the Individuals with Disabilities Education Act (IDEA).* These legislative acts ensure the right of students to be tested, at a school system's expense, if they are suspected of having a disability that interferes with learning. The law asserts that schools must make accommodations, within the *least-restrictive environment,* for students with learning disabilities (U.S. Department of Education, n.d.).
- ➤ *Section 504 of the Rehabilitation Act.* Relative to assessment, any instrument used to measure the appropriateness of a program or service must be measuring the individual's ability, not be a reflection of his or her disability (U.S. Department of Health and Human Services, 2006a).
- ➤ *Health Insurance Portability and Accountability Act (HIPAA).* HIPAA ensures the privacy of client records, including testing records, and the sharing of such information (APA, 2013c; Zuckerman, 2008). In general, HIPAA restricts the amount of information that can be shared without client consent and allows clients to have access to their records, except for process notes used in counseling.

The Counselor in Process:
Assessment as Holistic and Ongoing

Assessment of clients is much broader than simply giving an individual a test. In fact, one should generally "avoid using a single test score as the sole determinant of decisions . . ." And one should "interpret test scores in conjunction with other information about individuals" (JCTP, 2004, Section C-5). Thus, a thorough assessment will involve a number of different kinds of assessment procedures, such as formal tests, informal assessment instruments, diagnosis, and a clinical interview. This holistic process can help us obtain a broader and more accurate picture of the client than if we were to rely on just one test (Mislevy, 2004; Moss, 2004).

Assessment is also an ongoing process that begins the first moment the counselor and client meet. As the helping relationship continues and deepens, the assessment process tends to move from being counselor-centered, in the sense that the counselor provides the tools to assist the client in his or her own self-assessment process, to being client-centered, where the client learns how to assess himself or herself. Although the counseling relationship will eventually end, it is hoped that seeds have been planted for the client to continue with an ongoing and deepening self-assessment process throughout his or her life.

Summary

This chapter started by defining assessment and noted that testing was a subset of assessment. We noted that assessment includes such things as personality testing, ability testing, informal assessment, and the clinical interview, examined why testing and assessment are important, and stated that assessment is one additional way that counselors can come to understand the inner world of the client. In addition, we discussed how assessment can aid counselors in understanding the client's abilities and personality and can be useful in diagnosis, goal setting, treatment planning, program evaluation, and research. We also found that testing and assessment are an important function of counselors in all settings, noting that counselors provide a wide range of testing and assessment activities.

Throughout history, people have always been assessed. This chapter noted that the modern-day origins of assessment can be traced to the mid-1800s, when the assessment of individual differences and the use of the scientific method became popular. With changing demographics and the impact of the industrial revolution during the turn of the twentieth century, we saw the first need for the widespread use of tests, particularly vocational assessment. With the advent of World War I, the importance of assessment increased as ability and personality tests were developed to help with the placement of recruits. Soon, tests and assessment procedures of all kinds were used in many different settings. We noted that tests have been refined over the years and that new statistical models and computers have particularly improved the quality of tests.

Today, there are many different kinds of tests and assessment techniques, including ability tests, which comprise achievement and aptitude tests. Three kinds of achievement tests noted in this discussion include survey battery, diagnostic, and readiness. Some of the different kinds of aptitude tests highlighted were cognitive ability tests, intelligence tests, neuropsychological assessment, special aptitude, and multiple aptitude tests. We noted that personality tests measure temperament, habits, likes, disposition, and nature and identified three types: objective, projective, and interest inventories. We also identified a number of different kinds of informal types of assessment, such as observation, rating scales, classification methods, environmental assessment, records and personal documents, and performance-based assessment. The chapter also pointed out that the clinical interview is a type of assessment.

We noted that assessment procedures can be standardized and either norm-referenced or criterion-referenced; or nonstandardized and either norm-referenced or criterion-referenced. In putting meaning to test scores, it is important to examine an individual's score relative to his or her norm group and to understand what the score means to the individual taking the test. The chapter highlighted the fact that measures of central tendency (mean, median, and mode) and variability (range, interquartile range, and standard deviation) can assist in making comparisons between individuals who take the same test or between individuals who have taken different tests.

The chapter explained that in examining basic test statistics, one measure of variability is particularly important in understanding norm-referenced tests: the standard deviation. We also noted that the standard deviation helps convert raw scores to derived scores. We discussed the fact that derived scores, such as percentiles, T-scores, deviation IQ scores, ACT scores, SAT-type scores, NCEs, stanines, sten scores, grade equivalents, and idiosyncratic publisher test scores (scaled scores) are used because they are easier to interpret than raw scores.

Next, the text covered the statistical concept of the correlation coefficient and showed how it is important when examining some issues of test worthiness. We then went on to discuss four qualities of test worthiness. The first quality highlighted was validity, or whether or not a test measures what it is supposed to measure. We noted that face validity is not a real type of validity, and then we discussed three types of validity: content validity, criterion-related validity (concurrent and predictive) and construct validity (experimental, convergent, discriminant, and factor analysis). Then we defined reliability, or the ability of a test to accurately measure a trait or ability. Four types of reliability included test–retest, alternate forms (a.k.a., parallel or equivalent forms), split-half (a.k.a. odd-even), and internal consistency (Coefficient Alpha and Kuder-Richardson). The other two qualities discussed were cross-cultural fairness, (whether the test measures what it's supposed to measure in a consistent manner for all groups), and practicality (the ease of administration and interpretation of the test).

The chapter noted that today, there are many sources that can help find tests that have good reliability and validity, are practical, and have limited cultural bias. Some of these include publishers' resource manuals; professional journals; source books on testing, such as the *Buros Mental Measurement Yearbook* and *Tests in Print*; textbooks on testing; experts in schools and agencies; and the Internet. We also discussed the importance of writing a good assessment report and highlighted some potential problems in the writing of such reports.

Relative to multicultural and social justice issues, we pointed out that over the years, there have been problems with bias in assessment instruments and that in recent years, a number of standards have been developed to address these biases, such as AARC's

Standards for Multicultural Assessment. The discussion also pointed out the moral and ethical responsibility for counselors to address issues of bias and problems in testing.

Next, the chapter highlighted a number of ethical issues in the area of assessment, including identifying a number of guidelines for the ethical and professional use of assessment procedures, informed consent, invasion of privacy and confidentiality, competence in the use of tests (e.g., APA's "A, B, and C" system), technology and assessment, and others. Professional issues noted included the proper use of computer-driven assessment reports and identifying the ACA assessment division: the Association for Assessment and Research in Counseling (AARC).

We next went on to briefly discuss a number of legislative actions and their impact on testing, including the Americans with Disabilities Act, the Family Education Rights and Privacy Act (FERPA), the Carl Perkins Act, Civil Rights Acts, the Freedom of Information Act, PL94-142 and the Individuals with Disabilities Education Act (IDEA), Section 504 of the Rehabilitation Act, and the Health Insurance Portability and Accountability Act (HIPAA).

Finally, the chapter concluded by highlighting the fact that assessment is an ongoing, holistic process that includes a number of components, and that when a successful counseling relationship terminates, the client ideally will be able to continue the assessment process on his or her own.

Further Practice

Visit CengageBrain.com to respond to additional material that highlight the salient aspects of the chapter content. There, you can find ethical, professional, and legal vignettes, a number of experiential exercises, and study tools including a glossary, flashcards, and sample test items. Hopefully, these will enhance your learning and be fun and interesting.

Research and Evaluation

Christina Hamme Peterson and Ed Neukrug

> *Research has been maligned. Some criticize it, students fear it, and others approach it as if it were a virus, never coming too close to it. Unfortunately, many lose sight, or perhaps never gain the insight, that research "can be an exhilarating experience, analogous to adding pieces to a jigsaw puzzle."*

(Whiston, 1996, p. 622)

(Ed Neukrug) remember a graduate student coming to me, bewildered after not finding significant results on a study that she was conducting for her thesis. She had hypothesized that there would be a relationship between the number of years that one meditated and self-actualizing values; that is, the more you meditated, the more self-actualized you would be. She went to an ashram (a yoga retreat center) and had a number of meditators complete an instrument that measured their level of self-actualization, and then she collected information from these same individuals concerning how long they had been meditating. After collecting her data and performing a statistical analysis, she found no significant relationship. As she herself had meditated for years and was an ardent believer in meditation, she was convinced that she would find such a relationship; clearly, she was personally invested in the research. Upon finding no significant relationship, she said to me, "There must be something wrong with this research, because people who have meditated for years are more self-actualized than those who have just started meditating." I suggested there was nothing wrong with the research, but that perhaps she had a bias because of her own experiences with meditation. I explained that this does not mean that meditation does not affect people, but that for this population, using this instrument and research design, the evidence showed that no significant relationship existed. I went on to remind her that research is not how you feel something is, but what the results show. When she was able to see her own biases, she realized that perhaps I had a point.

A number of years ago, I was conducting research on the relationship between dogmatism, internal locus of control, and attitudes toward learning in graduate students. I dutifully collected my data and was hoping to do my statistical analysis soon when a colleague of mine pointed out that it might also be interesting to look at how students make meaning in their lives. He suggested a process by which he would interview a number of students who had participated in my study and attempt to find patterns and themes in their responses. He eventually hoped to distinguish students from one another based on their ways of making meaning and suggested that we could relate meaning making to the other attributes I was examining. I responded that his research seemed kind of soft. "How do you quantify interviews?" I asked. He was soon to teach me an important lesson about research: that research can be more than simply looking at numbers, and that research comes in many different forms. He was suggesting integrating a qualitative approach with my quantitative analysis—two very different ways of doing research.

A colleague and I once received a $70,000 grant to train helping professionals in the schools about substance abuse interventions. We ran a series of workshops and subsequently used a number of evaluation techniques to determine whether the training program had been worthwhile. These evaluation procedures served a number of purposes, including helping us examine what had been beneficial during the earlier workshops, assisting us in fine-tuning later workshops, helping us know the overall satisfaction of the participants with the total program, designing future training programs, and perhaps most significantly in this instance, producing evidence to show our funding source—the federal government, which was auditing us—that we were accomplishing our stated goals and that we were accountable.

Why should anyone do research and evaluation? Well, as you can see by the above examples, research and evaluation help us find answers to the questions we ponder, move us forward in our understanding of the world, help us show that what we are doing is worthwhile, are ways of expressing our creativity—and can even be interesting and fun.

This chapter will examine some of the more common research and evaluation techniques and, we hope, present them in a manner that is appealing and exciting. We will begin by defining the purpose of research and distinguishing between two major forms of research: quantitative and qualitative. We will also compare the value of different kinds of research. After surveying various research methods, we will offer an overview of evaluation methods and examine the relationship of evaluation to research. Finally, we will examine the multicultural, social justice, ethical, professional, and legal issues related to research and evaluation.

Research

The Purpose of Research

> *Research is formalized curiosity. It is poking and prying with a purpose. It is a seeking that he who wishes may know the cosmic secrets of the world and they that dwell therein.*
>
> (Hurston, 1942/2006, p. 143)

Best and Kahn (2006) describe research as "the systematic and objective analysis and recording of controlled observations that may lead to the development of generalizations, principles, or theories, resulting in prediction and possibly ultimate control of events" (p. 25). In other words, research analyzes information in order to give us knowledge about the present—knowledge that may help us to predict the future. Research comes in many forms and can be as varied as counting the number of times a child acts out during the day, surveying opinions of counselors, using intensive interviews to understand how moral development is established, or performing complex statistical analyses to determine which counseling skills are most effective.

Without research, knowledge remains stagnant, and new paradigms are unlikely to evolve (Kuhn, 1962). While our theories are interesting and are generally the basis for our research, theories hold little weight if they are not eventually grounded in research. Research validates what the counselor is doing and can suggest new avenues for approaching client change (Hays, 2010). Research is the basis for evaluation that enables us to know if the programs and workshops we are conducting are effective. Without research, we are an ethereal profession with our heads in the air and little or no means of showing that what we do is meaningful.

Who is the researcher? It's you, and me, and all individuals who rely on evidence to make sure that what we are doing is working. In fact, some have argued that all master's-level counselors are researchers in the sense that they are *practitioner–scientists*; they work with and collect information from clients (e.g., via clinical interviews) and use the information gathered, as well as information from science (e.g., journal articles) to make informed decisions about their clients (Houser, 2015).

Literature Reviews and the Statement of the Problem

Research offers us a mechanism to satisfy our innate curiosity about human nature. For instance, you have undoubtedly pondered the nature of emotional disorders and have wondered about effective ways to treat such problems. The researcher uses systematic methods to gather information in an effort to seek out plausible answers to these questions (Gay, Mills, & Airasian, 2012), and the practitioner uses the researcher's results.

So, where does the researcher start? At the beginning, of course, with a hunch or an educated guess about a topic of interest that the researcher would like to explore. Usually, the next step is for the researcher to examine prior research to see what has gone before (some *qualitative researchers* argue against conducting a literature review first—but more about this later). The examination of prior research is called the *review of the literature,* and it is generally begun by conducting a computerized search of abstracts in the fields of counseling, education, psychology, and other disciplines that might be relevant to the research. Although there are many electronic databases that are searchable, often through one's library, two particularly popular ones include *Educational Resources Information Center (ERIC)* and *PsycINFO.*

Emerging from a review of the literature is the *statement of the problem,* which places the research within its historical context, determines what research already exists on the topic, and discusses why the issue at hand is important. The literature review also limits the scope of what one is researching, explains how the research departs from past research, and points one in the direction of developing research questions, statements, and hypotheses that delimit the type of research that will be conducted (McMillan & Schumacher, 2010; Mertler & Charles, 2011). For example, examine the statement of the problem of ethical issues in counseling practices (see Box 13.1).

Once the statement of the problem is developed, the research design can be formulated. Generally, one's research design is based on a number of factors, including whether the researcher believes it is best to use quantitative research, qualitative research, or a mixed methods approach, and the kind of research that has previously been conducted, as evidenced in the literature review and statement of the problem.

BOX 13.1

Statement of the Problem

What constitutes ethical counselor behavior one year may not be ethical the next, especially in light of the fact that ethical codes change as a function of changing values in society, new evidence-based research, and the changing nature of professional associations (Ponton & Duba, 2009). The most recent ethics code of the American Counseling Association (ACA, 2014a) demonstrates how much a code can change by including a number of revisions that challenge counselors to work in new ways. For instance, the 2014 code includes new, stronger language prohibiting counselors from referring clients simply because of differences in personal values, extends confidentiality to include the time before and after an individual was a client, and provides standards on the ethical use of social media and other forms of technology with clients (Meyers, 2014; ACA, 2014a).

Making good ethical decisions depends upon knowledge of one's code, familiarity with models of ethical decision making, cognitive complexity of the counselor, and knowledge of problematic ethical situations (Corey, Corey, & Callanan, 2015; Hill, 2004; Neukrug, Lovell, & Parker, 1996). The problem is that as

ethical guidelines change, current and future counselors may not feel prepared to address ethical concerns in their practice adequately. Identifying how to help current and future counselors become more knowledgeable about and skilled at responding to difficult ethical issues has already partially been addressed by researchers in a number of ways. For instance, some have surveyed credentialing boards to assess the kinds of complaints and violations made against counselors (Neukrug, Milliken, & Walden, 2001; Saunders, Barros-Bailey, Rudman, Dew, & Garcia, 2007). This provides information as to what violations are most common and, therefore, should be covered in training. Others have surveyed counselors directly to identify those areas in which they may need additional training (Hermann, Legget, & Remley, 2008; Neukrug & Milliken, 2011).

Given the studies that have already been conducted, future research to address how counselors can feel more prepared to address ethical concerns might include investigations into effective and ineffective counselor responses to ethical challenges and what kind of ethics training leads to the greatest gains in self-efficacy and knowledge about what to do in ethics situations.

As you read the above statement of the problem, can you identify what the problem is? Also, how does the statement of the problem shape the research being suggested?

Distinguishing Between Quantitative and Qualitative Research

Quantitative research assumes that there is an objective reality within which research questions can be formulated and scientific methods used to measure the probability that certain behaviors, values, or beliefs either cause or are related to other behaviors, values, or beliefs. *Qualitative research*, on the other hand, holds that there are multiple realities and that one can make sense of the world by immersing oneself in the research situation in an attempt to understand and describe the phenomena being examined (Heppner, Wampold, & Kivlighan, 2008). Table 13.1 gives a summary of the distinguishing features of qualitative and quantitative research.

Qualitative and quantitative research approach the analysis of research problems differently. Thus, it is not surprising that their designs vary dramatically. Whereas quantitative research attempts to reduce the problem to a few very specific variables that can be experimentally manipulated, the aim of qualitative research is to make sense of the problem by analyzing it broadly within its naturally occurring context. Therefore, we will separately examine the types of research designs offered by the quantitative and qualitative researcher, while keeping in mind that some researchers attempt to combine these two approaches, and use a *mixed methods* approach (Gall, Gall, & Borg, 2007).

Quantitative Research Methods

As stated earlier, quantitative research assumes that there is an objective reality that can be verified only through the use of rigorous research methods and statistical analysis

TABLE 13.1   Distinctions Between Quantitative and Qualitative Research

	QUANTITATIVE	QUALITATIVE
Assumptions about knowledge	There is an objective truth that can be discovered through research and generalized to individuals who did not participate in the study. Knowledge is used to develop a hypothesis, which is set before the study starts.	Reality is socially constructed; there is no objective truth, only multiple realities. Often, what is found in one participant cannot be generalized to another. Knowledge and hypotheses emerge as data are collected and the study develops.
Data and methods used	Analytic approach dividing complex phenomena into parts. Data are numbers. Systematic, mathematical, statistical, and logical. Hypothesis testing and attempt to find answer to research questions. Deductive process.	Holistic approach describing complex phenomena in the natural state. Data are not numbers, but are words, observations, or other non-numeric sources of information. Philosophical and sociological. Multiple lenses to understand research question. Immersion in task with goal to have knowledge emerge. Inductive process.
Biases and validity	Bias is viewed as problematic, and objectivity is desired. Increased control of study to increase validity and reduce bias.	Bias is viewed as inevitable, and the subjectivity of researchers is recognized and described. Multiple data collection methods, sources, and researchers utilized to reduce the risk of capturing only a single perspective.
Goals and generalizability	To discover evidence and "truth" and generalize to a larger audience.	To describe culture, perceptions, and the lived experience in their complexity.
Researcher role	Detached, objective scientist. Researcher may intervene or manipulate.	Observer or participant observer often immersed in the research setting. Researcher does not intervene or manipulate.

of data. The researcher begins with a *hypothesis*, or a conjecture about the nature of human phenomena. Quantitative research then uses the *scientific method*, or a systematic process of observation, measurement, and experiment, to test the hypotheses, find possible answers to the research question being asked, or both. Two main types of quantitative research are experimental and nonexperimental research.

Although both experimental and nonexperimental research use the scientific method and a reductionistic approach to understanding the research problem, there are some crucial differences between these two types of designs. In *experimental research,* the researcher is manipulating the experience of the participants (the treatment) in some manner to show a cause-and-effect relationship between the experimenter's manipulation and specific outcome measures (Orcher, 2014). For example, a researcher might want to test the effects of rewards on treatment compliance. She would decide to form two groups: A group of patients that receives no rewards when taking their medication and a group that receives rewards when taking their medication. In this case, reward is the experience that the researcher manipulates by deciding which participants get the reward and which do not. *Nonexperimental research,* on the other hand, does not involve manipulation by the researcher; rather, it tends to look at relationships between variables or to describe the attitudes, beliefs, and behaviors of a group being surveyed (see Table 13.2).

TABLE 13.2 Summary of Experimental and Nonexperimental Quantitative Research Designs

| | EXPERIMENTAL | | | | | NONEXPERIMENTAL | |
	TRUE EXPERIMENT	QUASI-EXPERIMENT	SINGLE-SUBJECT	PRE-EXPERIMENT	EX POST FACTO (CAUSAL-COMPARATIVE)	CORRELATIONAL: BIVARIATE (EXPLANATORY/PREDICTIVE) MULTIVARIATE	SURVEY
Purpose	Show that X causes Y	Show that X causes Y	Show that X causes Y	Show that X causes Y	Show that X causes Y	Describe relationship; predict one variable from another	Assess opinions, beliefs, and attitudes
Number of groups	Two or more	Two or more	One or more individuals	One or more	Two or more	One	One
Manipulation of the independent variable	Yes	Yes	Yes	Yes	No	No	No
Design/Statistics	Manipulate treatment (X) to test for outcome (Y); inferential statistics in all but single subject designs				Examine differences of preexisting groups; inferential statistics (weak)	Examine relationship being correlated; descriptive statistics	Describe population, administer survey, analyze data; descriptive statistics
Methods of control for threats to internal validity	Random assignment	No random assignment; use other methods of control	Repeated measures to establish baseline	No random assignment; few other methods of control	No random assignment; use other methods of control	N/A	N/A
Strength of design for making cause-and-effect statements	Strong ——————————————→ Weak				Weak	N/A	N/A

Experimental Research

True Experimental Research.   In the realm of quantitative research, *true experimental research* designs are considered the crème de la crème, because they look, in a very controlled manner, for causal relationships between the variables being studied. In this type of research, the *independent variable*, or the variable being manipulated, is examined to determine if it has a direct effect on the *dependent variable*(s) or outcome measure(s).

In *true experimental research*, there is a comparison of outcomes between an experimental group and a control or comparison group and there is *random assignment* of subjects to those groups. An experimental group is a group that receives a treatment of interest to the researcher, while a control group receives no treatment, and a comparison group receives a different type of treatment than the experimental treatment (Fraenkel, Wallen, & Hyun, 2015). What distinguishes true experimental research from other types of experimental research is that participants in the study are assigned randomly to these groups so that each participant has an equal chance of being in any of the treatment groups. When random assignment is used, the researcher has greater certainty that participant characteristics such as gender, ability, attitudes, and prior experience will be roughly equivalent in each of the groups. This allows one to have confidence when attributing any differences found between the groups at the end of the study to the treatment, rather than to any preexisting differences between the participants.

One example of true experimental research would be a study of the effects of aerobic exercise (the independent variable) on stress (the dependent variable). Because aerobic exercise is the variable being manipulated, various levels of treatment (aerobic exercise) must be offered; and because this is true experimental research, there must be random assignment. Therefore, one design would be to assign 75 individuals randomly to three groups: a control group that does no aerobic exercise, a comparison group that participates in eight weeks of another, nonaerobic type of exercise (such as weight lifting), and an experimental group that participates in eight weeks of aerobic exercise.

Starting with the assumption that there would be no differences between these three groups, the researcher would develop a *null hypothesis* that states, "There will be no difference on measures of stress among individuals who participate in different types of exercise." When researchers use the null hypothesis, they hope to show that it is false; that is, the researcher wants to show that the treatment has caused differences between groups, thus demonstrating treatment effects. For instance, using the aerobic exercise example, if the researcher randomly assigns 75 individuals to three groups, the assumption is that prior to exercise (the treatment), these groups would look the same if their stress were measured. Therefore, following aerobic exercise (the treatment), any differences found between the groups would likely be due to the effect of the treatment, not other factors (see Figure 13.1).

Even if a treatment is completely ineffective, when measuring three groups of people on almost any characteristic, you are likely to find some differences between groups, just due to chance variables or fluctuations in scores. Therefore, when demonstrating that a treatment is effective, we are actually measuring the probability that these differences are due to the treatment and not due to chance or minor fluctuations. In fact, even in studies that showed that the probability was 999 out of 1,000 that the

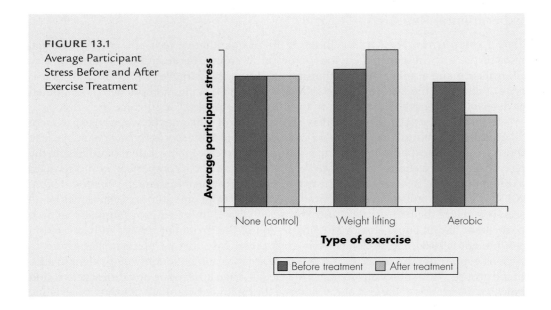

FIGURE 13.1
Average Participant Stress Before and After Exercise Treatment

results were due to the treatment, it could be that the results are spurious because you happened to hit that one time that variations were due to chance alone. It's kind of like playing the lottery. You know that you're not going to win, but once in a while, someone does! In research, you can be pretty darn sure that if the probability is 1 in 100, and your results are significant, the treatment has shown effects. However, it could be that you hit the lottery, but in this case, the lottery is not lucky, and you have found results that are not real. This is why researchers never speak of proving something, but instead talk in terms of the probability that the treatment was effective (Leary, 2012).

In some ways, the null hypothesis is used in our jurisprudence system. Criminal juries are operating from the null hypothesis, thus showing the probability that the criminal is guilty or not guilty. For instance, in a murder trial, the defendant goes to court with the presumption of innocence, which is really the null hypothesis: "The defendant did not commit murder." The prosecution attempts to disprove the null hypothesis by showing the probability that the defendant committed the crime. If there is evidence beyond a reasonable doubt, you have disproved the null hypothesis, which results in a finding of "guilty." On the other hand, if you have not convinced the jury of that probability, the defendant is found "not guilty," as opposed to "innocent." We are not working with proof, but with probabilities. This is why a certain number of people who are innocent will always go to jail, and a certain number of people will always be set free even though they are guilty. Science never gets to absolute truth, but perhaps, on occasion, it comes pretty close.

In doing true experimental research, there are a number of different kinds of design possibilities when deciding how to manipulate the independent variable and measure the dependent variable. You'll probably learn about those designs in a research class. However, regardless of the research design in use, in true experimental research, we randomly assign people to treatment groups and compare the groups on outcomes (see Figure 13.1).

Quasi-Experimental Research.   As with true experimental research, in conducting *quasi-experimental research*, the researcher is attempting to determine cause and effect, and there is manipulation of the independent variable; however, there is no random assignment (Heppner et al., 2008). Unlike true experimental research, instead of random assignment, quasi-experimental research examines already existing intact groups, giving one or more groups the treatment, while not giving the other groups the treatment. For instance, if a researcher wanted to see the effects of classroom guidance on bullying behaviors in 5th graders, he or she could select twelve fifth grade classes at the beginning of the school year and give classroom guidance activities related to bullying to six of those twelve. Then, the groups that received the treatment (classroom guidance) would be compared with the nontreatment groups.

Unfortunately, the lack of random assignment in quasi-experimental research often results in less credibility in determining whether differences are due to the effects of the treatment. As you might imagine, many factors could have differentially affected the treatment groups from the nontreatment groups, thus resulting in differences being found. One such factor may be the fact that there was not random assignment, so the groups may have differed initially, and what is found are differences based on selection rather than on treatment. For instance, in the example above, the classrooms that received the classroom guidance (treatment) may have started the year with fewer children who were likely to bully in the first place. As a result, bullying differences between the groups at the end of the year may have been due to differences in the children themselves rather than the treatment. Differences based on selection and factors other than the treatment (listed in Box 13.2) are called *threats to internal validity.*

Because the real world often does not provide opportunities to randomly assign individuals to treatment groups, quasi-experimental research and its use of intact groups is often used as an alternative to true experimental research (see Box 13.3). In such quasi-experimental designs, researchers use methods other than random assignment to control for threats to validity (Fraenkel et al., 2015). One such method is a *factorial design,* in which a preexisting difference between participants, such as bullying level, is treated as an independent variable. In a factorial design using the bullying example, all twelve classrooms would be assessed for prior bullying tendencies at the beginning of the study. Classrooms with high bullying tendencies would be divided into two groups: one that gets the guidance lessons (treatment) and one that does not. Similarly, classrooms with low bullying tendencies would be divided into a group that gets the treatment and one that does not. By ensuring that high and low bullying classrooms are in both the treatment and control groups, we eliminate preexisting bullying differences as a threat.

Single-Subject Experimental Research.   In some cases, counselors want to examine changes in a person or group after treatment but cannot use a control or comparison group. Because pre-experimental designs provide little information about cause and effect, counselors might use experimental single-subject designs (Foster, 2010). In these designs, participants serve as their own controls by providing at least three baseline

BOX 13.2
Threats to Internal Validity

In experimental research, there are many threats to internal validity that can result in researchers coming to false conclusions about their study if these threats are not controlled. The following are very brief descriptions of eight of these threats. A fuller understanding of them can be gained through a research course, a research text, and reading some of the classic texts that address these issues (e.g., Campbell & Stanley, 1963; Cook & Campbell, 1979). The eight threats include (Gay, Mills, & Airasian, 2012; Shadish, Cook & Campbell, 2002):

1. *Selection*, which includes the ways in which subjects are chosen and assigned to treatment groups, causes differences in those groups, thus clouding whether differences found are the result of the treatment or of selection.
2. *History*, in which external events occur during the research that affect the treatment and result in invalid conclusions.
3. *Maturation*, in which natural and developmental changes in subjects, such as growing older or gaining more experience, affect the results.
4. *Regression*, where there is a statistical tendency for extreme scores to move closer to the mean if tested a

second time. Therefore, regardless of the effect of the treatment, treatment groups with particularly high or low pretest scores may have scores that move toward the mean during post-testing, thus leading to false readings concerning the effect of the treatment.
5. *Attrition*, as when participants differentially drop out of treatment, thus leaving only the "better" or "worse" participants and results that are falsely attributed to the treatment.
6. *Testing*, in which exposure to a test can affect the results, such as when knowledge of the pretest affects the results of the post-testing.
7. *Instrumentation*, where changes in the instrument(s) can affect the results, such as when a more difficult pretest is used, thus leading to the false conclusion that there were gains in posttesting.
8. *Additive and interactive effects of threats to internal validity*, when two or more threats to internal validity are operating simultaneously and their joint or combined threats affect the results differently or more powerfully than each threat on its own.

BOX 13.3
A Failed Attempt at True Experimental Research

When I (Ed Neukrug) was living in New Hampshire, a colleague and I decided to conduct research on the effects of aerobic exercise on personality variables. After reviewing the literature, we found possible links between such exercise and the personality variables of self-actualization, depression, and anxiety. We approached our local YMCA, which was running a rather extensive aerobic exercise program. They agreed to let us talk with individuals who were about to start exercise for the first time. They also agreed to let these people have eight free weeks of membership at the Y if half of them (randomly chosen) would not start their exercise program for eight weeks. We found three instruments to measure anxiety, depression,

and self-actualizing values with the intent of comparing, at the end of eight weeks, the group that started aerobic exercise with the group that waited for eight weeks. We excitedly met with approximately 50 new exercisers. We told them our plans, and they looked at us and said, "Are you kidding? We want to start our exercise program now!"

Our good intentions obviously were not going to sway these individuals who were ready to get going with their exercise. Unfortunately for us, we were not able to implement our true experimental study. Instead, we had to consider using either a quasi-experimental or an ex post facto design, both of which would not be as powerful in showing treatment effects.

measures of the dependent variable before treatment (Gay et al., 2012). For instance, returning to the aerobic exercise example, if the researcher were working with a client who was struggling with anxiety and stress, he or she might design a study that examined the effects of aerobic exercise (the treatment) on anxiety and stress as measured by a short anxiety scale and the client's resting heart rate. Using what is commonly called an *ABA design*, the researcher would first obtain a baseline of the outcome measures (A), in this case anxiety and stress as measured on the anxiety scale and resting heart rate.

Over a few weeks, the researcher would take a number of *baseline* measurements and then introduce the treatment, aerobic exercise (B). From there, he or she would continue to measure anxiety and resting heart rate over the next few weeks as the client participated in aerobic exercise. Finally, the researcher would remove the treatment and again take baseline measures over the next few weeks (A again). Evidence that the treatment is working should be indicated by a reduction in anxiety and stress levels during the treatment and a return to higher levels after the treatment. Often, to show additional efficacy of the treatment, the design is extended and made into an ABAB design, where the study finishes during a treatment phase with the expectation that the outcome measures should again produce change (Heppner et al., 2008). Clearly, a study like this could also be done with a group of individuals, such as a family therapy group. Figure 13.2 shows an example of an ABAB design for aerobic exercise and its effect on anxiety and stress.

Pre-Experimental Research.   As in true experimental and quasi-experimental designs, the purpose of pre-experimental designs is to show a cause-and-effect relationship between the intervention and specific outcomes. Unlike the other experimental designs, however, pre-experimental designs do not have built in controls for threats to internal validity; therefore, it is very difficult to determine if the treatment is responsible for any differences in participants. One example of a pre-experimental design is the *one-shot case study design*, in which a single group gets the treatment and the result is measured (Kline, 2009). This is a design that is often used in classrooms, where we teach children and then we give them a test at the end of class. Unfortunately, because we have no comparison or control group and we have no pretest measure, we have no way to know if scores on the test are any better than they were at the beginning of class. In addition, even if the scores are better at the end of class than they would have been at the beginning, we don't know if that participant change is a result of what happened in class or is instead due to any of the threats in Box 13.2. For this reason, pre-experimental designs are seen as very weak designs.

Nonexperimental Research

Correlational Research.   *Correlational research* examines the relationship between two or more sets of scores and generally uses correlation coefficients in examining results. If you remember from Chapter 12, a correlation (r) between variables can range between -1 and $+1$ and indicates the strength of the relationships between variables. *A positive correlation* shows a tendency for one set of scores to be related to a second set of scores in the same direction. *A negative correlation* shows a relationship in opposite directions, and a correlation coefficient of 0 shows no relationship. For instance, if a correlation coefficient of .89 between height and weight was found, we would say $r = .89$ and that as height increases, so does weight. Alternatively, if we found that grades in graduate school had a mild negative correlation of $-.24$ with number of hours per week pursuing leisure activities, we would present the correlation as $r = -.24$ and say that as hours of leisure increase, grades decrease. Because correlational research does not show cause and effect and does not require random assignment, such research is generally easier to implement than experimental designs and is often used as preliminary research in an effort to check out a researcher's hunches. Two of the more frequently used types of correlation

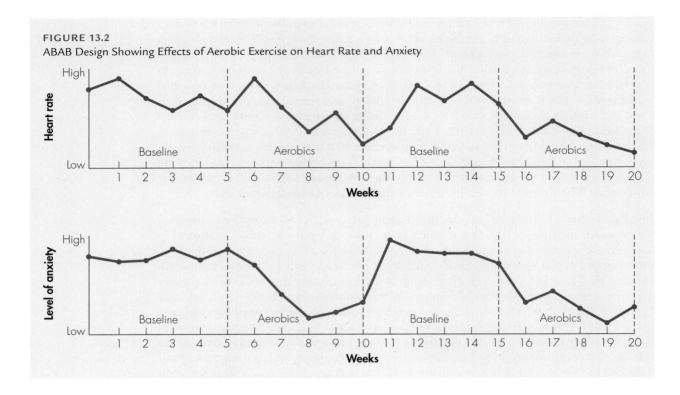

FIGURE 13.2
ABAB Design Showing Effects of Aerobic Exercise on Heart Rate and Anxiety

research include *bivariate correlational* studies, which explore the relationship between two variables; and *multivariate correlational* studies, which examine the relationship among more than two variables (Gall, Gall, & Borg, 2010; Mertler & Charles, 2011).

Bivariate correlational studies examine two selected variables that theory or past research suggests may be related to one another. Two types of bivariate correlation are *explanatory* and *predictive* (Creswell, 2012a; Fraenkel et al., 2015). In explanatory correlational research, you are merely examining the relationship between variables to try and explain a phenomenon. Often, these two variables are measured at the same time. For example, let's say that we were interested in examining the relationship between empathy and the strength of relationships with clients. If we could find an instrument to measure empathic responses and a second to measure the strength of the relationship between the counselor and client, we could be on the way to examining this relationship. Hypothetically, we could find hundreds of counselors, measure their empathic ability with clients using our empathic instrument, and then ask clients to complete an instrument that measures the strength of their perceived relationship with their counselor. We could then correlate scores on empathic ability with perceived strength of the relationship (see Figure 13.3). Figure 13.3 shows a hypothetical correlation of approximately .30, which reflects a moderate relationship between the two measures. Does empathy cause the strength of the relationship? No, but it is one factor that is related to it. Thus, such a study might be important in the training of counselors.

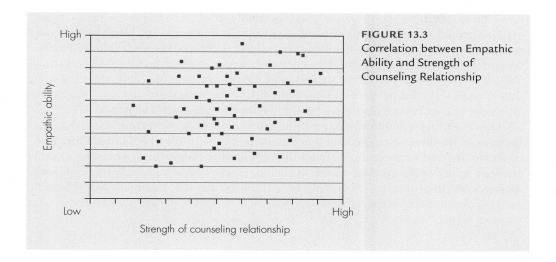

FIGURE 13.3
Correlation between Empathic Ability and Strength of Counseling Relationship

In contrast to explanatory correlational research, which simply examines the relationship between variables in the here and now, predictive correlational studies look at how one variable (called the *predictor variable*) might be able to predict an outcome on another variable (called the *criterion variable*). If the relationship between two variables is strong enough, it will be possible to predict a person's score on the criterion variable (graduate school GPA, for example) based on his or her score on the predictor (GRE score, for example). It must be made clear, however, that although one variable can fairly accurately predict another, a cause-and-effect relationship has *not* been established. For instance, scores on the GREs should be predictive of GPA in graduate school, or else they would not be useful for this purpose. Indeed, such scores have been shown to be moderately predictive of graduate school GPA in most subjects (Bridgeman, Burton, & Cline, 2009). However, GRE scores certainly do not cause a certain GPA in graduate school. Similarly, numerous studies have shown that the better the *congruence* or "fit" there is between personal characteristics and job environment (e.g., "social type" individuals fit better in helping professions), the higher the subsequent job satisfaction (Lent & Brown, 2013b; Rehfuss, Gambrell, & Meyer, 2012). This research suggests that using an interest inventory to identify personality type and matching personality types to specific job environments can lead to greater job satisfaction. Remember, however, that a study such as this does not show causation. For instance, it could be that individuals who have higher congruence scores are more mentally stable, brighter, or more skilled, thus leading to higher job satisfaction. Although we cannot assume a causal relationship, implications such as these can be critical. For instance, knowing that such a prediction exists for job satisfaction, if you were looking for a job, wouldn't you want to know if your personality type "fit" a specific occupational choice?

Multivariate correlational research is useful when you have more than two variables that you suspect are somehow related to one another. *Multiple regression*, one of the most commonly used types of multivariate correlational statistics, can tell you how a combination of scores predicts an outcome. For example, consider the relationship among empathic ability, being nondogmatic, and the ability to build an alliance, with client success in counseling. Hypothetically, one would hope that empathy, having a nonjudgmental attitude, and building an alliance with one's client would each be related to client success. By measuring these different variables, we can see the strength of the relationship of each variable with client success, and we can see how the combination of these three factors is related to client success. Empathy, being nonjudgmental, and building an alliance might each have respective correlations with success with clients of .32, .25, and .28. However, their combined relationship with success with clients might be .41, higher than any of the three alone, making the combination of the three a better predictor of success than any one variable alone. In addition to multiple regression, a number of other types of multivariate correlation are available, most of which use advanced statistics to determine their results. These include *discriminant analysis, factor analysis, differential analysis, canonical correlation,* and *path analysis.* But we'll let you learn about these in your research course!

Survey Research.   In *survey research,* a questionnaire is developed or an interview designed with the purpose of gathering specific information from a target population. Surveys can gather interesting information about the values, behaviors, demographics, and opinions of a specific population and are used in a myriad of business, educational, and social science arenas. In describing the data obtained, survey research uses basic *descriptive statistics* such as *frequency distributions, percentages, measures of central tendency,* and *measures of variability* (see Chapter 12). Often, charts and graphs are used to illustrate some of the data obtained.

A number of steps are usually followed when conducting survey research (McMillan & Schumacher, 2010), some of which include:

1. Defining the purpose and objectives of the survey
2. Determining the target population
3. Determining the response mode (snail mail, Internet, live interviews, phone)
4. Determining the resources needed (e.g., stamps, Web-based survey maker, etc.)
5. Developing the cover letter and instrument
6. Conducting a pilot study and making revisions
7. Collecting the data
8. Completing a follow-up of nonrespondents
9. Organizing the results
10. Distributing the results (e.g., by writing a journal article)

Although survey research can be quite interesting, it is not able to tell us the underlying reasons why we found what we found and often leaves gaps in our knowledge. For instance, in research that has been conducted on counselors' attendance in their own therapy, it was discovered that close to 80% of counselors had attended their own therapy. However, this information does not tell us the underlying reasons why they attended counseling. Do counselors attend therapy because they are more open to the experience, healthier, more dysfunctional, because they're required to in their programs, or other reasons? Therefore, survey research can be quite limiting, although sometimes quite intriguing.

Ex Post Facto (Causal-Comparative) Research.   Whereas experimental research involves the manipulation of variables, *ex post facto research*, sometimes called *causal-comparative research*, involves no manipulation of variables and compares already existing, intact groups. Ex post facto research is used when it is either impractical or impossible to manipulate the independent variable, such as when examining the differential effects of gender, personality type, or race, or when random assignment cannot be used (Heppner et al., 2008). Because groups are being compared in causal comparative, these research designs are often confused with experimental designs. The difference is that in causal comparative research, the researcher measures the dependent variable *ex post facto* ("after the fact").

For instance, let's say that we wanted to compare the scores on the National Counselor Exam (NCE) of students who graduated from CACREP-accredited counseling programs with the scores of those who graduated from non-CACREP-accredited programs. Obviously, we could not randomly assign students to graduate programs, and we cannot manipulate the independent variable, which is the type of graduate program attended. However, it would be relatively easy to obtain data from students, ex post facto, who already had attended these schools and who subsequently took the NCE. It would then be a simple process to run a statistical analysis of which students scored higher on the exam. And, in point of fact, the National Board for Certified Counselors (NBCC) does have these data available, and although they do not run comparative analyses, students from CACREP-accredited programs consistently do score higher on the certification exam.

Although ex post facto research is often more convenient than some experimental designs, there are inherent problems with this kind of research. For instance, because there is no manipulation of the independent variable and no random assignment, we cannot be sure exactly what is causing any differences that are found. For example, in the NCE example just discussed, there can be many, many explanations of why these differences are found. To name just a few that hypothetically could be true:

- ➤ Students who don't get into CACREP programs go to non-CACREP programs and are less prepared academically.
- ➤ Students who don't get into CACREP programs are more creative and care less about academics.
- ➤ CACREP programs are stuck in a curriculum that allows for no creativity.
- ➤ Non-CACREP programs teach "other" counseling-related topics not covered on the NCE.
- ➤ The faculty in CACREP-accredited programs are better teachers.
- ➤ The faculty in non-CACREP programs are more creative and don't need to focus on a specific curriculum.
- ➤ The faculty in CACREP-accredited programs teach to the test.
- ➤ Students in CACREP programs can take the test sooner, so their retention is better.
- ➤ On and on—you get the idea.

In an effort to control for such rival hypotheses as those identified above, researchers will sometimes attempt to match treatment groups on variables that may be confounding the results. For instance, in the hypothetical study above, students can be matched on GRE scores and graduate GPA to ensure that ability in both groups is similar. Also, students can be selected in a manner that ensures that both groups of students have taken the exam within the same amount of time since graduation. On the other hand, it might be more difficult to control whether or not faculty are teaching to the test. Therefore, this rival hypothesis, along with any others that might be identified, should be noted as possible *confounding variables* in any discussion of results. In addition, other rival hypotheses, not identified by the researcher, could be affecting the results. This is why researchers need to be very tentative when stating any conclusions in ex post facto research.

Qualitative Research Methods

Naturalistic–phenomenological philosophy is the basis of qualitative research (McMillan & Schumacher, 2010). This approach assumes that there are many ways in which reality can be interpreted and experienced by individuals. Rather than using the scientific method, as in quantitative research, qualitative research relies on the researcher to observe, describe, and interpret phenomena carefully within a natural setting or social context. For these reasons, qualitative research allows one to examine phenomena that quantitative research cannot explore, like our understanding of abstract concepts such as empathy and the spiritual nature of our lives (Hinson, 2011). As a result, the findings of qualitative research offer rich ways to apply research paradigms to clinical settings (Haverkamp, Morrow, & Ponterotto, 2005). Also, qualitative research can add important missing pieces of information that cannot be discovered through the reductionistic methods of quantitative research (Gall et al., 2007).

Whereas quantitative research relies on the deductive method of identifying variables, isolating them, and measuring them, qualitative research relies on the *case study method*, which focuses upon and deeply probes and analyzes events or phenomena. This approach uses a number of methods, often simultaneously, in an effort to allow *themes* and the meaning about the phenomenon being studied to emerge.

Qualitative research generally uses research questions as opposed to hypotheses to provide direction for the research. Although qualitative research can take many forms, four types often identified include *grounded theory, phenomenological approach, ethnographic research* and *consensual qualitative research (CSR)* (Hill, Thompson, & Williams, 1997; Houser, 2015) (see Table 13.3).

Grounded Theory

Developed by sociologists Glaser and Strass during the 1960s (Buckley, 2010; Houser, 2015), *grounded theory* can be described as a process used to generate a theory explaining the course, actions, or interactions of a phenomenon of interest. The process involves an inductive approach to data collection and analysis. The researchers collect information from the field, analyze the information and organize it into categories or themes, return to the field to collect more information with refined questions, and compare new information to themes that emerged from earlier data through *constant comparative analysis* (Strauss & Corbin, 1990). This process continues until the researchers reach *saturation*—in other words, until no new themes emerge from additional data. This exploration leads to the emergence of a theory that is grounded in the data. This contrasts with quantitative research, in which a hypothesis is developed from a literature review before the study

TABLE 13.3 Summary of Qualitative Research Designs

	GROUNDED THEORY	PHENOMENO-LOGICAL	ETHNOGRAPHIC	CONSENSUAL QUALITATIVE RESEARCH (CSR)
Purpose	To generate a theory explaining the course, actions, or interactions of a phenomenon of interest	To describe the lived experience of a phenomenon and the contextual factors that influence that experience	To describe and understand the shared values, beliefs, behaviors, and social patterns of a culture	To understand a phenomenon of interest in all its complexity
Method used to collect data	Individual interviews, focus group, observation, artifact and document reviews	Semistructured individual interviews are most common; focus group, observation, and artifact and document reviews	Observation is the primary source of data; ethnographic interviews, and artifact and document reviews	Semistructured individual interviews or questionnaires
Data questions	Questions asked of participants are changed and refined as study continues	Questions asked of participants may be changed and refined as study continues	Often begin with no clearly specified questions	Questions are established before study begins and do not change
Key distinguishing characteristics	Constant comparative approach of data analysis	A thick (complex and thoughtful) description in the participants' own words	Lengthy immersion in the field; key informants	Use of a research team instead of an individual; data analysis through consensus building and cross-analysis

begins and statistics are used to test that hypothesis or research question. In fact, grounded theorists often suggest not initially going to the literature for fear that it might cause bias in the interpretation of results.

For instance, let's say that we were interested in the research question: "How do counselors develop a theoretical orientation toward their careers?" We first would come up with a series of related questions that could be asked to counselors that would be the catalyst for exploring this subject, such as:

➤ When did you first consider a theoretical orientation?
➤ What experiences affected your choice of a theory?
➤ What's most important to you in picking a theory?
➤ How has your theoretical orientation changed over time?

After coming up with questions, we would prepare to interview counselors. For instance, we might come up with focus groups of counselors who had been in the field for a determined amount of time (e.g., 10 years) and begin to seek their responses to the questions, as well as additional questions that might emerge as the discussion unfolds. This process would happen through a series of steps that would include *preparing, data collection, note taking, coding,* and *writing.*

Preparing. This phase of research means that you reflect on your own biases and prepare to collect information from your participants. You are aware that meeting with individuals in and of itself will affect how they respond and you attempt to be respectful, nonjudgmental, and a good listener. You also attempt to be aware of how your own biases might shape your data collection process.

Data Collection.   This phase has to do with the process you use to obtain your information. As noted, focus groups are often a common method of collecting data, although other methods can be used (e.g., examining writings of individuals or observing in naturalistic settings). When interviewing others, it is here that we would use the list of questions developed earlier, recognizing that those questions will evolve as themes and new questions begin to emerge.

Note Taking.   Many grounded theorists do not take notes at all; instead, they rely on their memories to write down the most important elements after collecting data. However, others find no problem with note taking or even recording the interviews. In either case, this process should be as nonintrusive as possible and should allow participants to express their opinions.

Coding.   Coding has to do with identifying common themes among the various sources of data and giving them a code (discussed later in this chapter in the section "Statistics and Data Analysis in Quantitative and Qualitative Research"; also see Boxes 13.5 and 13.6). This helps to organize the data that you have collected. As individuals code, "core" categories will emerge that begin to point to broad themes evident in the data collection. In addition, *saturation* will occur when you realize that many individuals are referring to the same core themes. It is then that the coding process is nearing its end.

Writing.   During the note-taking and coding processes, the researcher is often *memoing*, which means that he or she is creating a memo about important themes that may be emerging. Also, during this process, the researcher begins to *sort* the different themes into major categories. As the final themes emerge, the researcher is ready to write up his or her findings. For instance, in examining how counselors come up with their theoretical orientation, the eventual theory might involve a series of stages that were uncovered through the interviews in the focus groups. The researcher would then identify and suggest these stages in his or her eventual write-up.

Grounded theory is a comfortable fit for counselors, as they are natural listeners and observers. However, it is painstaking and should not be considered a simple process of listening to different points of view. Instead, it is a systematic process that attempts to uncover underlying themes and theory relevant to an important research question.

Phenomenological Research

In many ways similar to the grounded theory approach, *phenomenological designs* are less involved with developing eventual theory and more interested in simply understanding and describing individuals' lived experiences of a phenomenon (Creswell, 2012b). For instance, let's say that a researcher was interested in understanding the experiences of younger siblings of children with special needs. In this case, he or she would have a *purposeful sample* of individuals who have an older sibling with special needs. Because the researcher wants to understand the phenomenon in all of its complexity and contradictions, he or she might deliberately select individuals whose experiences are likely to have been different from one another. Next, the researcher might conduct in-depth interviews with these individuals and ask them to describe what it has been like for them to be a younger sibling and to describe the contextual factors that influenced how they experienced the phenomenon (Creswell, 2012b). The researcher would observe the individuals carefully, be respectful of them, and ask follow-up questions if he or she thought that such questions would deepen the stories of the members and give *richer* (sometimes referred to as *thicker)* descriptions of what it has been like for them. The researcher would be constantly aware that his or her very presence is affecting their responses in some way, and would carefully try to *bracket* any biases he or she might have that might influence the data collection. The researcher might tape the interviews and transcribe them later and would also be interested in collecting other sources of information that might enlighten him or her further about the experiences of these individuals (e.g., diaries, personal journals, Facebook pages, parents' and or teachers' perspectives, etc.).

Data analysis in the phenomenological approach is similar to the grounded-theory approach, in the sense that the researcher would be identifying and coding themes and trying to find common elements in what the individuals experience and how they experience it. Whereas a grounded theory approach seeks to develop an explanation for the process of the phenomenon, phenomenology merely describes what the phenomenon is like for those who experienced it.

Ethnographic Research

The term *ethnography* refers to the description (*graphy*) of human cultures (*ethno*). Sometimes called *cultural anthropology,* ethnographic research was made popular by Margaret Mead, who studied aboriginal youths in Samoa by immersing herself with the people and their culture as she attempted to understand their lifestyle (Mead, 1961). Much ethnography also occurs in the United States, and more recent examples include a sixteen-month study of the culture of the homeless in Boston's Station Street Shelter (Desjarlais, 1997) and a spiritual ethnography of an African American gospel community (Hinson, 2011). Such research is characterized by the researcher's long immersion in the day-to-day lives of the group and often by the reliance on *key informants,* or individuals within the culture who can provide entrance into the group and can explain phenomena. The resulting ethnography is a description, analysis, and interpretation of cultural beliefs, behaviors, language, values, and social patterns.

The first step in conducting ethnographic research is to identify a group with a shared culture and a method of gaining access to that group. Conducting a literature review can help the researcher gain a better understanding of the culture or group being studied, although often the group is so unique that there is little or no research available. Next, the researcher decides on what method he or she wishes to use to immerse himself or herself in the culture of the population. Prior to entering the culture, the researcher should develop a plan for implementing his or her data collection methods. Three common methods

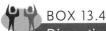

BOX 13.4
Disruptive Observation of a Third-Grade Class

While working in New Hampshire, I (Ed Neukrug) was once asked to "debrief" a third-grade class that had just finished a trial period in which a young, paraplegic boy with a severe intellectual disability had been mainstreamed into their classroom. During this trial period, these third graders had a stream of observers from a local university come into their classroom to assess their progress. Because this was not participant observation, the observers would sit in the back of the classroom and take notes about the interactions between the students. This information was supposed to be used later to decide whether it was beneficial to all involved to have the disabled student mainstreamed.

When I met with the students, they clearly had adapted well to the presence of this young boy who was disabled. Although the students seemed to have difficulty forming deep relationships with him, his presence seemed in no way to detract from their studies or from their other relationships in the classroom. However, almost without exception, the students noted that the constant stream of observers interfering with their daily schedule was quite annoying. Perhaps if participant observation were employed, where an observer interacted and was seen as part of the classroom, the students would have responded differently.

used in ethnographic research include *observation, ethnographic interviews*, and *collection of documents and artifacts*.

Observation. Ethnographers often will observe a situation or phenomenon and, using extensive notes, describe what they see. Although sometimes qualitative researchers may take a disengaged role when observing, more often they become *participant observers*. In this kind of observation, the researcher immerses himself or herself in the group and may even live with the group (Gall, et al., 2007; Houser, 2015). However, it is important not to interfere with the natural process of the group and to listen and take scrupulous notes so that the observer understands the unique perspective of the group. It is only in this manner that the observer can obtain a rich appreciation for the ways in which the group constructs reality. It is particularly important that the observer record what role and what effect observing the group may have had on the group (see Box 13.4).

Ethnographic Interviews. Ethnographic interviews constitute a second popular qualitative method of collecting data from a culture or group. Such interviews involve open-ended questions in an effort to understand how the interviewees construct meaning. Interviews may be informal, where a general topic is explored but without specific guidelines; guided, in which questions are outlined in advance; or standardized, in which the exact questions are determined prior to the interview, but the responses remain open-ended. Counselors are adept at doing ethnographic interviews because of their training in open-ended questioning. As with participant observation, it is important that the interviewer take scrupulous notes or record the interviews in order to obtain verbatim accounts of the conversations.

Documents and Artifact Collection. *Artifacts* are the symbols of a culture or group and can help the ethnographer understand the beliefs, values, and behaviors of the group. In this process, it is helpful if the researcher knows how the artifact was produced, where the artifact came from, the age of the artifact, how the artifact was used, and who used it. Interpretation of the meaning of artifacts should be corroborated from observations and through interviews.

McMillan and Schumacher (2010) suggest the following major categories of artifacts: personal documents, such as diaries, personal letters, emails and texts, and anecdotal records; official documents, such as internal and external papers and communications, records and personnel files, and statistical data; and objects that hold symbolic meaning of the culture (e.g., Native American headdresses).

Consensual Qualitative Research

Like the other qualitative designs, consensual qualitative research (CQR) emphasizes describing complex experience and behavior as they exist in their natural settings. Unlike the other designs, however, CQR uses a heavily standardized, replicable, and systematic process of data collection and analysis. The process is detailed and specific, but some key components that distinguish CQR research from other qualitative methods are a diverse research team, a defined sample and protocol, analysis through consensus building, and cross-analysis (Heppner et al., 2008; Hill et al., 1997).

Diverse Team.   The CQR method always requires a team of researchers. The assumption is that a single researcher may be subject to his or her own biases and thus be unable to see patterns in the data that are inconsistent with his or her worldview. For this reason, the first step in CQR is to establish a team of about seven people: three to five researchers to analyze the data, and one or two auditors to provide feedback on the analysis. As the object in team formation is to ensure that multiple perspectives are heard, care should be taken in selecting diverse team members.

Defined Sample and Protocol.   Both sample selection and the interview protocol are clearly defined at the beginning of the study. The researchers establish specific criteria for inclusion of participants in the study based on the research question and then select eight to fifteen participants who meet those criteria. In addition, after a review of the literature, a semistructured interview protocol (set of questions) is developed. All questions on the protocol will be asked of all participants. This is different from other methods of qualitative research, where the questions evolve as data are collected and the study develops.

Consensus Building.   Data analysis and coding into domains is conducted by each researcher independently at first. Then the team meets to build consensus on the coding, domains, and core ideas in each of the interview transcripts. The auditors review the data and provide feedback on the domains and core ideas that are incorporated into the researchers' coding of the data.

Cross-Analysis.   Finally, there is a quantitative element to CQR. After all the interviews are analyzed, the researchers look across cases to see in how many instances a category or theme is mentioned. This enables the researchers to determine if a category is *general* (meaning that it is common), *typical* (meaning that it occurs in half the cases), or *variant* (meaning that it is unusual).

Statistics and Data Analysis in Quantitative and Qualitative Research

Although a textbook such as this cannot go into detail about the various kinds of statistical and inductive analyses that can be used, suffice it to say that the proper use of analytic procedures is critical to the eventual interpretation of research studies and does not always occur in published studies (Thompson, 1995; Wester, et al., 2013). Whereas quantitative research uses statistics to analyze results, qualitative research uses a process called *inductive analysis*.

Quantitative Research

The general goal of quantitative research is to apply statistical procedures to a set of controlled variables to test research questions and hypotheses. The choice of which statistics are applied in quantitative research varies depending on the type of study you are conducting, but it more or less falls into two broad categories: *descriptive statistics*, which are used to summarize and describe results; and *inferential statistics,* which are mathematical procedures used to make inferences about a larger population from the sample you are studying. The following discusses a few of the more commonly used descriptive and inferential techniques.

Largely discussed in Chapter 12, descriptive statistics include measures of central tendency, such as the mean, median, and mode; measures of variability, such as range, variance, and standard deviation; derived scores, such as percentiles, stanines, T-scores, and DIQ scores; and measures of relationship, such as correlation coefficient. Descriptive statistics are often used with survey research.

With inferential statistics, we take the results from a sample and draw conclusions about the broader population. For example, if we find differences between treatment groups in our sample, we would like to know if those differences are due to the treatment and would likely be found in the broader population, or if they are merely due to chance and would not be found in the broader population. Although we can't know this for sure (unless we test everyone in the population), inferential statistics allows us to test the likelihood that those differences are due to chance and do not reflect real population differences. Some of the more common types of analyses include the *t*-test to measure differences between two means; the *analysis of variance (ANOVA),* to measure differences between two or more means; *factorial analysis of variance,* used when there is more than one independent variable and the researcher is interested in examining each independent variable and how they might interact; *multivariate analysis of variance (MANOVA),* used when two or more dependent variables are being examined; *significance of correlation coefficient*, used when examining whether the relationship between two variables is statistically significant; and *chi square*, which is used to compare whether the observed frequency of scores differs from the expected frequency of scores. Generally, experimental research and ex post facto research use inferential statistics that measure differences between means, while correlational research examines the degree of relationship between variables.

In recent years, the effect size of a study has become increasingly important in understanding the results of quantitative research. The term *effect size* refers to the practical significance of one's finding. For instance, in recent research conducted by Neukrug & Milliken (2011), significant differences were found between male and female counselors' views of whether certain counselor behaviors were ethical. For instance, males were more likely to believe that it was all right to persuade their clients not to have an abortion even though they want to. However, when you looked at the actual figures, the vast majority of males and females believed this to be unethical, despite this statistical significance. So although a statistical difference was found, the effect size in practice was small. Today, effect size is shown using a number of varied statistical procedures and should usually be referred to in published studies.

Qualitative Research

In contrast to quantitative research, which applies statistical procedures to numeric variables, qualitative data collection relies on a process called *inductive analysis* of nonnumeric data, which means that *themes* and categories emerge from data (McMillan & Schumacher, 2010). Thus, the researcher who is examining the data collected through the various methods mentioned earlier looks through the information for themes, ways of categorizing information, and ways of selecting important pieces of information. As this process continues, the researcher begins to see particular points emerge.

Often, qualitative researchers classify their data by a process called *coding*. This process breaks down large amounts of data into smaller parts that seem to hold some meaning regarding the research question. For instance, if involved in a study to determine what problems at-risk high school students might have in a specific school, a researcher might observe the youths; interview them; interview their teachers, school counselors, parents, and peers; and collect school records. Then, the researcher would go through all of these pieces of information and identify and code themes that seem to emerge from the data. For instance, Box 13.5 shows pieces of interviews with (1) an at-risk student ("John"), (2) one of his teachers, and (3) his school counselor, as well as (4) a summary of his student records. Each of these four segments of information is broken down into themes. Similar themes are coded in the box with the same superscript number.

The next step would be to place all similar themes (same coded numbers) together in a category that has a logical name (see Box 13.6). You can see in this box that a number of categories have emerged from this process. Then the researcher would continue this same process with a number of the identified at-risk students. Finally, the researcher would look at all the categories that emerged from all of the students interviewed and begin to look for similarities among students. It may be that some of the categories will merge with one another while other, new themes might emerge. For instance, if the researcher consistently sees at-risk youths using humor to avoid issues (item 9 in Box 13.6), it may end up as a subtopic of defensiveness (item 13 in Box 13.6). Eventually, the researcher would come up with a list of categories that represented the most relevant issues for at-risk students.

Issues of Quality in Research Studies

As you can see, qualitative and quantitative research designs take a very different approach to understanding the world, so you probably will not be surprised to learn

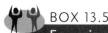

BOX 13.5
Emerging Themes through Data Analysis for an At-Risk Student

Segment of Verbatim Interview with John

I don't like school.[1] It's a waste of time.[1] The only thing it's good for is hanging out with my friends.[2] My dad never went to school, so why should I?[3] You don't learn nothing here anyway, nothing that's good for me. I don't care how I do on tests,[4] I just want to get some money[5] so I could buy some neat clothes. Then I could show off[6] to my friends and they would think I'm cool.[2] School sucks, I cut a lot[7]—I wish I could get out of here and get a job and make some money.[5] Can you get me a job?

Segment of Verbatim Interview with One of John's Teachers

John seems to be thinking of other things while in school and not interested in what's going on in class.[1] He is always talking to his friends in class, and seems to be in a clique[2]—that is, when he comes to school. He seems absent much.[7] He rarely does well on tests,[4] but I have noticed that he seems to do a little better if I let his mom know[8] that a test is coming up and when he's attending school consistently.[7] He always dresses very well and seems a little bit like a show-off.[6] He has a funny sense of humor,[9] although I would never laugh at his jokes in class because I don't want to reinforce his joking around. I think his scores in school are not reflective of how well he can do.[10] It's a shame. It's a wasted life.[11] I'm kind of sick of seeing this same pattern over and over again.

Documents and Records

a. Achievement test scores are low.[4]
b. Aptitude test scores are average.[10]
c. Records show that student seems to miss a lot of classes.[7]
d. An autobiography that he wrote for his counseling group seemed to show a number of painful events,[12] like his parents' divorce, that he may be covering up.[13]
e. He's gotten a number of detentions for "cutting up" in class.[9]
f. Poems he wrote in English were funny,[9] yet morbid about his future.[11]
g. A sentence-completion test he took with his counselor seemed to show an obsession with money.[5]

Segment of Verbatim Interview with John's School Counselor

John was in a group of students with high absenteeism, low grades, and an apathetic attitude toward school.[7,4,1] He was the jokester in the group.[9] He always had excuses for why he was absent.[6,13] On the one hand, he used his father as a role model for not having to finish school;[3] however, it seemed that his father is absent from his life and that he's hurt over this.[12] In general, I think his jokes are a way for him to gain attention [6,9] and cover up some inner hurts.[12] He's likable in many ways, but he's hard to reach.[13] He seems to have a wall around him.[13] His mother seems a source of comfort,[8] but his peer group is increasingly having more influence on him.[2] I'm concerned about his future.[11]

---

that different metrics are used to evaluate these two types of designs. For quantitative research, we look to see how well researchers controlled threats to internal and external validity. For qualitative research, there is less agreement on how to evaluate the quality of this research, but many look for evidence of the trustworthiness and credibility of the study, as described by Lincoln and Guba (1985).

Evaluating Quantitative Research

Internal Validity.   In quantitative research, internal validity represents the degree to which extraneous variables have been accounted for when drawing your conclusions. Briefly discussed earlier (see Box 13.2), studies that are more tightly controlled will have fewer threats to internal validity and therefore fewer rival hypotheses that may explain the data will be found. True experiments generally have greater controls than all other quantitative designs and thus best eliminate threats to internal validity. For this reason, with true experiments, we can be most confident that the independent variable (and not

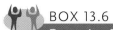

BOX 13.6

Emerging Themes from Data Analysis

1. Dislike of school: I don't like school. It's a waste of time. . . . Not interested in what's going on in class. . . . In a group of students with . . . an apathetic attitude toward school.

2. Peer relationships: The only thing school is good for is hanging out with my friends . . . [If I wore neat clothes, my friends would think] I'm cool. . . . He is always talking to his friends in class . . . seems to be in a clique. . . . His peer group is increasingly having more influence on him.

3. Dad as role model: My dad never went to school, so why should I? . . . Uses his father as a role model for not having to finish school. . . . Father is absent from his life.

4. Test performance: I don't care how I do on tests. . . . He rarely does well on tests. . . . Achievement tests scores are low. . . . In a group of students with . . . low grades.

5. Importance of money: I just want to get some money. . . . I wish I could get out of here and get a job and make some money. . . . An obsession with money.

6. Narcissism: [If I had the neat clothes], I could show off. . . . He always dresses very well and seems a little bit like a show-off. . . . Jokes are a way for him to gain attention.

7. Absenteeism: School sucks, I cut a lot. . . . He seems absent much. . . . [Does] better . . . when he's attending

school consistently. . . . Records show that student seems to miss a lot of classes. . . . In a group of students with high absenteeism. . . . He always had excuses for why he was absent.

8. Relationship with mom:. . . [Does] better [if his mom knows] a test is coming up. . . . His mother seems a source of comfort.

9. Use of humor: He has a funny sense of humor. [He cuts up] in class. Poems he wrote in English were funny. . . . His jokes are a way for him to gain attention.

10. Underachiever: His scores in school are not reflective of how well he can do. . . . Aptitude scores are average. [Achievement scores and grades are low.]

11. Sense of future: It's a shame. It's a wasted life. . . . Poems . . . were funny yet morbid about his future. . . . I'm concerned about his future.

12. Emotional pain: An autobiography . . . seemed to show a number of painful events. . . . His father is absent from his life and [he] hurts over this. . . . Jokes . . . cover up some inner hurts.

13. Defensiveness: An autobiography . . . seemed to show a number of painful events. . . . He may be covering up. . . . He always had excuses for why he was absent. . . . He's hard to reach. He seems to have a wall around him.

some other factor) caused any changes we saw in the dependent variable. By contrast, pre-experimental designs do little to eliminate these threats and so don't allow causal interpretation.

External Validity.   External validity, on the other hand, refers to the *generalizability* of the results, or whether conclusions of the research can be applied to the larger population or to different environments from those included in the study. The tight controls, homogeneous samples sometimes used, and reductionist methods of quantitative research sometimes make it difficult to generalize to the larger population. In order to control for threats to internal validity, quantitative researchers often reduce the amount of variability in the participants they select. Because participants and environments are tightly controlled, they may be quite different than individuals and environments in the broader context. This threatens external validity and makes it difficult to generalize the results to other people or environments.

Evaluating Qualitative Research

Good qualitative research provides evidence of trustworthiness and credibility. In other words, the researchers present good evidence that the findings accurately represent the experiences of the participants rather than the biases, motivations, or perspectives of the researcher. The following are some ways to ensure the credibility and trustworthiness of qualitative research (Best & Kahn, 2006; Christensen & Brumfield, 2010; McMillan & Schumacher, 2010):

➤ Conduct prolonged and persistent field work when gathering information.
➤ Use *triangulation*, or the use of multiple methods in obtaining information (e.g., observation, interviewing, document collection).
➤ Use language that participants understand.
➤ Describe information obtained in concrete terms.
➤ Use multiple researchers to lessen bias.
➤ Acknowledge and attempt to "bracket off" one's own biases so they don't interfere with data gathering.
➤ Mechanically record data, if possible, to ensure accuracy, and make transcripts available for review.
➤ Use an *informant* or a person who is familiar with the group, setting, or phenomenon to corroborate any evidence obtained.
➤ Have an outside *auditor* check for biases in the research process.
➤ Conduct *member checks* that ask individuals who are interviewed to review transcripts for accuracy, review summaries of conclusions, or both.
➤ Actively search for discrepant data or information that does not support a particular point of view, as such information offers a differing view of the "truth" of the situation.
➤ Describe participants and setting in enough detail that generalizability to other settings is apparent.

After data have been obtained and authenticated, the researcher must go through a rigorous process of reviewing the data, synthesizing results, and drawing conclusions and generalizations. The researcher's original research question(s) may have been changed by this point as he or she has gone through the involved process of reviewing the literature and analyzing sources of information. The final results of the research involve a logical analysis of the materials obtained, as opposed to a statistical analysis as we find in quantitative research. Also, the researcher needs to be careful not to get caught up in his or her point of view and should be open to offering opinions that both support and contradict the ultimate findings. See Box 13.7 to consider what trustworthiness methods were used in this hypothetical example that examines the development of a counselor's theoretical orientation.

Reading and Writing Research

It is likely that some readers of this book will be actively involved in doing research, while all of you will be reading research. Certainly, if you are to remain professionally astute, it is your obligation to read the professional journals that offer the most current research in our field. Although qualitative and quantitative research studies approach the attainment of knowledge differently, the manner in which results of the research are presented

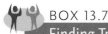

BOX 13.7

Finding Trustworthiness and Credibility in Qualitative Research

Below is a hypothetical example of qualitative research that examines the development of a counselor's theoretical orientation. After reading it, answer the questions that follow.

In conducting our research, we started by placing an ad in *Counseling Today*. The ad requested volunteers who had counseled for more than ten years and were going to the ACA's annual convention to meet with us and other volunteers in a focus group to discuss how they developed their theoretical orientation. At the conference, we ended with a purposeful sample that included six to eight counselors in each of four groups. We asked them a series of questions related to the main research question: "How did you develop your theoretical orientation?"

As they talked, we listened and tried to bracket any of our biases. Mostly, we were respectful and would periodically ask questions to encourage the conversation. We believe that we rarely, if ever, gave our opinions, but we did actively encourage discussion. Although many qualitative researchers do not record their sessions, we decided, for accuracy, that we would. From these recordings, we summarized what we believed to be the more salient points in each group. We asked for volunteers (member checkers) from each group to review our summary for accuracy. We then took the summaries and coded the responses into logical groupings. We asked a colleague to do the same, separately. After we separately coded the data, we met with our colleague and together, we

came up with a number of themes that seemed to run through all the groups. The themes showed a progression relative to how the counselors tended to develop their theoretical orientation:

1. *Ignorance:* Not realizing the importance of a theory
2. *Learning:* Realizing that theories drive the way that one does counseling
3. *Adherence:* Taking on one theoretical approach
4. *Being willing to experiment:* Desiring to incorporate other theoretical perspectives within the one main approach
5. *Becoming an expert:* Being willing to develop one's own personal theory based on a number of theoretical constructs

We asked an expert in counseling theory to review our work for biases, and then we decided to write up what we had found and submit it for publication.

Questions to Ponder:

1. What types of evidence of credibility and trustworthiness can you find in this study?
2. What additionally could have been done to increase the credibility and trustworthiness of this study?
3. How could biases have affected the results?
4. How generalizable is a study such as this?

---

is similar. Here are some of the major headings that are often used when writing research manuscripts (listed in the order that they appear):

Abstract. The abstract is a short summary of the article, generally fewer than 100 words.

Review of the Literature. The review of the literature examines past research that has been completed in the area being studied and elaborates on the statement of the problem. The review can be as short as one page or as long as ten and should justify the research hypothesis or research question.

Research Hypothesis or Research Question. Generally found at the end of the review of the literature, the hypothesis or research question defines the variables or what is being examined and defines the population to be studied.

Methodology. The methodology or procedures section is a description of how the study was conducted and is based on the type of research that was conducted. It may include one or more of the following: a description of the participants; statements about instruments used, including their reliability and validity (or credibility and trustworthiness); the sources of data; procedures employed in conducting the study; and procedures used in collecting the data. An individual should be able to replicate the study being presented based on the information in this section.

Results. Results describe the types of statistical analysis or data synthesis that were used, as well as an objective description in writing or through the use of charts, tables, and figures of results found.

Discussion, Implications, and Conclusions. This section describes how the results are related to the research question or hypothesis. Results should be related to past research, and possible reasons why the results were found should be discussed. Any methodological problems should be described in this section. Although authors have some liberty in this section to speculate about the results, they should do so tentatively. Often the author concludes this section by suggesting how the research might be applied to future studies.

References. Almost all educational and psychological publications require that manuscripts use the style of the *Publication Manual of the American Psychological Association* (APA, 2010b). If you learned referencing using a different style, this approach will initially seem foreign to you. Generally, the publication manual encourages simplicity in its approach, and you will quickly become used to its streamlined manner of citing and referencing. Without going into detail on how to reference, throughout all manuscripts, citations should be listed whenever a statement needs to be supported by past research, and all citations are listed at the end of the manuscript.

Evaluation

The Purpose of Evaluation

Although many research concepts are used in evaluation, the purpose of evaluation is generally different from the purposes of research (Leary, 2012). Whereas research tends to examine new paradigms to expand understanding and knowledge and how such knowledge can be applied to practice, program evaluation has to do with whether a program has achieved its goals and objectives and has been shown to have worth and value (Houser, 2015; Leary, 2012). Evaluation, therefore, serves the very practical purpose of enabling counselors to make informed decisions about program improvement, continuation, expansion, and dissolution (Fitzpatrick, Sanders, & Worthen, 2011; Royse, Thyer, & Padgett, 2010).

Formative and Summative Evaluation

There are two main types of evaluation, which have different purposes: *formative* and *summative* (Scriven, 1967, 1996). Formative evaluation is concerned with the collection of information that will guide improvement of the program. Typically done during the early stages of program development and implementation, formative evaluation results are provided to the program facilitator so that he or she can make the program better. On the other hand, summative evaluation is used to determine if a program should be continued, expanded, or eliminated. Often used to show accountability to funding agencies and agency administrators, summative evaluation is done after the program has been well established and is generally an involved and formal process that has a strong research design.

In both types of evaluation, evaluators may look at the program *process* or *outcomes* (Fitzpatrick, et al., 2011). Program process components are the activities and conditions of the program, and may include characteristics of the clients served, resources and materials provided, program location and environment, and the design of the activities themselves. Outcome components are the changes in program participants and other relevant community members or variables as a result of the program. These may be immediate results of the program, such as changes in knowledge and skills of participants, or long-term effects, such as changes in behavior or impacts on nonparticipants (Kirkpatrick & Kirkpatrick, 2006). For example, imagine that you have developed a holistic wellness program for expectant teenage mothers (Figure 13.4). One of the immediate outcomes of this program might be increased knowledge about the effects of drug and alcohol use on the fetus, but a longer term outcome would be delivery of a healthy baby.

One way to conduct formative evaluation is to ask for feedback from program participants. This is often done by asking participants to complete rating forms on the *process* components of the program and to write down any comments or suggestions they might have for program improvement. Data from rating forms can be easily collated and offer a quick and yet somewhat structured mechanism to obtain immediate feedback. The questions on the forms must be written in such a way, however, that if participants provide a low rating, the evaluator knows what to change. For example, if we ask participants to rate the instructor from poor to excellent, and the average rating is poor, the instructor still doesn't know what the participants dislike. Is he or she hard to understand, unprepared for class, poorly organized, not engaging, distant and cold, or something else? Rating forms, therefore, must be well designed to enable the program facilitator to use the feedback. For example, imagine you were going to do a formative evaluation of the drug and alcohol awareness class in your holistic wellness program (Figure 13.4). Some questions on your rating form might target specific instructor characteristics so that you can see what aspects of the instructor are strong and what areas need improvement (see Box 13.8).

Another way to conduct formative evaluation is to look at the outcomes of the program. If participants aren't changing in the way we expect as a result of the program, then we might have an idea as to what part of the program needs to be improved. Returning again to the holistic wellness program example (Figure 13.4), you might test participants' knowledge of the consequences of drug and alcohol use on the fetus. Then, if you found that participants understand the impact of heroin and alcohol, but still don't understand the impact of cigarettes, you might add more training in the program on tobacco use and its consequences.

As already mentioned, summative evaluation occurs after the program has been running for some time and improvements have been made. Only then do we evaluate the program to determine if it should be continued, expanded, or eliminated. In a summative evaluation, we are often comparing to other, alternative programs or to a control group that had no program. In these cases, we might look at process components

FIGURE 13.4

Simplified Evaluation Model for a Holistic-Wellness Program for Teenage Expectant Mothers

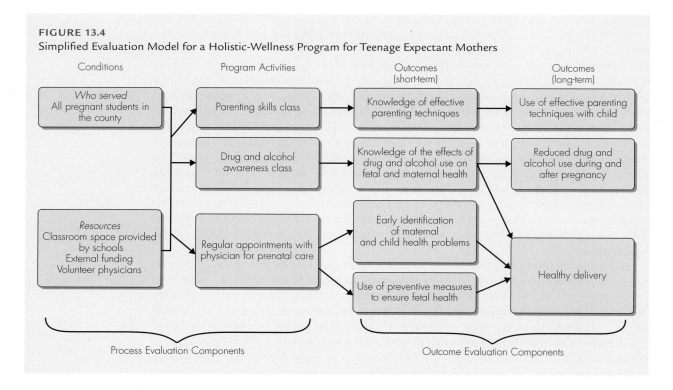

<!-- figure decorative icon -->

BOX 13.8

Sample Rating Form for Drug and Alcohol Awareness Class in Holistic Wellness Program

Describe your reaction to each of the following statements on a scale from 1 (*never*) to 5 (*always*)

The program instructor:	Never	Seldom	Sometimes	Usually	Always
1. was well prepared.	1	2	3	4	5
2. delivered material in a clear, organized manner.	1	2	3	4	5
3. stimulated intellectual curiosity.	1	2	3	4	5
4. showed respect for questions and opinions of participants.	1	2	3	4	5
5. allowed relevant discussion when appropriate.	1	2	3	4	5
6. was concerned that participants understood her.	1	2	3	4	5
7. was easy to talk to.	1	2	3	4	5
8. did not judge me.	1	2	3	4	5

(do participants in our holistic wellness program attend appointments with a physician more often than those who are not in the program?) or outcome components (do participants in our program have higher rates of healthy delivery than similar youths who do not participate?). In some cases, you might expect training programs to have some far-reaching effects, and this too can be an aspect of summative evaluation. For instance, in the holistic wellness program just discussed, some of the long-term outcome measures that we hoped to see from this training included reduced used of alcohol and drugs by participants after the child is born and higher rates of usage of effective parenting techniques. To obtain information like this would be a major undertaking and would involve large-scale assessment of graduates of the program. Although it would not be an easy project, these behaviors are measurable and could be an indication that our program was effective.

Summative evaluation will sometimes involve the use of specific research designs. For instance, in employing survey research, a university trying to decide if it should maintain its graduate counseling program might desire to survey all students who have graduated within the past five years, as well as their employers, in an effort to assess how effective they believe the counseling program was in preparing them to become counselors and might compare those results to surveys of non–counseling program graduates. Even true experimental designs can be employed in summative research. For example, if we wanted to determine if online instruction is an effective program for teaching empathy skills to counselor trainees, we might develop a true experimental design to compare the effectiveness of the online program with a classroom-based program. Forty students could be randomly assigned to each program. At the conclusion of the programs, each student would be asked to respond empathically to a role-played client. A statistical comparison of the empathy scores in the two programs can then be completed using a *t*-test, and the online program will be continued or eliminated based on how well its student empathy scores compared with those of the other program. Whatever technique is used in summative evaluation, you can see that it is often more involved than formative evaluation.

Multicultural/Social Justice Focus in Research

Bias in Research and Evaluation

> *Scientific inquiry cannot be value-free . . . for cultural and social values make knowledge possible. These values must, of course, be subject to examination and critique, ideally by those from outside the community who do not share those cultural assumptions.*

> (Goldenberg, 2006, pp. 2626–2627)

Researchers choose to study specific issues because of their preferences and biases (Eaves, 2010; Parham, 1993). They design studies based on their values. They include or exclude certain participants based on their biases, and they make conclusions that are at least somewhat a function of the prism through which they view the world. There is little

BOX 13.9
Female Genital Mutilation from a Qualitative Research Perspective

In recent years, there has been an uproar in many countries concerning the act of female genital mutilation (FGM), which occurs mostly in some parts of Africa, the Middle East, and the Far East (Robinson, 2014). The practice generally includes anything from a partial clitoridectomy to excision of the clitoris, the inner labia, and the skin of the outer labia. In some cases, the remaining skin is stitched, leaving a tiny opening that makes it difficult to urinate, leaves the women prone to infections, and acts as a kind of chastity belt (World Health Organization, 2014). The procedure, which typically occurs at around age 7, symbolizes the induction into adulthood, reduces or eliminates sexual pleasure, and often results in painful sexual intercourse. Despite laws against such FGM in the United States, in some cases, it is still practiced:

> Some immigrant populations remain steadfast in their belief that it is their right and duty to cut and mutilate the genitals of their daughters and granddaughters regardless of the laws of the land.
>
> (Raya, 2010, p. 305)

If one were to examine this procedure from a Western perspective, undoubtedly we would find this procedure distasteful, sexist, without purpose, oppressive, and abusive. In fact, even the term *female genital mutilation* carries with it Western inherent bias. The qualitative researcher, however, would ask the following questions:

1. When does the event occur in the culture?
2. Who is involved in carrying out this event?
3. What does this event symbolize for the culture?
4. How do the participants in this event view it?
5. Are the meanings to the event viewed in the same manner by all the participants?

getting around the fact that all research, to some degree, is biased as a result of the preferences of the researcher (Chang, Hays, & Gray, 2010).

Although quantitative research has brought us many advances, its so-called purity must be called into question when we realize that every decision that a quantitative researcher makes in designing, implementing, analyzing, and interpreting a study is a reflection of his or her personal biases. The subject matter that is chosen, the population to be examined, the kinds of designs that are chosen, and even the statistical analysis used can lead a researcher to certain conclusions that might differ from a researcher working with the same data who has a different worldview. Qualitative research questions and interpretation are similarly subject to the unique perspectives of the researcher, while also offering us a unique opportunity to conduct research that focuses on the worldview of the participants. Such research seems like a natural fit for counselors who are used to taking on a phenomenological perspective when working with clients (Duffy & Chenail, 2008). It allows us to peek inside the world of other groups and cultures in an effort to understand how individuals within that group or culture understand reality. For instance, examine Box 13.9, which discusses female genital mutilation, and ask yourself whether you could approach this subject in an unbiased fashion. Then consider the challenges that a qualitative researcher has when studying such a topic.

By bracketing his or her biases, an effective qualitative researcher can add much to our understanding of a culture or practice. For instance, reading a qualitative researcher's study on FGM could offer a counselor a broad understanding of the issues involved and why such practices have been important in particular cultures, and help the counselor have empathy for women who have undergone such a procedure. Although few if any of us would ever approve of such a procedure, qualitative research can help us understand the circumstances around the procedure and its meaning for the individuals within the culture.

Although qualitative research can offer a unique perspective on events, don't be misled into thinking that such research does not have its share of biases. It is the unique researcher who can enter a group or culture and truly leave his or her self behind (Chang et al., 2010). For this reason, qualitative research can surely be criticized as too subjective. Therefore, when conducting or reading quantitative or qualitative research, we must always keep in mind that even the seemingly purest of research studies will suffer from researcher bias. We must both learn from research and question it.

White Researchers Conducting Multicultural Research: An Unnatural Fit?

From 1932 to 1972, the U.S. Public Health Services examined the effects of untreated syphilis on African American men in Tuskegee, Alabama. This appalling research, known as "the Tuskegee Experiment," was one of a number of abuses against minorities and women that have taken place in the name of research. Thus, it is not surprising that some researchers have questioned whether White researchers should even perform multicultural research (Guthrie, 2003; McDonald & Chaney, 2003; Parham, 1993; Petersen, 2008). In an effort to reduce biases, Chang et al. (2010) suggest that researchers do the following:

a. obtain a skill for exploring each individual cultural perspective
b. be aware of their own cultural biases and be able to articulate, explore, and challenge the validity of their worldview
c. always remain aware of cultural differences, but without making them the major focus
d. be considerate of participants' ethnic, racial, and cultural views when developing methodology (p. 271)

Ethical, Professional, and Legal Issues

Ethical Issue: Code of Conduct

The ACA ethical code (ACA, 2014a) has a separate section on research and publication that emphasizes many important research issues (see Section G of the ethics code in the Appendix). Summarizing a few of these, we find the following:

➤ *Research responsibilities:* Research must be conducted in a manner that is consistent with federal and state laws, institutional policies, and scientific standards. It must be conducted in a manner that respects the rights of individuals and takes reasonable precautions to avoid emotional, physical, or social injury to participants.

➤ *Rights of research participants:* A number of key procedures must be in place to respect the rights of research participants. These include:

    ➤ *Informed consent:* Prior to consenting to participate in research, subjects must be told the purpose of the research, the procedures, any potential risks involved, the potential benefits, alternative procedures to the research, any limits to confidentiality, and the fact that they can withdraw from the study at any point.

➤ *Confidentiality:* All information obtained from research must be kept confidential, and procedures must be implemented to protect confidentiality.

➤ *Student/supervisee participation*: Students' participation (or lack of participation) in a faculty member's or supervisor's research should not affect their academic standing. If students choose not to participate, they should be given alternatives to fulfill the relevant requirements.

➤ *Managing and maintaining boundaries:* Researcher must maintain appropriate boundaries between himself or herself and the research participants. This includes, but is not limited to, refraining from having romantic relationships with participants.

➤ *Reporting results:* The researcher must "plan, conduct, and report research accurately" (ACA, 2014a, p. 16). There must be no misrepresentation of data or deliberate bias of results, and researchers must report results that may be undesirable or unfavorable to their goals.

Professional Issue: Standards in Research

ACA and the American Psychological Association (APA) have both set standards in conducting research through statements in their ethical codes (ACA, 2014a; APA, 2010a). In addition, research and program evaluation is one of the eight core content areas designated by the Counselor for Accreditation of Counseling and Related Educational Programs (CACREP) for counselor training programs. Thus, for programs to obtain accreditation, they must teach the specific areas identified by CACREP. Finally, although one division of ACA—the Association for Assessment and Research in Counseling (AARC)—specifically addresses research, all divisions are committed to research, as is reflected in their journals and the scholarship that they produce.

Legal Issues

Exclusion of Females and Minorities in Research

The National Institute of Mental Health (2001) and other agencies now require that females and minorities be included in all research unless there is a compelling reason not to include them.

Institutional Review Boards

Federal legislation now requires that all organizations that conduct research supported by federal funds have a human subjects committee or institutional review board (IRB) whose purpose is to ensure that there is little or no risk to research participants. Today, many institutions have adopted human subjects committees even if they do not receive federal funds. All researchers in those institutions are required to get IRB approval before conducting their research.

The Counselor in Process: Discovering New Paradigms

Whiston (1996) challenges all practitioners to come forth and risk leaping into the black hole called research. It's scary to dive in, but one comes out a scholar, as well as a better counselor. Counselors must see themselves as conductors of research, readers of research, and publishers of research. We cannot afford to be bound by our fears of research because this keeps us stuck in our inert former ways of understanding the profession of counseling. We must move forward toward new paradigms. Research and evaluation allow us to examine what we are doing, change what we have done, and adopt new and better ways of working with clients. We need to stop being fearful of conducting research; we need to embrace the reading of research; and we need to realize that research is not a virus to avoid, but rather a living process that offers us new directions for the future and new ways of defining who we are and how we work. Learn various ways of doing research and evaluation, apply them, and publish them. Become a true scholar in the helping professions. Give to both your clients and your peers, and make a contribution to knowledge.

Summary

This chapter examined research and evaluation. Relative to research, we noted that it is conducted to give us knowledge about the present—knowledge that may help us to make predictions about the future. We noted that research and evaluation help us find answers to the questions we ponder, move us forward in our understanding of the world, help to show us that what we are doing is working, and offer us new ways of approaching our work. We pointed out that some have used the term practitioner–scientist to describe the fact that all counselors use research in some fashion.

We pointed out that usually researchers examine a subject by conducting a literature review, which is an examination of prior research. Two databases often used in this process are ERIC and PsycInfo. Out of the literature review comes the statement of the problem, which helps to orient the research to its historical context, to its scope, and to research questions, statements, and hypotheses.

We noted that qualitative and quantitative research approach the process of attaining new knowledge differently, with each offering an important perspective. We explained that although evaluation has a different purpose than research, it will often employ research designs to complete its task.

Explaining the differences between quantitative and qualitative research, we noted that quantitative research assumes that there is an objective reality within which research questions can be formulated, as well as reductionist, scientific methods used in the pursuit of knowledge, while qualitative research holds that there are multiple ways of viewing knowledge and that the role of the researcher is to observe and describe phenomena carefully and to interpret them within a social context.

In examining quantitative research, we distinguished between experimental and nonexperimental research. Experimental research includes true experimental, quasi-experimental, single subject, and pre-experimental designs, all of which attempt to show cause and effect and manipulate the independent variable. Nonexperimental research includes correlation research (bivariate and multivariate), survey research, and ex post facto (causal-comparative) research. Nonexperimental research generally does not imply cause and effect; there is no manipulation of the independent variable.

In looking at qualitative research, we delineated the following kinds of research: grounded theory, phenomenological designs, ethnographic research, and consensual qualitative research. Noting that each employs the case study method of probing or analyzing an event, group, or phenomenon, we highlighted some of the differences. We noted that grounded theory attempts to develop theory from the exploration of a particular population or experience being examined. This process unfolds through a series of steps: preparing, data collection, note taking, coding, and writing. Phenomenological designs attempt to understand the experience of a phenomenon but are less interested in theory development. Ethnographic research, we noted, examines a group within its social context by having the researcher immerse himself or herself in the culture using observation, ethnographic interviews, and document and artifact collection. Consensual qualitative research uses a team of researchers to systematically collect and analyze qualitative data, with the intent of coming to consensus about the phenomenon under investigation.

In discussing some of the statistics that are used with quantitative research, we noted that descriptive statistics are used to describe characteristics of a sample and are often employed with survey research, while inferential statistics are mathematical procedures used to make inferences about a larger population from the sample that one is studying. Such statistics are generally used when one is examining group differences or relationships among treatment groups. We pointed out the importance of effects size, or the practical significance of research findings.

When organizing results from qualitative research, we noted that one generally relies on a process called inductive analysis, which means looking for patterns and categories that emerge from data. Thus, the researcher examines data from observation, interviews, artifacts, records, relics, and other sources and looks through the information for salient patterns and ways of categorizing information. Often, coding is used in this process.

In examining issues of quality when conducting research, we noted that quantitative research relies on an examination of a study's internal validity to show potential confounding variables and its external validity to show whether the research can be generalized to other populations. Whereas quantitative research examines the kinds of strict control one has over internal and external validity, qualitative research is more concerned with whether there is congruence between the researcher's understanding of events and the actual events that have taken place. Here, we often look at the credibility and trustworthiness of the information we obtained from our study. We pointed out a number of ways to show trustworthiness of our research (e.g., prolonged research, triangulation, bracketing, using an informant, using an outside auditor, member checks, etc.).

Although qualitative and quantitative research differ in their approach to understanding knowledge, they generally both start with a problem statement, a review of the literature, and a hypothesis or research question. After a study is complete, researchers respond to the hypothesis or research question by publishing their results. Generally, a publication includes an abstract; a literature review; the hypothesis or research question; the methodology; the results; the discussion, implications, and conclusions; and the references.

The last part of the chapter reviewed evaluation. We noted that unlike research that examines new paradigms, program evaluation examines the value and worth of a program and the extent to which a program has achieved its goals and objectives. Whereas formative evaluation is concerned with the assessment of a program during its implementation, summative evaluation involves assessment of the total training program in order to decide whether the program was worthwhile and whether it should be offered again. Formative evaluation can include informal assessment procedures, such as asking for verbal feedback or ratings on forms, and is an ongoing process as long as a program is being conducted. Summative evaluation, on the other hand, may involve more formal assessment procedures and may use research designs to show the efficacy of a program. Both formative and summative evaluation techniques are becoming increasingly important to the process of being accountable to administrators and funding agencies.

In this chapter, we stated that all research is biased. The subject matter that is chosen, the population to be examined, the kinds of design that are picked, and even the statistical analysis used can lead a researcher to certain conclusions. However, that does not mean that research is not important. On the contrary, research can enhance our understanding of the world, but we need to know its limits. The strict controls of quantitative research provide us with answers to many questions, but its extremely focused results often limit its generalizability. On the other hand, the less rigid structure of qualitative research offers a way of understanding how others come to define themselves and the culture in which they are embedded, but it can be criticized for being too subjective and easily subject to researcher bias.

As we neared the end of the chapter, we noted that a recent controversy has questioned whether White researchers should even perform multicultural research. We stated that researchers should obtain skills for working with people from cultures different from their own, be aware of their own cultural biases, remain aware of cultural differences, and be considerate of participants' cultural views when developing methodology.

We next highlighted a number of ethical, professional, and legal issues related to research and program evaluation. We noted that researchers must respect all research participants and ensure that no harm will occur to any person, ensure that research participants give informed consent, keep all information gained from research participants confidential, and report all findings accurately. In speaking to standards in the profession, we noted that in addition to the ethical guidelines requiring adherence to high standards in research, CACREP requires that counseling programs address specific content issues in the area of research and program evaluation. Two legal issues discussed were the importance of including minorities and women in research and the necessity of institutional review boards to ensure that no harm occurs to research participants. Finally, this chapter ended by noting the importance of diving into research and the benefits of becoming a conductor of research, a reader of research, and a publisher of research. We must be active researchers if we are to remain alive and forward-thinking in our profession and if we are going to be helpful to our clients and add knowledge to the world.

Further Practice

Visit CengageBrain.com to respond to additional material that highlight the salient aspects of the chapter content. There, you can find ethical, professional, and legal vignettes, a number of experiential exercises, and study tools including a glossary, flashcards, and sample test items. Hopefully, these will enhance your learning and be fun and interesting.

SOCIAL AND CULTURAL FOUNDATIONS IN COUNSELING

CHAPTER 14 **Theory and Concepts of Multicultural Counseling**

CHAPTER 15 **Knowledge and Skills of Multicultural Counseling**

Overview

The tragedy of 9/11 makes it clear that issues of class, race, ethnicity, religion, and culture are some of the most pressing concerns of the twenty-first century. These issues weigh heavily on the counselor and the counseling profession and they must be addressed. Thus, this section of the text offers two chapters that will examine the ever-important area of multicultural counseling.

The two chapters in this section are a natural complement to one another. Chapter 14 focuses on theory and concepts of multicultural counseling and is foundational to the understanding of this important area. With this basic grounding in place, you are ready to move on to Chapter 15, which zeroes in on the knowledge and skills necessary when working with diverse populations. Although the chapters differ in their general thrust, throughout both you will be presented with statistics on diversity, learn how discrimination and prejudice affect us all, be given the opportunity to examine your own cultural identity, and of course, gain some of the knowledge, skills, and attitudes that you will need to be an effective cross-cultural counselor.

Both chapters will present multicultural counseling as one of the most pressing issues in the mental health profession. Called by some a "fourth force" in the helping professions, multicultural counseling represents a major thrust for the counseling profession. As you read through these chapters, consider the importance that sensitivity and understanding toward different cultural groups can have for you, our profession, our country, and the world.

Theory and Concepts of Multicultural Counseling

There is an old story. We are each of us told in its tale. A child went to a rabbi and asked why God started with just Adam and just Eve. The child asked why God had not made everyone at once. The rabbi answered that God had made only Adam and only Eve so that no one of us could ever turn to another person and say, "Your father is not my father, your mother is not my mother, and we are neither brother nor sister." So this can never be said. By any of us. To any of us.

(Author Unknown)

When I was growing up in New York, the city was a world unto itself: the ethnic foods, the multicultured music, the people—oh, how I loved to watch the people. Walk down a Manhattan street and you can watch an endless sea of people, a sea that seems to change color as it flows by you, a sea whose shape transforms constantly; and, if you flow with it long enough, you can visit every part of the world. There is no question that New York gave me a multicultural perspective that many people don't have an opportunity to obtain. However, despite this exposure to a variety of cultures and ethnic groups, I never really got below the surface. I could taste the foods, I could see the people, and I could listen to the music, but that experience alone was still from a detached perspective. Even though I might see the brightly colored clothes of the Nigerian, I still didn't know that person. Even though I could taste the sushi, I didn't understand the world of the Japanese. And even though I could listen to the Latin music, I didn't really understand the people.

This chapter is about differences, similarities, and understanding one another. We will begin the chapter by suggesting a number of reasons why issues related to multicultural counseling must take a prominent place in the counseling profession today. We will review important definitions in the field and examine continued patterns of discrimination and prejudice that exist in the United States. By exploring models of racial and cultural identity development, as well as White identity development, we will try to understand how each of us has developed our own cultural identity and how that might affect the way that we view the world and work with clients. The chapter will highlight the importance of counselors understanding their own attitudes and beliefs, having basic knowledge of many cultures, and of knowing cross-cultural counseling skills if they are to work effectively with culturally different clients. Near the conclusion of the chapter, we will stress the importance of multicultural counseling training standards and examine some important ethical, professional, and legal issues.

What Is Multicultural Counseling?

Do counselors have the ability to understand a client who is from a different culture than their own? Can anyone, ever, truly understand the experience of another? Is it possible to connect with a client who is from a different culture or ethnic background? What additional skills must a counselor learn if he or she is to work effectively with clients from nondominant groups? These are some of the important questions that must be asked when defining multicultural counseling. And, as you might expect, based on how people respond to these questions, their definition of multicultural counseling will vary. For instance, McAuliffe (2013a) suggests that multicultural counseling "a consistent readiness to identify the cultural dimensions of clients' lives and a subsequent integration of culture into counseling work" (p. 6). Sue and Torino (2005) suggest that multicultural counseling (Figure 14.1):

> . . . can be defined as both a helping role and process that uses modalities and defines goals consistent with the life experiences and cultural values of clients, utilizes universal and culture-specific helping strategies and roles, recognizes client identities to include individual, group, and universal dimensions, and balances the importance of individualism and collectivism in the assessment diagnosis and treatment of client and client systems. (p. 6)

In addition to definitions of multicultural counseling, *Multicultural Counseling Competencies* have been developed by our profession and help drive the training of counselors (Arredondo et al., 1996; Roysircar, Arredondo, Fuertes, Ponterrotto, & Toporek, 2003). These competencies, which will be discussed in more detail later in the chapter, represent minimum standards needed by counselors if they are to work effectively with diverse clients, and delineate attitudes and beliefs, knowledge, and skills in three areas: (1) counselor self-awareness of assumptions, values, and biases, (2) knowledge of the world view of the culturally different client, and (3) familiarity with intervention strategies and techniques (see Figure 14.2).

FIGURE 14.1
One Way of Understanding
Multicultural Counseling

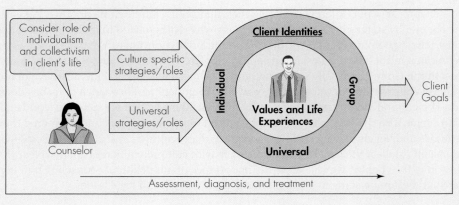

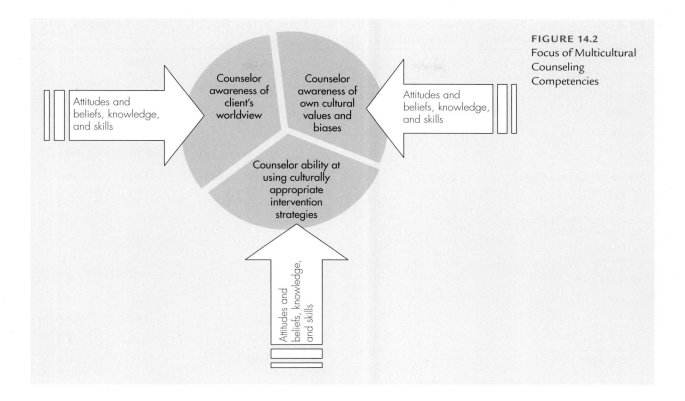

FIGURE 14.2
Focus of Multicultural
Counseling
Competencies

Why Multicultural Counseling?

Diversity in the United States

The most obvious answer to the question, "Why multicultural counseling?" is that the United States is the most diverse country in the world—a country that is truly a conglomerate of ethnicities, races, cultures, and religions. Examine Table 14.1, and you will see individuals from every race, culture, and ethnicity; individuals whose roots are from all parts of the globe; individuals with different sexual orientations; and individuals who embrace a wide range of religious affiliations. We live in a truly multicultural nation and thus are called to offer counseling services to individuals from many diverse backgrounds. However, besides the sheer number of individuals from diverse backgrounds, there are numerous other reasons why the profession must make special efforts at focusing upon multicultural counseling. Let's explore some of those.

Counseling Is Not Working for a Large Segment of Our Population

If you were distrustful of therapists, confused about the counseling process, or felt worlds apart from your helper, would you want to go to or continue counseling? Assuredly not.

TABLE 14.1   Number and Percentage of Individuals from Select Racial, Ethnic, Religious, and Sexual Identity Backgrounds in the United States

ETHNICITY/RACE*	NUMBER (MILLIONS)	%	RELIGION***	NUMBER (MILLIONS)	%
White, Not Hispanic	199.16	63.0	*Christian*	247.74	78.4
Hispanic	53.43	16.9	Protestant	162.11	51.3
Black or African American	41.41	13.1	Evangelical	83.11	26.3
Asian	16.12	5.1	Mainline churches	57.20	18.1
American Indian and Alaska Native (AIAN)	3.79	1.2	Historic Black churches	21.80	06.9
			Catholic	75.52	23.9
Native Hawaiian and other Pacific Islander (NHPI)	0.63	0.2	Mormon	5.37	01.7
			Jehovah's Witness	2.21	00.7
Two or more races	7.59	2.4	Orthodox[†]	1.90	00.6
White alone	246.26	77.9	*Jewish*[†]	5.37	01.7
			Buddhist[†]	2.21	00.7
			Muslim[†]	1.90	00.6
			Hindu	1.26	00.4
SEXUAL ORIENTATION**			*Other World Religions/ Faiths*	4.74	01.5
Bisexual[†]		1.8	*Unaffiliated*	50.88	16.1
Gay or Lesbian[†]		1.7	Atheist or agnostic	12.64	04.0
Transgender		0.3	Nothing in particular[†]	38.23	12.1

* SOURCE: U.S. Census Bureau (2014b). State and county quickfacts. Retrieved from http://quickfacts.census.gov/qfd/states/00000.html

** SOURCE: Gates, G. J. (2011). How many people are lesbian, gay, bisexual, and transgender? Retrieved from http://williamsinstitute.law.ucla.edu/wp-content/uploads/Gates-How-Many-People-LGBT-Apr-2011.pdf

*** SOURCE: Pew Research (2013). Religion and public life project: Religious landscape survey. Retrieved from http://religions.pewforum.org/reports (note: numbers based on 316 million).

[†] Numbers of bisexual, gay, or lesbian change dramatically from study to study; "Orthodox" includes Greek Orthodox (<.03%), Russian Orthodox (<0.3%) and Other Orthodox (<0.3%); "Jews," "Buddhists," and "Muslims" include various sects; Muslims are often undercounted as many mosques do not officially register; "Other World Religions/Faiths" include 0.7% Unitarians and other liberal faiths, 0.4% New Age, and < 0.3% Native American religions; "Nothing in particular" includes secular (6.3%) and religious unaffiliated (5.8%).

Unfortunately, this is the state of affairs for many diverse clients. In fact, it is now assumed that when clients from nondominant groups work with majority helpers, there is a possibility that the helper will (1) minimize the impact of social forces on the client, (2) interpret cultural differences as psychopathological issues, and (3) misdiagnose the client (Buckley & Franklin-Jackson, 2005; Constantine & Sue, 2005). Perhaps this is why a large body of evidence shows that diverse clients are frequently misunderstood, often misdiagnosed, find counseling and therapy less helpful than their majority counterparts, attend counseling and therapy at lower rates than majority clients, and tend to terminate from counseling more quickly than Whites (Evans, Delphin, Simmons, Omar, & Tebes, 2005; Sewell, 2009; U.S. Department of Health and Human Services, 2001). In addition, many people of color who seek counseling appear to feel more satisfied when seeing a counselor of their own cultural background. This is particularly disconcerting when we know that over 80% of counselors are White (Neukrug & Milliken, 2011), thus making it more difficult for clients of color to find counselors with whom they feel comfortable. Why is counseling not working for a good segment of our population? Often it is helper incompetence because the helper holds one or more of the following viewpoints (Buckley & Franklin-Jackson, 2005; Constantine & Sue; 2005; McAuliffe, Gómez, & Grothaus, 2013; Sue & Sue, 2013; Suzuki, Kugler, & Aguiar, 2005):

1. *Believing in the melting-pot myth.* Some believe this country is a melting pot of cultural diversity. However, this is not the experience of many diverse clients, who find themselves on the fringe of American culture, view themselves as different from the mainstream, and cannot relate to many of the values and beliefs held by the majority. In truth, most cultures want to maintain their uniqueness and are resistant to giving up their special traditions. Thus, the helper who assumes that clients should conform to the values of the majority culture may turn off some clients. Viewing the United States as a society with a myriad of diverse values and customs, or a *cultural mosaic*, more accurately represents the essence of diversity that we find today.

2. *Having incongruent expectations about counseling.* The Western (particularly American) approach to counseling and psychotherapy tends to contain a number of assumptions, including presuming that the counseling process should emphasize the individual; stressing the expression of feelings; encouraging self-disclosure, open-mindedness, and insight; and showing cause and effect. In addition, most helpers are not bilingual, approach counseling from a nonreligious perspective, and view the mind and body as separate. These beliefs and behaviors create barriers that result in diverse clients entering helping relationships with trepidation and feelings of disappointment, and sometimes being harmed by techniques that should not be used with them. For example, the Asian client who is proud of her ability to restrict her emotions may leave counseling feeling as if she disappointed her helper, who has been pushing her to express feelings.

3. *Deemphasizing social forces.* Although helpers may be effective at attending to clients' *feelings* concerning how they have been discriminated against, abused, or affected by other "external" factors, the same helpers will often deemphasize the actual influence that these social forces have on clients. Helpers often assume that most, if not all, negative feelings are created by the individual, and they often have difficulty understanding the power of social influences. The helper's negation of social forces results in an inability to build a successful relationship with a client who has been considerably harmed by external factors. For instance, the client who has been illegally denied jobs due to his disability may be discouraged when a helper says, "What have you done to keep yourself from getting a job?"

4. *Holding an ethnocentric worldview.* Ethnocentric helpers, or helpers who see the world only through their own lenses, tend to falsely assume that their clients view the world in a similar manner or believe that when their clients present a differing view of the world, they are emotionally disturbed, culturally brainwashed, or wrong. Although the importance of understanding a client's unique worldview is crucial to an effective helping relationship, it becomes particularly significant when working with diverse clients whose experience of the world may be particularly foreign to that of the helper. For instance, a helper may inadvertently turn off a client who is a Muslim by saying, "Have a wonderful Christmas."

5. *Ignorance of one's own racist attitudes and prejudices.* Of course, the helper who is not in touch with his or her prejudices and racist attitudes cannot work effectively with diverse clients and will often cause harm to those clients. Understanding our own stereotypes and prejudices takes a particularly vigilant effort, as many of our biases are unconscious. For instance, the heterosexual helper who unconsciously believes that being gay or lesbian is a disorder but consciously states that he accepts all sexual orientations may subtly treat a gay or lesbian client as if there is something wrong with him or her.

6. *Misunderstanding cultural differences in the expression of symptomatology.* What may be seen as "abnormal" in the United States may be usual and customary in another culture. The helper's lack of knowledge about cultural differences as they relate to the expression of symptoms can seriously damage a counseling relationship and result in misdiagnosis, mistreatment, and early termination. For instance, whereas many individuals from Anglo-European cultures would show grief through depression, agitation, and feelings of helplessness, a Latino/Latina might present with somatic complaints.

7. *Misjudging the accuracy of assessment and research procedures.* Over the years, assessment and research procedures have notoriously been culturally biased. Although advances have been made, one can still readily find tests that have cultural bias, and research that does not control adequately for cultural differences. One common problem in the use of assessment instruments is that individuals from different cultures may inadvertently be answering questions in a manner that would be considered "abnormal" by "American" (i.e., White Eurocentric) standards when they actually do not have an emotional disorder. For example, when an item on a test asks if a person "hears voices," a religious Latina client might answer "yes," thinking that she "talks to God"—a normal response in her culture. Although acculturated Americans might also "talk to God," they have learned to deny that they "hear voices" because that phrase implies psychopathology in traditional American culture.

8. *Ignorance of institutional racism.* Because institutional racism is embedded in society (and, some would argue, even within the helping professional organizations), it is likely that materials used by helpers will be biased and helpers will unknowingly have a skewed understanding of culturally different clients. Examples are plentiful. For instance, some diagnoses that have been listed in the *Diagnostic and Statistical Manual-5 (DSM-5)* may hold cultural biased; counseling approaches that have been given precedence in the professional journals

have been shown to be practically useless when working with clients from some cultures; and, until recently, training programs have not stressed multicultural issues. No doubt there are culturally biased statements in this text of which I am not aware.

In recent years, the emphasis on multicultural counseling has taken center stage, with increasing publications and great focus in counselor education programs (D'Andrea & Heckman, 2008a). As we continue to move forward as a profession, the need to continually focus and expand on different aspects of multicultural counseling will undoubtedly remain strong:

> . . . *cultural competency is more than a promise; it is a mandate for the counseling profession. As was the case decades ago when social activists stood up for civil rights and social justice against the forces of oppression, counselors are encouraged to stand up now for better training, more resources, less bias, and greater levels of professional proficiency.*
>
> (Arredondo, Tovar-Blank, & Parham, 2008, p. 267)

Some Definitions

In understanding differences within American society, it is important to distinguish among a number of terms, such as *culture, discrimination, microaggressions, ethnicity, minority, nondominant group, power differentials, race, religion, spirituality, sexism, heterosexism, sexual prejudice, sexual orientation, social class* (or *class* for short), *stereotypes, prejudice,* and *racism*. Understanding these terms gives all of us a common framework within which to communicate. The following are brief definitions of some of these terms.

Culture

Shared values, symbols, language, and ways of being in the world are some of the words and phrases I think of when reflecting on the word *culture*. Culture is expressed through common values, ideas, habits, norms of behavior, rituals, symbols, artifacts, language, customs, and worldviews (McAuliffe, 2013a; Sewell, 2009; Spillman, 2007). For instance, despite great diversity in the United States, most Americans share a similar cultural heritage because there is a shared language, symbols that most of us recognize, and patterns of behavior with which most are familiar. Traveling throughout this country, we find many symbols of a common culture (e.g., fast-food restaurants, music, laws, basic values, and shared language). Yet, even as I acknowledge this common culture, I am acutely aware of the bicultural, tricultural, or multicultural nature of many individuals in the United States. For instance, there are those who share the culture of urban gays and lesbians; of their racial, ethnic, and religious groups; of their gender; and of their region (e.g., "the South"). Culture can also change through time, as the group to which one identifies changes as that group's shared language and discourses that they use to define themselves change.

Discrimination and Microaggressions

Active, harmful, and conscious and unconscious acting out, is what I think of when I reflect on the words *discrimination* and *microaggression*. Whereas *discrimination* may result in active behaviors, such as unfair hiring practices focused on specific ethnic or cultural groups or gay bashing (Law, 2007; Lum, 2004), today, many do not view themselves as discriminatory. Instead, subtle, usually brief, and often unconscious behaviors that denigrate others, called *microaggressions,* are often directed toward individuals from diverse cultures (Nadal, 2011; Sue, 2010). Some examples include statements like, "you don't seem 'gay' (or 'Black,' or . . .)," "My ancestors made it in this country without anything—I don't see why your family can't," poor or slow service directed at diverse individuals at a restaurant or store, and differential treatment by individuals, such as police or others in positions of power. Such discrimination is probably more commonplace by those who "know" that outward discrimination is wrong and yet still carry with them subtle, embedded feelings of prejudice toward others—feelings that they would often be ashamed of if they were to let themselves be conscious of them.

Although we have undoubtedly made progress, there is still quite a bit of discrimination in the United States. For instance, the most recent hate crime statistics from the Federal Bureau of Investigation (FBI) indicate that of the 293,790 nonfatal violent and property hate crime victimizations, 51% were based on ethnicity, 46% on race, 34% on association with individuals having certain characteristics, 28% on religion, 26% on gender, 13% on sexual orientation, 11% on disability, and 7% on perceived characteristics (U.S. Department of Justice, 2014). Perceptions of Americans seem to verify the notion that as a country, we still discriminate, with fairly high percentages of Americans believing that the following groups face "a lot" of discrimination: gays and lesbians (64%), Muslims (58%), Hispanics (52%), Blacks (49%), women (37%), Jews (35%), evangelical Christians (27%), atheists (26%), and Mormons (24%) (Pew Forum on Religion and Public Life, 2009).

Ethnicity

Heritage, ancestry, and tradition are some of the things that come to mind when I reflect on the word *ethnicity*. More specifically, when a group of people share a common ancestry, which may include specific cultural and social patterns such as similar language, values, religion, foods, and artistic expressions, they are said to be of the same ethnic group (Jenkins, 2007). Ethnicity is not based on genetic heritage, as race is sometimes said to be, but on long-term patterns of behavior that have some historical significance and may include similar religious, ancestral, language, and cultural characteristics. Therefore, many (but not all) Jews share common ancestry, religion, and cultural practices, so Jewish people are often considered an ethnic group; on the other hand, people of Asian heritage may not share the same culture or ethnic background, given the diverse religious, political, historical, and cultural experiences of this region of the world.

Minorities and Nondominant Groups

Oppression of one group over another is my immediate reaction to the word *minority*. A *minority* is any person or group of people who are being singled out due to their cultural or physical characteristics and are being systematically oppressed by those individuals who are in a position of power. Using this definition, a minority could conceivably be the numerical majority of a population, as was the case for many years for Blacks in South Africa and as is the situation with women in the United States (Atkinson, 2004a; Macionis, 2014). In recent years, we have seen the counseling profession increasingly use the term *nondominant group* rather than *minority* because of the negative connotations that the word *minority* carries and because the term *nondominant group* suggests that there are social causes (the oppression by dominant groups) causing distress to other (nondominant) groups.

Power Differentials

Potential abuse, force, control, and *superior/underling* are some of the words and phrases that come to my mind when I think of the term *power differential*. Power differentials may represent greater disparities between people than culture, ethnic group, race, or social class (Kuriansky, 2008). Power can be a function of race, class, gender, occupation, and a host of other factors and can easily be misunderstood. Whether perceived or real, power can be abused. For instance, a professor may abuse his or her real power by sexually harassing a student. Or, in an example of perceived power, an action by a Latina supervisor might be resented as an abuse of power, but the same action by a White supervisor wouldn't be because of the belief by some that Whites should have power.

Race

Genetic heritage, skin color, and *ambiguity* are some of the words and phrases I think of when reflecting on the word *race*. Whereas the concept of culture has been based on such elements as shared, learned characteristics generally agreed upon by those in the culture, race has traditionally been defined as permanent physical differences as perceived by an external authority (Arthur, 2007). Although historically, this notion was based on genetics, this concept has been challenged in recent years. For instance, research on the human genome shows that humans share much more genetically than was at one time thought (National Human Genome Research Project, 2012). In fact, genetic differences between any two people are only 0.1% (1/1,000!). In addition, gene pools throughout the world, and especially in the United States, have become increasingly mixed due to migration, exploration, invasions, systematic rape as a result of wars and oppression of minorities, and intermarriage (see Box 14.1). Also, behaviorally, there seem to be more differences

BOX 14.1
What Race Are You Anyway?

Although most people tend to think of themselves as one race or another, take a look at what happened in this one study that genetically examined a group of students at Pennsylvania State University:

. . . about 90 students took complex genetic screening tests that compared their samples with those of four regional groups. Many of these students thought of themselves as "100 percent" white or black or something else, but only a tiny fraction of them, as it turned out, actually fell into that category. Most learned instead that they shared genetic markers with people of different skin colors.

("Debunking the Concept of Race," 2005)

within racial groups than among them (Atkinson, 2004b). With some sociologists saying that there are no races, others saying that there are 3, and still others concluding that there are as many as 200, the issue of race is cloudy and perhaps inconsequential. However, it is undeniable that race and the perception of race have had some effect at every level of society. At its best, race represents perceived differences, at its worst, those perceived differences become translated into real differences that result in oppression of "racial" groups. This is why I try avoiding the use of the word *race*.

Religion and Spirituality

Religion is seen as an organized or unified set of practices and beliefs that have moral underpinnings and define a group's way of understanding the world (Cipriani, 2007; Eriksen, Jackson, Weld, & Lester, 2013). In contrast, *spirituality* is seen as residing in a person, not a group, and defines the person's understanding of self, self in relationship to others, and self in relationship to a self-defined higher power or lack thereof. Because religion is concerned with values from an external referent group and spirituality has more to do with internal processes, there are important differences in how one would counsel a person who is struggling with religious concerns (e.g., value differences between self and a self-chosen religious group) versus how one would counsel a person who is struggling with spiritual concerns (e.g., finding meaning in life).

Sexism, Heterosexism, and Sexual Prejudice

Denigrating and consciously putting another person down due to his or her gender and/or sexual orientation are some of the things I think of when I hear the words *sexism, heterosexism,* and *sexual prejudice*. Whenever a person discriminates, denigrates, or stigmatizes another due to his or her gender, that person is said to be *sexist*. In a similar fashion, when a person discriminates, denigrates, or stigmatizes a person for nonheterosexual behaviors, that person is said to be *heterosexist*. The word *heterosexism* has become preferred over *homophobia*, as the latter implies there is a phobia or disorder within a person that makes the person act in a stigmatizing or denigrating fashion, whereas the former suggests that language and social institutions are at play in fostering such attitudes (Adam, 2007). Finally, *sexual prejudice* is a more inclusive term referring to negative attitudes targeted toward homosexual, bisexual, or heterosexual individuals (Herek, 2000).

Sexual Orientation

Szymanski (2013) suggests that *sexual orientation* (in contrast to *sexual preference*) is the gender toward which a person consistently has sexual feelings, longings, and attachments. Although all of you are probably familiar with the terms *gay, lesbian,* and *bisexual,* some other common terms that individuals sometimes confuse with *gay, lesbian,* and *bisexual* include *transgender, transsexual, cross-dresser, intersex,* and *asexual* (National Center for Transgender Equality, 2014). *Transgender* refers to a person who does not identify with his or her birth sex and lives in congruence with the sex to which he or she does identify. A transsexual strongly disidentifies with his or her sex and uses hormones, surgery, or both to realign his or her sex with gender identity, although this word has taken on less prominence in recent years. A *cross-dresser* is an individual who enjoys wearing clothes of the opposite sex (formerly called *transvestite*, but that is now considered derogatory by some). An *intersex person*, formerly called a *hermaphrodite*, is a person born with a combination of male and female genitalia. A person who is asexual has little or no sexual attraction toward others. Most important, it should be emphasized that those who are *transgender, transsexual, cross-dresser, intersex,* and *asexual* are not uniquely gay, lesbian, or bisexual.

Because a number of words like *queer* and *fag* have had negative conations over the years, some have recently started using words like these as a means of reclaiming power and defusing the negative connotations that they have come to hold. Finally, it should be emphasized that in 1975, the American Psychological Association (APA) stated that homosexuality was not a disorder and the American Counseling Association (ACA) has continually supported this statement.

Social Class

Money, power, status, and *hierarchy*—these are the words that come to mind when I think of the term *social class* (or just *class*). Class is based on a person's education, income, and wealth and represents the perceived ranking of an individual within society and the amount of power an individual wields (Macionis, 2014; Goodspeed-Grant & Mackie, 2013). An individual's social class may cut across a person's ethnicity, cultural identification, or race. Therefore, even though individuals may share a similar culture, ethnicity, or race, they may have little in common with one another due to differences in social class.

Prejudice, Stereotypes, and Racism

Generalizing, falsehoods, irrational fears, and anger are things I think of when I consider the words *prejudice, stereotypes,* and *racism*. Generally, all three of these words are related to preconceived ideas or attitudes people have toward others. Whereas *prejudice* has to do with judging a person or a group based on preconceived notions about the group (e.g., gays are no good; therefore, I hate John because he's gay), *stereotyping* is the rigidly held belief that most or all members of a group share certain characteristics, behaviors, or beliefs (e.g., Asians are intelligent people, or Native Americans are alcoholics) (Jennings, 2007; Lum, 2004). *Racism* has to do with believing one race is superior to another (e.g., Whites are better than Blacks) and is considered a social construction that leads to prejudice, stereotyping, and discrimination (McAuliffe et al., 2013).

Political Correctness, or "Oh My God, What Do I Call Him?"

Hispanic, Latino, Latina, Black, African American, Brown person, Oriental, Asian American, Chinese American, Japanese American, Native American, Indian, Eskimo, Inuit, Aleut, Native American, American Indian, Asian Indian, Jew, Hebrew, Jewish American, Protestant, WASP, Muslim, Moslem, Islamic, Born again, Fundamentalist Christian, Christian, Catholic, White, Caucasian, European American, American, gay, homosexual, heterosexist, straight, heterosexual, bisexual, lesbian, queer, transgender, transsexual, cross-dresser, transvestite, disabled person, individual with disability, mentally retarded, individual with an intellectual disability, handicapped person, physically challenged, and on and on.

Did I offend anybody? I hope not, but in these days of political correctness, finding the correct term to refer to a person is often difficult. Not only that, but even once you find the "correct" term, you are bound to offend somebody.

Although there is great variety in how individuals prefer to be addressed, it is often for a specific reason. For example, words like *Hispanic* and *Negro* are associated with a long history of oppression for people who have historically been labeled as such by their oppressors. More than simple "political correctness," naming conventions can represent a way for people to reclaim their identity and should be taken seriously. That said, the next paragraph describes some terms that have been used recently.

For Americans with African heritage, the term *African American* is generally used, although *Black* is still acceptable and even preferred in some circles. *Asian American* refers to any of a number of individuals with heritage from Asia and the Pacific Islands, including approximately 50 distinct subgroups that differ in language, cultural identity, and histories (Social Security Administration, n.d.). *Hispanic*, the word that the U.S. Census Bureau uses, refers to Mexican Americans, Puerto Ricans, Cuban Americans, individuals with Central and South American heritage, and individuals with roots from Spanish-speaking countries in the Caribbean. However, not all individuals from these countries are comfortable with the word *Hispanic*, as it refers to anyone with Spanish roots and connotes a history of colonialism. Thus, in recent years, the words *Latino or Latina* have become preferred by many. Islam is a religion whose followers are called *Muslim* (less commonly *Moslem*). Homosexuals, today, generally use the term *gay* for men and *lesbian* for women, although as noted earlier, some have now moved to the word *queer* to define their sexual orientation. The term *straight* is becoming less acceptable to describe heterosexuals because of the implication that it is better than another type of orientation (e.g., "on the straight and narrow"), and, as already noted, *heterosexist* is now the preferred term over *homophobic*. Individuals who have been born in this country and identify with their cultural or ethnic background often place the word *American* following their heritage. Therefore, it is not unusual for us to find individuals referring to themselves as "Irish American," "Italian American," "Arab American," and so forth. On the other hand, individuals who are naturalized citizens tend not to use the word *American* following their country of origin. For instance, a colleague of mine who was raised in Mexico and became a U.S. citizen refers to herself as "Mexican." Rather than saying *handicapped* or *disabled person*, generally people now say "individual with a disability" (notice the importance of placing the word *individual* prior to the word *disability*), although some prefer the term *physically challenged*. Finally, the term *mentally retarded* has been replaced with the term *intellectual disability* in the *DSM*-5 (American Psychiatric Association, 2013a). Thus, we will be seeing the term *mentally retarded* used less frequently in the years to come.

Although it is not within the scope of this text to detail the accepted nomenclature for all cultural groups, I have attempted to use commonly accepted terms throughout Chapters 14 and 15. Of course, people vary in how they wish to be addressed, and it's always good to ask a client what he or she likes to be called. In either case, making an effort to use terms correctly shows our sensitivity to individuals from diverse cultures.

Conceptual Models Toward Understanding Cultural Identity

Every person is in certain respects is like all other people, like some people, and like no other person.

(paraphrased from Kluckhohn & Murray, 1948, p. 35)

The following briefly describes a number of models to help us understand how individuals come to make sense of the world relative to their cultural identities. Here, we will describe the existential model of identity, the tripartite model of personal identity, developmental models of racial/cultural identity, and a White identity development model.

Existential Model of Identity

One of the first attempts to understand the individual from a cross-cultural perspective was done by the existential therapists, who believed, and continue to believe, that the individual can be examined in a number of spheres (Binswanger, 1963; van Deurzen, 2002). Using German words from the early existential philosophers, they suggested that *Eigenwelt* is our psychological world, or how we come to understand ourselves; *Mitwelt* means common experiences that we share through our culture; *Umwelt* is grounded in our biology and has to do with how we experience the world around us; and *Überwelt* is the manner in which we relate to our spiritual self, or to the unknown. According to existentialists, we all share concerns relative to each of these domains, and it is only through empathy and understanding that we can come to know each individual in these four essential domains. These domains are fluid, in the sense that they influence each other, and thus we see dashes in the lines on Figure 14.3 representing this notion.

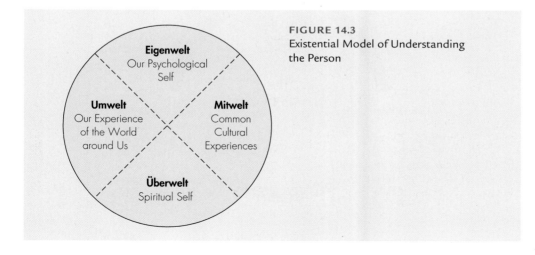

FIGURE 14.3
Existential Model of Understanding the Person

Tripartite Model of Personal Identity

Perhaps borrowing from the existential model of cultural identity development, Sue and Sue (2013) suggest that we understand our clients in three spheres: the *Individual Level,* which represents the clients' uniqueness; the *Group Level,* which is related to aspects of the person that can vary based on the cultural and ethnic groups to which the clients belong; and the *Universal Level,* which is related to common experiences, such as "(a) biological and physical similarities, (b) common life experiences (birth, death, love, sadness, etc.), (c) self-awareness, and (d) the ability to use symbols such as language" (p. 39) (see Figure 14.4).

Developmental Models: Cultural/Racial and White

In contrast to the more static tripartite and existential models of cultural identity, *cultural/racial developmental models* examine how individuals from cultural and racial groups pass through unique stages as they become increasingly aware of their cultural selves (Ponterotto, Casa, Suzuki, & Alexander, 2010; Sue & Sue, 2013). These models tend to view movement from an early conformity stage, through appreciation of their unique identity, to a final stage of universal acceptance. Like many development models, all individuals can pass through all stages, but not all people are afforded the nurturing

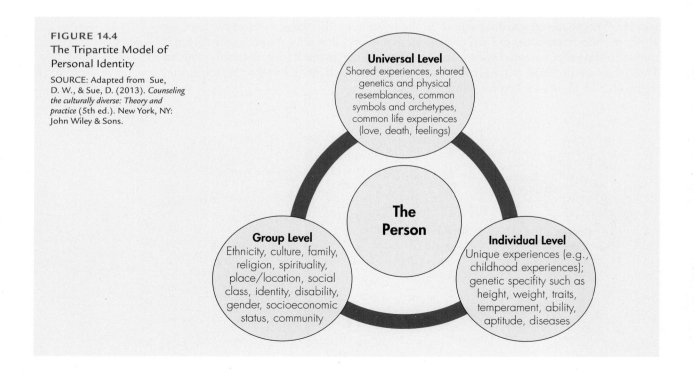

FIGURE 14.4
The Tripartite Model of Personal Identity

SOURCE: Adapted from Sue, D. W., & Sue, D. (2013). *Counseling the culturally diverse: Theory and practice* (5th ed.). New York, NY: John Wiley & Sons.

Universal Level
Shared experiences, shared genetics and physical resemblances, common symbols and archetypes, common life experiences (love, death, feelings)

The Person

Group Level
Ethnicity, culture, family, religion, spirituality, place/location, social class, identity, disability, gender, socioeconomic status, community

Individual Level
Unique experiences (e.g., childhood experiences); genetic specifity such as height, weight, traits, temperament, ability, aptitude, diseases

and educational environment that allows them to do so. One such model, which we'll look at here, is McAuliffe's Racial Identity Development for People of Color (RIDPOC).

The RIDPOC Model.   Although culture-specific models of racial and cultural identity development have been created (e.g., African American development, Native American development), McAuliffe, Gómez, & Grothaus (2013) offer a generic five-stage model of racial/cultural identity that synthesizes some of the more popular models. With the RIDPOC model, McAuliffe et al. (2013) note that a stage in the model represents a general tendency, or overall focus of behavior, relative to an individual's culture or race. Short descriptions of the five stages follow (see Table 14.2). If you are a person of color, see whether the model resonates with you as you read through the stages.

White Identity Development.   As with cultural/racial identity development models, White identity development models also suggest stage progression, in that they propose specific stages that Whites are likely to pass through as they become increasingly cross-culturally aware (D'Andrea & Daniels, 1991, 1999; Helms, 1984, 1999; Helms & Cook, 1999; Sabnani, Ponterotto, & Borodovsky, 1991). Two such models presented in Table 14.3 include Helms's model, which speaks to Whites in general; and the model of Sabnani et al., which speaks specifically to White graduate students in counseling. Research has supported the notion that such models reflect the deepening awareness and understanding of multicultural issues that individuals gain as they are exposed to experiences that increase their understanding of multiculturalism (Hays, Chang, & Havic, 2005; Middleton et al., 2005). If you are White, see whether the models resonate with you as you read through the stages.

Sabnani et al. (1991) describe a number of variations in the ways that students can move through the stages. A few examples are shown in Figure 14.5. For instance, Student A is stuck in stage 1. As the student is confronted with multicultural issues (perhaps in a course on multicultural counseling), he or she retreats to stage 1 behavior, preferring denial about racism and prejudice in society. The change process is too fearful for him or her. Student B moves through the first three stages, does not feel a strong need to retreat into his own culture in stage 4, and moves on to stage 5, where he or she can feel good about his or her own culture while having an understanding of and appreciation for others. Student C, on the other hand, feels a need to retreat as he or she is rejected by some minority individuals (stage 4). This student becomes angry, upset, and discouraged; moves away from cross-cultural contact; and needs time to reflect on his or her experiences. This student does not understand that individuals from diverse backgrounds are dealing with their own identity issues, which leads some of them to reject Whites, even Whites with good intentions. Some stage 4 students will eventually move out of their shells and have an easy transition to stage 5. Others, however, such as Student D, may poke their heads out as they consider moving on to stage 5, but because they continue to struggle with feelings of rejection and anger, quickly move back to stage 4. Keep in mind that because this is a developmental model, it is assumed that any White student, if given a conducive environment, can move to the higher stages.

TABLE 14.2   McAuliffe's Model of Racial Identity Development for People of Color

Stage 1: Conformity. In this stage, persons of color do not see culture/race as important and tend to conform to the dominant views of culture/race. Some may denigrate their own culture/race and highly value the lifestyle, achievements, and characteristics of the dominant group. Others may simply place little importance on culture/race. These individuals tend to prefer White counselors.

Stage 2: Dissonance and Beginning Appreciation. As individuals begin to gain positive experiences about people of color through the media, reading, and role models, they begin to question the negative views they had about their culture/race. This newfound awareness leads to confusion or dissonance about how they once viewed their culture/race and move toward a positive experience of their culture/race. In this stage, it is suggested that counselors should offer clients positive readings, symbols, and role models from the clients' culture/race.

Stage 3: Resistance and Immersion. As the name implies, in this stage individuals of color are immersed in their own cultural group and increasingly mistrustful of and angry at Whites. They see the dominant group as the cause of most of their problems and feel an increasing pride in their own culture/race and the struggles they have gone through. They tend to see only the positive qualities of their culture/race and are mistrustful of White counselors.

Stage 4: Introspection and Internalization. As individuals move out of total immersion in their own culture/race, they become increasingly introspective about cultural and racial issues in general. As some encounters with Whites are positive, they begin to let go of the dualistic thinking of Stage 3 that suggested that their culture/race was good and that the White culture/race was the cause of all of their problems. Although they continue to recognize the positive qualities of their own culture/race, they can also see the positive qualities of other cultures/races. Here the counselor supports the more complex thinking and the newfound introspection of the client.

Stage 5: Universal Inclusion. This final stage is when individuals see that all people can experience oppression, even Whites. They have moved out of the black-and-white thinking that was central to the earlier stages and toward a desire to promote social justice for all individuals. They have an interest in all cultures/races and want to embrace aspects of all cultures/races into their own understanding of the world. Counselors in this stage can work side-by-side with almost all of their clients and share complex views of the world.

TABLE 14.3   White Identity Models

HELMS (HELMS, 1984; 1999; 2005; HELMS & COOK, 1999)	SABNANI, PONTEROTTO, & BORODOVSKY (1991)
Stage 1: Contact. Here, Whites are unaware of themselves as racial beings, oblivious to social and cultural issues and White privilege, and naïve concerning how race affects themselves and others.	*Stage 1: Pre-exposure.* White graduate students show naiveté and ignorance about multicultural issues and sometimes believe that racism does not exist or that, if it does, only to a limited degree. Racism is generally thought of as over, and students in this stage do not understand more subtle, embedded racism.
Stage 2: Disintegration. In this stage, Whites begin to acknowledge that racism exists. Believing that society is unjust leads to a sense of confusion and disorientation as past beliefs are being challenged. Some may feel anxiety and guilt over racism and may overly identify with those from other cultures, while others may act paternalistically toward them.	*Stage 2: Exposure.* Students enter this stage when first confronted with multicultural issues, such as when students discuss multicultural counseling in class, or take a course on the subject. Increasing awareness of embedded racism in society leads to feelings of guilt over being White and depression and anger over the current state of affairs. This stage is highlighted by conflict between wanting to maintain majority views and the desire to uphold more humanistically oriented nonprejudicial views.
Stage 3: Reintegration. This stage is a backlash to the confusion and disorientation in Stage 2, and many Whites retreat back to protecting their privileged status and maintaining the status quo. Feelings of anxiety and guilt are now transformed to anger and fear of individuals from nondominant groups.	*Stage 3: Prominority/Antiracism.* Here, students often take a strong pro-minority stance, are likely to reject racist and prejudicial beliefs, and sometimes will reject their own Whiteness in an effort to assuage the guilt felt in Stage 2. Students in this stage tend to have an intense interest in diverse cultural groups and are likely to have an increasing amount of contact with individuals from different cultures.
Stage 4: Pseudoindependence. Not comfortable with racism, these individuals have an intellectual acceptance and curiosity regarding individuals from nondominant groups. However, these individuals have not taken personal responsibility regarding their own racism and tend to see others as responsible for racism.	*Stage 4: Retreat to White Culture.* Students retreat into their own culture as they experience rejection from some individuals from nondominant groups. Intercultural contact is ended because they feel hostile toward and fearful of those from nondominant groups. The cozy home of the students' culture of origin is feeling quite safe at this point in time.
Stage 5: Immersion. Individuals in this stage have a need for more information about others and are eager to gain a deeper understanding of how they have been socialized to embrace racist attitudes. These individuals have a need to find a new and more compassionate definition of *White.*	*Stage 5: Redefinition and Integration.* Students develop a worldview of multiculturalism and are integrating it into their identity. They are able to feel good about their own identity and roots and also have a deep appreciation of the culture of others. Here, they are able to expend energy toward making deeply rooted structural changes in society.
Stage 6: Emersion. Here, the individuals reach out and embraces a new community of Whites that can move toward a deeper understanding of race and White identity.	
Stage 7: Autonomy. This person is cognitively complex, able to understand life from multiple perspectives, able to understand his or her White privilege, is humane and humanistic, and willing to fight all forms of racism and oppression. This person has a multicultural or multiracial transcendent worldview.	

Working with Diverse Clients in the Helping Relationship

Understanding our clients is certainly a critical first step in working with them, and that allows us to view them from a perspective that we may not have had before. However, after understanding our clients, it is critical that we have some ways to apply this understanding. Two ways of working with clients include using the *RESPECTFUL* acronym and applying the *Multicultural Counseling Competencies.*

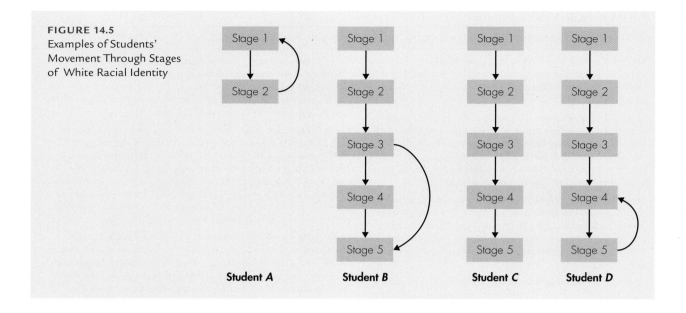

FIGURE 14.5
Examples of Students' Movement Through Stages of White Racial Identity

Using the RESPECTFUL Acronym

In Chapter 1, we suggested that one method of understanding clients is to address a number of areas, represented by the RESPECTFUL acronym. Feeling comfortable asking their clients about the following aspects of their lives makes it easier for the counselor to work effectively with the client.

R – religious/spiritual identity
E – economic class background
S – sexual identity
P – level of psychological development
E – ethnic/racial identity
C – chronological/developmental challenges
T – various forms of trauma and other threats to one's sense of well-being
F – family background and history
U – unique physical characteristics
L – location of residence and language differences

Lewis, Lewis, Daniels, & D'Andrea, p. 54

Using the Multicultural Counseling Competencies

In addition to the RESPECTFUL acronym, the *Association for Multicultural Counseling and Development (AMCD)*, ACA, and other counseling associations have endorsed the *Multicultural Counseling Competencies*. Discussed briefly earlier in the chapter, these competencies delineate attitudes and beliefs, knowledge, and skills in three areas: (1) counselor self-awareness of assumptions, values, and biases; (2) knowledge of the worldview of the culturally different client; and (3) familiarity with intervention strategies and techniques (Arredondo, 1999; Sue & Sue, 2013) (see Figure 14.2). Let's examine each of these next.

Attitudes and Beliefs

The effective cross-cultural counselor has an awareness of his or her own cultural background and has actively pursued gaining further awareness of his or her own biases, stereotypes, and values. Although the effective cross-cultural counselor may not hold the same belief system as his or her client, he or she can accept differing worldviews as presented by the helpee. In other words, differences are not viewed as pathological, or anything to be concerned about (Sue & Sue, 2013). Being sensitive to differences and tuned into his or her own cultural biases allows the effective cross-cultural counselor to refer a client from a nondominant group to a counselor of the client's own culture when a referral will benefit the helpee. Unfortunately, examples of how mental health professionals have failed clients who are culturally different from themselves as a result of their own biases and prejudices are common (Sue & Sue, 2013) (see Box 14.2).

Knowledge

The effective cross-cultural counselor has knowledge of the group from which the client comes and does not jump to conclusions about the client's ways of being. In addition, he or she shows a willingness to gain greater depth of knowledge of various cultural groups. This counselor is also aware of how sociopolitical issues, such as racism, sexism, and heterosexism, can negatively affect clients. In addition, this counselor knows how different theories of counseling carry values that may be detrimental for some clients in the counseling relationship. This counselor understands how institutional barriers can affect the willingness of clients from nondominant groups to use mental health services.

 BOX 14.2
Lack of Awareness of Own Biases and Prejudices

The following offers a few situations where a client's biases, prejudices, or insensitivities can lead to a rupture in the counselng relationship. Consider them, and if possible, discuss them in class:

1. The counselor who "jokingly" says to a client who is having trouble focusing, "I'll have to get you on some Ritalin." Although distasteful at any point, this statement is particularly inappropriate with this client, whose son is a child who struggles with a learning problem. The client ends up feeling as if the counselor is insensitive.
2. The counselor who encourages his client to be "more manly" so that he could have a more satisfying relationship with his wife. Meanwhile, the client secretly identifies as a female, and now he feels as if he cannot share this secret with his counselor.
3. The counselor who has pro-life or pro-choice literature in his or her office. When a woman comes in with a difficult pregnancy, this literature could make her feel like she cannot share her dilemma.
4. The atheistic counselor who dismisses her client's conflict between her religious beliefs and her same-sex attractions. Instead the counselor suggests the client change her religion. This, in effect, shuts down the client's desire to talk about her problem.
5. The counselor who has a client whose parent is in the last stages of hospice care and the client is considering on assisting his parent with suicide due to the pain she is in. The counselor says to the client, "I cannot discuss that, as it is against the law." This has the effect of ending the conversation and leaving the client feeling as if she has no one to talk to.

BOX 14.3

Lack of Knowledge: Blackbirds Sitting in a Tree

A White female elementary school teacher in the United States posed a math problem to her class one day. "Suppose there are four blackbirds sitting in a tree. You take a slingshot and shoot one of them. How many are left?" A White student answered quickly, "That's easy. One subtracted from four is three." An African immigrant youth then answered with equal confidence, "Zero." The teacher chuckled at the latter response and stated that the first student was right and that, perhaps, the second student should study more math. From that day forth, the African student seemed to withdraw from class activities and seldom spoke to other students or the teacher. . . .

If the teacher had pursued the African student's reasons for arriving at the answer zero, she might have heard the following: "If you shoot one bird, the others will fly away." Nigerian educators often use this story to illustrate differences in worldviews between United States and African cultures. The Nigerians contend that the group is more important than the individual, that survival of all depends on interrelationships among the parts. . . . (from Sue, 1992, pp. 7–8)

Unfortunately, lack of knowledge of a cultural group can cause counselors and others to jump to incorrect conclusions (see Box 14.3).

Skills

The cross-culturally effective counselor is able to apply, when appropriate, generic interviewing and counseling skills and also has knowledge of and is able to employ specialized skills. This counselor also has knowledge of and understands the verbal and nonverbal language of the client and can communicate effectively. In addition, the culturally skilled helper appreciates the importance of having a systemic perspective, such as an understanding of the impact of family and society on clients; being able to work collaboratively with community leaders, folk healers, and other professionals; and advocating for clients when necessary. What happens when a counselor does not have the appropriate skills when working with a culturally diverse client? Most likely, the client will drop out of counseling early, feel discouraged and dissatisfied with counseling, have little success in counseling, or a combination of all three (see Box 14.4).

BOX 14.4

Lack of Awareness of Skills

A female [Asian] client complained about all kinds of physical problems such as feeling dizzy, having a loss of appetite, an inability to complete household chores, and insomnia. She asked the therapist if her problem could be due to "nerves." The therapist suspected depression since these are some of the physical manifestations of the disorder and asked the client if she felt depressed and sad. At this point, the client paused and looked confused. She finally stated that she felt very ill and that these physical problems were making her sad. Her perspective was that it was natural for her to feel sad when sick. As the therapist followed up by attempting to determine if there was a family history of depression, the client displayed even more discomfort and defensiveness. Although the client never directly contradicted the therapist, she did not return for the following session. (Tsui & Schultz as cited in Sue & Sue, 2008, p. 366)

If this counselor had the appropriate knowledge and skills, he would have known that for Asian clients, the mind and body are inseparable, and physical complaints are a common and acceptable means of expressing emotional problems. An appropriate response to this client would have been to focus on the somatic complaints and suggest physical treatments prior to working on emotional problems. (Sue & Sue, 2008)

As you can see by the example in Box 14.4, there is a close connection between our beliefs about culturally diverse clients, our knowledge base regarding such clients, and our effective use of skills.

Multicultural/Social Justice Focus

Multicultural Counseling as the "Fourth Force"

> *Multiculturalism is not competing with humanism, behaviorism, or psycho-dynamic perspectives but rather demonstrates the importance of making the cultural context central to whichever psychological theory is being applied.*

> (Pedersen, Crethar, & Carlson, 2008, p. 223)

In 1996, Pius K. Essandoh wrote an article that raised the possibility that multicultural counseling could be representing a new paradigm in the counseling profession—a *fourth force*, following the first three forces in our profession: psychoanalysis, behaviorism, and humanistic psychology. Today, there is little doubt that his prediction was correct (Ratts, 2009). For instance, one study showed that between 1990 and 2001, 102 multicultural-centered articles were published in the *Journal of Counseling and Development* alone (Arredondo, Rosen, Rice, Perez, & Tovar-Gamero, 2005). And since that time, the rate of articles in this area has increased. Another study demonstrated that in the past twenty years, there have been 75 articles that researched the *multicultural counseling competencies* (Worthington, Soth-McNett, & Moreno, 2007). Also, one other study showed that there has been a large increase in the number of multicultural counseling outcome research articles (D'Andrea & Heckman, 2008b). In addition, texts and coursework on multicultural counseling have increased tremendously.

Despite these strides, many suggest that we are just at the beginning of this journey (e.g., Arredondo, Tovar-Blank, & Parham, 2008; Atkinson & Israel, 2003; D'Andrea & Heckman, 2008a). They advocate for better and more focused training, for research that more effectively examines the efficacy of different approaches to multicultural counseling, for counselors to look increasingly at their own resistance to working with clients of color, and for our profession to spend more time devising mechanisms that can highlight and reinforce this new paradigm. Clearly, we have come a long way, but we still have a way to go.

Social Justice and the Advocacy Competencies?

> *Social justice counseling includes empowerment of the individual as well as active confrontation of injustices and inequality in society because they affect clientele as well as those in their systemic contexts.*

> (Crethar, Rivera, & Nash, 2008, p. 270)

It used to be that multicultural counseling was solely focused on how to counsel diverse clients. However, it has become abundantly clear that being culturally competent includes

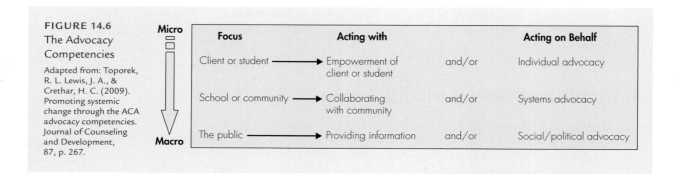

FIGURE 14.6
The Advocacy Competencies

Adapted from: Toporek, R. L. Lewis, J. A., & Crethar, H. C. (2009). Promoting systemic change through the ACA advocacy competencies. Journal of Counseling and Development, 87, p. 267.

advocating for your clients and for causes. As is evidenced by the recent *Advocacy Competencies* (Toporek, Lewis, & Crethar, 2009), counselors have a calling to periodically step out of the safety of their offices and work for systemic change—change that will help our clients in broad and significant ways, such as being a voice for our client when they are discriminated against or advocating for a law that will better the conditions of nondominant groups and those with mental health problems. Unfortunately, many of us are used to sitting around and letting others do the work. Next time you have a chance, don't just sit there—take a stand, do something, advocate, push for change.

The *Advocacy Competencies* are relatively new and encompass three areas of competence (client/student, school/community, and public arena), each of which are divided into two levels: whether the counselor is "acting with" the competency area or "acting on behalf" of the competency area (e.g., acting with the client to empower him or her to obtain needed services, or "acting on behalf" of the client to assist him or her in obtaining needed services) (see Figure 14.6). Some are suggesting that advocacy is so important we should call it the "fifth force" in counseling (Ratts, 2009).

Ethical, Professional, and Legal Issues

Standards and Multicultural Counseling

Increasingly, every standard, competency, and guideline within the counseling profession has increasingly addressed multicultural issues. Thus, whether it is the CACREP (2009) standards or the upcoming 2016 CACREP standards, the CPCE or NCC exam, or assessment standards (Neukrug & Fawcett, 2015; see Chapter 12), we increasingly see the infusion of multicultural issues interspersed within them. One standard that has made great strides in the infusion of multicultural issues is the ACA ethics code. In fact, the most recent ACA code of ethics (ACA, 2014a) finds cross-cultural issues addressed throughout (see Table 14.4). In addition to what is highlighted in Table 14.4, the code also discusses bartering, receiving gifts, being knowledgeable about appropriate referrals, issues related to the rights of parents and guardians, competence, being nondiscriminatory, reporting assessment results, and other topics (see Appendix A).

TABLE 14.4   Select Subsections That Address Diversity in the ACA 2014 Code

A. Counseling Relationship	**A.2.c. Developmental and Cultural Sensitivity.** Counselors communicate information in ways that are both developmentally and culturally appropriate. Counselors use clear and understandable language when discussing issues related to informed consent. When clients have difficulty understanding the language that counselors use, counselors provide necessary services (e.g., arranging for a qualified interpreter or translator) to ensure comprehension by clients. In collaboration with clients, counselors consider cultural implications of informed consent procedures and, where possible, counselors adjust their practices accordingly.
	A.4.b. Personal Values. Counselors are aware of—and avoid imposing—their own values, attitudes, beliefs, and behaviors. Counselors respect the diversity of clients, trainees, and research participants and seek training in areas in which they are at risk of imposing their values onto clients, especially when the counselor's values are inconsistent with the client's goals or are discriminatory in nature.
B. Confidentiality, Privileged Communication, and Privacy	**B.1.a. Multicultural/Diversity.** Counselors maintain awareness and sensitivity regarding cultural meanings of confidentiality and privacy. Counselors respect differing views toward disclosure of information. Counselors hold ongoing discussions with clients as to how, when, and with whom information is to be shared.
C. Professional Responsibility	**C.5. Nondiscrimination.** Counselors do not condone or engage in discrimination against prospective or current clients, students, employees, supervisees, or research participants based on age, culture, disability, ethnicity, race, religion/spirituality, gender, gender identity, sexual orientation, marital/partnership status, language preference, socioeconomic status, immigration status, or any basis proscribed by law.
E. Evaluation, Assessment, and Interpretation	**E.5.a. Proper Diagnosis.** Counselors take special care to provide proper diagnosis of mental disorders. Assessment techniques (including personal interview) used to determine client care (e.g., locus of treatment, type of treatment, or recommended follow-up) are carefully selected and appropriately used.
	E.5.b. Cultural Sensitivity. Counselors recognize that culture affects the manner in which clients' problems are defined and experienced. Clients' socioeconomic and cultural experiences are considered when diagnosing mental disorders.
	E.5.c. Historical and Social Prejudices in the Diagnosis of Pathology. Counselors recognize historical and social prejudices in the misdiagnosis and pathologizing of certain individuals and groups and strive to become aware of and address such biases in themselves or others.
	E.8. Multicultural Issues/Diversity in Assessment. Counselors use with caution assessment techniques normed on populations other than that of the client. Counselors recognize the effects of age, color, culture, disability, ethnic group, gender, race, language preference, religion, spirituality, sexual orientation, and socioeconomic status on test administration and interpretation, and they place test results in proper perspective with other relevant factors.
F. Supervision, Training, and Teaching	**F.2.b. Multicultural Issues/Diversity in Supervision.** Counseling supervisors are aware of and address the role of multiculturalism/diversity in the supervisory relationship.
	F.7.c. Infusing Multicultural Issues/Diversity. Counselor educators infuse material related to multiculturalism/diversity into all courses and workshops for the development of professional counselors.
	F.11.a. Faculty Diversity. Counselor educators are committed to recruiting and retaining a diverse faculty.
	F.11.b. Student Diversity. Counselor educators actively attempt to recruit and retain a diverse student body. Counselor educators demonstrate commitment to multicultural/diversity competence by recognizing and valuing the diverse cultures and types of abilities that students bring to the training experience. Counselor educators provide appropriate accommodations that enhance and support diverse student well-being and academic performance.
	F.11.c. Multicultural/Diversity Competence. Counselor educators actively infuse multicultural/diversity competency in their training and supervision practices. They actively train students to gain awareness, knowledge, and skills in the competencies of multicultural practice.
	F.11.c. Multicultural/Diversity Competence. Counselor educators actively infuse multicultural/diversity competency in their training and supervision practices. They actively train students to gain awareness, knowledge, and skills in the competencies of multicultural practice.
H. Distance Counseling, Technology, and Social Media	**H.5.d. Multicultural and Disability Considerations.** Counselors who maintain websites provide accessibility to persons with disabilities. They provide translation capabilities for clients who have a different primary language, when feasible. Counselors acknowledge the imperfect nature of such translations and accessibilities.

SOURCE: American Counseling Association. *ACA code of ethics*. Retrieved from http://www.counseling.org/docs/ethics/2014-aca-code-of-ethics.pdf?sfvrsn=4.

Infusion of Multicultural Counseling into Training Programs

As CACREP has required programs to address Social and Cultural Issues within their curriculum, most counselor training programs now offer a separate course on cross-cultural counseling, weave multicultural perspectives throughout their counseling program, or both (Arthur & Achenbach, 2002). This emphasis in training has led to a number of interesting ways for students to become increasingly culturally competent. For instance, one method commonly used by faculty is to have students participate in an immersion activity that allows them time to experience and reflect on another culture (e.g., spend a few weeks attending an all-Black church) (DeRicco & Sciarra, 2005; Hipolito-Delgado, Cook, Avrus, & Boham, 2011).

The *triad model* (Pedersen 2001; Seto, Young, Becker, & Kiselica, 2006) has the client, the counselor, an *anticounselor*, and a *procounselor* all meet together during an interview. The procounselor and anticounselor give continual and immediate positive as well as critical feedback to the counselor in an effort to increase the counselor's ability to understand the client's perspective, recognize client resistance, recognize the counselor's defensiveness, and learn how to recover from mistakes that the counselor might make during the interview.

Ancis and Marshall (2010) suggest that during field placements, supervisors could potentially discuss the impact that a counselor's culture has on relationships with clients, provide a respectful and safe environment for counselors to discuss cross-cultural issues, and develop a relationship of interpersonal depth that can enable discussions of power dynamics in the supervisory relationships.

No doubt there are dozens of activities that can be introduced into a program to enhance cross-cultural competence. As you go through your program, consider the kinds of activities that you are being asked to participate in and reflect on whether you think they have increased your knowledge of clients from cultures different from your own.

Association for Multicultural Counseling and Development

In an effort to supply leadership for helping professionals in the area of multicultural counseling, the *Association for Multicultural Counseling and Development (AMCD)*, a division of ACA, provides workshops, graduate program training standards in multicultural counseling, and publications, such as the *Journal of Multicultural Counseling and Development*. If you have a particular interest in multicultural counseling, training, and research, you might consider joining AMCD (go to www.multiculturalcounseling .org/).

Knowledge of Legal Trends

In just about every chapter of this textbook, you will find mention of some legislative initiative that addresses multicultural concerns, and every year, new laws are passed and old ones are amended. Counselors need to have intimate knowledge of the law and how it affects the clients from nondominant groups if they are to (1) assist the client in advocating for his or her rights; (2) be an advocate for the client; (3) campaign for legislative initiatives on the local, state, and national levels; and (4) protect themselves from potential malpractice suits.

The Counselor in Process: Working with Culturally Different Clients

Becoming expert in the attitudes and beliefs, knowledge, and skills about clients from cultures of which we have had little contact does not occur overnight—not even when we have finished our counseling program. It is an active and ongoing process that occurs throughout our careers. If it is to occur at all, however, we must be open to learning about others and to discussing differences among ourselves and others; by actively putting ourselves in situations conducive to it, we can absorb knowledge about other cultures. No one is expecting you to suddenly be expert on all cultures. However, faculty members and clients alike expect you to be open to learning about other people's backgrounds and histories, and they are hoping that you have, or will develop, an attitude of humility and curiosity when it comes to increasing your cross-cultural competence.

Summary

This chapter reviewed theoretical and conceptual issues related to multicultural counseling. We started by noting that there is not one hard-and-fast definition of multicultural counseling. We first suggested one definition that stated that multicultural counseling is a consistent readiness to identify the cultural dimensios of clients' lives and a subsequent integration of culture into counseling.work. A second definition suggest that multicultural counseling encompasses a client's individual, group, and universal identities. With this definition in mind, we stated that the counselor should take into account individualism and collectivism in making assessment, diagnosis, and treatment decisions. This definition also highlighted the importance of culture specific and universal techniques in reaching client goals. We then pointed out that Multicultural Counseling Competencies have been developed by the profession to help in the training of counselors, and that such training is often focused on attitudes and beliefs, knowledge, and skills in three areas: (1) counselor self-awareness of assumptions, values, and biases; (2) knowledge of the worldview of the culturally different client; and (3) familiarity with intervention strategies and techniques.

We next discussed some of the reasons why multicultural counseling has become so important. We first pointed out the fact that we live in the most diverse country in the world and offered some statistics highlighting this fact. Despite being a multicultural nation (or perhaps because of it), we noted that many clients from nondominant groups are misdiagnosed, dissatisfied with counseling, and drop out of counseling at high rates. We then noted why nondominant clients sometimes have been poorly served by counselors, including the fact that some counselors (1) view this country as a melting pot instead of a cultural mosaic, (2) have incongruent expectations about counseling, (3) deemphasize social forces, (4) have an ethnocentric worldview, (5) are ignorant of their own prejudices, (6) are unable to understand that the expression of symptomatology is often a function of culture, (7) misjudge the accuracy of assessment and research instruments, and (8) are unaware of how institutional racism affects the counseling process.

In an effort to give us common ground on which to communicate, a number of words and terms were defined in this chapter. Thus, we defined culture, discrimination, microaggressions, ethnicity, minority, nondominant group, power differentials, race, religion, spirituality, sexism, heterosexism, sexual prejudice, sexual orientation, social class (or just class), prejudice, and racism. We also discussed words and terms that are generally used to describe various cultural groups in the United States.

In this chapter, a number of conceptual models were described, which were designed to help us better understand our work with clients from diverse backgrounds. We first briefly described the existential model of identity, which includes understanding our client in four realms: *Eigenwelt*, our psychological world; *Mitwelt*, our common experiences; *Umwelt*, our experience of the world around us; and *Überwelt*, our spiritual self. Next, we described the tripartite model of personal identity, which suggests that we understand our clients in three spheres: the Individual Level, which represents the client's uniqueness; the Group Level, which is related to aspects of the person that can vary based on the cultural and ethnic groups to which the client belongs; and the Universal Level, which is related to common experiences (e.g., physical similarities, life experiences, and self-awareness).

Offering a developmental perspective, we suggested that a number of models have been developed to help us understand how individuals from different ethnic/cultural groups come to understand their ethnic identity development. This can help counselors gain increased empathy for their clients and also help them understand their own development. First, we presented McAuliffe's Racial Identity Development for People of Color (RIDPOC) model, which offers a five-stage structure of racial/cultural development, including conformity, dissonance and beginning appreciation, resistance and immersion, introspection and internalization, and universal inclusion. We then highlighted two models of White identity. Helms's model includes the following stages: contact, disintegration, reintegration, pseudoindependence, immersion, emersion, and autonomy. Sabnani et al. focus on stages that White graduate students might typically pass through during graduate school. The stages in this model include pre-exposure, exposure, prominority/antiracism, retreat to White culture, and redefinition and integration.

As the chapter continued, we looked at how the RESPECTFUL acronym and the Multicultural Counseling Competencies are both important to our ability to work effectively with clients from diverse backgrounds. Relative to the competencies, we highlighted how culturally competent counselors have (1) an awareness of their assumptions, values, and biases, (2) the knowledge needed about their clients' culture so that they can better understand their clients, and (3) a repertoire of skills or tools that can be effectively applied to clients from diverse backgrounds.

Focusing on multicultural and social justice issues, we noted that multicultural counseling has become the "fourth force" in the counseling profession, following psychoanalysis, behaviorism, and humanistic psychology; and that some are suggesting that advocacy be called the "fifth force." We pointed out that even though great progress has been made, we still have a way to go in the training of culturally competent counselors. We also noted that today, multicultural counseling includes social justice action, and that counselors must advocate for clients if it seems like such advocacy would benefit the client. We showed how the Advocacy Competencies could help in this effort.

Relative to ethical, professional, and legal issues, we noted that standards in counseling, such as CACREP standards, the NCC and CPCE exams, and assessment standards, have increasingly infused multicultural issues. We then particularly took note of the changes in the ACA ethics code and highlighted some parts of the code that speak to multicultural issues and multicultural counseling.

We then went on to note that today, most counseling programs offer a separate course on social and cultural issues and also infuse multicultural issues into most of their classes. We discussed how many programs require an immersion activity to help students understand individuals from diverse backgrounds, and we highlighted Pedersen's triad model and the importance of supervisors addressing multicultural issues in the supervisory relationship.

As the chapter neared its conclusion, we highlighted the Association of Muliticultural Counseling and Development (AMCD), which is a division of ACA, and noted that counselors should have intimate knowledge of how laws differentially affect clients from nondominant groups. We concluded the chapter by acknowledging that becoming culturally competent does not happen overnight—it's a lifelong process that counselors should approach with humility and curiosity.

Further Practice

Visit CengageBrain.com to respond to additional material that highlight the salient aspects of the chapter content. There, you can find ethical, professional, and legal vignettes, a number of experiential exercises, and study tools including a glossary, flashcards, and sample test items. Hopefully, these will enhance your learning and be fun and interesting.

I've learned that people will forget what you said, people will forget what you did, but people will never forget how you made them feel.

—Maya Angelou

Within our borders, there are a large number of cultural/ethnic groups, each with its own unique story. Each story reflects the group's identity and offers us a picture of how it has been assimilated into the broader culture that we call the United States. For instance, when originally writing this chapter, I was astounded and ashamed by the number of slaves who died coming over to this country and how Japanese people were interned in the United States during World War II. I was reminded of the strong nationalism felt by many Latinos/Latinas and of the uniqueness of each American Indian tribe. I realized that most gays do not live a "gay and lesbian lifestyle," and that there are some very distinct skills one may want to consider when counseling women and when counseling men. I was taken aback by the number of hate crimes that continue to be perpetrated against nondominant groups, and I was reminded of the many, many different religions across this land, each of which holds deeply different beliefs. Finally, I found that each of us has special needs that can be addressed in the counseling relationship if the counselor wants to take the time to find out what those needs are.

Although we should not assume that a person from a nondominant group necessarily shares the perceived characteristics of that group, we should realize that knowledge about different groups could assist us in understanding individuals who share a common story. The fact is that most of us are blind to the history and cultural values of many of the cultural/ethnic groups outside our own sphere. Therefore, this chapter is designed to give you a taste of the history and culture of some diverse groups, while stimulating your interest in multicultural counseling. We cannot touch on all diversity in the United States, for that would require much more than one chapter. However, we can spend a little time focusing on some of the groups of people that have been most obviously discriminated against. Finally, by noting special issues and identifying counseling strategies unique to the groups identified, we will attempt to offer you ways in which you can optimally work with clients from diverse groups.

After discussing a number of cultural/ethnic groups, we will examine the debate in the profession concerning whether one need be knowledgeable about all cultures when doing counseling. Near the end of the chapter, we will discuss the ethical code of the American Counseling Association (ACA), its relevance to cross-cultural counseling, and ethical decision making from a cross-cultural perspective. We will conclude the chapter by considering the future of cross-cultural counseling. But first, let's look at just how diverse we are!

The Changing Face of America

The United States is the most diverse country in the world and is becoming increasingly more so. In fact, today, well over one-third of Americans are racial and ethnic minorities, and nondominant groups are expected to become the majority by the year 2043 (U.S. Census Bureau, 2014a). In fifty years, the makeup of the United States will be quite different than it is today (see Figure 15.1).

The changing demographics highlighted in Figure 15.1 are a function of a number of factors, including higher birth rates of culturally diverse populations, the fact that most immigrants no longer come from Western countries, and immigration rates that are the largest in U.S. history. Of legal immigrants today, 48% are White, 46% have Hispanic or Latino/Latina roots, 25% are Asian, 9% are Black, 16% report some other race, and 2% percent report being of two or more races. In recent years, the great majority of immigrants have been Latin American (53.6%) and Asian (26.8%) (Migration Policy Institute, 2014). Today's immigrants have a tendency to want to assert their cultural heritage rather than be swallowed up by the Western-based American culture. To a large degree, this has always been the case, as Italian Americans, Irish Americans, Jewish Americans, German Americans, and others all developed their own communities and maintained their unique heritages when they first came to this country. After all, there is some sense of safety when you live with those who are familiar in a new, yet strange land.

Changes in the racial, ethnic, and cultural makeup of Americans bring with them changes in the religious composition of the country. As increasing numbers of Asians, Latinos/Latinas, and people from the Middle East arrive at our shores, we will more frequently encounter religions that were previously rare in this country. But diversity in religion is not only brought to us by our immigrants. Although the United States is a country that is largely Christian, diversity within Christianity is now greater than ever. From a multitude of generic and mainline Christian faiths, to Roman Catholics who are

FIGURE 15.1

Changes in Population by Race/Cultural Background

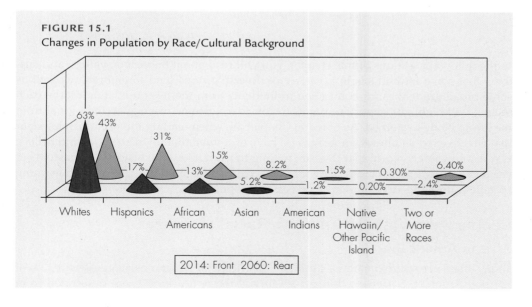

increasingly varied in their beliefs, to Eastern Orthodox members, Mormons, Christian Scientists, Seventh-day Adventists, Amish, Mennonites, and on and on. Christian religion in the United States is a religious mosaic in and of itself.

In addition to the changing ethnic, cultural, and religious diversity in the United States, today there are also changes in sex-role identity. The macho male is no longer considered the model for maleness, while expectations concerning the role of women in the workplace and as childcare providers have changed dramatically. Also, in the United States today, we see increased awareness and increased acceptance of sexual minorities, such as those who are gay, lesbian, bisexual, and transgender. Whereas in the past, many individuals felt a need to hide their sexual preference for fear of discrimination, today an increasing number of gays, lesbians, and bisexuals feel comfortable being open about their sexual orientation. In addition, changes in federal, state, and local laws, as well as a gradual move toward more tolerance of differences, have given us an increased sensitivity to and awareness of a number of groups, including individuals who are HIV positive, the homeless and the poor, older persons, individuals with mentally disorders, people who are physically challenged, and others. Let's spend a little time examining each of these groups.

Understanding and Counseling Select Culturally Diverse Groups

> *Imagine a future in which all girls and boys are able and encouraged to form an identity free of sexist, racist, classist, ableist, and heterosexist prejudices and expectations; in which all girls and boys are equally supported to explore their emotional, relational, spiritual, cultural, intellectual, and vocational needs, talents, and capacities, and a future in which girls and boys, women and men, feel safe and free from exploitation, violence, and victimization and are encouraged to thrive within environments of mutual support and encouragement.*
>
> (Kees et al., 2005, p. 381)

In the following sections of this chapter, you will read about behaviors, values, and customs that some individuals in a variety of diverse groups tend to embrace, as well as some broad guidelines for counseling individuals from these groups. In addition, each section will highlight important points to consider when counseling an individual from the group being examined. As noted in Chapter 14, when reading this section, remember that effective cross-cultural counselors (1) have examined their own attitudes and beliefs; (2) are knowledgeable, in that they are willing to learn about the history and customs of various groups; and (3) are facile with many counseling skills and are open to learning specific counseling skills applicable to varying populations.

People from Varying Cultural/Racial Heritages

African Americans

Today, there are approximately 42 million Americans of African heritage—about 13% of the population (U.S. Census Bureau, 2014b). Of these, nearly 90% are descended from slaves. Conditions in the ships that brought the slaves were deplorable, and it is estimated that 6 to 10 million Africans died during the passage (Allen & Turner, 1988). By 1790, 19% of the U.S. population was of African heritage, with this percentage dropping after slave trading was made illegal in 1809. By 1860, 90% of African Americans lived in the South and tended to remain there following the Civil War, becoming sharecroppers or working for White farmers. Restrictive work laws and lack of education made it difficult for Blacks to leave the South, and it wasn't until the early 1900s that they began to move to urban centers in the North, where there were hopes of better educational and career opportunities and freedom from increasing violence toward Blacks in the South. More recently, however, there has been a reversal of this trend, with better-educated Blacks moving to the South to obtain higher-level jobs.

It was not until the *1964 Civil Rights Act* that we finally saw an end to some of the more overt discrimination in the United States, including the remnants of *Jim Crow laws*, which promulgated "separate but equal" status for African Americans in the United States (Evans, 2013). These laws, which usually resulted in separate but *unequal* conditions, seemed like a far cry from the underlying moral principles for which our country stood. Despite the passage of the Civil Rights Act and the repeal of the Jim Crow laws, other laws restricting access to education, work, and recreational facilities and generally supporting segregation continued in some states until the early 1970s. With racism and prejudice being endemic throughout American society, it was necessary in 1991 to pass an extension of the *Civil Rights Act* to protect minority workers, particularly African Americans, from discriminatory practices in employment. There is no question that African Americans have been particularly oppressed in this country—and we are all still paying the price for this oppression.

Today, African Americans continue to be confronted with discrimination, as is apparent when we realize that 46% hate crimes are due to race, and that a large portion of these are perpetrated against African Americans (U.S. Department of Justice, 2014). However, most racism, prejudice, and discrimination against African Americans today manifests itself in much more subtle, covert, and unconscious ways (e.g., microaggressions). Although, a large number of African Americans have now assimilated into the middle class, more subtle forms of oppression are responsible for a large underclass of African Americans who continue to have little opportunity for upward mobility in American society (Evans, 2013). We must all take responsibility for the continued oppression and discrimination against African Americans in today's society and work collectively to end it.

Perhaps more than any other cultural group, African Americans' values are differentially affected as a function of their social class, experiences with racism and other forms of oppression, and the degree to which they have been exposed to African heritage. However, some commonalities may exist among many African Americans. Generally, African Americans are group-oriented and value cooperation and interdependence, especially in relation to the extended family and the community (Sue & Sue, 2013). The extended family can be varied and is particularly important, and family matters tend to be kept within the family or extended family (Blackburne, 2011; McGoldrick, 2005). In addition, African Americans as a group tend to value their churches more than other cultural groups, and counselors should understand why some African Americans may more readily seek counseling from a pastor than a mental health counselor (American Psychiatric Association, 2014b; Evans, 2013; Williams, 2013).

Relative to counseling, exposure to discrimination and racism may justifiably make some African Americans guarded, defensive, and minimally verbal with White counselors and mistrustful of the mental health system (American Psychiatric Association, 2014b; Evans, 2013). Perhaps it is not surprising that African Americans are more likely to use mental health services less frequently, drop out of treatment early, and be misdiagnosed more often than Whites. Finally, African Americans vary widely in their connectedness to their roots, and counselors must assess the role that cultural background plays in seeking mental health treatment and when working with an African American client (Williams, 2013).

Latinos/Latinas/Hispanics: People of Central American, South American, and Caribbean Origin

Collectively, people of Central America, South America, and from various islands in the Caribbean are called *Hispanic* or *Latinos/Latinas*. Today, there are over 53 million (16%) Latinos/Latinas in the United States, 65% of whom have their origins from Mexico, 9.4% from Puerto Rico, 3.8% from El Salvador, 3.6% from Cuba, 3.0%, from the Dominican Republic, 2.3% from Guatemala, and the rest from the remaining Hispanic/Latina/Latino countries (U.S. Census Bureau, 2013). Although *Hispanic* is the official word used by the U. S. government, some have felt that it has been too closely associated with colonial heritage and prefer the word *Latino* or *Latina* (Delgado-Romero, Nevels, & Capielo, 2013). In addition, when counseling Latinos/Latinas, it is best to have knowledge of the client's country of origin or ancestry, as most would culturally identify with their country of heritage in contrast to the broader culture that the word *Hispanic* implies (Casas, Raley, & Vasquez, 2015).

Because much of California was a northern province of Mexico, a large number of Mexicans became citizens of California when it achieved statehood in 1850 (Allen & Turner, 1988). Other Mexican Americans first emigrated here in the mid-1800s, traveling north from Mexico to the Southwest and West in search of gold in California, good grazing land for cattle, and economic prosperity. A second wave of Mexican immigrants arrived here in the late 1800s and early 1900s, with many moving to California. Today, over 50% of the Mexican American population of the United States lives in California.

Most Puerto Ricans settled in the United States during the twentieth century. In 1898, following the Spanish-American War, Puerto Rico became a territory of the United States. In 1917, Puerto Ricans were given citizenship, and in 1952, Puerto Rico became a commonwealth of the United States. Over the years, many Puerto Ricans have moved to New York City, where there were hopes of a better life, and more recently, there has been a large migration of Puerto Ricans west in search of better employment opportunities. Although Puerto Rico has one of the best economies of Latin America, it lags far behind the economy in the 50 states.

Most Cubans came to the United States in the late 1950s and early 1960s following Fidel Castro's overthrow of the Cuban dictatorship of Fulgencio Batista. Cubans came to the United States out of fear of persecution and imprisonment and out of ideological differences with the communist regime. The vast majority of Cubans settled in southern Florida, although there are sizable communities in New York, Chicago, and Los Angeles.

In the United States today, there is a sizable group of Americans of Spanish descent who arrived here from Central and South America. Many of these people settled along the Rio Grande, although during the 1800s, many migrated to New Mexico, Arizona, and Colorado. Finally, due to political turmoil in their countries of origin, many people from Central America have migrated to the United States between the 1960s and now.

Although a sizable number of Latinos/Latinas have done well in the United States, there continues to be a disproportionate number of Latinos/Latinas who are poor and have had a difficult time acculturating. A number of reasons account for this. For instance, many Latinos/Latinas have not established roots in this country due to the proximity of their countries of origin, the lack of economic opportunity today compared to what was available to past immigrants, the ability to make frequent trips back to their countries of origin, and the fact that sharing a common language with other Hispanics makes it easier to maintain a Latino/Latina culture (Axelson, 1999).

Despite many differences, there are certain values and customs that are shared by most Latinos/Latinas. For instance, the extended family is emphasized and interdependence is valued over independence. Also, the family tends to be patriarchal and follow traditional sex roles. In addition, in Latino/Latina culture, individuals are respected based on their age, socioeconomic status, gender, and perception of the individual's importance. Finally, many Latinos/Latinas deeply embrace traditional Catholic values while at the same time believing in *cultural fatalism* (*fatalismo*), or the belief that life is out of one's control (Delgado-Romero et al., 2013; Sue & Sue, 2013).

When working with Latino/Latina clients, it is crucial that the counselor understands the client's unique values, behaviors, symbols, and even language, all of which are functions of the client's country of origin. At the same time, the counselor should assess the degree to which some of the common qualities may motivate the Latino/Latina client.

People of Asian and Pacific Island Origin

Americans of Asian and Pacific Island origin include fairly large numbers of Chinese, Filipinos, Japanese, Koreans, Asian Indians, Vietnamese, and native Hawaiians, and smaller numbers of Laotian, Thai, Samoans, and Guamanians. In 1965, major changes in immigration laws created more equity in who could immigrate to the United States and resulted in an increase in Asian and Pacific Island immigrants from almost 50 countries and ethnic groups from this area of the world (U.S. Environmental Protection Agency, 2011).

To escape poverty, many Chinese people immigrated to the United States during the California gold rush of the mid-1800s. However, Whites ousted many Chinese people from the mines, and a large number ended up taking low-paying farm and blue-collar jobs. Because of prejudice and poor working conditions, many Chinese people dispersed to Midwestern and Eastern cities. In addition, the development of Chinatowns represented a haven for many of the Chinese. Today, many Chinese people have moved out of the Chinatowns, and these areas now generally house the poorer Chinese.

In the late 1800s, a large number of Japanese, Asian Indians, and Koreans settled in California, and like the Chinese, took low-paying farm jobs. During World War II, almost 120,000 West Coast Japanese Americans (70,000 of which were U.S. citizens) were forcibly removed from their homes and placed in internment camps. California, Oregon, and

Washington were deemed more vulnerable to attack by the Japanese, and some believed that those of Japanese descent would be loyal to Japan if these parts of the country were attacked (and may even be working to help that happen). In 1943, some of the Japanese who were interned were able to leave the camps if they promised not to live on the West Coast. Many moved to the Midwest, while others chose to remain in the camps until the end of the war, when they were allowed to resettle on the West Coast. Realizing the racism behind the forced encampment, in 1988, President Ronald Reagan signed the Civil Liberties Act, which formally apologized for the internments and paid $20,000 to the Japanese Americans who were placed in internment camps, or their heirs.

When the Spanish-American War ended in 1898, the United States set up colonial rule in the Philippines. Although this takeover of the Philippines was not met calmly by the Filipino people, it did lead to a large influx of Filipinos to this country. Many went to Hawaii and worked as sugar growers. In the 1920s and 1930s, many Filipinos moved to California and Alaska, some to take low-paying jobs and others to pursue an education. In addition, until recently, Filipinos who enlisted in the U.S. armed services for a specified length of time could obtain citizenship, and many therefore relocated to naval cities such as San Diego, California, and Norfolk, Virginia.

Following the wars in Korea and Vietnam, large numbers of Koreans and Vietnamese people immigrated to this country. A sizable number of Korean immigrants were war brides, war orphans, and professionals, whereas many Vietnamese immigrants were refugees from the Vietnam War and were brought to this country following the fall of South Vietnam to the North Vietnamese.

Although some general customs are shared among people of Asian and Pacific Island origin, as with Hispanics, there is great variability in the customs and traditions among the varying countries. A few of the similar values include the fact that children tend to be obligated to parents and place them first; family members are highly interdependent; families are generally patriarchal and sons are highly valued; guilt and shame are used to control the behavior of family members; individuals are restrained and pride themselves on their ability to control their feelings; there is formality in social relationships; the mind and body are seen as one; emotional distress should be handled on one's own; the needs of others should be placed above one's own; and physical complaints are often an accepted way of expressing psychological problems (Kim & Park, 2013; Sue & Sue, 2013).

When working with an Asian client, it is important to have knowledge about the client's country of origin. Differences in language, social behavior, economic development, and history are vast and should not be underestimated because they greatly affect the Asian client's way of living in the world. On the other hand, a counselor should also assess the degree to which some common qualities, as noted above, may be embraced by the Asian client.

Native Americans

In the United States, Native Americans consist of two major groups: American Indians and Alaskan Natives. About 5.2 million (1.6%) Americans report being Native American. Of these, 3.8 million (1.2%) report being only Native American, while the rest report being Native American and one other race (U.S. Census Bureau, 2009a, 2014b). Of these, most report being from one or more of ten American Indian tribes, while another 120,000 are Alaskan Native (U.S. Census Bureau, 2006). These groups have dramatically different histories and cultural values and should not be confused with one another.

Approximately 10,000 years ago, people from Siberia crossed over the Bering Strait land bridge to what is now Alaska. Some of these people headed westward toward the Aleutian Islands and are now called *Aleuts,* whereas others headed north and east and are now called *Inuits* (Eskimos). Alaska, which was owned by Russia, sent Russian Orthodox missionaries to bring Christianity to Alaskan Natives. Today, there are approximately 57,000 Inuit (Eskimo), 23,000 Tlingit-Haida, 22,000 Alaska Athabascan, and 18,000 Aleut (U.S. Census Bureau, 2006).

Prior to the colonization of North America, American Indians were numerous, with estimates ranging between 1 and 18 million (Thornton, 1996). However, due to disease brought by the Europeans and the wars they initiated, a large percentage died or were killed. Today, six tribes account for about 40% of the close to 5 million Americans who identify as American Indians: mostly Cherokee, Navajo, Latin American Indian, Choctaw, Sioux, and Chippewa. Although American Indians are a diverse group, as is evidenced by the fact that they speak a total of 252 languages, there are many commonalities among tribes (Garrett, 2004):

> . . . a prevailing sense of "Indianness" based on common worldview and common history seems to bind Native Americans together as a people of many peoples. Although acculturation plays a major factor in Native American worldview, there tends to be a high degree of psychological homogeneity, that is, a certain degree of shared cultural standards and meanings based on common core values . . . (p. 148)

Approximately 22% of American Indians live on reservations where living conditions are not good, and social problems, which can be traced to the uprooting of their civilization, are severe (Garrett, 2004). Social problems include high rates of poverty, unemployment, suicide, and substance abuse; poor health care; malnutrition; shortened life expectancy; and limited educational opportunities (Herring, 2004). American Indians also have higher rates of emotional illness, most likely related to their serious social problems. Unfortunately, American Indians tend to underutilize available mental health services.

Although many Native Americans have acculturated to broader societal customs, some of their traditional values include humility, generosity, patience, living by the clock of Mother Nature, "being" or living with the flow of life energy and connectedness to others, and spirituality (harmony, connection, and listening to one's life rhythm) (Garrett et al., 2013). American Indians tend to view mental health problems from a spiritual and holistic perspective (Garrett, 2004; Juntunen & Morin, 2004). Such problems are seen as an extension of the community, and thus the community is often actively involved in the healing process. In this process, the use of ceremony, storytelling, and metaphor are important for understanding the individual.

As with Latinos/Latinas and Asians, it is important to understand the unique language and cultural traditions of the tribe with which the Native American has been affiliated (Rayle, Chee, & Sand, 2006). In addition, as many Native Americans have acculturated, it is important when counseling Native Americans to assess how much their culture of origin continues to influence their lives.

Counseling Individuals from Different Cultures

As you can tell from the preceding sections, traditions and values vary considerably as a function of cultural group, and even within cultural groups. Thus, it is difficult to ascribe one specific approach to working with a broad range of groups such as these. However, there are some common ingredients that we can take into account when working with African Americans, Asian Americans, Latinos/Latinas, and Native Americans:

1. *Have the right attitudes and beliefs, gain knowledge, and learn skills.* Be prepared to work with clients with varying cultural heritages by embracing the appropriate knowledge, skills, and beliefs prior to meeting with them.
2. *Encourage clients to speak their own language.* Make an effort to know meaningful expressions of the client's language. When language becomes a significant barrier, refer the client to a counselor who speaks the client's language.
3. *Assess the cultural identity of the client.* Use the racial/cultural identity models in Chapter 14 to assist you in knowing how to work with clients. For example, a client who has acculturated and has little identification with his or her culture of origin is very different from a client from the same culture of origin who is a new immigrant.
4. *Check the accuracy of your interpretation of the client's nonverbals.* Don't assume that nonverbal communication is consistent across cultures. Ask the client about his or her nonverbals when in doubt.
5. *Use alternative modes of communication.* Use appropriate nonstandard forms of communication, such as acting, drawing, music, storytelling, collage making, etc., to draw out clients who are reticent to talk or have communication problems.
6. *Assess the impact of sociopolitical issues on the client.* Examine how social and political issues affect your client and decide whether advocacy of client concerns can be helpful to the client's present problems.
7. *Encourage clients to show you culturally significant and personally relevant items.* Have clients bring items to sessions (e.g., books, photographs, articles of significance, culturally meaningful items, and the like) to help you to better understand them and their culture.
8. *Vary the helping environment.* When appropriate, explore alternative environments to ease the client into the helping relationship (e.g., take a walk, have a cup of coffee at a quiet restaurant, initially meet your client at his or her home, and so forth).

Religious and Spiritual Diversity in the United States

The United States continues to be a highly religious country, with 92% of Americans stating they believe in God and 78% identifying as Christian (see Chapter 14, Table 14.1) (Newport, 2011). Despite the fact that there has been an increase in the numbers of individuals who state that religion is not very important to them (19% today, compared to 5% in 1952), religion remains a critical piece of the fabric of U.S. society. Although most Americans who affiliate with a religious group today are Christian, there are a wide variety of Christian sects. In addition, there are increasing numbers of other religions (e.g., Buddhist, Hindu, Muslim) in the United States today, partly as the result of changing immigration patterns. With 8 out of 10 Americans saying that religion is a fairly or very important aspect of their lives, it is clear that counselors must understand the diversity of religious beliefs in this country.

As one might expect, there is a relationship between religious affiliation and social class, culture, ethnicity, race, and political attitudes (Macionis, 2014), although one should be careful not to stereotype a person too readily based on his or her religious affiliation. Religion can be divisive, such as when wars are started over sectarian differences and individuals are oppressed because of their religious beliefs. However, for many within a specific cultural group, religion can be a unifying factor and offer a sense of community, direction, and strength (Eriksen, Jackson, Weld, & Lester, 2013). In addition, religion has offered answers to questions about life's meaning and has been an important factor in focusing world attention on the importance of assisting those in need. In this spirit, many counseling theorists believed that religions fashioned God, and God's image, to be the perfect reflection of what we all should strive for in life (Neukrug, 2011).

Although religion and spirituality are often used synonymously, Eriksen et al. (2013) suggest that religion is "the organized set of beliefs that encode a person or group's attitudes toward, and understanding of, the essence or nature of reality" (p. 456), while spirituality is "mindfulness about the existential qualities of life, especially the relationship among self, other, and the world" (p. 457). With the great diversity of religious and spiritual beliefs in this country, and knowing that religious affiliation is closely aligned with cultural factors, it is a sad statement that in many texts and articles on multicultural counseling, religion and spirituality have been given little or no mention. With this in mind, we will briefly examine five religions (covered in alphabetical order) and then offer general guidelines when counseling individuals with strongly held religious and spiritual beliefs.

Christianity

Founded 2,000 years ago on the teachings of Jesus of Nazareth, adherents of Christianity now include close to 2 billion people (approximately 33% of the world's population). Starting as a Judaic movement, followers of Jesus believed him to be the Christ, "the chosen one," fulfilling God's promise of salvation. Although Judaism eventually rejected Jesus as the Christ/Messiah, Christianity was born, and the teachings of Jesus were consolidated into what we now call the "New Testament" or "Christian Scriptures." Over the centuries, interpretation of the Gospel (the "good news" of Jesus) by religious scholars and leaders has varied greatly. Thus, throughout the world, we have seen the development of many different Christian religious groups that have ranged from conservative to liberal in their interpretations of the Gospel. Differences among Christians' values and beliefs can vary dramatically with respect to a number of core issues that may affect the counseling relationship, such as beliefs around marriage and divorce, sexuality, abortion and birth control, views on counseling, and spiritual practices (Eriksen et al., 2013). Therefore, some understanding of a person's particular religious background and spiritual orientation is important when counseling individuals who hold strong Christian beliefs.

Finally, differences among Christian churches and between Christian religions and non-Christian religions have led to tensions among people throughout the world. On the other hand, Christianity has also brought people together in a common worship of Jesus as part and whole of the Holy Trinity, along with God the Father and the Holy Spirit. And, based on Christian beliefs, many Christian churches have understood their mission to include helping others by housing the poor, counseling the weary, feeding the hungry, and bringing unity among people.

Buddhism

Founded in the sixth century BCE in India, Buddhism is based on the Tripaka, which are teachings of Gautama Siddhartha, who, after becoming enlightened, became known as the Buddha. Also of significance in Buddhism are comments about the Buddha's writings, called the sutras. Four truths of Buddhism include (1) the truth of suffering; (2) the cause of suffering, which is desire; (3) the cessation of suffering, which is the renunciation of desire; and (4) the way that leads to the cessation of suffering (Tsering, 2005). Related to these truths, Buddhists believe that what we understand to be reality is an illusion, that one lives and is reborn due to attachment to an illusory self, and that nirvana is reached when, through meditation, you can transcend attachment to the illusory self. The actual practice of Buddhism varies greatly depending on the sect to which the person belongs. Although Buddhists represent 6% of the world's population, in American culture, Buddhism continues to be misunderstood.

Hinduism

The collection of traditions known today as Hinduism began to develop around 1500 BCE, when Aryan invaders of India intermingled their religious practices and beliefs with those of the native Indian people. The sacred texts include the Veda, Upanishads, Bhagavadgita, Mahabharata, and Ramayana. These texts are mythological and philosophical commentaries about life. Although the religion speaks of many gods, heroes, and saints, Hindus believe in one principle—that these many gods are aspects of a single divine unity. Hindus believe that people are born and reborn based on their *samsara*, or separation from the divine, and that one's karma, or total way of acting and being, can be improved through pure actions and meditation. Through these pure acts, one can eventually become closer to the divine. Hindus believe that reincarnation is the road to unity with the divine and that it answers many perplexing questions, such as why there are so many personalities in this world. Although Hindus represent 13% of the world's population, Hinduism is misunderstood and considered strange by many Americans, just as Buddhism is.

Islam

Fully 18% of the world is Islamic, and yet this mostly nonauthoritarian and egalitarian religion continues to be confusing for most Americans. Following the beliefs established in 622 by the prophet Muhammad, Muslims accept Allah (God) as the merciful, kind, and all-powerful creator of the universe. Humans are seen as the highest creation of God, good by their very nature, although they are capable of forgetting their true nature and being misled by Satan. However, Muslims believe that if people forget their true nature, they can repent, return to a state of remembering, and go to Paradise. Two of the major texts of Islam are the Koran, which is said to be the true word of God given by the angel Gabriel to Muhammad, and the Hadith, traditions that developed from the life and teachings of the prophet. Muslims have five duties, or pillars, to which they should adhere: to profess their faith to Allah, to pray five times a day, to give a portion of their material wealth to charity regularly, to fast daily until sundown during the month of Ramadan, and to attempt to make at least one pilgrimage to Mecca.

In the United States, Muslims have obtained an undeserved negative reputation. This has been particularly so since the tragedy at the 9/11 attacks at the World Trade Center and the Pentagon, which led some Americans to wrongfully view the majority of Muslims and Arabs as terrorists. Certainly, the vast majority of Muslims are peace-loving and in sync with the teachings of Muhammad as depicted in the Koran. Finally, it should be noted that although a large percentage of Arabs are Muslim, Muslims are found around the world, and only a small percentage are Arab. Also, not all Muslims are religious, and a counselor should not assume that a Muslim client is religious any more than he or she would assume that a Christian is devout.

Judaism

A monotheistic religion that coalesced around 1300 BCE, Judaism is based on the Hebrew Bible, which includes the five books attributed to Moses (called the Torah), the writings of the prophets, and the writings of the ancient historians, kings, and wisdom-teachers. Later writings, called the Talmud, are interpretations by teachers (known as *rabbis*) and judges of the early writings, and they are also used as a basis for knowledge and worship. Adherence to Jewish laws varies from those who are very orthodox to those who are very liberal, although the majority of Jews in the United States fall somewhere in the middle. Some of the major holidays include Rosh Hashanah, the New Year; Yom Kippur, the Day of Atonement for one's sins; Hanukkah, the Festival of Lights; and Passover, which celebrates the liberation of Jews from slavery in Egypt and is symbolic of liberation in general. Finally, the bar mitzvah is another major Jewish ceremony, which celebrates a boy entering adulthood at age 13 (the corresponding ceremony for girls is called the *bat mitzvah*).

The Jewish people have faced a particularly long history of oppression. Despite the fact that the Jewish religion is peaceful and forward-thinking and that Jewish individuals have fully assimilated into American society, false stereotypes of Jews continue, and prejudice and discrimination against Jews is still evident. In fact, although fewer than 2% of Americans are Jewish, hate crime statistics indicate that 61% of all religious hate crimes and close to 12% all hate crimes have been committed against Jews (U.S. Department of Justice, 2012).

Counseling Individuals from Diverse Religious Backgrounds

A client's religious beliefs and spiritual orientation may hold the keys to understanding the underlying values that motivate him or her. To help guide counselors in working with clients around religious beliefs and spirituality, the *Association for Spiritual, Ethical, and Religious Values in Counseling (ASERVIC)*, a division of ACA, has developed fourteen

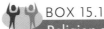

BOX 15.1
Religion as Projection of Self

My wife was raised Catholic, and I was raised Jewish. We have two daughters. When my oldest child was still an infant, I remember telling a therapist I had been seeing how Jewish my daughter seemed and that I thought my wife would see her in this light also. After reflecting on this for a moment, he gave me one of those looks that said, "Yeah, get real—you best check this out," but his only comment was "Uh huh." As soon as I got home, I asked my wife, "Do you see Hannah as Jewish?" She laughed and said, "No, I think she seems Catholic." I was quickly reminded how so much of our inner experience is projected onto the world.

competencies built around six core values. In working with clients, counselors can be guided by these points (ASERVIC, 2009, "Spiritual Competencies"):

Culture and Worldview

1. The professional counselor can describe the similarities and differences between spirituality and religion, including the basic beliefs of various spiritual systems, major world religions, agnosticism, and atheism.
2. The professional counselor recognizes that the client's beliefs (or absence of beliefs) about spirituality, religion, or both are central to his or her worldview and can influence psychosocial functioning (see Box 15.1).

Counselor Self-Awareness

3. The professional counselor actively explores his or her own attitudes, beliefs, and values about spirituality, religion, or both.
4. The professional counselor continuously evaluates the influence of his or her own spiritual and religious beliefs and values on the client and the counseling process.
5. The professional counselor can identify the limits of his or her understanding of the client's spiritual and religious perspective and is acquainted with religious and spiritual resources, including leaders, who can be avenues for consultation and to whom the counselor can refer.

Human and Spiritual Development

6. The professional counselor can describe and apply various models of spiritual and religious development and their relationship to human development.

Communication

7. The professional counselor responds to client communications about spirituality and religion with acceptance and sensitivity.
8. The professional counselor uses spiritual and religious concepts that are consistent with the client's spiritual and religious perspectives and that are acceptable to the client.

9. The professional counselor can recognize spiritual and religious themes in client communication and is able to address these with the client when they are therapeutically relevant.

Assessment

10. During the intake and assessment processes, the professional counselor strives to understand a client's spiritual and religious perspective by gathering information from the client, other sources, or both.

Diagnosis and Treatment

11. When making a diagnosis, the professional counselor recognizes that the client's spiritual and religious perspectives can (a) enhance well-being, (b) contribute to client problems, (c) exacerbate symptoms, or any combination of these.
12. The professional counselor sets goals with the client that are consistent with the client's spiritual and religious perspectives.
13. The professional counselor is able to (a) modify therapeutic techniques to include a client's spiritual and religious perspectives, and (b) utilize spiritual and religious practices as techniques when appropriate and acceptable to a client's viewpoint.
14. The professional counselor can therapeutically apply theory and current research supporting the inclusion of a client's spiritual and religious perspectives and practices.

Gender Differences in the United States and Gender-Aware Therapy

The words *sex* and *gender* are often confused, and the meanings of those terms are critical to any conversation about gender differences. Whereas one's sex is biologically determined, one's gender includes the social, cultural, and psychological roles that are assumed by a person based on his or her sex (Trepal, Wester, & Notestine, 2013). In recent years, controversy has emerged over whether differences between men and women are biological, sociological, or even relatively nonexistent (Else-Quest, Hyde, & Linn, 2010; Harkins, Hansen, & Gama, 2008; Hyde, 2005; Petersen & Hyde, 2010; Trepal, Wester, & Notestine, 2013). Although some may argue about whether "real" differences exist, it is clear that men and women are treated differently in society, and how they respond to cultural expectations varies dramatically. Research, as well as commonly held assumptions, reveal many differences based on gender, some of which are listed in Table 15.1 (Anderson, 2009; Harkins, Hansen, & Gama, 2008; Sue & Sue, 2013; Trepal, Wester, & Notestine, 2013).

Whether working with a man or a woman, knowledge of gender bias can allow a counselor to be effective at what some have labeled *gender-aware therapy* (Matthews, 2015). Such therapy considers gender central to counseling, views problems within a societal context, encourages counselors to actively address gender injustices, encourages the development of collaborative and equal relationships, and respects the client's right to

TABLE 15.1   Some Common Differences Between Men and Women

➤ Women are more nurturing, more compassionate, more relational, less focused on "doing" and more on "being" in relationships.	➤ Men tend to seek counseling less frequently than women and have a more negative attitude toward the helping process.
➤ Women have more difficulty expressing anger than men.	➤ Men are more restrictive emotionally, less communicative, less affectionate, and less comfortable with sad feelings, collaboration, self-disclosure, and intimacy.
➤ Women struggle more with self-esteem and depression than men.	➤ Men tend to be more comfortable with angry feelings, aggression, and competitiveness.
➤ Women earn less money for doing the same work as men.	➤ Men are sometimes ostracized for expressing feelings, especially those considered to be traditionally feminine feelings, and yet criticized for not being more sensitive.
➤ Job and advancement opportunities are fewer for women.	
➤ Women are more frequently sexually harassed on the job and at other places.	➤ Men are criticized for being too controlling and self-reliant and made to feel inadequate if they do not take control.
➤ Women are physically abused by their spouses or partners at alarming rates.	➤ Men are socialized to be more aggressive and individualistic and thus are more prone to accidents, suicide, early death through wars, and other acts of violence.
➤ Single and divorced women and their children live below the poverty level at alarming rates.	➤ Men are encouraged to be competitive and controlling (take charge), and yet these very behaviors lead to increased stress and are likely to play a factor in the shorter life expectancy of men in comparison with women.
➤ Assumptions about the abilities of girls and women may prevent females from realizing their potential.	
➤ Women tend to be more comfortable with expression of sad feelings, intimacy, and nurturing behavior and less comfortable with the expression of anger and assertive behavior.	➤ Men are socialized not to be engaged in child rearing, and yet also are criticized for being distant fathers.
➤ Women tend to be more socially compassionate and hold more traditional moral values.	➤ Men have biological problems unique to them (e.g., prostate cancer, prostatitis, higher rates of stress-related diseases, and testicular cancer).
➤ Women, on average, tend to be less comfortable in competitive situations.	➤ Men are placed in a position of being in charge of others, which sometimes results in the oppression of women. Such oppression not only harms women but also harms men's psyche.
➤ Women are more frequently misdiagnosed than are men when seeking mental health services.	
➤ Women are sometimes torn between their roles as nurturer and child-care provider and their place in the world of paid work.	➤ Men commit the vast majority of crimes, and a particularly high percentage of violent crimes.
➤ Nearly all cases of complaints made against therapists for sexual exploitation are from women complaining about male therapists.	➤ Men have higher rates of substance abuse.
➤ Women have biological problems unique to them (e.g., premenstrual syndrome, breast cancer, pregnancy, ovarian cysts, ovarian cancer).	

choose the gender roles appropriate for himself or herself regardless of their political correctness (Kees, 2005; Mejia, 2005). Let's look at two variations on gender-aware therapy: feminist therapy and counseling men.

Feminist Therapy

Feminist therapy had its basis in the feminist political movement of the 1960s and 1970s, which sought to offer women a new vantage point that was not based on traditional gender role expectations (Pusateri, 2015). Broadly, feminist theory recognized the impact of gender, the oppression of women, and the influence of politics. Feminist therapy understood that as a function of a male-dominated society, women were often devalued, and therefore, awareness of gender issues and the battle to decrease oppression against women and other minorities through social justice actions became significant principles of feminist theory.

Today, the overarching goal of feminist therapy is the empowerment of female clients (Brown & Bryan, 2007). Several components comprise feminist theory and the empowerment of women (Pusateri, 2015). The first is viewing the person as a political entity. Specifically, this refers to the fact that no client is an isolated individual but one who is affected by the political and social environments. Historically and currently, women and minorities have been at a disadvantage politically, and one focus of feminist therapy is to encourage these marginalized clients to find their voice and create societal change.

A second guiding principle is recognition of the power and authority that the counselor holds in the relationship. The feminist counselor actively seeks to establish a therapeutic alliance that is collaborative and effectively balances the relationship's power dynamics (Brown, Weber, & Ali, 2008). The third critical component is to focus on wellness (Brown & Bryan, 2007). Feminist helpers do not see problems arising from psychopathology, otherwise termed the "disease model." On the contrary, they tend to view problems as a function of external factors; that is, symptomatic behaviors are seen as coping responses to societal and political stress and oppression.

In addition to the three critical components, the American Psychological Association (APA, 2007) adopted the *Guidelines for Psychological Practice with Girls and Women*, which should be integrated into the practice of feminist therapy, and include three sections: (1) Diversity, Social Context, and Power, (2) Professional Responsibility, and (3) Practice Applications (see Table 15.2). Finally, in the actual practice of feminist therapy, 12 steps are offered that take into account the critical components of feminist therapy and the APA guidelines in counseling:

1. *Have the right attitudes and beliefs, gain knowledge, and learn skills.* Be prepared to work with women by embracing the appropriate knowledge, skills, and beliefs prior to meeting with them (e.g., know and incorporate the APA guidelines in Table 15.2).
2. *Ensure that the counseling approach you use has been designed specifically for women or adapted for women.* Conduct an inventory of your theoretical approach for any inherent sexist leanings it may have. Discard it or adapt as necessary.
3. *Establish a collaborative and egalitarian relationship, give up your power, and demystify the counseling process.* Recognize the importance that power plays in all relationships and attempt to equalize the counselor-client relationship. This can be done by downplaying the "expert" role, encouraging women to trust themselves, and using appropriate self-disclosure. The counselor and client should work toward a relationship that focuses on cooperatively created actions and objectives.
4. *Identify social and political issues related to client problems and use them to set goals.* Help women understand the nature of the problem within its sociocultural context and see how the unique dynamics of women tend to cause them to internalize these issues. For instance, it is common for abused women to blame themselves for the abuse. Help them see that they are not responsible and help them set goals to break free of the abuse.
5. *Use a wellness model and avoid the use of diagnosis and labels.* Diagnosis and labels can be disempowering to women and tend to focus treatment toward psychopathology. A wellness orientation that uplifts women can help them get in touch with their strengths.

TABLE 15.2 APA Guidelines for Psychological Practice with Girls and Women

SECTION 1: DIVERSITY, SOCIAL CONTEXT, AND POWER

Guideline 1: Psychologists strive to be aware of the effects of socialization, stereotyping, and unique life events on the development of girls and women across diverse cultural groups (p. 35).

Guideline 2: Psychologists are encouraged to recognize and utilize information about oppression, privilege, and identity development as they may affect girls and women (p. 37).

Guideline 3: Psychologists strive to understand the impact of bias and discrimination upon the physical and mental health of those with whom they work (p. 39).

SECTION 2: PROFESSIONAL RESPONSIBILITY

Guideline 4: Psychologists strive to use gender and culturally sensitive, affirming practices in providing services to girls and women (p. 46).

Guideline 5: Psychologists are encouraged to recognize how their socialization, attitudes, and knowledge about gender may affect their practice with girls and women (p. 50).

SECTION 3: PRACTICE APPLICATIONS

Guideline 6: Psychologists are encouraged to employ interventions and approaches that have been found to be effective in the treatment of issues of concern to girls and women (p. 52).

Guideline 7: Psychologists strive to foster therapeutic relationships and practices that promote initiative, empowerment, and expanded alternatives and choices for girls and women (p. 55).

Guideline 8: Psychologists strive to provide appropriate, unbiased assessments and diagnoses in their work with women and girls (p. 58).

Guideline 9: Psychologists strive to consider the problems of girls and women in their sociopolitical context (p. 60).

Guideline 10: Psychologists strive to acquaint themselves with and utilize relevant mental health, education, and community resources for girls and women (p. 62).

Guideline 11: Psychologists are encouraged to understand and work to change institutional and systemic bias that may impact girls and women (p. 64).

SOURCE: American Psychological Association (2007). *Guidelines for psychological practice with girls and women.* Washington, D.C.: Author.

6. *Validate and legitimize a woman's angry feelings toward her predicament.* As women begin to recognize how they have internalized social and political issues, they begin to understand how they have been victimized. Helpers should assist women in combating feelings of powerlessness, helplessness, and low self-esteem and help them identify their strengths.

7. *Actively promote healing through learning about women's issues.* Helpers should encourage women to learn more about women's issues. This can be done by providing written materials, suggesting seminars to attend, and providing a list of women's groups or women's organizations that support women's issues.

8. *Provide a safe environment to express feelings as clients begin to form connections with other women.* As female clients gain clarity regarding their situation, they see how society's objectification of women has led to fear and competition among women. This newfound knowledge will lead to a desire to have deeper, more meaningful

connections with other women. Helpers can validate feelings of fear and competition with other women that result from such objectification. As these feelings dissipate, women will move toward a strong and special connection with other women. At this point in counseling, helpers should consider the possibility of referring clients to a women's support group.

9. *Provide a safe environment to help women understand their anger toward men.* As women increasingly see that a male-dominated society has led to the objectification of women, they will begin to express increasing anger toward men. However, helpers can assist clients in understanding the difference between anger at a man and anger at a male-dominated system. Slowly, women will see that some men can be trusted.

10. *Help clients deal with conflicting feelings between traditional and newfound values.* As women develop newfound feminist beliefs, they become torn between those beliefs and values that do not seem congruent with those beliefs (e.g., wanting to stay home to raise the children). Helpers should validate these contradictory feelings, acknowledge the confusion, and assist clients in exploring their contradictory belief systems.

11. *Facilitate integration of the client's new identity.* Helpers can assist clients in integrating their newfound feminist beliefs with their personal beliefs, even those personal beliefs that may not seem to be traditionally feminist. Clients are able to feel strength in their own identity development and no longer need to rely on an external belief system.

12. *Say goodbye.* It is important to help women move on with their newfound identity, and helpers should encourage women to try being in the world without counseling. Counseling can always be resumed in the future if needed.

Counseling Men

> *In order for us to be able to "hold" others we have to imagine ourselves being held by our fathers, perhaps the first male we wanted to hold and be held by.*
>
> (Osherson, 1986/2001, p. 195)

Although the concerns of men are generally quite different from those of women, they are no less important, especially in light of the fact that compared to women, men are more reluctant to seek counseling and have a more negative attitude toward the helping process (Berger, Levant, McMillan, Kelleher, & Sellers, 2005; Evans, Duffey, & Englar-Carlson, 2013). As with women, men need to feel supported in counseling and not feel judged for having their own issues—issues that are common to the male experience and that cut across all racial, ethnic, and cultural groups (see Table 15.1). As with women, counselors need to be aware of men's issues and have empathy for a man's situation. A number of ideas can be incorporated into a set of guidelines when working with male clients (Englar-Carlson & Kiselica, 2013; Good & Brooks, 2005; Greer, 2005; McCarthy & Holliday, 2004; Mejia, 2005; Wexler, 2009):

1. *Have the right attitudes and beliefs, gain knowledge, and learn skills.* Embrace the appropriate knowledge, skills, and beliefs prior to meeting with a male client.

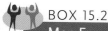

BOX 15.2
Men Expressing an Array of Feelings

Close your eyes for a moment and imagine a person running into a burning apartment building to save the lives of children. Stay focused on that image, and let it sink in. Now, close your eyes again and imagine two young children snuggling and being taken care of by their parent. The parent makes "cooing" sounds to get the attention of the infant and show the infant love. Imagine this in your mind's eye.

If you imagined a man running into the building and a woman snuggling with her children, you are probably like many Americans. Our imaginations reinforce our stereotypes. And we tend to see nurturing as a compassionate behavior and running into a building to save lives as a brave behavior. Both are important, and perhaps reflect societal stereotypes of gender specific behaviors. But, in reality, can't we all be nurturing parents and brave heroes? In counseling, men may present with some traditional male behaviors, but are capable of expressing many feelings—if given the time!

2. *Accept men where they are, as this will help build trust.* Men, who are often initially very defensive, will work hard on their issues once they can trust the counselor.

3. *Don't push men to express what may be considered "softer feelings."* Don't push a man to express feelings, as you may force him out of the helping relationship. Men tend to be uncomfortable with certain feelings (e.g., deep sadness, feelings of incompetence, feelings of inadequacy, feelings of closeness), but more at ease with "thinking things through," problem solving, and expressing some feelings, such as anger and pride (see Box 15.2).

4. *Early on in therapy, validate the man's feelings.* Validate whatever feelings a man expresses, and remember that to protect their egos, men may initially blame others and society for their problems.

5. *Validate the man's view of how he has been constrained by male sex-role stereotypes.* Help to build trust by validating a man's sense of being constrained by sex-role stereotypes (e.g., he must work particularly hard for his family) and validate the positive aspects of masculinity.

6. *Have a plan for therapy.* Collaborate with men and together, build a plan for therapy. Men like structure and a sense of goal directedness, even if the plan is changed later on.

7. *Begin to discuss developmental issues.* Introduce male developmental issues so a man can quickly examine concerns that may be impinging upon him (e.g., midlife crises) (Levinson, 1978).

8. *Slowly encourage the expression of new feelings.* As you reinforce the expression of newfound feelings, men will begin to feel comfortable sharing what are considered to be more feminine feelings (e.g., tears, caring, feelings of intimacy).

9. *Explore underlying issues and reinforce new ways of understanding the world.* Explore underlying issues as they emerge (e.g., childhood issues, feelings of inadequacy, father–son issues).

10. *Explore behavioral change.* As insights emerge, encourage men to try out new behaviors.

11. *Encourage the integration of new feelings, new ways of thinking, and new behaviors.*

12. *Encourage new male relationships.* Encourage new male friendships in which the client can express his feelings while maintaining his maleness (e.g., a men's group).

13. *Say goodbye.* Be able to say goodbye and end the relationship. Although some men may want to continue in counseling, many will see it as a time-limited means to a goal.

Differences in Sexual Orientation

In his famous studies of the 1940s, Alfred Kinsey found that 50% of the men he surveyed had some sexual history with other males during their adult life, 13% had more homosexual than heterosexual experiences, 8% were exclusively homosexual for three years of their lives between the ages of 16 and 55, and 4% were exclusively homosexual throughout their lives (Kinsey, Pomeroy, & Martin, 1948; Kinsey, Pomeroy, Martin, & Gebhard, 1953). Kinsey also found that most individuals were not purely homosexual or heterosexual but rather fell on a continuum between homosexual and heterosexual feelings and sometimes identified themselves as bisexual. Although some have questioned Kinsey's results (Cole, Gorman, Barrett, & Thompson, 1993), there is little doubt that his research helped to change the mental health professions' belief that homosexuality and bisexuality were disorders toward the current view that they, like heterosexuality, are simply sexual orientations (Chiang, 2008).

Although surveys today suggests that about 3.5% of Americans currently identify as gay, lesbian, or bisexual (see Chapter 14, Table 14.1), this percentage is likely much higher if you take into account those gays who have not come out, bisexuals who identify as heterosexual, and others who had once lived a gay or bisexual lifestyle and now identify as heterosexual. In either case, determining percentages is less important than approaching every individual with dignity and respect, regardless of their sexual orientation. No matter what the number of gays, lesbians, bisexuals, or heterosexuals there are in society, the most current research suggests that sexual orientation is determined very early in life, most likely related to biological and genetic factors, may be influenced by sociological factors, and has little if anything to do with choice (Saravi, 2007).

Meanwhile, views about gays, lesbians, and bisexuals have changed dramatically in the United States. Today, 66% of Americans believe that gay and lesbian relationships should be legal, compared to 27% in 1996; 58% believe gay and lesbian relationships are morally acceptable, compared to 40% in 2001; and 42% believe that gays and lesbians are born with their sexual orientation as compared to 13% in 1977 (Gallup, 2014). However, we still have some work to do, as the most recent FBI hate crime statistics indicate that about 19% of all hate crimes were perpetrated against individuals due to their sexual orientation, with the vast majority of those directed toward male homosexuals (U.S. Department of Justice, 2014).

In the counseling profession, a recent survey of counselors found that 94% of counselors believe that homosexuality is not a pathology (one has to wonder about the other 6%) (Neukrug & Milliken, 2011). This compares to 86% in a 1993 study (Gibson & Pope, 1993), so clearly, the counseling profession has done its job in training counselors about the normality of homosexuality. However, stating that being gay or lesbian is not a pathology does not mean that one necessarily feels comfortable working with gays, lesbians, and bisexuals. Perhaps this is why the American Psychological Association endorsed guidelines for psychotherapy for lesbian, gay, and bisexual clients ("Guidelines for…," 2000). And, this is probably why ACA found it necessary to develop a statement against *sexual orientation change efforts* (SOCE), such as conversion or reparative therapy (efforts to change a person from homosexuality to heterosexuality):

> *Considering all the above deliberation, the ACA Ethics Committee strongly suggests that ethical professional counselors do not refer clients to someone who engages in conversion therapy or, if they do so, to proceed cautiously only when they are certain that the referral counselor fully informs clients of the unproven nature of the treatment and the potential risks and takes steps to minimize harm to clients.*

(Whitman, Glosoff, Kocet, & Tarvydas, 2006, interpretation section, para. 10)

So, keeping in mind that many of us still hold biases, let's take a look at some points to consider when counseling individuals who are gay, bi, or lesbian.

Counseling Gay, Bisexual, and Lesbian Individuals

A number of important points regarding the counseling of gay, bisexual, and lesbian individuals have been highlighted by many authors, some of which are summarized below (e.g., Pope, 2008; Szymanski, 2013; Sue & Sue, 2013; Ward, Dahlhamer, Galinsky, & Joesti, 2014):

1. *Have the right attitudes and beliefs, gain knowledge, and learn skills.* Be prepared to work with gay, lesbian, and bisexual clients by embracing the appropriate knowledge, skills, and beliefs prior to meeting with them.
2. *Have a gay-, lesbian-, and bisexual-friendly office.* Make sure that your intake forms are gay, lesbian, and bisexual friendly. Some counselors may choose to have literature in their office that promotes a gay friendly atmosphere. Others may just want to ensure that there are not heterosexist materials in the office.
3. *Help gays, lesbians, and bisexuals understand and combat societal forms of oppression.* Oppression and discrimination of gays, lesbians, and bisexuals is rampant throughout American culture, and it is important that gays, lesbians, and bisexuals understand how it affects them, what they can do to combat it, and how they can gain a sense of empowerment despite it.
4. *Adopt an affirmative and nonheterosexist attitude.* The importance of adopting an attitude that affirms your client's right to his or her sexuality cannot be stressed enough, as so many individuals (including counselors!) have embedded biases and stereotypes about gays and lesbians.
5. *Don't jump to conclusions about lifestyle.* There is no "one" gay, lesbian, or bisexual lifestyle, and counselors should not jump to conclusions about how their clients live their sexuality.
6. *Understand the differences among people who are gay, lesbian, and bisexual.* Although lumped together here, and often confused as embodying many of the same characteristics, there are great differences among gay, lesbian, and bisexual individuals. For instance, bisexuals are sometimes ostracized by heterosexuals and even by gays and lesbians. Moreover, identity development for gays, lesbians, and bisexuals is considerably different.

7. *Know community resources that might be useful to gays and lesbians.*
8. *Know identity issues.* Be familiar with the identity development of gays, lesbians, and bisexuals, especially as it relates to the coming-out process (e.g., Morrow, 2004; Szymanski, 2013).
9. *Understand the complexity of sexuality.* People express their sexuality in different ways. For instance, gay and bisexual men are generally more sexually active than lesbians. Also, the expression of sexuality in men and women sometimes differs, with women being more focused on relationship issues.
10. *Understand the idiosyncrasies of religious views of homosexuality.* Some religions view being gay, lesbian, or bisexual as sinful, while others are empowering of different sexual orientations. Also, how an individual adheres to the beliefs of his or her religious sect can vary dramatically. For instance, one Catholic might view his being gay as sinful, while another might see it as being normal.
11. *Recognize the importance of addressing unique issues that some gays, lesbians, and bisexuals may face.* Although the research is mixed, there is some evidence that lesbian, gay, and bisexual people may have higher somewhat incidents of smoking, drinking, psychological stress, and some other health issues than heterosexuals. Know the prevalence of these and other issues within the specific population and the unique ways of treating them in counseling.

Individuals Who Are HIV Positive

Today, over 1 million people in the United States are living with HIV, and about one in six of them don't know it (Centers for Disease Control, 2013). It is also estimated that about 50,000 new cases of HIV arise each year, about 15,000 individuals die of the disease each year, and that close to 636,000 Americans have died since the disease was first identified. AIDS continues to spread in this country, and an estimated 35.3 million children and adults worldwide are living with HIV (UNAIDS, 2013). With 10% of the world's population, and 67% of the world's cases of AIDS, sub-Saharan Africa has been most affected by the AIDS epidemic. With access to drugs to slow the disease difficult to obtain in some Third World countries, it is clear that this epidemic has had a personal and economic cost to people throughout the world.

The response of social services to the AIDS epidemic has varied and includes programs that offer support and counseling groups for HIV-positive individuals and their families, assisting HIV-positive individuals with the disclosure process, programs for children who have AIDS, prevention and education programs, helping individuals learn to live with a chronic illness, and hotlines to respond to questions about AIDS (Barstow & Lum, 2011; Dahlbeck & Lease, 2010; Kalichman et al., 2007; Yarhouse, 2003). Workshops and articles about the AIDS virus and how to counsel individuals who have tested HIV positive are now commonplace at conferences and in professional journals. As we work toward finding a cure for HIV and AIDS, the counselor will increasingly play an important role in offering education and prevention activities about the disease, counseling individuals who are HIV positive, dealing with issues related to disease process and mortality, and advocating for HIV treatment programs. As sexual activity with an HIV-positive individual is potentially life-threatening, counselors who are in a helping relationship with HIV-positive clients may be challenged with knowing when it is ethical to break confidentiality when there is "foreseeable risk" of a person who might be unwittingly exposed to the disease by their client (see ACA, 2014a, Section B.2.c).

Counseling Individuals Who Are HIV Positive

A number of challenges face the counselor who works with an individual who is HIV positive or who has AIDS. Some points to consider when counseling an individual who is HIV positive include the following:

1. *Have the right attitudes and beliefs, gain knowledge, and learn skills.* Be prepared to work with HIV-positive individuals by embracing the appropriate knowledge, skills, and beliefs prior to meeting with them.
2. *Know the cultural background of the client.* Keep in mind that HIV-positive individuals are found in all cultures, races, and ethnic groups. Counselors need to remember that a client's background may change how the counselor works with him or her.
3. *Know about the disease and combat myths.* Knowledge helps fight fear. Armed with knowledge, counselors can become advocates for the HIV-positive person.
4. *Be prepared to take on uncommon counselor roles.* Realize that the counselor may need to be an advocate, caretaker, and resource person for the client—roles in which the counselor has not always been comfortable.
5. *Be prepared to deal with unique treatment issues.* Be prepared to deal with unique problems, including feelings about the loss of income from the loss of work or the high cost of medical treatment, depression and hopelessness concerning uncertain health, changes in interpersonal relationships when others discover the client is HIV positive (rejection, pity, fear, and so forth), and the probability that the client may have friends and loved ones who are HIV positive or have died of AIDS if he or she is part of a high-risk group.
6. *Know the implications of working with someone who has a long-term, manageable disease.* As treatment for HIV and AIDS has improved, it is now seen by many as a chronic disease. Know the psychological drawbacks (and benefits—yes, there can be some) of knowing that one may be HIV-positive for many years to come.
7. *Deal with your own feelings about health and mortality.* Be able to deal effectively with your own feelings about living with a chronic disease, as well as mortality issues.
8. *Understand the legal and ethical implications of working with individuals who may pose a risk to others or may be considering end-of-life decisions.* Ethical codes, such as the ACA code (ACA, 2014a), address the complicated issues of working with individuals who may pose a risk of transmitting a disease to others and when it may be appropriate to counsel an individual on end-of-life decisions. Sometimes the codes contradict legal dictates. Counselors need to know both their ethical codes and the law and come to a wise decision on how to work with individuals who may be involved in such dilemmas.
9. *Offer a "strength-based" approach to treatment.* Help clients focus on what is positive in their lives and the possibilities that exist for them instead of focusing on the diagnosis and the dread of the disease.

The Hungry, the Homeless, and the Poor

It is estimated that over 600,000 people are homeless in the United States on any particular day and about 3.5 million Americans experience homelessness in a given year, with close to 40% of them being children (National Coalition for the Homeless, 2009; U.S. Department of Housing and Urban Development, 2013). Although homelessness has existed throughout history, the faces of the homeless have changed dramatically. Today, the homeless include children who have run away from home, single-parent families, intact families who have no place to live, poor single men and women, and the deinstitutionalized mentally ill. In addition, the homeless of today are more likely not to have shelter, are younger, are less apt to find employment, and are heavily overrepresented by minorities. In addition, up to 35% of homeless who are sheltered have a chronic substance abuse issue and 26% have a severe mental illness (SAMHSA, 2010). Despite these statistics, resources to serve these individuals have remained minimal.

In past years, being poor did not necessarily mean that one was at greater risk of being homeless, but today, being poor is often one step away from not having a roof over one's head. The number of poor Americans is about 43 million, a little over 14.3% of the population (Maccartney, Bishaw, & Fontenot, 2013). In addition, a staggering 16 million children—22% of all children in the United States—live in poverty (National Center for Children in Poverty, 2014). Also, poverty is associated with race and ethnicity, as can be seen in Figure 15.2.

Poverty is somewhat more prevalent in the cities and the southern and western regions of the United States (U.S. Census Bureau, 2009b). In addition, poverty is related to educational level, as the more educated have lower poverty rates. Although the *McKinney-Vento Homeless Assistance Act* provides mental health services, substance abuse treatment, outreach services, emergency food and shelter, housing, health care, education, job training, and child care, the outlook for this section of society seems bleak ("History of the McKinney Act," 2014).

FIGURE 15.2
Poverty as a Function of Race and Ethnic Groups

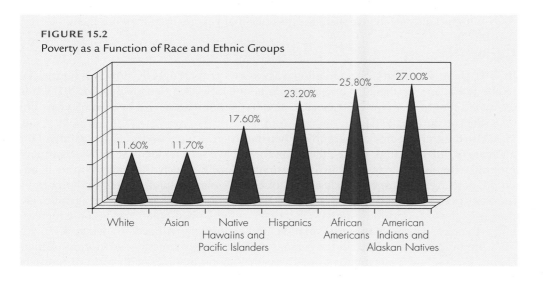

Counseling the Homeless and the Poor

A number of unique points should be considered when counseling the homeless and the poor (APA, 2014b; Barstow & Lum, 2011; Dykeman, 2011; McBride, 2012; Sun, 2012):

1. *Have the right attitudes and beliefs, gain knowledge, and learn skills.* Be prepared to work with the homeless and the poor by embracing the appropriate knowledge, skills, and beliefs prior to meeting with them.
2. *Focus on social issues.* Help clients obtain basic needs such as food and housing, as opposed to working on intrapsychic issues.
3. *Know the client's racial, ethnic, and cultural background.* Be educated about the cultural heritage of clients because a disproportionate number of the homeless and the poor come from diverse racial, ethnic, and cultural groups.
4. *Be knowledgeable about health risks.* Be aware that the homeless and the poor are at much greater risk of developing AIDS, tuberculosis, and other diseases, and be able to do a basic medical screening and have referral sources available.
5. *Be prepared to deal with multiple issues.* Be prepared to deal with mental illness, chemical dependence, and other unique problems because up to 50% of the homeless are struggling with these problems.
6. *Know about developmental delays and be prepared to refer if needed.* Know how to identify developmental delays and have potential referral sources because homeless and poor children are much more likely to have delayed language and social skills, be abused, and have delayed motor development.
7. *Know psychological effects.* Be prepared to deal with the client's feelings of despair, depression, and hopelessness as a result of being poor, homeless, or both.
8. *Know resources.* Be aware of the vast number of resources available in your community and make referrals when appropriate.
9. *Be an advocate and stay committed.* Because the homeless and the poor are often dealing with multiple issues, and because a high percentage of them have mental illness, advocating for their unique concerns and being committed to them is particularly important, as you give them the message that you are truly there for them.

Older Persons

In 1900, about 4% of the U.S. population was over 65 years of age. By 1960, this figure rose to about 9%, and by the 2010 census, it was about 15% (U.S. Census Bureau, 2011). It is estimated that by the year 2030, close to 20% of the population will be over 65 years old (U.S. Census Bureau, 2008).

With these changing demographics, there has been an increased focus on treatment for and care of older persons. Across the country, we have seen an increase in day-treatment programs for older persons and in long-term-care facilities such as nursing homes. In addition, housing that is specially designed for older persons, senior centers, and programs for older persons offered through religious organizations and social service agencies are now prevalent around the country. Of course, as the United States has become increasingly diverse, so has our aging population, and counselors will need to be familiar with both the unique concerns of older persons and the race, ethnicity, and culture of their clients. With a high percentage of older persons having mental health concerns and yet attending counseling at low rates, counselors will become increasingly important in treating this population (World Health Organization, 2013).

Counseling Older Persons

Older persons have a number of problems and concerns that need to be addressed when they are counseled (Anderson, Goodman, & Schlossberg, 2012; Barstow & Lum, 2011; Myers & Harper, 2004; Stickle & Onedera, 2006). Below are some guidelines for working effectively with older clients:

1. *Have the right attitudes and beliefs, gain knowledge, and learn skills.* Counselors' own stereotypes and biases may affect their prognosis of clients from this population. Be prepared to work with older clients by embracing the appropriate knowledge, skills, and beliefs prior to meeting with them.

2. *Adapt your counseling style.* Adapt your counseling style to fit the needs of the older client. For instance, for the older person who has difficulty hearing, the counselor may use journal writing or art therapy. For clients who are not ambulatory, the counselor may need to have a session in the client's home. In addition, certain types of counseling, such as group and life review therapy, seem particularly advantageous with older persons if used appropriately.

3. *Build a trusting relationship.* Spend time building a trusting relationship. Remember that older persons seek counseling at lower rates than other clients, and those who do seek counseling may be less trustful of therapy, having grown up in a generation when counseling was much less common.

4. *Be knowledgeable about issues that many older persons face.* There are a number of issues that are more prevalent within the geriatric population, including loss and grief, depression, elder abuse, sleep disturbance, health concerns, identity issues, substance abuse, dementia, and others. Be knowledgeable of and assess for these issues.

5. *Know about possible and probable health changes.* Be aware of the many potential health problems common to older persons and have readily available referral sources. Predictable changes in health can lead to depression and concern about the future. Unpredictable changes in health can lead to loss of income and a myriad of emotional problems.

6. *Have empathy for changes in interpersonal relationships.* Changes in relationships may result from such things as retirement; the death of spouses, partners, and friends; changes in one's health status that prevent visits to and from friends; and relocations, such as to a retirement community, retirement home, or nursing home.

7. *Know about physical and psychological causes of sexual dysfunction.* Be aware of the possible physical and psychological causes of sexual dysfunction in older persons. As individuals age, it is fairly common for both men and women to have changes in their sexual functioning. Remember that regardless of age, we are always sexual beings.

8. *Involve the client's family and friends.* As social networks change, it may become important to involve family and friends in treatment planning. Families and friends can offer great support to older persons.

With an increasing number of older persons in the United States, it is likely that more mental health providers who are trained in geronotological counseling will be needed. Unfortunately, there has been little emphasis on this important area within the counseling profession, and few counselors are actually choosing to work with older persons (Schweiger, Henderson, McCaskill, & Clawson, 2012; Stickle & Onedera, 2006). Perhaps it's time for the counseling profession to place more emphasis on this important area.

The Chronically Mentally Ill

In 1950, there were well over half a million individuals with severe mental illness hospitalized in inpatient psychiatric hospitals (Stroup & Manderscheid, 1988; Treatment Advocacy Center, 2014). Although fewer than 50,000 individuals are hospitalized today, the number of psychiatric facilities that offer in-service treatment has decreased, and there is now a shortage of beds necessary for these individuals.

Unfortunately, the reduction in the number of inpatients is not the result of the sudden increase in mental health of Americans, but the consequence of a number of important events since the 1950s. In fact, about one-fourth to one-fifth of adult Americans are diagnosed with a mental disorder every year, with the types of disorders varying dramatically (National Institute of Mental Health, n.d.) (see Figure 15.3).

There are many reasons for deinstitutionalization of psychiatric patients. First, the development of new psychotropic medications, such as antipsychotics (e.g., Abilify and

FIGURE 15.3
Percentage of Adults with Select Mental Disorders Per Year

SOURCE: National Institute of Mental Health (n.d.). *The numbers count: Mental disorders in America.* Retrieved from http://www.nimh.nih.gov/health/publications/the-numbers-count-mental-disorders-in-america/index.shtml.

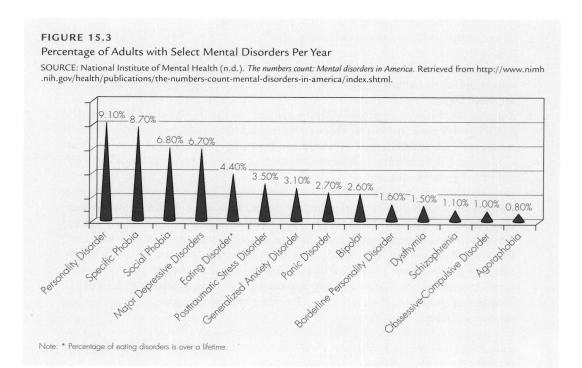

Note: * Percentage of eating disorders is over a lifetime.

Haldol), mood-stabilizing drugs (e.g., Lithium), antidepressants (e.g., Prozac, Zoloft, and Elavil), and anti-anxiety agents (e.g., Valium, Tranxene, and Xanax), has made the management of severe emotional conditions possible outside the inpatient setting. Second, the passage of the *Community Mental Health Centers Act of 1963* funded the establishment of mental health centers and made it possible for many with severe emotional problems to obtain outpatient mental health services for free or at low cost (Neukrug, 2013). Third, the proliferation of social service programs introduced through the *Great Society* initiatives of President Lyndon Johnson created a wide range of social service agencies, many of which serve the multiple needs of the chronically mentally ill. Finally, in 1975, the Supreme Court decision of *Donaldson v. O'Connor* stated that a person who is not dangerous to self or others could not be institutionalized against his or her will at inpatient psychiatric hospitals (see Box 2.3 in Chapter 2).

Unfortunately, many of the chronically mentally ill find themselves on the streets and homeless, with some sources stating that as many as 26% of all homeless people may have severe psychiatric problems (SAMHSA, 2010). Counselors who will be working with the chronically mentally ill will need to understand psychiatric disorders, psychotropic medications, and the unique needs of the chronically mentally ill, such as dealing with homelessness, continual transitions, difficulty with employment, and dependent family relationships.

Counseling the Chronically Mentally Ill

As just noted, a large percentage of Americans will have a mental disorder every year. However, most of these individuals will live functional and relatively normal lives and learn how to live with or be able to overcome their mental health problem. However, some of those individuals will become chronically mentally ill and will suffer throughout their lifetimes with a mental disorder, which leads to severe debilitation. The following treatment guidelines are focused on working with such individuals (Barstow & Lum, 2011; Garske, 2009; Kliewer, McNally, & Trippany, 2009; Walsh, 2000; Wong, 2006):

1. *Have the right attitudes and beliefs, gain knowledge, and learn skills.* Be prepared to work with mentally ill clients by embracing the appropriate knowledge, skills, and beliefs prior to meeting with them.
2. *Help the client understand his or her mental illness.* Give clients complete, up-to-date knowledge about their mental illness. Many do not have an understanding of their illness, the course of the illness, and the best methods of treatment.
3. *Help the client work through feelings concerning his or her mental illness.* Mental illness continues to be stigmatized in this society, and clients are often embarrassed about their disorder. Support groups and a nonjudgmental attitude can go a long way in normalizing the view that clients have of themselves.
4. *Ensure that clients attend counseling.* Increase the chances of clients coming to counseling by calling the day before, having a relative or close friend assist the client in coming to counseling, or having counselors develop specific strategies to help clients make their appointments (e.g., putting Xs on a calendar). Clients will miss appointments due to denial about their illness, embarrassment about seeing a counselor, problems remembering, or not caring.

5. *Ensure that clients comply with medication instructions.* Be vigilant about encouraging clients to take their medication and assess its functionality. Clients will discontinue medication due to forgetfulness, denial about the illness, the false belief that they will not have a relapse and don't need the drugs anymore because they feel better (i.e., the medication is working), and because the dosage is too small or too large.

6. *Ensure accurate diagnosis.* Diagnose clients accurately to ensure proper treatment planning and the appropriate choice of medication. Accurate diagnosis can be ensured through testing, clinical interviews, interviews with significant others, and appropriate use of supervision.

7. *Reevaluate the client's treatment plan and do not give up.* Be committed to working with clients and reevaluate treatment plans as often as necessary. Individuals who are chronically mentally ill are some of the most difficult clients to work with. Progress, if any, is slow, and it is easy for both the client and the counselor to become discouraged.

8. *Involve the client's family.* Ensure adequate family involvement and have the family understand the implications of the client's diagnosis. Families can offer great support to clients with mental illness and can be a window into the client's psyche.

9. *Know resources.* Have a working knowledge of resources, as the mentally ill are often involved, or need to become involved, with many other resources in the community (e.g., Social Security disability, housing authority, and support groups).

People with Disabilities

According to the U.S. Census Bureau (2012), nearly 56.7 million (18.7%) of all Americans have a disability. Of people 15 years or older, 30.6 million (12.6%) have limitations related to walking or using stairs, 19.9 million (8.2%) have difficulty with select physical tasks like lifting, grasping, reaching, and pulling; 15.5 million (6.4%) have difficulty with instrumental activities of daily living, such as taking medication, bathing, going to bed, preparing meals, and doing housework; 15.2 million (6.3%) have a mental disability such as a learning disability, Alzheimer's or dementia, an intellectual disability, a developmental disability, or other mental disability; 14.9 million (6.2%) have a sight, hearing, or speaking disability; and 9.4 million (3.9%) have problems with activities of daily living such as dressing, bathing, eating, toileting, etc. In addition, you are more likely to be unemployed if you have a disability and are more likely to have a disability if your median income is lower than the national average (Brault, 2012). But as troubling as the above facts are, it is even more unsettling to know that the worst mistreatment of people with disabilities is the reaction that many get from others, for many individuals with disabilities are feared, ignored, stared at, infantilized, treated as intellectually inferior, accused of faking their disability, or pitied.

A number of federal laws have had an impact on the ability of individuals with disabilities to receive services. The *Education for All Handicapped Children Act of 1975 (PL94-142)* and the subsequent *Individuals with Disabilities Education Act (IDEA)* ensure the right to an education within the least restrictive environment for all children who are identified as having a disability that interferes with learning (U.S. Department of Education, n.d.). The *Rehabilitation Act of 1973* ensures access to vocational rehabilitation services for adults with disabilities who are in need of employment (U.S. Department of Health and Human Services, 2006a). The *Americans with Disabilities Act of 1992* ensures that individuals with disabilities cannot be discriminated against in job application procedures, hiring, firing, advancement, compensation, fringe benefits, job training, and other terms, conditions, and privileges (U.S. Equal Employment Commission, n.d.).

Counseling Individuals with Disabilities

As federal laws have increasingly supported the right to services for individuals with disabilities, the counselor has taken an increasingly active role in the treatment and rehabilitation of such individuals (Barstow & Lum, 2009; Kelsey & Smart, 2012; Martin, 2007; Smart, 2009). Some treatment guidelines for working with the individual who has a disability include the following:

1. *Have the right attitudes and beliefs, gain knowledge, and learn skills.* Be prepared to work with clients who have a disability by embracing the appropriate knowledge, skills, and beliefs prior to meeting with them.
2. *Have knowledge about the many disabling conditions.* To be effective, a counselor should understand the physical and emotional consequences of the client's disability.
3. *Help clients know their disabilities.* Help clients understand their disabilities, the probable course of treatment, and the prognosis. Such knowledge allows them to be fully involved in the counseling process.
4. *Assist the client through the grieving process.* Help clients pass through stages of grief as they deal with their loss and move toward acceptance. Similar to the stages of bereavement (Kubler-Ross & Kessler, 2005), it is usual for a client to experience denial, anger, negotiation, resignation, and acceptance.
5. *Know referral resources.* Be aware of potential resources in the community (e.g., physicians, social services, physical therapists, experts on pain management, vocational rehabilitation). Individuals with disabilities often have a myriad of needs.
6. *Know the law and inform your client of the law.* Know the law to ensure that the clients are receiving all necessary services and not being discriminated against. In addition, clients often feel empowered when they know their rights.
7. *Be prepared to do, or refer for, vocational and career counseling.* Be ready to conduct career counseling or to refer a client to a career counselor. Often, when faced with a disability, clients also must face a career transition or transitions.
8. *Include the family.* Whenever possible and reasonable, include the client's family in the treatment process, as they can offer support, assist in long-term treatment planning, and help with the client's emotional needs.
9. *Be an advocate.* Individuals with disabilities often face prejudice and discrimination. Advocate for clients by knowing the law, fighting for clients' rights, and assisting clients in fighting for their own rights.
10. *Empower your clients.* Avoid being overly sympathetic and having low expectations, and listen and support your client. Assume that your client knows what is best for him or her.

Multicultural/Social Justice Focus

Is All Counseling Multicultural?

First counselor asserts: "All counseling is multicultural, for everyone is different and just because you're African American, Asian, or Hispanic, have a disability, are homeless or mentally ill, or whatever, doesn't mean you're more different than the person I counsel who comes from the same background as me but still has some different values than I have."

Second counselor retorts: "You do not understand what it's like to be culturally different. To assert that all counseling is multicultural just shows your ignorance. Clearly, some individuals have roots in their unique culture, are dramatically different from you, and you had better learn about their unique culture if you are to work with them effectively."

At the beginning of Section VI, you were asked to consider whether a person can truly understand a client from a different culture. Now that you've read Chapters 13 and 14, you may want to consider whether you agree with the first counselor, that all counseling is multicultural, or with the second counselor, that some groups' cultural differences are great and one must have basic knowledge of these groups and skills to work with clients from these groups.

I'll let you decide where you stand, but my answer to this challenge lies somewhere in the middle. Is it necessary to gain knowledge and skills about different cultural and ethnic groups? I say, "Yes," because to have empathy and understanding of others, we need to be able to understand fully the world in which the client lives. However, knowledge of specific cultures can also lead to stereotyping, generalizing, and not fully seeing the uniqueness of the client. Perhaps we have to have the knowledge and skills, and also treat the individual as a unique person just like any other person:

> *No single counseling theory, construct, or tradition adequately suits all of the cultural groups in the United States . . . Therefore, it is unrealistic to expect there to be a prescription for culture-specific interventions. Instead, culturally alert counseling consists of counselor vigilance about the impact of culture on people accompanied by a set of some culturally alert practice. In fact, many existing counseling approaches can be used, but in a culturally intentional way.*

> (McAuliffe, 2013b, p. 545)

Client-Counselor Match Versus Cultural Competence

The research on counseling outcomes when client and counselor are matched based on any of a number of ethnic, cultural, or gender demographics is relatively new and somewhat mixed. However, overall, it does seem to indicate that when client and counselor are matched, outcomes tend to be better (see Dana, Gamst, Der-Karabetian, & Kramer, 2001; Gamst, Dana, Der-Karabetian, & Kramer, 2004; Kim, Ng, & Ahan, 2009; Whitfield, Venable,

& Broussard, 2010). Sue and Lam (2002) note that counselor-client match is probably most important for unacculturated ethnic minorities. In addition, sometimes what appears to be a cultural match actually is not. For instance, a highly acculturated, middle-class, male, African-American counselor may have difficulty relating to a poor African-American male client. In this case, although culture is matched, social class and acculturation are not—both of which may be more important factors. In the long run, it appears that what might be most important is the counselor's cultural competence—that is, whether the counselor has gained the necessary knowledge and skills about the client's culture to work effectively with him or her and is able to demonstrate to the client that he or she is understood (McAulife, Gómez, & Grothaus, 2013; McAuliffe, Grothaus, Paré, & Wolf, 2013).

Ethical, Professional, and Legal Issues: Making Wise Ethical Decisions

Although ethics codes in the mental health professions, including the ACA (2014a) code, tend to include many statements that focus on diversity, their use can be problematic for counselors, as counselors are sometimes challenged to either follow the code and disregard the cultural context of the client, or respect the cultural context of the client and disregard the code (Pedersen, 2008). This is because despite the efforts to make the codes cross-culturally sensitive, they still tend to reflect the dominant values of the society in which they were created. Consider, for example, the following situation:

> You are working with a first-generation Somali client who tells you she is planning to take her teenage daughter on "vacation" to Somalia with one goal being to have her daughter undergo a partial clitoridectomy—the removal of part of her clitoris (see Turkewitz, 2014). You realize that federal law bans this practice, as well as the transport of young girls for this purpose. However, your client believes that it is an important ritual that speaks to the value of her culture and her religion. What do you do?

In the above scenario, you realize your legal obligation and you understand your ethical responsibility to ensure the safety of the girl, but you may also be conflicted, as you have a sense of the importance of the ceremony to your client. In addition, your values are different from your client's, and your ethics code says that your values should not interfere with your efforts to counsel the client. So, what do you do?

Although I'll let you decide on the decision in this scenario, you can see that clearly, ethical decision making is complex. On the one hand, we must carefully use our ethical codes and understand our legal obligations. But how do we reconcile with our ethical and legal obligations with our attempts to understand the cultural differences of our clients. In addition, what is our obligation to our own value system, such as our sense that this practice is a way of oppressing women? In the end, when making ethical decisions, we must make careful, wise choices based on all the evidence. Such wise decisions often involve a deeply self-reflective process, as well as the attainment of as much knowledge as possible of the situation at hand.

The Counselor in Process: The Ongoing Process of Counseling the Culturally Different

Despite the fact that throughout this text, we have stressed specific methods of working effectively with clients, it should be emphasized that counseling methods are not fixed. This is particularly true in the realm of multicultural counseling, as new approaches to working with clients from diverse backgrounds are quickly finding their way into the professional literature. For instance, international counseling theories, which have been largely ignored by American counselors and psychotherapists and which sometimes approach counseling in ways that vary greatly from what we are used to, are now being researched (Gerstein, Heppner, Aegisdóttir, Leung, & Norsworthy, 2009). This is particularly important because counseling theories are almost exclusively centered around Western values (Neukrug, 2011). As counselors, we must continue to find the best ways to assist all individuals. We must continue to examine new treatment approaches, explore new counseling theories, and be open to an expansive view of counseling all individuals. Perhaps we can learn from Mahatma Gandhi, who noted:

> *I do not wish my house to be walled on all sides and my windows stuffed. I want the cultures of all lands to be blown about my house as freely as possible.*

Summary

In this chapter, we examined the changing face of the United States and noted that this country is becoming increasingly diverse, as evidenced by the fact that by 2043, the majority of Americans will be from nondominant groups. We then highlighted a number of diverse groups, starting with a discussion of people from varying cultural and racial heritages. We first presented some background information about African Americans, Latinos/Latinas/Hispanics, Asian Americans, and Native Americans. In addition, while encouraging the reader not to overgeneralize, we examined some common customs, values, and behaviors held by many individuals within each of these groups. Also, we highlighted important issues that should be addressed in the counseling relationship with these groups and presented specific suggestions for working with individuals from these groups.

In addition to examining people from varying cultural/racial heritages, we explored a number of other groups because of their unique needs and their tendency to face discrimination. We discussed diversity in religious affiliation and spiritual beliefs, differences between women and men, differences in sexual orientation, and the special issues of individuals who are HIV positive, homeless and poor, older persons, the mentally ill, and individuals with disabilities. Two specific standards that were pointed out included the ASERVIC competencies concerning religion and spirituality, and the APA Guidelines for the Psychological Practice with Girls and Women.

For each diverse group discussed, we highlighted some of the major issues that individuals within that group are likely to face. For instance, we discussed the importance of recognizing the differences among religions in the United States and throughout the world; the sociopolitical and psychological differences between men and women; some of the myths about and biases against gays, bisexuals, lesbians, and transgender individuals; the physical and emotional needs of individuals who are HIV positive; the unique characteristics and needs of many individuals who are homeless, poor, or both; the interpersonal, psychological, and physical changes that face many older persons; the changes in the treatment of the mentally ill over the years; and the emotional, physical, psychological, and legal concerns of individuals with disabilities. For each of these groups, we talked about the importance of having the correct attitudes and beliefs, knowledge, and skills and highlighted important issues of that group while noting some important counseling concerns. We offered specific steps for working with these groups in the helping relationship.

As we neared the end of this chapter, we reminded you of the debate in the field concerning the definition of multicultural counseling, and asked you to decide where you stand. We noted that some assert that all counseling is multicultural and that being culturally sensitive and culturally appropriate by gathering specific knowledge of ethnic and cultural groups can lead to stereotyping and gross generalizations. In contrast, we noted that others assert that knowledge of a client's cultural background is essential if we are to understand and work effectively with that client. We concluded that in order to gain empathy for the culturally different client, it may be important to learn about cultures. However, we also warned that the counselor be vigilant in not stereotyping a client.

Next, we discussed the fact that outcome research on matching client and counselor demographics is a bit mixed, although overall, it does seem that client-counselor match by culture, ethnicity, or both seems to have stronger client outcomes than when clients and counselors are not of similar backgrounds. We also suggested that regardless of whether there is a cultural or ethnic matching of clients and counselors, it is critical that the counselor has gained the necessary knowledge and skills to be an effective cross-cultural counselor and whether the client feels understood by the counselor.

The next part of the chapter examined ethical, professional, and legal issues relative to diversity. We noted that following an ethics code explicitly can sometimes be problematic if what is stated in the code conflicts with the client's culture. This, we noted, could create a dilemma for the counselor—should the counselor follow the code or be respectful of the client's cultural context? We offered one example of this potential dilemma and encouraged counselors to make wise, reflective, and thoughtful decisions when faced with such a conundrum.

Finally, the chapter concluded by noting that the theories and skills important to the multicultural counseling relationship will continue to change in the future, perhaps more rapidly than in other counseling disciplines. We highlighted the importance of staying current with these changes if we are to be effective with clients from diverse backgrounds.

 ## Further Practice

Visit CengageBrain.com to respond to additional material that highlight the salient aspects of the chapter content. There, you can find ethical, professional, and legal vignettes, a number of experiential exercises, and study tools including a glossary, flashcards, and sample test items. Hopefully, these will enhance your learning and be fun and interesting.

SELECT SPECIALTY AREAS IN COUNSELING

CHAPTER 16 **School Counseling**

CHAPTER 17 **Clinical Mental Health Counseling**

CHAPTER 18 **Student Affairs and College Counseling (Postsecondary Counseling)**

Overview

The three chapters in this section represent the most frequently chosen specialty areas of today's counseling students. Chapter 16 focuses on elementary, middle, and high school counseling. Chapter 17 examines a large array of agency and private practice settings, and Chapter 18 examines a wide range of settings in which a counselor might work in higher education. Throughout these chapters, the same format is used, and it includes a broad definition of what the specialty area encompasses, a brief history of the specialty area, some typical functions and roles of counselors in that specialty area, the theoretical basis by which counselors in the specialty area work, and examples of settings where we find the counselor in the specialty area. As with all previous chapters, we conclude with a discussion of multicultural/social justice issues; ethical, professional, and legal concerns; and some thoughts about "the counselor in process."

Many of you may have already decided the specialty area that best suits you. For you, these sections will likely offer a little more depth about your chosen career goal as they highlight foundational components of each specialty area. For the rest of you, I believe these chapters will help you choose the specialty area that you want to pursue. By understanding the philosophical basis and practical implications of each specialty area, your choice about your future specialty area in counseling will hopefully become clearer. In either case, I hope you find the following chapters interesting and enlightening.

School Counseling

By Emily Goodman-Scott and Ed Neukrug

When I (Emily Goodman-Scott) was young, I was curious about pursuing a career in education, but I didn't see myself as a classroom teacher or administrator and didn't know much about other opportunities. After completing a bachelor's degree, I worked as a special education autism teacher and immediately felt at home in the K-12 school environment. I particularly enjoyed being on the school leadership team and meeting regularly with my students' parents. I didn't feel compelled to teach long term, and I explored other professional opportunities.

One day, I shadowed a school counselor at a Title 1, urban elementary school. What a day—I don't think we sat down once! I watched this school counselor advocate for resources for students and families struggling with homelessness, create student behavior plans, conduct individual and group counseling, consult with teachers and administrators, and meet with parents and students to create individualized student plans of study for middle school and plan for the upcoming transition. After enjoying the hectic and inspiring day, I knew school counseling was my home.

I completed a master's degree in counselor education with a strong school counseling professional identity and had the privilege to work as a school counselor at a new school in the suburbs of the diverse Washington D.C. Metro area. There, I designed a school counseling program from infancy, using the ASCA National Model as my guide. Opening a new school required a lot of time, but it was gratifying to help build a school community from the ground up.

Even with an optimal school counseling job and a fantastic school and district, I saw a disconnect between the school counseling training from my master's program and how I was actually perceived and utilized as a school counselor. There were drastic budget cuts early in my school counseling career, which included discussions of cutting school counseling positions. I spent time advocating for and educating others about the school counselor's role, both inside my school and with local policymakers. I remember my principal telling me: *School counselors are so busy advocating for others, they often don't advocate for themselves.*

I saw firsthand that school counselors can make a big difference serving students, schools, and communities . . . but I also saw that not everyone understood the role of the school counselor. Although I loved my school counseling job, I decided I wanted to serve students, schools, and communities in a new capacity: as a school counselor educator. In this role, I could prepare school counselors for their future jobs, as well as contribute to the field through research, leadership, and service. Although the profession has made great gains in the last several decades, there is still work to do.

This chapter will explore the world of the school counselor. You will first be given some brief definitions of school counseling and then be presented with a synopsis of the history of school counseling. This will be followed by a description of the functions and roles of the school counselor and some of the theories school counselors use in their work. Next, we will examine the settings and the kinds of work school counselors do in elementary, middle, and high schools, as well as at the district and state levels. The chapter will conclude by discussing multicultural/social justice, ethical, professional, and legal issues in school counseling.

What Is School Counseling?

The school counselor's roles are many and varied and sometimes much more involved than most people think (see Table 16.1). One moment a school counselor might be chatting with a student about his college application, and the next moment engrossed with a sobbing student that is threatening to kill herself. Over the last few decades, school counseling has changed its emphasis from providing services for some students to implementing a comprehensive school counseling program (CSCP) that serves *all* students. The American School Counselor Association (ASCA) suggests that in addition to asking the question, "What do school counselors do?" school counselors now must also answer the question, "How are students different as a result of what we do?" (ASCA, 2012). So, who is the school counselor? ASCA's role statement for school counselors states:

> *Professional school counselors are certified/licensed educators with a minimum of a master's degree in school counseling, making them uniquely qualified to address all students' academic, career, and personal/social development needs by designing, implementing, evaluating and enhancing a comprehensive school counseling program that promotes and enhances student success. Professional school counselors are employed in elementary, middle/junior high and high schools; in district supervisory positions; and counselor education positions. Professional school counselors serve a vital role in maximizing student success (Lapan, Gysbers, & Kayson, 2007; Dahir & Stone, 2012). Through leadership, advocacy, and collaboration, professional school counselors promote equity and access to rigorous educational experiences for all students. Professional school counselors support a safe learning environment and work to safeguard the human rights of all members of the school community (Sandhu, 2000), and address the needs of all students through culturally relevant prevention and intervention programs that are a part of a comprehensive school counseling program (Lee, 2001).*

> (ASCA, n.d., para. 1–2)

In 2013, the American Counseling Association (ACA) School Counseling Task Force defined school counseling in relation to the larger counseling field:

> *Counseling is a professional relationship that empowers diverse individuals, families, and groups to accomplish mental health, wellness, education, and career goals. Using counseling theories and techniques, school counselors accomplish these goals by fostering educational and social equity, access, and success.*

TABLE 16.1 Examples of the Many Roles and Functions of the Professional School Counselor

➤ A student is sent to the counselor by his second-grade teacher with a note that reads,"Tomas hasn't been himself. He's not getting his work completed and doesn't seem to be paying attention. Would you please talk with him and see what might be going on?"

➤ The high school counselor notes the disproportionally low number of students of color, students receiving special education services, and students receiving free and reduced lunches enrolled in AP or IB classes and rigorous coursework. She states her concern at the school leadership team meeting, advocates for collaboration with feeder schools to address this situation, and works toward making the system more equitable.

➤ Some third graders are immersed in a group for students whose parents are deployed in the military.

➤ Checking in on the new faculty, the school counselor notes that a first-year seventh-grade teacher is struggling with classroom management in one of his classes. The school counselor offers to consult with the teacher.

➤ James, a quiet third-grade boy, comes to school with bruises on his upper arms. He reveals to the school counselor that his father punches him and hurts him.

➤ A school counselor conducts a series of classroom guidance lessons on harassment, bullying, and the role of bystanders for the sixth-grade classes. The school counselor consults and collaborates with the sixth-grade faculty teams and administrator to implement school safety measures and enhance the school climate.

➤ Jamal, a twelfth-grade student, asks his counselor to write a college recommendation letter.

➤ The school counselor is part of the Response to Intervention team examining services for English Language Learners (ELL) schoolwide and for those ELL students who have low test scores.

➤ Two fifth-grade students who were arguing on a school bus begin to push and shove one another. The bus driver tells them to go to the counselor or they will be disciplined. The counselor works with the students to mediate their concern and also has them join a social skills/conflict resolution skills group.

➤ Concerned about the high rate of ninth-grade retention, the school counselor collaborates with the school improvement team to implement a prevention plan that includes classroom guidance lessons on study skills, time management, and test-taking skills (with small groups for those needing additional assistance); establishing a peer tutoring program; and coordinating the training, supervision, and services offered by volunteer mentors from the community.

➤ Rachel, a fourth-grade student, requests to see the counselor to talk about a problem in one of her classes. In the middle of the conversation, she blurts out that her parents have just separated, and she begins to sob.

➤ Concerned about the discrepancies in the number of disciplinary referrals along racial or ethnic lines, a school counselor decides to meet with principals and teachers to develop a plan to address this issue.

➤ A parent shares with the school counselor that his daughter is receiving treatment for substance abuse and asks the counselor to coordinate in-school services with the substance abuse treatment agency.

➤ A student approaches the school counselor with concerns about being pregnant and not wanting her parents to know.

➤ A middle school counselor and a high school counselor are asked to join a districtwide task force seeking to increase the number of students completing high school and attending a postsecondary institution.

➤ The parent of an eighth grader comes to see the counselor with concerns over the violence in her community and how it might affect her son. The counselor connects her with resources in their community, including a community advocacy group to which the counselor belongs.

➤ Your school system's school counseling director asks all of the counselors to examine aggregated and disaggregated high-stakes test scores in their building and then develop a plan to assist students with low test scores.

➤ Two seventh graders approach the school counselor with a concern that their friend has been cutting and sometimes burning himself on a regular basis.

➤ The school counselor works with the tenth-grade language arts faculty to develop a career guidance curriculum that fits into the language arts curriculum.

➤ A group of eleventh-grade girls comes to the school counselor concerned about sexually transmitted diseases.

➤ A group of several elementary school counselors work together to provide peer supervision. They decide to assist and support each other as all of them apply for Recognized ASCA Model Program (RAMP) status, a national recognition of a fully implemented school counseling program.

➤ A teacher asks the counselor how to interpret the achievement test scores for her classes.

➤ The school counselor works with a first-grade teacher to implement behavior plans and classroom management/instructional changes for students struggling in her class.

> *The professional school counselor serves as a leader and an assertive advocate for students, consultant to families and educators, and team member to teachers, administrators, and other school personnel to help each student succeed.*
>
> (as cited in Erford, 2015, p. 2)

In order to become a school counselor, typically one must have a master's degree in school counseling, similar to master's degrees in other counseling specialty areas. The preparation program requirements range from having one distinctive course in school counseling (along with practicum and/or internship experiences in the schools) to having most of the classes geared specifically to school counseling. In many programs, students who are in the school counseling "track" are asked to focus their projects on school counseling as they take all of their courses. At this time, approximately 55% of school counseling master's programs in the United States are accredited by the Council for Accreditation of Counseling and Related Programs (CACREP) (T. Kimbel, personal communication, March 19, 2014). Some states offer a K-12 school counseling credential, whereas others have separate credentialing for elementary, middle, and high school counselors. In a handful of states, school counselors are required to have teaching certificates and experience, although the trend has been to eliminate this prerequisite.

Although school counseling is commonplace today, this was not always the case. Let's review the history of school counseling and then take a more extensive look at the roles and functions of school counselors.

A History of School Counseling

Early Developments

Although societies throughout the world have long provided means and methods to support or train their youth to assume adult roles, the systematic provision of counseling and guidance to young people appears to be an American innovation (Erford, 2015). Against the backdrop of the Industrial Revolution and the progressive education movement, vocational guidance interventions attempted to assist young people in their moral or character development and to negotiate the work environment (Schmidt, 2013). Early efforts included George Merrill's vocational guidance program at the California School of Mechanical Arts in San Francisco in 1895, Jesse B. Davis's initiation of a systematic guidance program at Central High School in Detroit in 1898, and the work of Anna Y. Reed in Seattle schools and Eli Weaver at Boys High School of Brooklyn (Baker & Gerler, 2008).

From the start, school counselors' roles and functions have been responsive to the influential social, political, and economic concerns of the times. At the beginning of the twentieth century, the first school counselors, then called *vocational counselors*, were trained in response to an increased need for vocational guidance (Gysbers & Henderson, 2012). Society was becoming more complex, and individuals struggled to find their place in a rapidly changing world. Recognizing the need to train experts in vocational guidance, Frank Parsons organized the Boston Vocational Bureau in 1908, which trained teachers and others in vocational guidance. Parsons, who developed the *trait-and-factor* approach to vocational guidance, believed that successful vocational choice was based on (1) an understanding of self (e.g., abilities, interests, and basic personality dynamics); (2) knowledge of the principles of success and of occupational information; and (3) the ability to make a reasoned vocational choice based on one's understanding of self and one's knowledge of the world of work (Schmidt, 2013).

Parsons (1909/2009) was very concerned about the counseling process, and many of his ideas were ahead of his time. For instance, he believed that counselors should possess the following qualifications:

1. A practical working knowledge of the fundamental principles and methods of modern psychology.
2. An experience involving sufficient human contact to give them an intimate acquaintance with human nature in a considerable number of its different phases; they must understand the dominant motives, interests, and ambitions that control people's lives, and be able to recognize the symptoms that indicate the presence or absence of important elements of character.
3. An ability to deal with young people in a sympathetic, earnest, searching, candid, helpful, and attractive way.
4. A knowledge of requirements and conditions of success, compensation, prospects, advantages, and disadvantages, etc., in different lines of industry.
5. Information relating to courses of study and means of preparing for various callings and developing efficacy therein.
6. Knowledge of scientific method analysis and principles of investigation by which laws and causes are ascertained, facts are classified, and correct conclusions drawn. (pp. 94–95)

Widely recognized as the *founder of vocational guidance,* Parsons helped to identify and launch a new profession, *guidance counseling* (Pope & Sveinsdottir, 2005). His work, along with the efforts of Merrill, Davis, Weaver, Reed, and others, greatly influenced American education and was an impetus for the spread of vocational guidance to school systems around the country (Erford, 2015; Gysbers & Henderson, 2012; Schmidt, 2013) (see Chapter 2). Although Parsons died at a relatively young age in 1908, his efforts were responsible for the first use of school counselors: teachers who added vocational counselor duties to their full-time job. This eventually led to the first required certification for guidance personnel, which was mandated in New York State in 1926. Counseling, at least vocational counseling, was establishing itself in the schools.

Developments in the area of assessment came on the heels of the vocational guidance movement. Soon, psychometrics was to become a crucial piece of vocational guidance, as it was the vehicle to help students and others identify their abilities and interests. Guidance work in schools was also influenced in these early decades by the burgeoning mental hygiene movement with its emphasis on individual adjustment and mental health (Baker & Gerler, 2008; Gysbers & Henderson, 2012).

As vocational guidance spread throughout the United States, individuals began to advocate for a broader approach to school counseling that attended to a large variety of students' psychological and educational needs (Erford, 2015). For instance, advocates like John Brewer (1932) suggested that guidance be seen in a total educational context and that guidance counselors be involved in a variety of functions in the schools, including adjustment counseling, assistance with curriculum planning, classroom management, and, of course, occupational guidance. During the 1930s and into the 1940s, school guidance workers often used E. G. Williamson's *directive approach* to counseling, which promoted setting goals, overcoming obstacles, and achieving a satisfactory lifestyle (Schmidt, 2013).

During the 1940s, the directive approach was overshadowed by the *nondirective*, relationship-oriented, humanistic approaches of Carl Rogers and others (Gysbers & Henderson, 2012). The humanistic philosophy was to affect all of counseling, and it soon seeped into the training of school counselors. The days where school counselors were seen as only providing vocational counseling within a directive and didactic framework were clearly gone. Now, within a humanistic framework, they would provide a broad spectrum of counseling services that included mental health counseling, consultation, coordination of services, and, of course, the more traditional guidance functions.

Modern-Day School Counseling: Becoming a Profession

Several factors led to the rapid expansion of school counseling and the emergence of school counseling as a recognized profession. The United States increasingly prioritized employment and vocational counseling as a result of the Great Depression in the 1930s and World War II veterans seeking employment in the 1940s. Thus, the federal government passed the 1946 *Vocational Education Act*, which provided federal funds to support guidance, counseling, and counselor training and leadership at the local and state levels (Gysbers & Henderson, 2012). For the first time, the federal government funded counseling and guidance in schools.

During the 1950s, the school counseling field was further defined by the creation of professional counseling organizations and ethical standards for preparation and practice (Erford, 2015). In 1953, the *American School Counselor Association (ASCA)* became the fifth division of the *American Personnel and Guidance Association* (today, the *American Counseling Association, or ACA*). Over the years, ASCA has shaped the direction of school counseling through discussion, debate, conferences, and the publication of role statements, journals, position papers, ethical standards, and more recently, a national model for school counseling. Also during the 1950s, the *Association for Counselor Education and Supervision (ACES)* and the *National Career Development Association (NCDA)*, two other ACA divisions, were founded. These associations have significantly contributed to the development of school counseling by highlighting school counseling issues, developing interest networks, establishing accreditation procedures, offering program sessions at conferences, supporting legislative initiatives, and collaborating with ASCA (Baker & Gerler, 2008). During the 1950s, the term *guidance counselor* was widely used to label school counselors (Erford, 2015).

In 1957, the Soviet satellite Sputnik "launched" a new round of Cold War competition between the United States and the Soviet Union. Suddenly, Americans were jolted into believing there was a great need for more trained scientists so that we could beat the Soviets to the moon. There was public criticism of education and its failure to supply trained individuals for careers identified as vital to the national well-being. As a direct result, the *National Defense Education Act (NDEA)* of 1958 was passed to help create and define counseling positions within the public schools. This act allocated funds for training institutes to quickly graduate secondary school counselors. Those counselors were then charged with the task of identifying young people who had math and science talent and to encourage these students to pursue further studies in the sciences. Although the goal of the NDEA was to train vocational counselors, the humanistic and mental health orientation of school counseling was firmly embedded into counselor training, and before long, these guidance counselors were also providing individual and group counseling, as well as consulting with parents and school staff.

In the middle and late 1960s, school counseling expanded further with the passage of the *Elementary and Secondary Education Act* and amendments to the *Vocational Education Act*. These acts focused on the implementation of specialized programs beyond the traditional college-bound and vocationally oriented students to include services for students from families with low income, school dropouts, and those having severe academic problems, as well as promoting elementary school counseling (Erford, 2015). These acts and others directly stimulated growth in many other areas of the school counseling profession, including performance standards for school counselors, criteria for the credentialing of school counselors, and the strengthening of accrediting bodies, such as those established by state departments of education. All of these developments launched a new era in the guidance and counseling profession (Gibson & Mitchell, 2008).

The vision for the school counseling profession broadened in the 1960s, 1970s, and 1980s. As a result of the Civil Rights Movement and greater diversity in society and the schools, the field placed greater emphasis on multicultural counseling (Erford, 2015). In addition, during these decades, counseling graduate programs taught developmental theory and school counselors incorporated human development concepts into their work with students (Havighurst, 1972). Then, in the late 1960s and 1970s, professional leaders proposed a change in school counseling implementation. Rather than school counselors primarily providing ancillary counseling, consultation, and guidance services to *some* students with the highest needs, school counselors were tasked with systematically providing a developmentally appropriate, goal-oriented, accountability-based program of counseling and guidance services to *all* students and the school as a whole (Erford, 2015; Gysbers & Henderson, 2012). ASCA endorsed the guidance and counseling program model in 1974 (Gysbers & Henderson), which has been known by several names, including CSCPs, comprehensive developmental guidance programs, and similar variations. Although leaders created the concept of CSCPs decades ago, it took many years for the model to become widespread, something counseling leaders are still working on today.

Recognizing the evolution of the profession, in 1990 the ASCA Governing Board unanimously voted to call the profession *school counseling* and the programs that school counselors offered *school counseling programs* (ASCA, 2005a). This shift signified the changing direction of school counseling over the years.

Educational Standardization, High-Stakes Testing, and the Achievement Gap

In the last several years, school counselors have undergone a major shift in how they do business (Martin, 2015). This is a result of a number of initiatives that have had a major impact on school counseling: high-stakes testing, educational standardization, and the achievement gap. During the 1990s, many states developed learning standards whose purpose was to ensure that all children succeeded in school. These standards, as reflected in children's scores on statewide high-stakes testing, were an attempt to make sure that all children were meeting minimum competencies in the schools. Increasingly, school personnel were being held accountable for the test scores of all the children in their classes. Although the standards emphasized "all" children, the most significant impact was upon students of color, students from families with low income, English language learners, and children with disabilities, as these children had traditionally done most poorly on standardized tests. This achievement gap needed to be eliminated if children were to succeed.

In 2001, President George W. Bush signed the *No Child Left Behind (NCLB) Act,* which declared that within the next twelve years, each state needed to demonstrate that all students achieved proficiency in reading/language arts and math as reflected in scores on standardized tests (U.S. Department of Education, 2001). Although many states had statewide learning standards, competencies, and tests to measure student achievement, NCLB dictated requirements for all states. The goal of this federal law was to close the achievement gap by ensuring that all students had fair and equal access to education. However, NCLB placed particular pressure on the lower-performing school districts, which tended to be located in poorer neighborhoods (Baker, Robinson, Danner, & Neukrug, 2001; Neukrug & Fawcett, 2015). Many school districts in high-poverty areas found themselves struggling to focus limited resources on bringing up achievement test scores while also trying to maintain other needed resources (Holcomb-McCoy, 2007).

Transforming School Counseling in the Twenty-First Century

The educational emphasis on high-stakes testing had quite an impact on the role of the school counselor. New initiatives for school counseling were developed, as reflected by publications and projects sponsored by the *Education Trust* (2006), and ASCA, including the *ASCA National Model* (2012).

In the wake of high-stakes testing and accountability, school counselors have become an integral part of the educational team to ensure that all students are achieving (Martin, 2015). No longer can counselors be on the sidelines of education, supporting the educational process. No longer can they see themselves as separate from teachers and administrators, or as running miniature mental health clinics in the schools. Instead, school counselors are being asked to demonstrate that the services they provided assist teachers and students in creating a more effective learning environment—an environment that allows children to learn in ways that would be reflected on achievement test scores. Table 16.2 presents this new vision of the school counselor and compares it with the way that school counselors have been trained in the past.

This redefinition of school counseling was the result of grants funded by the *Education Trust* and a new model for developing and implementing CSCPs called, as noted earlier, the *ASCA National Model.* Let's take a quick look at each of these.

TABLE 16.2   Transformation of the Role of the Professional School Counselor

PRESENT FOCUS	NEW VISION
Mental health issues	Academic and student achievement
Individual student concerns and issues	Whole school and system concerns and issues
Clinical model focused on student deficits	Academic focus, building on student strengths
Providing service , one-to-one and small groups	Leading, planning, and developing programs
Primary focus on personal/social	Focus on academic counseling, learning and achievement, supporting student success
Ancillary support personnel	Integral members of educational team
Loosely defined role and responsibility	Focusing on mission and role identification
Record keeping	Use of data to effect change
Sorting, selecting course placement process	Advocating inclusion in rigorous preparation for all, especially students from low-income and minority families
Work in isolation or with other counselors	Teaming and collaboration with all educators in school in resolving issues involving the whole school and community
Guarding the status quo	Acting as a change agent, especially for educational equity for all students
Involvement primarily with students	Involvement with students, parents, education professionals, community, and community agencies
Little or no accountability	Full accountability for student success, use of data, planning and preparation for access to wide range of postsecondary options
Dependence on the system's resources for helping students and families	Brokering services for parents and students from community resources/agencies as well as the school system's resources
Postsecondary planning with interested students	Creating pathways for all students to achieve high aspirations

SOURCE: Martin, P. J. (2015). Transformational thinking in today's schools. In B. T. Erford (Ed.), *Transforming the school counseling profession* (4th ed., pp. 45–65). Boston, MA: Pearson, p. 55.

The Education Trust

Arguing that school counselors were not trained for the twenty-first century, during the late 1990s and into the new millennium, the Education Trust funded major grants to a number of universities across the country to help them develop plans that would transform their school counselor training programs (Martin, 2015). Their model emphasized training counselors as educational leaders who can become advocates for all students as they focus on fostering academic achievement and career aspirations. In addition, this model saw school counselors as an integral part of the educational system, not an ancillary service, and believed that counselors should play a crucial role in helping all students achieve academically. The Education Trust has been a major impetus in transforming the role of school counselors. Their model influenced the development of the ASCA National Model.

The ASCA National Model

Recognizing that school counselors were being left on the sidelines during the discussions of educational reform, ASCA published the *National Standards for School Counseling*

Programs (Campbell & Dahir, 1997), which contained the standards and competencies (knowledge, attitudes, and skills) that students were expected to gain in the academic, career, and personal/social domains as a result of participating in a CSCP. These standards were revised in 2004 as the *ASCA National Standards for Students,* and again in 2014 as the *ASCA Mindsets and Behaviors for Student Success: K-12 College- and Career-Readiness Standards for Every Student.*

ASCA collaborated with the Education Trust and leaders in the field of school counseling to develop a CSCP model that all school counselors could use as a framework for designing and implementing a school counseling program. The result was the ASCA National Model, first published in 2003 then revised in 2005 and 2012 (ASCA, 2012). This innovative model (see Figure 16.1) has four systems: *foundation, delivery, management,* and *accountability.* Central to each of these systems is the belief that school counselors must be leaders, advocates, collaborators, and systemic change agents.

In an effort to further define school counseling and clarify the school counselor's role in implementing a CSCP, ASCA created competencies and codes for school counselors aligned with the National Model. The organization's *Ethical Standards for School Counselors* (ASCA, 2010) outlines expectations for ethical school counseling practice. In addition, ASCA created *School Counselor Competencies* (ASCA, 2012), which describes school counselors' knowledge, abilities, skills, and attitudes in implementing a CSCP and meeting students' academic, career, and personal/social needs.

FIGURE 16.1
The ASCA National
Model Graphic

SOURCE: American School
Counselor Association.
(2005a). *The ASCA national
model: A framework for school
counseling programs* (2nd ed.).
Arlington, VA: Author, p. 20.

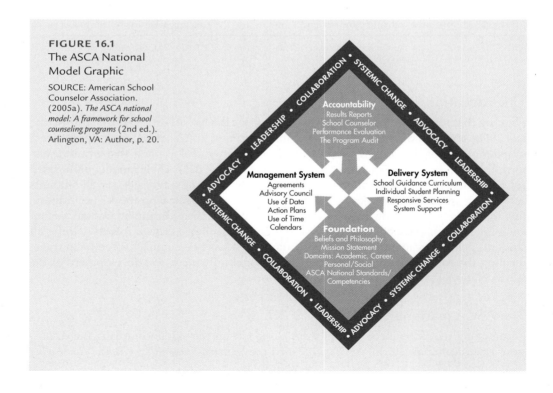

Recent History: College and Career Readiness

NCLB has been criticized for using a one-size-fits-all approach by heavily focusing on test scores rather than student growth and progress (The White House, n.d.b). In the last couple of years, most states have been granted waivers from implementing NCLB (U.S. Department of Education, 2014b). These states must continue to demonstrate student achievement and closing achievement gaps, but can have greater flexibility to adapt interventions for the unique needs of each school. In exchange for these NCLB waivers, states must create a plan for college and career focused standards, teacher and principal development and evaluation, and continue to implement interventions to decrease the achievement gap and improve student achievement.

In 2010, a group of state leaders and educational groups introduced the *Common Core State Standards*, rigorous math and English language arts student standards that had a particular emphasis on students being prepared for future college and careers (ACA, 2013d). Almost all states have adopted these standards, which brings consistent course content across states, and more attention on preparing K-12 students to be ready for colleges and careers. In fact, many high school students are now required to have educational and career plans.

President Barack Obama aims that by the year 2020, the United States will have the highest percentage of college graduates in the world (The White House, n.d.a). In 2014, both U.S. Secretary of Education Arne Duncan and First Lady Michelle Obama named school counselors as an integral part of assisting all students to be college- and career-ready.

How has this increased emphasis on college and career readiness affected school counselors? School counselors are being asked to assist in removing student barriers to college and career access and promote college and career readiness for all K-12 students. School counseling–related organizations, such as the *College Board* and their affiliated *National Office for School Counselor Advocacy*, have resources to help school counselors with their college and career readiness mission. In addition, the most recently revised 2014 ASCA student standards place greater emphasis on student college and career preparation and are aligned with competencies such as the Common Core State Standards.

The school counseling profession has grown and evolved dramatically over the years, from its meager beginnings at the turn of the century, to its slow inclusion in the schools, to its rapid expansion as a result of Sputnik and the NDEA, to its broader humanistic, developmental, and comprehensive focus in recent years, to the widespread implementation of CSCPs such as the ASCA National Model. As the National Model is now central to what school counselors do, it will be discussed in detail in the next section.

Roles and Functions of School Counselors: The ASCA National Model

The ASCA National Model has revolutionized the profession by clarifying school counselors' roles and providing a unified professional identity. The National Model explains the school counselors' roles by focusing on activities that counselors should and should not be performing (see Box 16.1), providing a consistent professional vision for the field,

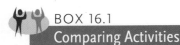

BOX 16.1
Comparing Activities

Appropriate Activities for School Counselors

- ➤ Individual student academic program planning
- ➤ Interpreting cognitive, aptitude, and achievement tests
- ➤ Providing counseling to students who are tardy or absent
- ➤ Providing counseling to students who have disciplinary problems
- ➤ Providing counseling to students as to appropriate school dress
- ➤ Collaborating with teachers to present school counseling core curriculum lessons
- ➤ Analyzing grade-point averages in relationship to achievement
- ➤ Interpreting student records
- ➤ Providing teachers with suggestions for effective classroom management
- ➤ Ensuring student records are maintained as per state and federal regulations
- ➤ Helping the school principal identify and resolve student issues, needs, and problems
- ➤ Providing individual and small-group counseling services to students
- ➤ Advocating for students at individual education plan meetings, student study teams, and attendance review boards
- ➤ Analyzing disaggregated data

Inappropriate Activities for School Counselors

- ➤ Coordinating paperwork and data entry of all new students
- ➤ Coordinating cognitive, aptitude, and achievement testing programs
- ➤ Signing excuses for students who are tardy or absent
- ➤ Performing disciplinary actions or assigning discipline consequences
- ➤ Sending students home who are not appropriately dressed
- ➤ Teaching classes when teachers are absent
- ➤ Computing grade-point averages
- ➤ Maintaining student records
- ➤ Supervising classrooms or common areas
- ➤ Keeping clerical records
- ➤ Assisting with duties in the principal's office
- ➤ Providing therapy or long-term counseling in schools to address psychological disorders . . .
- ➤ Coordinating schoolwide individual education plans, student study teams and school attendance review boards
- ➤ Serving as a data entry clerk

SOURCE: American School Counselor Association (2012). *The ASCA National Model: A framework for school counseling programs* (3rd ed.). Alexandria, VA: Author, p. 45.

recommending a data-driven decision-making process to guide services and demonstrate student impact, closing the achievement gap and advocating for social justice and equity in the schools, and connecting school counselors' goals to the school's mission.

The ASCA National Model, which has received the endorsement of the major players in the school counseling profession, is now taught in counselor education programs and being adopted by states and school systems across the nation.

A comprehensive school counseling program is an integral component of the school's academic mission. Comprehensive school counseling programs, driven by student data and based on standards in academic, career, and personal/social development, promote and enhance the learning process for all students. The ASCA National Model ensures equitable access to a rigorous education for all students, identifies the knowledge and skills that all students will acquire as a result of the K-12 comprehensive school counseling program, is delivered to all students in a systemic fashion, is based on data-driven decision making, and is provided by a state-credentialed school counselor (ASCA, 2012, pp. xii).

The model identifies four elements that are critical to the development and implementation of a comprehensive school counseling program: *foundation, management, delivery,* and *accountability.* Four overarching themes critical to the implementation of the four systems are also identified, including *leadership, advocacy, collaboration,* and *systemic change* (shown earlier in the chapter in Figure 16.1). The following is a summary of the four elements, followed by a summary of the themes.

The Four Elements: Foundation, Management, Delivery, and Accountability

Foundation

The foundation lays the groundwork for the National Model. Here, school counselors define the program with vision and mission statements, as well as program goals. Student and school counselor competencies and standards are housed in the foundation system, including the *ASCA School Counselor Competencies* (ASCA, 2012), the *Ethical Standards for School Counselors* (ASCA, 2010), the *ASCA Mindsets and Behaviors for Student Success* (2014), and related student standards, such as relevant Department of Education state standards. When implementing the ASCA National Model, school counselors should begin by developing the foundation.

Management

The management system is comprised of tools and assessments to assist school counselors to organize, implement, and evaluate their CSCPs, as well as collaborate with and report information to stakeholders. School counselors use self-assessments to determine the degree of CSCP implementation (*School Counseling Program Assessment*) and how they spend their time (*Use-of-Time-Assessment*). Tools for working with stakeholders include the *Annual Agreement* between the school counselors and supervising administrators, which outlines school counselors' responsibilities and goals. The management system provides recommendations for meeting with an *advisory council* of stakeholders to provide feedback on CSCP design and implementation. Data collection, analysis, and interpretation are crucial for assessing the impact that school counselors and school counselor–run CSCPs have on students and schools. The types of and uses for data are described in the management system. School counselors create *action plans* to design strategies for meeting CSCP goals and use *lesson plans* to thoughtfully plan for giving and evaluating classroom lessons. Finally, *calendars* are developed annually to purposefully plan for and advertise CSCP activities.

Delivery

The method that school counselors use to serve students and schools is outlined in the delivery system. The ASCA National Model recommends school counselors spend 80% of their time engaged in a combination of direct and indirect services, as shown in Figure 16.2. Direct services are face-to-face services *with* students, such as utilizing school counseling core curricula through teaching lessons and facilitating student workshops

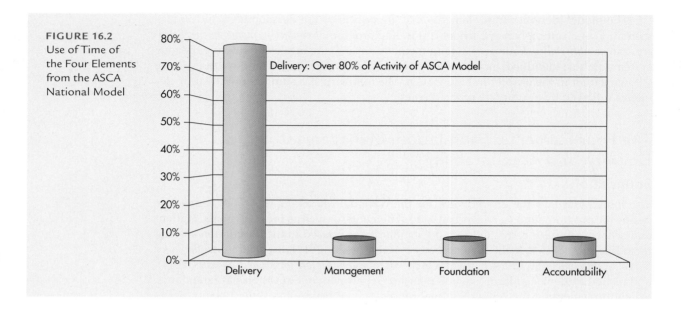

FIGURE 16.2
Use of Time of the Four Elements from the ASCA National Model

and activities; individual student planning, including advising and appraisal; and finally through responsive services, such as counseling and crisis response. School counselors conduct indirect services *for* students, usually by interacting with others such as teachers, parents, administrators, community members. Examples of indirect services are consultations, collaborations, and referrals. The majority of school counselors' time should be spent delivering services directly and indirectly to students. Since the ASCA National Model is a framework, school counselors can adapt their implementation for the unique needs of their school.

Accountability

The accountability system in the ASCA National Model addresses the question *How are students different as a result of the CSCP?* According to ASCA (2012), "school counselors use data to show the impact of the school counseling program on student achievement, attendance, and behavior and analyze school counseling program assessments to guide future action and improve future results for all students" (p. xiv). School counselors collect and evaluate data to create program goals, determine student progress and close the achievement gap, assess and evaluate programs, and determine the effectiveness of school counseling programs (Kaffenberger & Young, 2013). The ASCA Model provides a tool used by supervising administrators to evaluate school counselors' job performance (*School Counselor Performance Appraisal*). In addition to gathering and interpreting data to guide school counseling decisions, it is imperative that school counselors communicate findings to key stakeholders, which is described in the accountability system.

The Themes: Leadership, Advocacy, Collaboration, and Systemic Change

According to the ASCA National Model (2012), school counselors engage in the four themes of leadership, advocacy, collaboration, and systemic change to support every student's academic achievement and preparation for postsecondary opportunities.

Leadership

The effective school counselor is a leader in the schools and embraces qualities that include being collaborative, facilitative, professional, empowering, and encouraging (Gorton & Alston, 2012). If school counselors want to transform counseling programs into the new paradigm identified in ASCA's National Model, and if they desire to contribute significantly to lessening the achievement gap, they will increasingly take on leadership roles in the schools (DeVoss & Andrews, 2006). This involves the orchestration of services as they collaborate with stakeholders (Holcomb-McCoy, 2007). It means that school counselors can no longer isolate themselves from the mission of the educational system; instead, they must be essential players and voices within that system (Dahir & Stone, 2012). Leadership also involves being multiculturally responsive (Grothaus, Crum, & James, 2010).

Advocacy

Gordon (2006) noted that, "educational opportunity and academic achievement are directly tied to the social divisions associated with race, ethnicity, gender, first language, and social class" (p. 25). In order to counteract this inequitable status quo, being an advocate for student success has been identified as an essential role for school counselors (Howard & Solberg, 2006; McAuliffe, Grothaus, Paré, & Wolf, 2013; Ratts, DeKruyf, & Chen-Hayes, 2007). To paraphrase an old adage: *When we're not engaging in advocacy, we're part of the problem.* School counselors advocate for equity in access, support, and resources to ensure that all students are able to achieve academic success, acquire career and college readiness skills and knowledge, develop desirable personal/social attitudes and skills, and have viable postsecondary options. When advocating, school counselors may work directly with students or advocate on behalf of students while working with school staff, the community, and larger educational system to identify and remove barriers to student success (ASCA, 2012).

Collaboration

School counselors collaborate with colleagues, family members, and community partners to ensure that all students have access to rigorous academic preparation and receive the support necessary to be successful. "Through school, family and community collaboration, school counselors can access a vast array of support for student achievement and development that cannot be achieved by an individual, or school, alone" (ASCA, 2012, p. 6). School counselors should be especially attentive to collaborating with families, as research clearly indicates that enhanced family involvement in schools is related to a host of improvements for students (Bryan & Henry, 2008; Grothaus & Cole, 2010; Van Velsor & Orozco, 2007).

Systemic Change

Schools are like a family system: the individuals within the system are connected (ASCA, 2012), and school counselors must examine the school as a whole system. School counselors are in a unique and critical position to understand the systemic needs of schools because they are one of the few individuals in the school to examine systemwide data, and because they are collaborators who work with all the stakeholders in the school. School counselors are charged with challenging inequitable policies and systems and promoting equity for all students (ASCA, 2012; Grothaus & Johnson, 2012; Holcomb-McCoy, 2007). "Without a systemic approach that uses strategic interventions and multilevel approaches, school counseling programs struggle to align with the mission of schools and the educational program . . . many environmental factors affecting student development and achievement are beyond student control" (Lee & Goodnough, 2015, p. 70).

ASCA National Model Implementation

Although huge changes have occurred in school counselors' roles and functions as the result of the National Model and education reform efforts, these changes haven't occurred overnight. In the last several years, researchers found that school counselors are indeed performing job activities aligned with CSCP, such as the ASCA National Model; however, school counselors continue to perform other nonrecommended job activities as well (Goodman-Scott, in press; Rayle & Adams, 2008; Scarborough & Culbreth, 2008). Although CSCPs, are implemented in many schools and states (Burnham & Jackson, 2000; Martin, Carey, & DeCoster, 2009; Rayle & Adams, 2008), there remains a need to advocate for implementing this revolutionary school counseling approach in all schools. When implementing CSCPs such as the ASCA National Model, there are several factors to consider, such as the student benefits, suggested student ratios, RAMP designation, data-driven initiatives, and principal collaborations. We will wrap up this section by looking at each of these.

Student Benefits of CSCP Implementation

How do CSCPs, like the National Model, benefit students? CSCP implementation has been associated with students being better prepared for college and careers, as well as higher achievement scores (Carey, Harrington, Martin, & Stevenson, 2012; Sink, Akos, Turnbull, & Mvududu, 2008; Sink & Stroh, 2003). Not only that, but also students in schools with CSCPs reported higher grades and a more positive school climate (Lapan, Gysbers, & Sun, 1997), as well as feeling safer and having better relationships with teachers (Lapan, Gysbers, & Petroski, 2001). Implementing CSCPs have been related to better student attendance, graduation, retention suspension, and truancy rates (Burkard, Gillen, Martinez, & Skytte, 2012). Many researchers and practitioners speak highly of fully implemented CSCPs such as the ASCA National Model.

Student Ratios

When implementing CSCPs, like the National Model, the number of students assigned to each school counselors, known as the *student-to-school-counselor ratio,* is important. ASCA recommends 250 students for every school counselor (ASCA, 2012); however, the national average is actually 471 students (U.S. Department of Education, 2012)—nearly double that! California has the highest average caseload, with 1,016 students, while Wyoming's average is the lowest, at 200 students. Lower student-to-school-counselor ratios have been associated with higher student attendance and lower discipline and suspension rates (Carey, Harrington, Martin, & Stevenson, 2012; Lapan, Whitcomb, & Aleman, 2012). Lower ratios can be especially meaningful in schools in high-poverty areas, as lower ratios have been related to greater high school graduation rates, higher attendance rates, and fewer discipline referrals (Lapan, Gysbers, Stanley, & Pierce, 2012).

RAMP Designation

A growing national trend has been schools achieving the *Recognized ASCA Model Program (RAMP)* designation. This involves schools completing a rigorous refereed review process to determine whether the school counseling program is comprehensive, data driven, serves all students, and fully incorporates the four elements and four themes of the ASCA National Model (ASCA, 2013). As of 2013, nearly 500 schools nationwide have achieved the RAMP designation.

Data-Driven Implementation

Utilizing data is a tremendous part of implementing the ASCA National Model and CSCPs. In recent years, school counselors have been called on more and more to use data to inform their practice and demonstrate how students are affected by the school counselor and the school counseling program (ASCA, 2012; Dimmitt, Carey, & Hatch, 2007; Hatch, 2014; Kaffenberger & Young, 2013). School counselors can use data to determine school needs, set related goals, create an action plan for reaching goals, implement the action plan, assess outcomes, and share results with stakeholders. The *Center for School Counseling Outcome Research and Evaluation (CSCORE)* and the annual Evidence-Based School Counseling conference are both dedicated to promoting evidence-based practices in school counseling.

Principal Collaborations

Finally, a key component of implementing CSCPs, such as the ASCA National Model, is collaborating with school administrators. School counselors are often hired, supervised, and evaluated by school administrators, such as the building principal. Principals may not always understand the role of the school counselor, which can result in school counselors being assigned a range of job activities not aligned with the ASCA National Model (Clemens, Milsom, & Cashwell, 2009; Kimbel & Goodman-Scott, 2011). School counselors should build a collaborative relationship with their supervising administrators and use data to advocate for the implementation of CSCP-relevant job activities. Tips for creating a strong relationship with principals include meeting at the start of every school year and regularly throughout the school year; discussing and signing the annual agreement every year, which outlines the school counselor's roles and responsibilities; and learning about the principal's priorities and incorporating them into the school counseling program (Goodman-Scott, 2011).

Theory and Process of School Counseling

Because school counselors are involved in such a wide range of tasks, they need many theories and processes to perform the job adequately. Thus, school counselors need to know about a wide range of theories to implement such programs as the ASCA National Model. These include knowledge of *counseling theory, career development theory, human development theory,* and *systems theory,* discussed in the next sections.

Counseling Theory

In Chapter 4, we identified a number of counseling theories, all of which can be used to some degree when working with students. For instance, *humanistic theory* gives the school counselor the counseling skills necessary to understand the inner world of children, and *cognitive* and *behavioral theories* can be used by counselors who want to set specific goals that are focused on changing behaviors or cognitions. Although school counselors are trained in all of these theoretical approaches, due to time constraints on the job, they tend to practice theoretical approaches that lend themselves to short-term or brief-treatment modalities. Therefore, *behavioral, cognitive, reality therapy, solution-focused,* and *narrative approaches* are often used (Dahir & Stone, 2012; Murphy, 2008; Winslade & Monk, 2007). Although humanistic approaches can be unwieldy because of the amount of time they take, being empathic, the critical component of this type of approach, has been an important tool for building relationships with stakeholders.

Career Development Theory

A number of career development theories can be successfully applied in the schools. However, perhaps the most important approach in this context is the use of a developmental theory such as that of *Super's Lifespan Development Approach,* as it helps the school counselor devise career programs that are appropriate to children's age levels. Once such programs are devised, a number of other theories can be applied, so long as they are appropriate to the age level. For instance, developmental theory is the basis for devising career awareness programs for elementary school children, as this theory reminds us that young children are just beginning to explore the world of work; *trait-and-factor* and *personality theories* can be applied in middle school as children begin to examine who they are and what talents they possess; and *social cognitive career* and *constructivist theories* are important to high school students as they begin to examine the realities of work or college and to look at how they understand the world. Infusing multicultural responsiveness into any career theory appears vital, as studies have shown that some children begin to foreclose prematurely on career possibilities as early as age six or seven due to stereotypes based on gender, race, ethnicity, and social class (Jackson & Grant, 2004).

Human Development Theory

Knowledge of theories of normal and of abnormal development is crucial if school counselors are to understand how children develop over their lifespan. Thus, knowledge of *physical* and *cognitive development* helps school counselors identify those students who may be developmentally delayed or gifted. Knowledge of *moral development* helps school counselors understand why some children are self-reflective and humble, while others can be narcissistic and aggressive. *Lifespan development approaches*, such as that of Erik Erikson, can help the school counselor determine if a student is progressing normally and identify appropriate interventions if needed. Theories of *personality development* can help a school counselor understand why a student might be exhibiting what some call abnormal behavior. Such theory makes sense out of what sometimes appears to be nonsensical acting out. Still other developmental theories help us understand the sometimes dualistic world of the child and adolescent and reminds us that these seemingly black and white thinkers can, and hopefully will, grow into complex adults.

Systems Theory

Section III of this textbook introduced the concept of *systems theory* as it applies to family counseling, group counseling, and consultation and supervision. Clearly, knowledge of all three of these systems is a critical piece of the school counselor's job. Knowing how children "fit" into their family and understanding the complex dynamics of the family are basic to working with children and parents/guardians. Being able to work effectively with groups of children and having insight into the sometimes-intricate interactions that can occur are both critical if the school counselor is to work effectively in groups. In addition, school counselors can effectively plan CSCPs, seek resources, consult and advocate when they understand the complexity of the school as a system, the dynamics of the school system, as well as local and state policies and politics affecting education and their school. As Erford, House, and Martin (2007) suggest, "An appropriate mantra for professional school counselors might be: 'Fix the system, not the student' " (p. 12). Finally, understanding that administrative and clinical supervision impacts the counselor, and all with whom the counselor interacts (e.g., students, parents, staff, teachers, administrators), are additional important activities that the effective school counselor should embrace (Gysbers & Henderson, 2012; Virginia School Counselor Association, 2008).

Settings for School Counselors

School counselors are employed at the elementary, middle, and high school levels and serve as directors, supervisors, and counselor educators (ASCA, n.d.). Of all the counseling students graduating from CACREP-accredited programs, approximately 40% specialize in school counseling; and of these, approximately 32% work in elementary schools, 27% work in middle schools, and 41% work in high schools (Schweiger, Henderson, McCaskill, Clawson, & Collins, 2012). School counselors at the K-12 level provide comprehensive, developmental, preventive, multiculturally responsive services that address students' academic, career, and personal/social development (ASCA, 2012).

As a result of school counseling programs, all K-12 students should gain knowledge, attitudes, and skills on a wealth of academic, career, and social/emotional topics (ASCA, 2014). The recommended topics include learning strategies, self-management skills, and social skills, including the following:

- ➤ Critical thinking skills
- ➤ Creativity
- ➤ Time management
- ➤ Organizational and study skills
- ➤ Self-directed learning
- ➤ Media and technology skills
- ➤ Goal setting
- ➤ Choosing challenging coursework
- ➤ Making informed decisions
- ➤ Participating in enrichment and extracurricular activities
- ➤ Responsibility
- ➤ Balancing multiple activities
- ➤ Personal safety skills
- ➤ Independence
- ➤ Self-discipline
- ➤ Self-control
- ➤ Delaying immediate gratification for long-term rewards
- ➤ Strategies for reaching goals
- ➤ Coping skills
- ➤ Managing transitions and change
- ➤ Overcoming barriers to learning
- ➤ Perseverance
- ➤ Ethical decision making and social responsibility
- ➤ Professionalism
- ➤ Effective communication and listening
- ➤ Creating and maintaining positive relationships with peers and adults
- ➤ Leadership and teamwork
- ➤ Empathy
- ➤ Collaboration and cooperation
- ➤ Advocacy skills
- ➤ Assertiveness (ASCA, 2014)

School counselors at all grade levels can present these topics through classroom lessons, small and large groups, and school activities.

The ASCA National Model recommends that school counselors spend 80% of their time in direct and indirect services to students. Within that framework, school counselors have the flexibility to implement the model differently to meet the unique needs of their school and grade levels. With that in mind, let's examine what school counselors do as a function of their setting.

Elementary School Counselors

The elementary years of school life comprise the formative phase of child development. During this time, children are building their academic self-concept as they address issues of competence and confidence toward learning. They are also working on decision making, communication skills, and developing values. In addition, they are beginning to develop social relationships and examine their position in their family. Box 16.2 offers the perspective of an elementary school counselor who is being asked to transition to using the ASCA National Model.

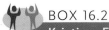

BOX 16.2
Kristina: Elementary School Counselor

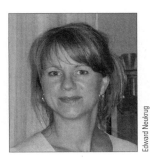

Edward Neukrug

I have been an elementary school counselor for the past fourteen years. I chose counseling as my profession because of my deep interest in psychology and my desire to understand the inner world of people and how they change and develop. My decision to work as a school counselor came about as a result of becoming a mother and wanting a work schedule that would allow me time with my children.

As a school counselor working with children in pre-kindergarten through grade 5, my days are very busy and my responsibilities are varied. I do individual counseling, small group counseling, and classroom guidance. I also work with teachers, school administrators, parents, and social service agencies. The goal of all my work is to help children be successful in school. The nature of my role is proactive and preventative in that I help to promote the academic, social, emotional, and career development of each student. Typical issues I deal with include study skills, peer relationships, self-esteem, family changes, behavior problems, school anxiety, feeling awareness, attention difficulties, learning differences, bullying, motivation, conflict mediation, character development, decision making, and problem solving. However, in helping children with such various developmental and situational concerns, working in a school setting requires my overriding focus [to] be on school achievement.

The ASCA national model has become quite important over the past few years. The guidance department for my school system is working to adopt and implement its philosophy and principles. One way that the model has impacted my role as a school counselor is that there is now a greater emphasis placed on data, accountability, leadership, and systemic change. For example, whereas before I hoped that I was helping children and believed that I was because of their self-reports, as well as feedback from parents and teachers, I now need to show the effectiveness of my role with hard data. However, this can be difficult because of time constraints brought on by being one counselor for 400 to 600 students and because of the very nature of counseling, as well as the many variables that affect an individual student's school success. Despite such changes, I love my job and feel energy and fulfillment working with children. As I change and grow along with the field of school counseling, I anticipate becoming more effective and hope to have more positive impact on the children I serve.

Middle School Counselors

As children move into adolescence, they face a multitude of developmental tasks highlighted by a need to understand their interests, their abilities, the world of work, their peer relationships, their sexuality, and a variety of life roles (see Box 16.3). Ultimately, they are beginning to define who they are—beginning to obtain a sense of self and a unique identity. At this point in their lives, they often are increasingly relying on feedback and reinforcement from their peers rather than from parents or guardians. Social relationships become paramount. Box 16.4 offers the perspective of a middle school counselor who is being asked to change the way he works by using the National Model.

High School Counselors

As students enter high school, they are taking an important step toward adulthood as they aim for career and college readiness and begin to have increased clarity as to how they define themselves. High school students are better able to describe their values, their skills, and their abilities. At the same time, they increasingly are influenced by their peers, and they will face important life decisions regarding such things as alcohol and drugs,

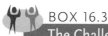

BOX 16.3
The Challenges of Middle School

Reggie and Sam, two sixth graders, have come to the counseling office to participate in a conflict mediation session. For the past three months, Sam has been continually teasing Reggie about his size, and Reggie recently started a fight over it. Prior to the meeting, however, the school counselor met with Reggie and Sam's teacher to get an "inside view" of what was going on with them and to find out how they are doing in school. The counselor also examined the test scores and records of Reggie and Sam and noticed that in the past few months, Reggie's grades have dropped precipitously.

The counselor facilitates a discussion between the two students, and after 10 minutes, which was more like bantering back and forth, Sam offers an apology to Reggie and says he won't tease him any longer. Shaking his head in disbelief, Reggie says, "You've said this before! What did I ever do to you?" Reggie looks dejected, perhaps on the verge of tears. "What do you think is going on, Sam?" the counselor asks. Slowly, Sam replies, "Kids have been teasing me about being learning disabled, and I can take it, why can't he!" The counselor spends a few moments having Reggie and Sam discuss

their feelings, and a resolution occurs when Reggie and Sam shake hands and agree to leave each other alone. The counselor requests two more meetings with Reggie and Sam, which they agree to.

Following the meeting, the counselor decides to conduct a needs assessment of students, teachers, and parents to get a handle on how much bullying is occurring in the school. The counselor will consider conducting psychoeducational groups and other schoolwide activities if bullying seems to be a systemwide problem. Also, the counselor will check with the teacher to see if Reggie's test scores begin to improve.

This exchange demonstrates the changes that begin to unfold during the middle school years and how some students respond to them. Faced with many transitions, the middle school years can leave children harboring great feelings of anger, hurt, or both. The vignette shows the importance of paying attention to academics, consulting with the teacher, having a systemic perspective, and providing needed preventive measures (e.g., schoolwide bullying programs) when necessary.

sexual behavior, and developing meaningful relationships with others. These students will be facing important decisions about their future. Box 16.5 offers the perspective of a relatively new high school counselor as she describes her roles, duties, and vision for her profession and position.

School Counselor Supervisors and Educators

In addition to serving at the elementary, middle, and high school levels, school counselors are district- and state-level supervisors, as well as counselor educators. District and state supervisors oversee school counseling in their respective school districts and states and perform a range of job activities such as facilitating professional development, collaborating with stakeholders and decision-makers, and advocating for school counselors implementing CSCPs. Supervisors often have school counseling experience, but this is not always the case. More and more often, these supervisors are required to have a certification in school administration. Counselor educators typically have doctorates and teach in master's and doctoral programs to prepare future school counselors and school counselor educators, as well as providing research and services to the field. In some states, district supervisors collaborate with state supervisors, counselor educators, and professional counseling organizations to support the profession. Box 16.6 offers the perspective of a school counseling district supervisor from an urban school district regarding her vision of the roles and responsibilities of professional school counselors.

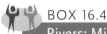

BOX 16.4
Rivers: Middle School Counselor

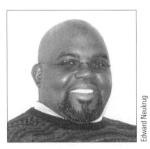

Edward Neukrug

I always felt like I had a calling—a calling to help others. My father was a minister and my mom was a counselor—not by degree, but because everyone would come to her to talk about their problems. It was an endless stream of people, seeking her out. My mom's two sisters married my dad's two brothers, and we all lived together for a while until everyone could afford to live on their own. That's how my family was—always helping each other. So, with my dad's values, my mom's behaviors, and the constant message that it was important to care for others, there was no choice for me—I had a calling to be there for others.

My calling led me on the path to becoming a math teacher. It was my way of helping others learn. But even as a teacher I found myself counseling—students always came to me, and faculty too sought my advice and counsel. After twelve years of teaching, I knew I had to do more. I considered administration, but ultimately counseling pulled me toward that field. I soon obtained my master's degree in counseling and became a middle school counselor. And that's where I am today—at the same middle school for more than 15 years.

I believe that counseling is a calling—you can have all the book learning in the world, but if somewhere inside you, you don't have that calling, you're not going to be much of a counselor. It's a service and you are looking to the higher good—the best in people. And my calling was to work with children—it seems like the best fit for me.

What do I do? Well, I work on schedules, do individual counseling and group counseling, including grief groups, groups to assist students academically, first-generation college-bound groups, groups on bullying, and suicide prevention groups. I also do classroom guidance for academic planning, career decision-making, testing, and behavior management. In addition, I coordinate testing programs, deal with attendance and truancy issues, deal with gangs, help students with issues around their sexuality, and more . . .

The ASCA Model and the Education Trust initiatives have certainly put the focus on having ALL children achieving at high levels. However, I feel we have always been proactive in our school. We look at each report card and find students having difficulty with classes. We meet with parents, teachers, and concerned others when students are having academic problems. We coordinate mentor and volunteer mental health programs. We are always trying to make sure that students achieve at their highest level. And, as an African American, I try to make sure that I am reaching out to as many African American students as possible—to act as a mentor and a model. I always try to keep in mind that the next child I touch could be the one who ends up turning his or her life around.

And oh yes, I am a minister also. I run a small church on the side with its focus being to help individuals in the poorest section of the city. My life is pretty full!

Multicultural/Social Justice Focus

Creating a Multicultural School Environment

American schools are becoming increasingly diverse, yet they still appear to lag in serving students of color, students from families with low income, English language learners, students receiving special education services, and students who are lesbian, gay, bisexual, and transgendered (Grothaus, Crum, & James, 2010; Holcomb-McCoy, 2007; Kosciw, Greytak, Bartkiewicz, Boesen, & Palmer, 2012).

As a result of students' needs, these changing demographics, and an increased focus on multiculturalism, equity, and social justice, school counselors are challenged to make schools more responsive to students and stakeholders with diverse cultural affiliations (Bemak & Chung, 2008; Cholewa & West-Olatunji, 2008; Day-Vines & Terriquez, 2008; Ford, Moore, & Whiting, 2006; Grothaus & Johnson, 2012). School counselors are expected to "specifically address the needs of every student, particularly students of

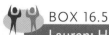

BOX 16.5
Lauren: High School Counselor

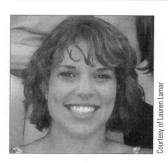

Courtesy of Lauren Lamar

From early on, I knew that I wanted to work with youth. I thought about becoming a teacher, a child psychologist, a social worker, even a family lawyer. In college, I majored in psychology and volunteered in a program working with teenagers facing many challenges, but I still did not know what the right career was for me.

After I graduated from college, I did some research and I learned about the counseling program at a local university. School counseling appealed to me because we're in the perfect position to help children and youth in a proactive manner. I also liked that school counselors have the opportunity to impact the lives of all students, not just the high achievers or the ones who are getting into trouble. High school students are so multidimensional. In many ways they are still children, but they are also coming into their own, becoming adults. As a school counselor, I'm able to play a part in that development.

Every day is different in a high school, which is one of the things that I love about it. Emergencies that require my attention can come up at any time. This can be challenging, but I am never bored. A typical day for me begins about 30 minutes before the students arrive. I check my messages and I prepare to see students.

During the day, I meet with students about a variety of topics, including academic issues, college planning questions, [and] social and personal concerns. I write letters of recommendation, help students with college applications, collaborate and consult with parents, teachers, and administrators. I conduct classroom guidance on academic, career, and personal/social topics and work with students in small groups. I am often involved in child study team and student support team meetings, as well as parent-teacher conferences. Additionally, I collect data to track my effectiveness in working with students and see how I'm spending my time. I also coach both swimming and field hockey at my high school. I find that it allows me to get to know students who are not on my caseload and to learn even more about my students outside of my office.

I have been a high school counselor for two and a half years, and I absolutely love my job. I work with a tremendous and incredibly supportive group of counselors. Most importantly, though, by acting as an advocate I can make an enormous difference in the lives [of] my students. Many of my students come from populations that are typically underserved in the school setting. To work toward closing the achievement gap, I promote enrollment in rigorous courses and arrange for the support students need to succeed. I advocate for the students and their parents with teachers, administrators and even college admissions officers. I see myself as an agent of change. I collaborate with my colleagues to support equity for all students in school and to help all students succeed. At the end of the day, there is nothing more rewarding than knowing that I have been able to have lasting positive impact on the life of a student.

culturally diverse, low social-economic status, and other underserved or underperforming populations" (ASCA, 2005a, p. 77). Yet there is some evidence that school counselors have lower expectations for students from some cultural groups (Auwarter & Aruguete, 2008). Improving our own multicultural competence and the cultural responsiveness of our schools and communities is an ongoing journey that can begin with looking within and acknowledging that our "own practices are cultural in origin, rather than the 'only right way to do things'" (Dimmock & Walker, 2005, p. 190). Today's school counselors are called to develop a positive multicultural atmosphere and to promote social justice and equity in many ways, some of which are delineated in Table 16.3.

Assessing Multicultural Competence

One way that school counselors can ensure that they are creating a multicultural environment is to do a systematic analysis of their school. Holcomb-McCoy (2007) offers a

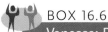

BOX 16.6
Vanessa: District Supervisor of School Counseling

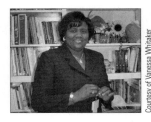

Courtesy of Vanessa Whitaker

From early on, I've had a love and a passion for helping others. When I was 10, I received a present that helped me realize my love for education—a black-board and a box of chalk. I spent hours "playing" school. I loved teaching and guiding my students through lessons. I wanted them to be happy and well adjusted.

During that time, I also witnessed the unfair treatment of a student in my class. One boy looked disheveled and hungry most of the time. When he was required to read aloud, he was ridiculed by teachers and students. This seemed to embarrass and hurt him. I would go to bed at night feeling sad and thinking of ways to help him. I realized that I wanted to be a teacher so that I could help others, especially those who were considered outcasts and treated unfairly.

Years later, as a fourth-grade teacher, I discovered that even students who initially struggled could learn and excel when they were shown respect and knew that somebody cared about them and wanted them to do their very best. I taught as many social and personal skills as I did academic skills. This helped me to realize how important relationships are to learning.

In 1985, I was selected to participate in a program that provided training to become a professional school counselor. I loved my time as a school counselor. I had an opportunity to practice both of my passions—teaching and helping others! During the ensuing years, my school district afforded me the opportunity to work at all levels and to coordinate programs at the district level. I organized professional development,

coordinated meetings, and supported the school counselors. Gradually, my supervisor gave me more responsibilities and, when she announced her retirement, urged me to apply for her position. I started supervising school counselors for Newport News Virginia Public Schools in 1997.

As the supervisor of school counseling, I am responsible for providing leadership for the school counseling programs in our district. I support our professional school counselors to serve successfully as educational advocates so that every student can graduate college-, career-, and citizen-ready and prepared to succeed in this global society. I support school counselors in their work to remove barriers that prevent students from succeeding. That support takes the form of professional development, coaching, management, assisting with accountability systems, and providing resources. I work to help school counselors implement best practices that have been proven to impact student success while using the framework of the ASCA National Model.

One of the most meaningful aspects of my job is helping counselors concentrate on issues, strategies, and interventions that will help close achievement and opportunity gaps. I hold them accountable to demonstrate their impact on student achievement and to share the results data with school stakeholders. I look forward to the day when all the administrators, teachers, parents, and community members realize the difference that school counselors can and do make to promote the lifelong success of students.

When empowered, professional school counselors collaborate with others and serve as agents of change in the educational system, they can create opportunities for all students to realize their dreams. Then and only then will that passionate, impressionable 10-year old realize her dreams.

---

checklist of 51 items across nine categories to help the school counselor do this. The categories, which are based on "theme analysis" of multicultural issues in school counseling, are as follows:

- ➤ Multicultural counseling
- ➤ Multicultural consultation
- ➤ Understanding racism and student resistance
- ➤ Multicultural assessment
- ➤ Understanding racial identity development
- ➤ Multicultural family counseling
- ➤ Social advocacy
- ➤ Developing school–family–community partnerships
- ➤ Understanding cross-cultural interpersonal interactions

TABLE 16.3 Elements to Creating a Multicultural Environment and Promoting Social Justice

1. Raising awareness that culture is a powerful and pervasive influence on students, stakeholders, and our own attitudes and behavior.
2. Being actively involved in the community in which your school is located by engaging in networking, advocacy, and knowing available cultural resources (Griffin & Farris, 2010; Vera, Buhin, & Shin, 2006).
3. Participating in and leading multicultural workshops/trainings for the school and community stakeholders.
4. Making the school counseling program accessible, including being available at times that parents/guardians are able to see you. Also, ensuring that your school and school counseling office and materials are accessible for persons with disabilities. Communicating and assessing (through a translator if necessary) with students and stakeholders in their preferred language.
5. Creating a welcoming, inclusive school climate where cultural richness is celebrated.
6. Promoting use of inclusive language and recognition of multiple cultures (e.g., using *humankind* as opposed to *mankind*; celebrating various holidays, not just those of Christian or European-American origins; have school decor represent the contributions of multiple cultures).
7. Promoting inclusive curriculum and culturally aware teaching and classroom management strategies that are more salient to students' lives.
8. Working to improve cross-cultural relationships in your school and community, not just between racial/ethnic groups, but also with regard to social class, ability/disability, sexual orientation, and other factors.
9. Broaching the topic of culture when counseling, consulting, doing classroom guidance, and other school counseling practices; this can send a signal that these topics are important and open for discussion if they are salient.
10. Adapting your counseling and consultation techniques to be culturally sensitive.
11. Helping students to "code-switch," to make situationally intelligent decisions about language and behavior for various circumstances (Day-Vines & Day-Hairston, 2005). Also, train faculty and staff to be culturally sensitive and skilled (e.g., not emphasizing the terms *proper* or *correct* English, which implies that a student's home language is improper; instead, request that students use *school* or *formal* English).
12. Creating a multicultural advisory committee, with representative membership from the school and community, to examine and offer advice on all aspects of the school experience (e.g., curriculum, teaching methods, and inclusive climate).
13. Consulting cultural informants—people who are familiar with the cultures represented in your school.
14. Assisting schools in developing mechanisms for hiring individuals from diverse backgrounds.
15. Examining disaggregated school data for evidence of inequity (e.g., disproportionate numbers of some groups of students receiving behavioral referrals, inequitable representation in gifted programs and those receiving special education services, disparate graduation rates for different student groups). Collaborating with stakeholders to change school policies and practices that maintain the inequitable status quo.
16. Asking questions (Holcomb-McCoy, 2007) about the curriculum, the school climate, faculty/staff attitudes, and actions, such as:
    a. Are adults encouraging all students?
    b. Do we have an accurate and representative curriculum?
    c. Is there equity in access to opportunities, available resources, and teacher quality?
    d. Do we have adult role models for our diverse student body?
    e. Are there student and faculty friendships across racial, ethnic, ability, sexual orientation, and social class groups?
    f. Is the discussion of "–isms" safe and encouraged?
    g. Who is included in the decision-making process?
    h. How can we make a given situation more equitable and democratic?
17. Collaborating with community organizations that promote positive goals for youth and families.
18. Previewing practices, programs, and policies that have been successful elsewhere (e.g., see the Education Trust website: http://www.edtrust.org/).
19. Assisting others to be successful self-advocates.
20. Advocating with your federal, state, and local legislators and policy makers.
21. Being persistent. Addressing the source of peoples' concerns about your ideas/proposals and creating allies for positive change.
22. Performing evaluations to improve; celebrating the changes that your efforts produce.
23. Recognizing the need for self-care and support in this challenging enterprise.

Adapted from Virginia School Counselor Association (2008).

Ethical, Professional, and Legal Issues

Ethical Issues

Ethical Standards in School Counseling

School counselors are responsible for upholding professional ethics, which both ASCA and ACA describe in their ethical codes/standards (ACA, 2014a; ASCA, 2010). The *ASCA Ethical Standards for School Counselors* outlines ethical expectations, including school counselors' ethical responsibilities to students, parents/guardians, colleagues and associates, the school, the community, oneself, the profession, as well as maintaining the ethical standards. ASCA also lists steps to take when encountering ethical dilemmas.

Confidentiality: Ethical and Legal Implications

When working with minors, student confidentiality is a complicated issue (see Box 16.7). Although school counselors' primary *ethical* responsibility is to maintain student confidentiality, *legally* counselors typically are obligated to reveal information about counseling sessions if a parent/guardian requests such information (Remley & Herlihy, 2014). Further, parent/guardian permission is usually legally required before minors can begin counseling services. It is important that school counselors inform students of these legal limits to confidentiality, as well as suspected child abuse, court orders, and serious and imminent harm to the student or others (ASCA, 2010). The context surrounding confidentiality is also important, as laws and mandates often vary by state, school district, and student age and developmental level (Stone, 2013). We recommend that school counselors proactively discuss student confidentiality with parents, school administrators, and teachers before providing counseling services to students. Often, these stakeholders will respect the confidentiality of the counseling relationship if they are assured that the counselor is looking out for the best interests of the child and the family.

Professional Issues

ASCA and ACA

ASCA strives to provide, in the words of its motto, "One Vision, One Voice" for the school counseling profession. Supporting and representing school counselors from around the

BOX 16.7
Student Sues School System for Revealing Sexual Orientation to Parents

A federal judge in Santa Ana, California, ruled that a lesbian high school student could move forward on her suit against the school district that she attends because the principal had allegedly violated her privacy rights and revealed to the student's mother that she was a lesbian. Apparently, the principal and others had witnessed the student hugging and kissing her girlfriend on numerous occasions. The student had been disciplined for this behavior, and the lawsuit claimed discrimination because heterosexual couples had apparently not been disciplined. This case brought up interesting conversations surrounding students' privacy, schools' disclosures, and parents' rights to information ("Girl can sue. . .," 2005).

world, this organization has approximately 30,000 members (J. Cook, personal communication, July 14, 2014). ASCA does a tremendous amount for school counseling, including providing training to implement the ASCA National Model, sponsoring conferences and professional development workshops, developing and maintaining an ethical code, creating position statements on a number of important issues facing school counselors, assisting in accreditation and credentialing initiatives, advocating for legislative initiatives, supporting evaluation and research, sponsoring liability insurance, and publishing a magazine entitled the *ASCA School Counselor* and a journal entitled *The Professional School Counselor.*

With nearly 55,000 members (D. Brown, personal communication, July 14, 2014), ACA is a professional and educational organization that supports and promotes the counseling field and corresponding specialties within the field, such as school counseling. In 2013, the ACA School Counseling Task Force developed a definition of school counseling based on the 20/20 definition described in Chapter 2 (Erford, 2015).

ASCA is one of the largest and most active ACA divisions. However, there has been friction between ACA and ASCA in the last couple of decades. During the 1990s, ASCA considered leaving ACA (Hubert, 1995). Some of its members felt that ASCA could address the unique needs of school counselors better as an independent association. As a result, ASCA is a semi-independent ACA division. In addition, ASCA did not endorse the *20/20 Vision,* such as the definition of counseling (see Chapter 2). As a result, ASCA was subsequently excluded from being a full member of the 20/20 commission (Kaplan, Tarvydas, & Gladding, 2014). Both ASCA and ACA advocate for school counselors and offer deep discounts for student memberships and conference registrations. We encourage students to join both associations, as well as their related state-level associations.

Specialty Certification in School Counseling

Although school counseling credentialing (certification or licensure) on the state level has been around longer than any other counselor credential, national certification was not initiated until 1992, when the *National Certified School Counselor (NCSC)* credential became established (Paisley & Borders, 1995). In 1994, this certification became affiliated with the *National Board for Certified Counselors (NBCC).* In addition to the NCSC, the *National Board for Professional Teaching Standards (NBPTS)* has developed a certification process that was finalized in 2004. This certification requires credentialing and three years as a school counselor as well as a two- to three-year performance-based assessment that demonstrates proficiency in a wide range of school counseling skills. Although this certification process is expensive, some school counselors may be reimbursed for the cost, offered salary incentives for becoming certified, or both. If you would like to compare these two certification processes, ASCA has developed a chart that highlights their differences (see ASCA, 2005b).

Youths Experiencing Trauma, Mental Health Concerns, Substance Abuse, and Other Issues

The shock of hearing about children being shot in schools has awakened us to the problems that many of our youths face today. One result of this new awareness is that school counselors are increasingly being asked to play a role in working with youths dealing with one or more significant concerns (Erford, Lee, & Rock, 2015). Nearly 20% of the students in U.S. schools have diagnosable mental health and behavioral disorders, yet only 20% of those students receive treatment. A few of the many roles that the counselor has taken on in this capacity include designing and implementing prevention efforts (e.g., bullying prevention and drop-out prevention); facilitating resiliency characteristics in students; promoting a welcoming, supportive, culturally responsive, and inclusive school climate; leading the efforts to prevent and manage crisis situations; assessing suicidal ideation and other threats of violence; coordinating with community resource providers; collaborating to develop safety programs in the schools; assisting students in dealing with bullying, abuse, or harassment; and performing grief counseling for students, families, and school staff.

Salaries and Job Outlook of School Counselors

Currently, there are about 262,300 educational, vocational, and school counselors, and the employment of school counselors in the near future is expected to grow "as fast as average," according to the Occupational Outlook Handbook (U.S. Department of Labor, 2014–2015b). The number of and need for school counselors has decreased slightly in the last couple of years, which may be the result of budget cuts and changes in state-mandated school counseling. Salaries of school counselors are almost always based on the salaries of teachers who have master's degrees. As of May 2012, the median salary of school counselors was $53,610.

Legal Issues
Public Law 94-142, IDEA, Section 504, RTI, and the ADA

Passed in 1975, *PL94-142*, along with the recent reauthorizations and expansions of the law referred to as the *Individuals with Disabilities Education Act (IDEA)*, has greatly affected the role of the school counselor. These laws ensure the right of students to be assessed, at the school system's expense, if the student is suspected of having a disability that interferes with learning. In addition, they assert that schools must make accommodations, within the least-restrictive environment, for any student from age 3 through age 21 who qualifies in one of the thirteen categories for receiving special education services; that is, students must be taught in regular classrooms whenever possible and reasonable (Baditoi & Brott, 2011). The importance of knowledge in this area should not be underestimated, and most school counseling programs now offer required coursework in understanding how to work with students with disabilities (Milsom & Akos, 2003). School counselors are also involved with *Response to Intervention (RTI)*, a data-driven and multiple-level approach to help students struggling with academics (ASCA, 2008).

School counselors play an active role in the implementation of these laws by referring students for testing, consulting with parents and teachers, and advocating and consulting with special education and RTI teams. These teams can develop RTI plans, *individual education plans (IEPs)* specific to the educational goals of the student, and *504 plans,* to ensure access to education when it may otherwise be limited due to physical or mental impairment. PL94-142, the IDEA, along with section 504 of the *1973 Rehabilitation Act* and parts of the *Americans with Disabilities Act (ADA)* are all important laws that aid children with disabilities to gain an education within the least-restrictive environment.

Parental Rights to School Records

The *Family Educational Rights and Privacy Act (FERPA),* passed in the mid-1970s, allows parents access to the educational records of their children and to decide how those records are shared. However, an amendment to FERPA was passed in January 2013, allowing schools to disclose students' educational records to specific organizations, such as state agencies, without parental consent. Under specified conditions, FERPA excludes counseling notes from the category of educational records (Stone, 2013). Remley, Hermann, and Huey (2003) suggested that school counselors keep case notes in their offices and do not allow other school personnel access to those notes, in order to abide by FERPA regulations. However, counselors need to be aware that their confidential notes can be subpoenaed, and they may have to reveal their notes, testify about them in court, or both, if requested by the court to do so.

Suspected Child Abuse

With close to 900,000 substantiated cases of child abuse being reported every year, and with a school counselor frequently assessing dozens of children a year, reporting suspected child abuse is clearly an important issue for school counselors (Bryant & Milsom, 2005). Today, all states require school counselors and teachers to report suspected child abuse (Hermann, Remley, & Huey, 2010). Each counselor needs to be aware of the specific procedures for reporting suspected child abuse in his or her state, which is often described by each state's Department of Social Services or similar organizations.

The School Counselor in Process: Adapting to the Twenty-First Century

> *Without that commitment to the process of change, a school counselor will not be able to effectively serve as a catalyst in student lives and a significant change agent in the educational community.*
>
> (Allen, as cited in Hopkins, 2005, "Counselors Make a Difference," para. 3)

The evolution of school counseling has been dramatic. We've moved from a vocational guidance focus to an emphasis on developing and implementing comprehensive school counseling programs while advocating and collaborating to ensure equity for all students, and preparing students to be college- and career-ready. School counseling today covers a wide range of services (ASCA, 2012). The school counselor of tomorrow can expect to see even more changes. Increased interactions with culturally diverse students, greater emphasis on the use of data, greater use of technology, increased career options for students, and increased involvement of families are a few of the opportunities and challenges facing school counselors in the future. Thus, counselors will need to become increasingly adaptable as their roles and functions continue to change and expand. This will require counselors to examine what they are doing and how they can respond to the everyday needs of students, parents and guardians, teachers, administrators, and community stakeholders, all while proactively providing prevention programming and being able to handle crises that will occur on a frequent basis. The counselor who is comfortable with change will survive and flourish.

First Lady Michelle Obama attended the annual American School Counselor conference in 2014 and said:

> School counseling should not be an extra or a luxury . . . School counseling is a necessity to ensure that all our young people get the education they need to succeed in today's economy . . . [School counselors] think about the extraordinary ripple effect of your work, because it's real. I want you to think about the impact you have not just on every child whose life you transform, but on the family that child will raise, on the business where that child will work, on the community that child will one day serve. I want you to think about how long after those kids graduate your work lives on in their hearts and minds, and in the hearts and minds of everyone they touch.

If you are reading this chapter, you are likely considering becoming a school counselor. Welcome aboard. You are entering a rewarding, multifaceted, and evolving profession with the potential to make a difference in the lives of many. Our profession has advanced a great deal in the last century, but progress is still needed. What will be your role in moving the profession forward? How will you affect students, schools, and communities?

Summary

This chapter discussed the unique specialty area of school counseling. We began by briefly defining school counseling, noting that its purpose is to offer a comprehensive school counseling program that promotes and enhances student achievement for all students by assisting them with their academic, career, and personal and social development. We noted that today's school counseling is developmental and preventative and that the services offered by the school counselor are interwoven throughout the school's total educational program.

We offered some background information on the emergence of school counseling, noting that its origins date back to the beginning of the twentieth century when there was an increasing need for vocational guidance. Frank Parsons and others were highlighted as instrumental in defining vocational guidance. Although the school counseling profession was initially slow to expand, it diversified and began to define itself more clearly during the 1930s, thanks to the influence of such individuals as E. G. Williamson and John

Brewer. During the 1940s, the humanistic psychology and education movement shifted the focus of school counseling from a directive, didactic approach to an approach that focused more on the importance of the relationship between the student and counselor and was more facilitative than directive. In addition, school counseling at this time took on a greater mental health focus.

The decade of the 1950s, with the launch of Sputnik and the subsequent passage of the *National Defense Education Act (NDEA)*, saw a great increase in the need for school counselors. The 1960s included continued expansion of school counseling and an increased focus on comprehensive school counseling programs (CSCPs). Increased professionalism and diversity were the major thrusts of school counseling in the 1970s and 1980s; and, as we moved into the 1990s, school counseling expanded its comprehensive developmental and preventative focus and also emphasized cultural competence and advocacy for equity and success for all students.

As the chapter continued, we noted that high-stakes testing, such as those that resulted from state learning standards as well as the federal *No Child Left Behind (NCLB) Act*, demanded that all students must meet minimum educational competencies. Such testing has challenged the traditional role of the school counselor, who tended to be seen as someone delivering an ancillary service that did not address students' educational concerns directly. We also noted that such testing, as well as grants from the Education Trust, led to a new paradigm in counselor training that was epitomized by the ASCA National Model. This model is now being taught throughout the country in counselor education programs and has been adopted by many school systems.

Subsequently, we briefly defined the ASCA National Model, which identifies four elements that are critical to the development of a school counseling program: foundation, management, delivery, and accountability. Four overarching themes crucial to the implementation of the four systems were also identified: leadership, advocacy, collaboration, and systemic change. In addition, we outlined key factors instrumental in implementing CSCPs, such as the ASCA National Model, including: student benefits, suggested student ratios, the Recognized ASCA Model Program (RAMP) designation, data-driven initiatives, and principal collaborations. Also, we highlighted the importance of a number of theories to the practice of school counseling. We briefly discussed how counseling theory, theories of human development, career development theory, and systems theory are all used in multiple ways when working with children.

Some of the roles and functions of elementary, middle, and high school counselors, as well as district- and state-level school counselor supervisors, were discussed. We also offered a window into the lives of typical elementary, middle, and high school counselors, as well as a school district director of school counseling. We highlighted some of the challenges and opportunities facing school counseling as we become more responsive to multicultural issues. We suggested that school counselors should particularly focus on lessening the achievement gap, reducing barriers to success, advocating for equity for all students, sensitizing the total school community to multicultural issues, ensuring that educational materials are not biased, striving to understand how students interpret their environment, and establishing a CSCP.

As the chapter neared its conclusion, we featured a number of ethical, professional, and legal issues. First, we described ASCA's ethical standards. Next, we highlighted the ethical and legal implications of student confidentiality as applicable to school counseling. We then discussed a number of important professional issues, including brief descriptions of ASCA, ACA, and their relationship, the specialty certifications in school counseling offered by NBCC and NBPTS, the importance of working with youths experiencing any number of serious concerns, and the salary average and the job outlook for school counselors. A brief description of laws affecting school counseling included PL94-142, the IDEA, section 504 of the *Rehabilitation Act*, Response to Intervention (RTI), the ADA, FERPA, and child abuse laws. Finally, the chapter ended by stressing the need for school counselors to remain flexible in the face of the many changes that will occur in the schools as we move forward.

Further Practice

Visit CengageBrain.com to respond to additional material that highlight the salient aspects of the chapter content. There, you can find ethical, professional, and legal vignettes, a number of experiential exercises, and study tools including a glossary, flashcards, and sample test items. Hopefully, these will enhance your learning and be fun and interesting.

I'm working at a crisis center, and a client tells me he's being followed by the Mob. They want to kill him, he states. He asks me what he should do, and I say, "Why don't you call the FBI, or the State Police?" He calls the State Police, and they want to see him. I drive him out to the State Police barracks, thinking the whole way, "This guy is paranoid." We get there. The cops talk with him for half an hour. They come out and tell him to lie down in the back of my car so no one will see him. My heart drops. "He's not paranoid?" I think, "Oh my God!" They tell me to take the back roads back to the crisis center!

I'm working at a mental health center with a client who had been hospitalized for depression a few years back. I've been seeing her for a few months and have built a fairly solid relationship with her. At the end of the session, she tells me, "You know, when I was hospitalized, one of the staff molested me."

I'm at the same mental health center. I've been seeing a client for about a year. She's been psychotic, on and off, for a number of years and is pretty stiff in the way she interacts with people. She's on some heavy-duty antipsychotic medication. She sees me once every three weeks for a check-in. Suddenly, at the end of a session, she looks at me and tells me that she had an abortion ten years ago. Her psychotic episodes started about ten years back. This certainly seems to be an interesting coincidence. I decide to see her weekly. She begins to share her guilt about the abortion, and within a couple of months, she's practically off her medication. Now, I wouldn't say that she is back to normal, but she certainly is doing better! What a success! Ironically, a month later, she dies in the middle of the night—but perhaps she found a bit more peace in her life. Life is certainly unpredictable.

I'm in private practice, and it's a Friday afternoon. I'm seeing one of my last clients of the day, looking forward to going away on a weekend trip to the country. He's a 15-year-old I've been seeing for a while. At the end of the session, he blurts out that he was molested when on a recent vacation. There goes my weekend trip, as I have to act on this immediately—I need to deal with his parents, the law, and him.

My girlfriend and I have just broken up. It's my birthday. I'm very depressed. I go to my part-time job at a small counseling center. A new client walks in. She immediately tells me it's her birthday and that she and her husband have just split up. Is this a coincidence, or what? I wonder if I can get through the session.

So you want to work as a mental health counselor? It can be fun. It can be boring. It can be scary. It can be sad, and it can be exhilarating. It's the best of jobs and the worst of jobs. Let's see what it's all about.

This chapter is about working in *clinical mental health counseling*. We'll start by defining this counseling arena. Then we'll offer a brief overview of the history of this specialty area. This will be followed by an overview of some of the places you can find clinical mental health counselors. We will examine some of the theories used by counselors in these settings and some typical roles and functions of the clinical mental health counselor. We'll present some special issues currently impinging on the clinical mental health counselor and offer information on current salary ranges. As we near the end of the chapter, we will examine some multicultural and social justice issues, as well as some ethical, professional, and legal issues in the area of mental health counseling. We'll conclude the chapter with some thoughts about the changing nature of mental health counseling.

What Is Clinical Mental Health Counseling?

Probably the best place to start in describing *clinical mental health counseling* is to examine the course content and field placements needed in such programs. Today, all counseling programs accredited by the *Council for the Accreditation of Counseling and Related Programs* (CACREP, 2009) must provide content knowledge in eight areas: professional orientation and ethical practice, social and cultural diversity, human growth and development, career development, helping relationships, group work, assessment, and research and program evaluation. Clinical mental health counseling programs must also offer course content in psychopathology, diagnosis, assessment psychopharmacology, treatment planning, crisis counseling and trauma, psychosocial history, report writing, marriage and family, program development, addictions, case conceptualization, and evidence-based treatment, among many other topics. In addition, a 100-hour practicum and 600-hour internship are required. Although in the recent past, the CACREP standards have supported a 48- and then a 54-credit clinical mental health counseling program (sometimes called *agency counseling* or *community counseling*), CACREP's current standards support a 60-credit clinical mental health counseling degree program.

Despite the fact that the clinical mental health counseling degree is generally viewed as the specialty area most appropriate for becoming a *Licensed Professional Counselor (LPC),* in most states, one can become an LPC regardless of specialty area (see Box 17.1).

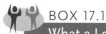 BOX 17.1

What a Long, Strange Road It's Been

My master's degree was in counseling with a specialization in student affairs and college counseling, and my internship was at a college-affiliated crisis center. Subsequent to obtaining my master's degree, I worked at a drug and alcohol abuse storefront crisis center. A couple of years later, I obtained a job as an outpatient therapist at a community mental health center. After obtaining my doctorate in counselor education, I taught counseling and later worked part time as an associate school psychologist and as a school counselor in New Hampshire. During this time, I received clinical supervision, and I eventually obtained licensure as a psychologist. Moving to Virginia,

I applied for licensure as a psychologist. The Virginia psychology licensure board denied me, saying my field was counseling, not psychology. I then happily applied for and obtained licensure as an LPC. Thus, despite my original degree in college student development counseling, I was able, with some additional training, to freely move into a number of different settings and obtain a variety of different credentials. Although it has become increasingly more difficult to obtain certification and licensure in closely related fields like psychology or school psychology, it remains true that with a bit more additional training, one can generally move from one counseling specialty area to another.

Although it hasn't been a straight path to get where we are today, the field of counseling is stronger than ever. It will be interesting to see where we are in 2025.

A History of Clinical Mental Health Counseling

The Beginning of the Mental Health Movement

As noted in Chapter 2, the fields of psychiatry and clinical psychology arose around the turn of the twentieth century. It was at that time that one's emotional state was seen as having "psychological origins," in contrast to physical or demonic ones. *Freud's psychoanalytic approach* was one major impetus for this new way of viewing emotional problems and drastically changed the manner in which mental disorders were conceptualized and treated. It was also during this period that sanitariums began to experiment with more humane methods of hospitalization (Smith & Robinson, 1995).

The early 1900s saw the beginning of *vocational guidance*. This movement, along with the development of the first *assessment instruments*, was to have an impact on the eventual role of counseling in the mental health field. Testing went hand in hand with vocational guidance, and both testing and vocational guidance were concerned with understanding the uniqueness of the person. This focus was to become a hallmark of counseling and psychotherapy in general.

During the 1930s, the federal government began to earmark small amounts of money for mental health treatment, especially for research in mental health. As the decade continued, one could see a new mindset sprouting in the United States. Influenced by psychoanalysis, vocational guidance, an increasingly humane attitude toward mental illness, and *existential philosophers and psychologists* (some of whom emigrated from Europe) (Neukrug, 2015), this country was beginning to accept the concept that mental health services were a necessary and important aspect of living in a civilized world. But traditional psychoanalysis was seen as too long-term and mostly used by the rich; vocational guidance was too limited, too short-term, and too directive in its approach; and existential philosophy was viewed as too ethereal. However, a merging of these three approaches seemed just right.

As the 1940s neared, a new approach to counseling and psychotherapy evolved—one that encapsulated many of the precepts of psychoanalysis, counseling, existentialism, and American take-charge philosophy. This approach was optimistic and relatively short-term as opposed to psychoanalysis, and it was founded on the belief that if people worked hard enough, they could change. Not surprisingly, it was during this time that we saw the beginnings of *self-help groups* like Alcoholics Anonymous and groups to assist new immigrants adjusting to American life, groups that affirmed the idea that individuals can change.

As a byproduct of World War II, evaluation techniques to determine who was emotionally fit to enter the military became much more sophisticated. In addition, the recovery rates of individuals who had emotional problems that resulted from the war were very high. Mental health providers were suddenly becoming more assured about their ability to treat individuals (Hershenson, Power, & Waldo, 2003). It was on the heels of these successes that the *National Mental Health Act* was passed in 1946, which gave states funding for research, training, prevention, diagnosis, and treatment related to mental health disorders.

During the late 1940s, the *National Institute of Mental Health (NIMH)* was created by Congress. NIMH supported increased research and training in the mental health field and was the impetus for the 1955 *Mental Health Study Act*. This act established the *Joint Commission on Mental Illness and Health*, which made a number of far-reaching recommendations around increased funding and services for mental health and mental illness. Partly as a result of this act, the 1950s saw the expansion and acceptance of mental health services around the country. It was also at this time that we began to see the widespread use of psychotropic medication. During the late 1950s and continuing into the 1960s, a number of new (and at the time revolutionary) approaches to counseling began to take shape.

Expansion of Mental Health Services

The 1960s saw great upheaval in American society. There was unrest in the "ghettos," and the country was in bitter turmoil over the Vietnam War. The civil rights movement was growing in momentum. Out of this turmoil came landmark civil rights, economic, and social legislation (Kaplan & Cuciti, 1986). One such legislative initiative was the *1963 Community Mental Health Centers Act*, which funded the establishment of mental health centers in communities throughout the nation. These centers would provide short-term inpatient care, outpatient care, partial hospitalization, emergency services, and consultation and education services. This made it possible for individuals with a wide range of mental health concerns to obtain free or low-cost mental health services. Although the intended 3,000 mental health centers never came to fruition, hundreds were in fact established and became an essential part of treatment for tens of thousands of people nationwide (Geller, 2000; Sharfstein, 2000).

The late 1960s and early 1970s saw a number of federal laws passed that expanded the scope of community mental health centers and funded substance abuse treatment. In 1975, the Supreme Court decision in *Donaldson v. O'Connor* led to the deinstitutionalization of tens of thousands of state mental hospital patients who had been hospitalized against their will and who were not in danger of harming themselves or others (see Chapter 2, Box 2.3). Many of these former patients would receive services at the newly established local community mental health centers. The 1970s also saw the passage of a number of important legislative acts that would have a direct impact on individuals with disabilities. One major legislative initiative was the *Rehabilitation Act of 1973*, which ensured access to vocational rehabilitation services for adults if they met three conditions: having a severe physical or mental disability, having a disability that interfered with their ability to obtain or maintain a job, and having feasibility of employment with their disability. This act increased the need for highly trained rehabilitation counselors.

With the election of President Jimmy Carter in 1976, there was an increased focus on the importance of mental health treatment, and, in the late 1970s, Carter authorized the expansion of mental health services. Near the end of this decade, we saw the establishment of the *American Mental Health Counseling Association (AMHCA)*, the first division of the *American Counseling Association (ACA)* to be focused solely on mental health counseling and mental health concerns (Colangelo, 2009). Although legislative actions of the 1970s brought with them increased diversification of the counseling field and resulted in large numbers of counselors settling into a variety of community counseling agencies, the boom period of the 1970s was soon to end with the election of Ronald Reagan.

Carter's defeat by Reagan in 1980 led to the reduction or elimination of some mental health programs and a move toward federal *block grants*. Block grants had the effect of allowing states to decide which programs to fund, and this resulted in less money for some programs, particularly mental health centers (Hershenson et al., 2003). Despite this temporary setback, the 1980s and 1990s saw a slow but steady expansion and diversification in the field of counseling and a settling-in phase in our profession. Counselors during these decades could be found in almost any mental health setting. In addition, it was during these decades that we began to see counselors working in settings where they had not been found before, such as family service agencies, prisons, substance abuse treatment centers, gerontological settings, hospitals, business, and industry.

Beginning in the 1980s and into the twenty-first century, we saw a dramatic changes in the delivery of mental health services as *managed care*, such as *health maintenance organizations (HMOs)*, increasingly became the primary health insurance providers (Harrington, 2013; Kongstvedt, 2013). Previously, clients who had medical insurance generally had their choice as to the type of counseling services they desired, as well as to which licensed professional they could see. However, in an effort to save money, HMOs carefully monitored which services would be allowable and oversaw which providers a client could see (Dasenbrook, 2014).

Recent Events

In 2009, California became the last state to pass a counselor licensure law (Shallcross, 2009). With licensure being the first important step toward counselors becoming *independent providers* and obtaining *third-party reimbursement*, this was no small feat. Today, most mental health counselors can become providers for the vast array of most managed care and health insurance companies (Walsh & Dasenbrook, 2009, 2010). In fact, these days, LPCs, who generally have a degree in clinical mental health counseling, are the primary providers for mental health counseling. This is partially due to the advocacy work of ACA, AMHCA, and the *National Board for Certified Counselors (NBCC)*, which have worked hard to ensure that clinical mental health counselors are included as providers in a wide variety of insurance plans, such as TRICARE, the large health care organization for U.S. military families (ACA, 2014e; NBCC, 2013b).

The expansion of counseling services provided by mental health counselors will likely be affected by the passage of the Affordable Care Act (more colloquially known as "Obamacare"). In fact, the Affordable Care Act mandates mental health services and substance use disorder services for all insurance providers, and it is expected that 62 million additional Americans will now be extended such coverage (AMHCA, 2013b).

With expanding numbers of individuals having insurance coverage and the overseeing of counseling services by the insurance companies, we have seen an increased use of diagnosis and of psychotropic drugs. Although there are benefits and drawbacks to the diagnostic and statistical manual (see Table 17.1, as well as Table 10.2 in Chapter 10), it is clear that mental health counselors need a working knowledge of this classification (Patureau-Hatchett, 2009).

Closely related to the use of DSM is an increased willingness on the part of counselors to refer clients for *psychotropic medication*. With persuasive evidence that some emotional disorders are genetically linked ("Cross-disorder group...," 2013; Keneally, 2014), and with research now showing that the treatment of some problems is best facilitated

TABLE 17.1 Drawbacks and Benefits of a Diagnostic and Statistical Manual Diagnosis

DRAWBACKS	BENEFITS
➤ Objectifies and depersonalizes the person, as we view him or her in a dispassionate manner, much like watching a rat in a maze. ➤ Labeling can lead to a self-fulfilling prophecy, whereby the individual is seen as the diagnosis, is treated in a manner consistent with that diagnosis, and therefore is reinforced for that diagnostic label. ➤ Provides clinicians with a common language that enables them to discuss clients as if they were not real people with real concerns. ➤ Creates artificial categories that we "buy into," and thus we believe that such diagnoses exist. In fact, some suggest that such diagnoses are a social construction and thus a function of the values of society.	➤ Offers us a way of understanding the person more deeply, as we are challenged to make a thorough assessment of the client. ➤ By understanding the diagnostic label and by knowing the research in the field, we can better match presenting problems with treatment plans and use of medication, thus leading to better therapeutic outcomes. ➤ Offers clinicians a common language by which they can consult with one another and jointly come up with more effective treatment decisions. ➤ Provides clear-cut diagnostic categories from which research designs can be generated and new treatments found.

through a combination of therapy and psychotropic medication, it is becoming evident that counselors will need to learn how to use such medications (Kalat, 2013; Ninnemann, 2012; Schatzberg & Nemeroff, 2009). To fail to do so will undoubtedly find the counselor out of sync with the rest of the mental health field. In addition, it may leave the counselor open to ethical misconduct charges and possible malpractice suits, since in some cases, not using medication may be viewed as practicing incompetent therapy.

As community counseling agencies have become more prevalent, and as licensure has taken hold in every state, the number of counseling programs that offer degrees in clinical mental health counseling has increased. Whereas most students in counseling programs used to specialize in school counseling, slightly more students today graduate from CACREP-accredited clinical mental health counseling programs (44%), compared to school counseling programs (39%) (Schweiger, Henderson, McCaskill, Clawson, & Collins, 2012). Of all students who graduate from CACREP-accredited programs, many find jobs in one or more of the following settings: 1% in counselor education, 5% in assisted living facilities, 6% pursue advanced education, 6% in church ministry, 6% in hospice, 6% in private practice, 6% in corporate settings, 8% in government, 9% in churches, 10% in criminal justice settings, 11% with the developmentally disabled, 11% in middle schools, 12% in private practice, 13% as higher-education staff, 13% in elementary schools, 14% in teaching, 17% in high schools, 35% in agencies, and 18% in "other" places. You can see by the above breakdown that a large percentage of these graduates are working in clinical mental health jobs.

Roles and Functions of the Clinical Mental Health Counselor

In light of the diversity of agencies in which clinical mental health counselors are found, it is clear that they may be actively involved in tasks that vary dramatically. However, there are a number of roles and functions in which most clinical mental health counselors participate, including (AMHCA, 2013c; CACREP, 2009; O*NET, 2013):

➤ *Assessment and diagnosis:* Conducting interviews with clients and making diagnoses in an effort to afford accurate treatment goals

➤ *Case manager:* Participating in a broad range of activities that help to run a practice or agency, such as completing paperwork, conducting evaluations, conducting follow-ups, doing billing, practicing time management, and so forth

➤ *Counseling and therapy:* Providing counseling and therapy individually, in groups, or with couples and families

➤ *Consultant:* Providing consultation for parents, colleagues, and professionals working with clients in need

➤ *Cultural competence.* Providing counseling and consultation for individuals from diverse backgrounds and continually updating one's attitudes and beliefs, knowledge, and skills about nondominant groups

➤ *Crisis, disaster, and trauma work:* Having knowledge about and being prepared to work with individuals who have experienced a crisis in their lives, have been exposed to a disaster, and have been traumatized in some manner during their lives

➤ *Ethical and legal issues.* Practicing within the parameters of one's ethical guidelines, and responding appropriately to legal issues

➤ *Evaluation.* Ensuring that client outcomes are measured and that the counselor's work is ameliorating client problems

➤ *Maintaining records:* Keeping client information regarding treatment accurate and ensuring its confidentiality

➤ *Psychoeducational activities:* Providing formal educational/informational activities for clients and the public in order to assist clients or their loved ones, with the mental health issues that they are experiencing or may experience

➤ *Providing primary, secondary, and tertiary services.* Participating in a wide range of counseling activities that range from education and preventive services, to working with nonsevere mental health problems, to working to control severe mental health concerns (see Figure 17.1)

➤ *Social justice advocate.* Championing and defending clients' causes and clients' rights and organizing client and community support in order to provide needed services

➤ *Supervisee/supervisor:* Participating in supervision in order to sharpen skills, and provide others with supervision to assist them in improving their skills

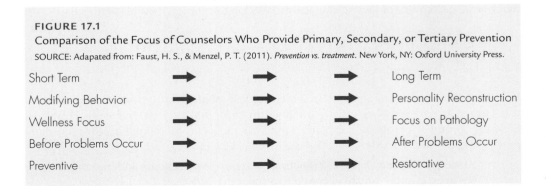

FIGURE 17.1

Comparison of the Focus of Counselors Who Provide Primary, Secondary, or Tertiary Prevention

SOURCE: Adapted from: Faust, H. S., & Menzel, P. T. (2011). *Prevention vs. treatment*. New York, NY: Oxford University Press.

Short Term	→	→	→	Long Term
Modifying Behavior	→	→	→	Personality Reconstruction
Wellness Focus	→	→	→	Focus on Pathology
Before Problems Occur	→	→	→	After Problems Occur
Preventive	→	→	→	Restorative

> *Testing*: Providing testing to clients in order to develop a more accurate diagnosis, provide a more focused treatment plan, provide information to those who need it (e.g., schools, courts, or lawyers), and to increase client insight

Theory and Process of Clinical Mental Health Counseling

Because clinical mental health counselors are found in many different settings with varying client populations, they emphasize different roles and functions and may adapt varying theoretical approaches to match their setting. For instance, a counselor who works in an agency that mandates a maximum of ten sessions per client will likely use one of a number of brief-treatment modalities. The counselor who mostly works with couples and families will choose any of a number of couples and family models when working with his or her clients. An LPC in private practice may choose from any of a number of theoretical approaches based on his or her personal leanings, and a counselor who mostly conducts career counseling will choose from any of a number of career development approaches when working with his or her clients. Therefore, defining a general theoretical approach that most mental health counselors would take is impossible.

Although it is impossible to identify a specific theoretical approach applicable to all clinical mental health counselors, there are some common principles to which most clinical mental health counselors would agree. For instance, the AMHCA Standards of Practice (2011) suggests that the scope of practice of clinical mental health counselors includes: "application of principles of psychotherapy, human development, learning theory, group dynamics, and the etiology of mental illness and dysfunctional behavior to individuals, couples, families and groups, for the purpose of promoting optimal mental health, dealing with normal problems of living and treating psychopathology" (p. 2). Hershenson et al. (2003) suggest that the following seven principles govern the ways in which counselors deliver services at all agencies:

> Respecting the client
> Providing a facilitative environment that fosters client progress
> Helping clients actively define goals to promote growth and development
> Empowering clients and helping them understand that counseling is an educational process that involves client learning
> Focusing on client strengths, not weaknesses
> Focusing on both the person and the context (environment)
> Using techniques that have been shown to be valid through prior research

Settings Where You Find Mental Health Counselors

The spread of the community mental health movement has led to the growth of counseling in a wide variety of agencies and settings and provide employment for clinical mental health counselors (AMHCA, 2013c). The following settings represent some of the more prevalent places where you are most likely to find clinical mental health counselors.

Career and Employment Agencies

Counselors today can be found at college counseling or college career management centers, state employment offices, vocational-rehabilitation offices, and private agencies that offer career and employment counseling (Ferguson's Careers in Focus, 2008). Such counselors typically assist individuals in the process of choosing or changing a career or educational path (Bureau of Labor Statistics, 2014). Usually, such work involves assessing clients' interests and aptitudes and helping to bring self-knowledge to clients concerning their career development process. In addition to AMHCA (www.amhca.org), one of the largest divisions of ACA, individuals who work in these settings often join one or both of the following ACA divisions: the *National Career Development Association* (NCDA; http://ncda.org) and the *National Employment Counseling Association* (NECA; www.employmentcounseling.org).

Community Mental Health Centers

Counselors have been working in mental health centers since they were first established more than 50 years ago (Garner, 2008; West, Hosie, & Mackey, 1987). Although a major function of the mental health center is to assist individuals with severe emotional problems, the kinds of services they offer vary greatly. Today, many community mental health centers provide a wide range of services, and counselors can be found working in any of these service areas (Centers for Medicare and Medicaid Services, 2013). They include:

1. Short-term inpatient services
2. Outpatient services
3. Partial hospitalization (day treatment)
4. Emergency services
5. Consultation and education
6. Special services for children
7. Special services for older persons
8. Preinstitutional screening (e.g., for admission to a state mental hospital)
9. Follow-up care for mental hospitals
10. Transitional care from mental hospitals
11. Alcoholism services
12. Drug abuse services

Because community mental health centers offer such a wide range of services, they often employ hundreds of clinicians, including psychiatrists, psychologists, counselors, social workers, psychiatric nurses, and human service professionals (Garner, 2008). The responsibilities of clinicians at mental health centers vary and include such activities as clinical assessment, consultation, education, prevention, referral, retention and education, individual, group, couples, and family counseling. Because there are a variety of different kinds of clinicians at mental health centers, it is not unusual for clinicians to work as a team. For instance, for a new client who enters the system, one clinician might conduct the intake interview, the psychiatrist might meet with the client for a medication assessment, and the case might be presented at a team meeting in order to determine which clinician might work best with this particular client.

As federal money for mental health centers has dried up, mental health centers have had to go elsewhere to secure funding. Thus, mental health centers have obtained grants from organizations like the United Way, and they rely on third-party billing for reimbursement of services. Because licensing is generally needed for insurance reimbursement, mental health centers have increasingly hired individuals who are licensed and who are eligible to receive third-party reimbursements.

Although clinical mental health counselors may be members of a variety of professional associations, many counselors who are employed at mental health centers belong to AMHCA, which is one of the largest divisions of ACA. AMHCA has a long history of advocacy for mental health issues and legislation.

Correctional Facilities

In 2013, approximately 7 million Americans—about 3% of adults residing in the United States—were in jail, on probation, or on parole, and of these, a majority were people of color (Bureau of Justice Statistics, 2013, 2014). With most prisoners being undereducated, abused as children, abusers of drugs and alcohol, and from dysfunctional families, the need for counseling is paramount. It is not surprising that counselors today find themselves performing multiple functions when working with those who are incarcerated. Some of these functions include counseling, assessment, crisis intervention, consultation, vocational training, assisting with day-to-day adjustment problems, preparing reports (e.g., sentencing, probation, and correction violations), testifying in court, maintaining contact with family members, and making referrals to outside agencies when the incarcerated individual is released from prison (Crighton & Towl, 2008; Hershenson et al., 2003; Sun, 2013).

With so many incarcerated individuals being addicted to drugs and alcohol, it is no wonder that in addition to AMHCA, many correctional counselors join the *International Association of Addictions and Offender Counselors (IAAOC)*, a division of ACA (www.iaaoc.org).

Family Service Agencies

Because of a historically strong emphasis on family issues and community advocacy in the social work profession, many family service agencies were originally established by social workers. This resulted in social workers being the clinicians of choice for many family service agencies, and these agencies continue to be one of the largest employers of social workers (Ritter, Vakalahi, & Kiernan-Stern, 2009). However, as counselors began to include couples and family counseling in their repertoire of skills, they have increasingly been hired by such agencies (O*NET Online, 2012). These agencies often receive partial funding through such organizations as United Way and through government grants. In addition, these agencies also receive payments via clients' insurance companies or directly from clients on a fee-for-service basis. Although many of these agencies have a religious affiliation (e.g., Catholic or Jewish Family Services), religion usually does not play a major role in acceptance of clients for counseling (Male, 1996). Counselors who work in such agencies have a full range of responsibilities, including conducting intake interviews, providing case management, offering consultation and education, and providing individual, group, and family counseling. In addition to AMHCA, individuals who work for family service agencies are often members of the *International Association of Marriage and Family*

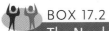

In an effort to understand some of the needs of older Americans, I visited a local community center that had organized senior services. This included meals at reduced prices; educational activities, such as guest speakers on a variety of topics; and social activities, such as movies, travel to local theater productions, and so forth. At the center, I had lunch with Irving, Lasard, Izzi, Jeanette, Max, Joe, and some other senior citizens, with their average age being about 80 years old. We had an informal discussion about a number of issues facing older Americans. Although there was some debate concerning the amount of federal subsidies that should be

given to seniors, some of their major issues seemed clear. For instance, all of them felt that seniors were entitled to safe and secure housing, access to good medical care, having their transportation needs met, healthy meals, and having federal assistance in the delivery and implementation of these programs. Most of this group felt that they had spent a lifetime of hard work and now deserved something in return.

Finally, it was clear that many of these seniors were dealing with losses in their lives—losses of spouses, friends, and relatives. Clearly, this psychological component was not being attended to by any of the existing available services.

Counselors (IAMFC, www.iamfconline.org), a division of ACA, the *American Association of Marriage and Family Therapists* (AAMFT; www.aamft.org), or both.

Gerontological Settings

As the population of individuals over 60 years old continues to rise (U.S. Census Bureau, 2011), so does their need for mental health services (Goodman, Schlossberg, & Anderson, 2006; Stickle & Onedera, 2006; Walsh, Currier, Shah, Lyness, & Friedman, 2008). Whereas older persons have traditionally been less amenable to counseling than younger people, this trend is likely to end as the baby boomers age (Maples & Abney, 2006). It is, therefore, not surprising that across the country, we have seen an increase in day-treatment programs for older persons at community mental health centers, long-term care facilities such as nursing homes, housing settings that are specifically geared toward older persons, senior centers, and programs for older persons offered through religious organizations and social service agencies (Ritter, Vakalahi, & Kiernan-Stern, 2009).

When working with older persons, both prevention and treatment become important, and counselors will often be found assisting older persons with developmental challenges and with situational crises such as loss of a spouse (Ferguson's Careers in Focus, 2008; Gladding & Newsome, 2014; Walsh et al., 2008). Counselors often have to assist older persons in dealing with the negative stereotypes placed on them by society, as well as the psychological and physiological changes that they face as a result of aging. Issues of loneliness, physical illnesses, loss and bereavement, and expected developmental changes of growing older are some of the things that counselors will confront when working with older clients (see Box 17.2). Although both individual and family counseling can be a means of treatment, some suggest that group counseling may be particularly effective when working with older persons (Gladding & Newsome, 2014; Thomas & Martin, 2006).

With some graduate programs offering emphasis areas in the counseling of older persons (Schweiger et al., 2012), it is clear that this area of counseling has gained quite a bit of importance. In addition to AMHCA, individuals who have an interest in gerontological settings often join the division of ACA known as the *Association for Adult Development and Aging* (AADA; www.aadaweb.org).

HMOs, PPOs, and EAPs

Ironically, although *health maintenance organizations (HMOs)* and *employee assistance programs (EAPs)* have cut into the ability of private practitioners to make a living (see the discussion in the section "Private Practice Settings," later in this chapter), they have provided another possible place of employment for clinical mental health counselors (Harrington, 2013; Ritter, Vakalahi, & Kiernan-Stern, 2009; Schweiger et al., 2012). For instance, some HMOs have designated clinicians for whom they provide office space, and subscribers must see one of these clinicians unless they receive special authorization to see someone else. HMOs such as these will often hire master's-level counselors. Other HMOs will select specific private practices to which they will refer, and counselors are often one of the many kinds of clinicians that may be found in these practices. Finally, due to the overseeing of clinicians' work that generally is handled by HMOs, some will hire counselors to review the casework of other clinicians.

Preferred provider organizations (PPOs), which are a type of HMO, are another source of employment for counselors (Banning, 2013, Harrington, 2013). PPOs are organized to provide discounted rates to members, and they feature gatekeepers who will refer clients to designated providers, although a client can go outside the PPO, with the PPO paying for a portion of the services.

Some businesses now hire counselors as part of their EAPs. EAP counselors provide education and prevention on such topics as substance abuse and stress reduction, assess employee problems, and sometimes provide short-term counseling. EAP counselors will often provide referrals to a wide range of community services, such as mental health centers, substance abuse agencies, lawyers, and private practice clinicians. Counselors who work for HMOs, PPOs, and EAPs will often join AMHCA.

The Military and Government

The military and government are unique work settings that offer a wide range of counseling opportunities. The general goals of counselors who work for the military or government is to encourage and deliver guidance, counseling, and educational programs for those in the armed services, employees of government agencies, and their families (ACEG, 2014). Such counselors assist military or government personnel with the identification of educational or training programs related to advancement within the military or government or helping people transition to a new career; provide prevention and psychoeducational programs (e.g., substance abuse); and conduct individual, group, and family counseling for military or government employees or their dependents. These individuals often work for a military family service center or an outpatient department of a military hospital or clinic, or serve as an in-house government employee, somewhat similar to an EAP counselor (see Box 17.3 for one example of such a person).

With an increased awareness and focus on mental health concerns of military members and their families (Military OneSource, 2014) and the recent approval for counselors to obtain TRICARE reimbursement (see the discussion in the section entitled "Recent Events," earlier in this chapter), career opportunities to work with this particular population may increase in the future. In addition to AMHCA, counselors who work for the military or government often join the *Association for Counselors and Educators in Government*

BOX 17.3
Meichell: A Military Counselor

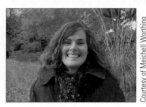

Courtesy of Meichell Worthing

I was raised in what some might call a typical military family. We moved every couple of years, changing schools thirteen times in a 12-year period. I always loved school and am fond of the adventure of moving to different places and experiencing different cultures. However, for every place that I was able to thrive in military life, my two brothers suffered educationally and emotionally, both dropping out in early high school. Both received special education services, but something was missing. No one was dealing with what it meant for them to be military kids. Many marriages also succumb to the pressures and end in divorce, which was the case with my parents' marriage.

There is a special shell type of emotional exterior that military families create around themselves in order to withstand the many losses they endure. Every deployment is a loss of time, memories, shared joys, and pains between husband and wife, parent and child, and general family wholeness. This often makes it hard to understand what is happening in the inner lives of these families. It takes special care and understanding of this organism that is its own culture.

I started out as a special education major in undergrad hoping to help children like my brothers. However, something was missing for me, and I made a drastic change to psychology my senior year. While exploring graduate studies, I met my husband, a Navy sailor, and found myself marrying into the Navy (ironically, something I said I would not do!). I began work on a graduate degree in counseling while my husband left for his first 1-year tour in the Middle East. After receiving my license, I opened my private practice. It was around this time that I was introduced to a consultant program sponsored by the Department of Defense. I serve as a contracted counselor to provide extra support on various military installations to both military personnel and their families. I also see military families in my private practice. It is rewarding to serve in this capacity having been raised in the military lifestyle/culture and continuing in this culture as the wife of a serviceman.

Why do I counsel military families? It is essential that these families have people in their communities that care about their struggles, are clinically trained, easily accessible, and willing to help them maintain strong families in the midst of constant change. Service men and woman deserve the best care and the secure knowledge that their families are emotionally cared for while they risk everything for the greater good of their country.

(ACEG), which initially was called *Military Educators and Counselors Association (MECA)*. ACEG is a division of ACA (http://acegonline.org/).

Pastoral, Religious, and Spiritual Counseling Agencies

Some counselors who obtain a degree in mental health counseling are interested in working in settings that have a religious or spiritual orientation. In fact, religious and spiritual issues seem to be an increasingly important aspect of counseling for many counselor trainees and counselors in general, despite the fact that they do not always infuse spiritual or religious issues within counseling sessions (Cashwell et al., 2013; Osborn, Street, & Bradham-Cousar, 2012).

Some who do pastoral counseling are ministers who may have had some coursework in counseling and sometimes pursue a master's degree in counseling. Others who have a strong religious orientation will obtain a degree in counseling and then seek out employment in a setting that fosters their particular point of view (e.g., Christian counseling agencies). These individuals tend to integrate the basic precepts of their religious viewpoints with what they've learned in graduate school (see Box 17.4 for one example). Obviously, at times, this makes for some interesting ethical and moral dilemmas, such as the pro-life Christian counselor whose counselor education training has taught him or her to respect the client's right to make decisions for himself or herself, including those

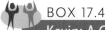

BOX 17.4
Kevin: A Christian Counselor

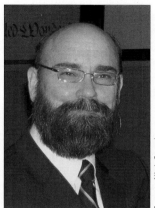

Courtesy of Kevin Coward

Let me start by saying that what I am doing as a vocation now was never considered in my earlier years. After a stint in the Navy in the late 1970s. I went into the ship repair industry and worked successfully in the field of electrical engineering for over 14 years. Subsequently, in the early 1990s. I went through a bitter divorce. Broken at a soul level, very alone and in deep despair, I sought out counsel with the minister at my church. Disappointed in his response, I went to a "Christian counselor." Even though I brought up my spirituality, I was dealt with very clinically—no prayer, no reference to biblical context, and no mention of Jesus as Healer, which are part of my core Christian beliefs. At that moment, a seed was planted to do something about this for others who might face a similar situation. I prayed long and hard and found what I

consider to be my calling by God: I wanted to help broken and shattered people by becoming a Christian counselor. I walked away from my prestigious career and simply followed this path. My quest led me to receive my master's degree in counseling, become an ordained minister, and obtain my license as a professional counselor, which allowed me to be employed as a pastoral counselor with a local church.

For the past 5 years, I was on staff with a large private Christian agency providing clinical counseling, within a Christian framework, to individuals, couples, and families who desire this perspective. Currently, I have opened a private practice of my own. By "Christian-based," I mean that I operate from a Christian worldview and recognize that the broken and shattered are all spiritual beings created to be in a relationship with God and with each other. By "clinically sound," I mean that I strive to constantly learn more in our field of expertise, counseling. This is partly why I am a member of the American Association of Christian Counselors and the International Society for the Study of Trauma and Dissociation. I diligently pursue knowledge on an ongoing basis to advance my deeper understanding of others so that I can provide effective interventions filtered through the Spirit of God.

---

clients who might want to have an abortion. Besides pastoral and religious counselors, an increasing number of counselors have integrated a spiritual viewpoint into their counseling orientation (Shaw, Bayne, & Lorelle, 2012). These counselors tend be driven less by religious convictions and more by the belief that that spiritual issues are primary to understanding a client's way of constructing meaning in their lives.

Pastoral counselors who are affiliated with a church, synagogue, temple, or mosque can often be found ministering at these settings. Religious counselors are often found in private practice groups that offer their particular religious bent, while counselors with a spiritual orientation can be found in all kinds of agency/mental health settings. In addition to AMHCA, pastoral counselors or counselors with a spiritual orientation might join the *Association for Spiritual, Ethical, and Religious Values in Counseling* (ASER-VIC; www.aservic.org) which is a division of ACA, and/or the *American Association of Pastoral Counselors* (AAPC; www.aapc.org).

Private Practice Settings

Now that every state has LPCs or its equivalent (ACA, 2011), there has been, and will continue to be, a rise in the number of counselors who are in private practice. Today, many private practice counselors can be found conducting individual, group, couples, and family counseling for individuals with "normal" life problems (primary and secondary prevention).

However, private practice counselors are increasingly found working with those who are seriously impaired (tertiary prevention), although additional training in psychopathology, psychopharmacology, and assessment is sometimes needed to work with this population. With mandates from the Affordable Care Act that insurance companies have to provide counseling and substance abuse services, it is likely that private practice will provide an additional venue for many counselors who are drawn to this type of setting.

Being in private practice has a number of advantages, including the fact that the counselor is independent; has choices of where he or she wants to work, when he or she works, fees, and type of work he or she provides; and can practice his or her preferred theoretical approach to therapy (Harrington, 2013). However, before jumping into private practice, one should also consider the fact that the counselor is completely responsible for all finances related to the practice, may not be able to get reimbursed from some insurance companies, may have difficulty getting networked and obtaining clients, and has to face the sometimes lonely world of the private practitioner. In addition, private practitioners need to ensure that they give clients a *professional disclosure statement*, have clients provide *informed consent*, deal with billing and insurance company issues, address privacy issues and confidentiality concerns related to the *Health Insurance Portability and Accountability Act (HIPAA)*, maintain proper records, and have a transfer plan (called a "*professional will*"), in case the counselor becomes incapacitated (Brennan, 2013).

Today, private practitioners often do other activities in addition to counseling (Dasenbrook, 2014; Hodges, 2012; Neuer, 2013). This helps them become networked and expands their revenue-earning ability. As a result, many private practice clinicians may also be found doing such things as coaching, community organizing, marital and divorce mediation, parent education, consultation and training in business and industry, stress management and biofeedback, educationally oriented seminars and workshops, supervision, evaluations for adoption and custody, and professional writing Private practice counselors often join AMHCA (see Box 17.5).

Rehabilitation Agencies

In the United States today, 56.7 million (18.7%) of all Americans have a disability (U.S. Census Bureau, 2012). Of people 15 years or older, these disabilities include limitations related to walking or using stairs; difficulty with select physical tasks like lifting, grasping, reaching, and pulling; difficulty with instrumental activities of daily living, such as taking medication, bathing, going to bed, preparing meals, and doing housework; mental disabilities, such as a learning disability, Alzheimer's or dementia, an intellectual disability, a developmental disability, or other mental disability; a seeing, hearing, or speaking disability; and problems with activities of daily living, such as dressing, bathing, eating, and toileting.

Individuals with disabilities are often counseled by those trained in clinical mental health counseling or in rehabilitation counseling at one of the following settings: state departments of vocational rehabilitation, community-based rehabilitation programs, in educational settings, Veterans Administration (VA) hospitals, independent-living facilities, and private rehabilitation agencies (Parker & Patterson, 2012). Whereas state vocational rehabilitation agencies and VA hospitals obtain federal or state funding (or both), private agencies mostly rely on insurance reimbursement, workers' compensation, and

BOX 17.5
Chevette: An LPC in Private Practice

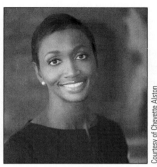

Courtesy of Chevette Alston

There is no magical story as to how I became a counselor; I am one of those rare people who knew from an early age that the mental health field was my area of interest. And perhaps like many in our profession, my path has taken some twists and turns.

I first worked with minority clients as a university counselor. I quickly realized that the word *minority* was inclusive of a number of areas, including ethnicity, culture, gender, socioeconomic status, and more. As a relatively young counselor, I tended to use one theoretical approach with all my clients. It didn't yet occur to me to vary my approach based on the unique needs of the individuals with whom I was working.

My next job was at a local community college where I worked for a federally funded student support program called the Open Door Project, whose purpose was to provide academic and counseling services to help students stay in college. Here I saw a variety of clients, some struggling with financial issues, which at times took priority over the desire to stay in college. Others were first-generation college students who struggled partly because there was no "culture of college" in their family of origins, and they did not have the advantage of family members that understood their experience or could give them helpful advice on how to study, testing skills, or other tips that would lend to successful college completion. It was here that I began to change my "generic" approach to counseling and learned to meet the client "where he or she was."

Today, I am in private practice. As I've grown as a counselor and professional, I've moved toward the idea that it is critical to have a broad base of knowledge and apply theories and techniques based on client needs and available resources. For example, clearly a middle class minority has different needs and resources from a minority who lives in subsidized housing. Although on the surface they may come from the same minority group, their backgrounds and available resources are dramatically different. To treat them the same would make little sense. And of course, all persons, regardless of where they come from, have their own unique concerns that are important to them and that are critical for me to understand.

As I look over my life as a counselor, I can see how my approach to counseling has changed as I have held various jobs and as I have matured as a professional. I am excited to see where I will be in the next 10 years.

other client-related methods of payment. In these settings, counselors often provide a wide range of services for their clients. For instance, they may

➤ Provide individual and group counseling to help clients adjust to their disability
➤ Evaluate clients' abilities, interests, experience, skills, health, and education
➤ Develop a treatment plan in consultation with other professionals, such as doctors, therapists, and psychologists
➤ Create rehabilitation or treatment plans based on clients' values, strengths, limitations, and goals
➤ Arrange for clients to obtain services, such as medical care or career training
➤ Help employers understand the needs and abilities of people with disabilities, as well as laws and resources that affect people with disabilities
➤ Assist clients in creating strategies to develop their strengths and adjust to their limitations
➤ Locate resources, such as wheelchairs or computer programs, that help clients live and work more independently
➤ Monitor clients' progress and adjust the rehabilitation or treatment plan as necessary
➤ Advocate for the rights of people with disabilities to live in the community and work in the job of their choice (U.S. Department of Labor, 2014–2015a, "Duties")

In providing these services, the rehabilitation counselor often employs individual and group counseling techniques and coordinates community services for clients (Leahy, Muenzen, Saunders, & Strauser, 2009; Parker & Patterson, 2012). Because of the wide range of disabilities with which the rehabilitation counselor works, it is often important that a team approach be taken when working with clients.

As new medical procedures make it possible for individuals to live longer with disabling and chronic health conditions, it is likely that we will see an increase in the number of individuals with disabilities. This will result in the need for additional services in which we will likely find the rehabilitation counselor taking an active role (Garner, 2008).

The rehabilitation counselor straddles two professional associations: the *American Rehabilitation Counseling Association* (ARCA; www.arcaweb.org), which is a division of ACA; and the *National Rehabilitation Counseling Association* (NRCA; http://nrca-net. org). Like many of ACA's divisions, ARCA has moved to a semi-independent state from its parent association, and one can now either join ARCA on its own or in conjunction with ACA.

Residential Treatment Centers

Increasingly, we are finding counselors working in residential treatment centers which tend to have a rehabilitative focus, provide a live-in setting for the duration of treatment, and provide counseling services (Blau, Caldwell, & Lieberman, 2014; Ellis, 2009). Today, residential treatment centers service many different people, including those who are incarcerated, individuals with physical disabilities, individuals with mental illness, the developmentally delayed, substance abusers, delinquent youths, and individuals with eating disorders, to name just a few.

The many kinds of services provided in such settings vary, but they often include individual and group counseling, family counseling, vocational counseling, medication management, client advocacy, assistance with reentry into the community, and consultation and referral to other professionals when the individual is ready to reenter the community (Blau et al., 2014; U.S. Department of Health and Human Services, 2006b). Because of the wide range of clients who may be served in residential treatment centers, as with vocational rehabilitation settings, a team approach involving a number of specialists and group treatment planning is often used. In addition to joining AMHCA, counselors who work at residential treatment centers often join the professional association that is most similar to the focus of the clientele with whom the counselor works. For example, counselors who work at residential centers for those with disabilities might join NRCA (see http://nrca-net.org) or ARCA (www.arcaweb.org); see Box 17.6.

Substance Abuse Settings

The substance abuse statistics in the United States are eye-opening (U.S. Department of Health and Human Services, 2013b). For instance, for individuals aged 12 and older, it was found that in 2012, 52.1% used alcohol, 23% binged, 9.2% used an illicit drug, 7.3% used marijuana, 6.5% used alcohol heavily, and 2.6% used psychotherapeutic drugs for nonmedical reasons. In addition, although 9% of Americans need treatment for drugs or alcohol, only about 1% are receiving it (National Institute of Drug Abuse, 2014).

BOX 17.6
Don—A Counselor at a Residential Treatment Center

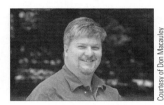

Courtesy of Don Macauley

I have always been interested in what makes people tick, which made a career in counseling a natural fit for me. Fresh out of getting my undergraduate degree in sociology, I volunteered as a co-facilitator of poly-substance abuse groups. Running these groups allowed me to develop basic group facilitation skills in an often challenging and intimidating environment. Empowered by my developing skills, I packed my bags and headed into the woods as a group leader in a youth wilderness program. I lived alongside troubled adolescents in the sweltering heat of summer and bitter cold of winter. This allowed me to not only appreciate but also experience many of the struggles the residents were facing being away from home, battling the elements, and processing difficult emotions.

After leaving the wilderness program, I worked as a unit staff member in a residential treatment facility while returning to school to earn my master's degree in community agency counseling

[now called clinical mental health counseling]. I completed my internship in the university's counseling center, where I was exposed to a diverse student population presenting a wide variety of issues that required me to be aware of my own cultural beliefs, attitudes, and perspectives. Upon graduation, I became a case manager for a local youth shelter, where I learned about family struggles and how different household roles influence family dynamics. I became increasingly interested in understanding the intricacies of youth and family issues. After becoming an LPC, I became an in-home clinician and had the unique opportunity of viewing families from within their own surroundings. Seeing some of the decrepit environmental conditions was an integral piece in identifying and understanding the stressors leading to family dysfunction.

In my current position at a residential treatment center for at-risk youth, I have been able to draw on my previous counseling experiences and thoroughly develop my counseling skills. This experience continues to teach me the value of empathy and unconditional positive regard, as well as the importance of maintaining a family systems perspective when working with at-risk youth.

Drug and alcohol abuse today can be found in the inner cities and in middle-class America. It not only affects the users but also has a great impact on family members and society (Fisher & Harrison, 2013; Woititz, 2002). There is little question that substance abuse is related to many of the problems facing our nation, including violent crime, problems on the job, and changing morals. As you might expect, the widespread abuse of substances provides an array of work settings for counselors, including hospital detoxification (detox) units, halfway houses, and drug and alcohol treatment centers (SAMHSA, n.d.).

Counselors who work in substance abuse treatment centers provide individual counseling, group counseling, and periodic couples and family counseling (O*NET Online, 2010). In addition, educational programs may be a part of this counselor's role as he or she attempts to bring increased awareness to the client and his or her family concerning the role that drugs and alcohol may play in their lives. In addition to joining AMHCA, many individuals with a focus on substance abuse will join the *International Association of Addictions and Offender Counselors* (IAAOC; www.iaaoc.org), a division of ACA.

Youth Services Agencies

Today, many state-assisted youth services programs employ master's-level counselors. Employment opportunities in such programs range from counselors who work with foster children, delinquent youth at residential treatment centers, children at mental health centers and child and family services agencies, juvenile offenders at state correctional systems, and other clients. Youth counselors provide a full range of services, including intake interviewing, assessment, guidance activities, consultation and referral with other mental health professionals, and individual, group, couples, and family counseling (Thompson & Henderson, 2010). With the increase in youth violence in the schools and the recognition of youth mental health needs, the importance of providing counseling services to youth has become clear (McWhirter, McWhirter, McWhirter, & McWhirter, 2013; Mellin, 2009; SAMHSA, 2013). Because of its focus on children, some counselors who work with youth are members of the *American School Counselors Association* (ASCA; www.schoolcounselor .org), while many simply decide to join AMHCA (www.amhca.org).

Counselors in Other Settings

In addition to the settings listed above, counselors can be found at many other community agencies, including crisis centers, psychiatric hospitals, hospices, group homes, women's shelters, and departments of social services, to name just a few (see Ferguson's Careers in Focus, 2008; Garner, 2008; Hodges, 2012). A degree in counseling is versatile and provides the counselor with a wide range of opportunities for employment. In fact, one might find the counselor in any setting where helping others is crucial. If you are considering a job in counseling, review the agencies listed above, but keep your options open.

Multicultural/Social Justice Focus

Counseling and the Diverse Client

Unfortunately, when it comes to counseling clients from nondominant groups, we have not done our job well, as such clients are:

➤ sometimes struggling with psychological disorders that is the result of perceived racism

➤ frequently misunderstood, misdiagnosed, find therapy less helpful than Whites, attend therapy at lower rates, and are more likely to terminate therapy

➤ often uncomfortable when working with a counselor who is not of the same culture

➤ often exposed to Western-based counseling theories that may not be congruent with their way of being in the world

➤ sometimes matched with counselors who have not had training in cultural competent counseling

➤ sometimes matched with counselors who are ethnocentric and even discriminatory, often through the use of microaggressions (see Chou, Asnaani, & Hofmann, 2012; D'Andrea & Heckman, 2008b; Evans, Delphin, Simmons, Omar, & Tebes, 2005; Sewell, 2009; Sue, 2010; Office of Minority Health, n.d.).

Clinical mental health counselors must heed these concerns if they are to work effectively with the increasingly large numbers of clients from nondominant groups who will require services in the decades to come.

Assessment Bias: Testing and DSM-5

When assessing clients through testing, it is of particular importance to understand the nature of bias in tests and to remember that counselors' biases can lead to misinterpretation of test scores, even when the tests are designed to be cross-culturally fair (Neukrug & Fawcett, 2015). Similarly, when assessing a client for a clinical diagnosis, counselors should consider the possibility that a diagnosis may be culturally predisposed, thus leading to the likelihood that individuals from some cultures will be misdiagnosed (American Psychiatric Association, 2013c; Kress, Eriksen, Rayle, & Ford, 2005).

The American Psychiatric Association (2013c) has attempted to combat potential problems with diagnosis of clients from nondominant groups by asking clinicians to understand cultural differences as a function of symptomatology (see the section "DSM-5 and Cultural Sensitivity," in Chapter 10). Thus, clinicians should be aware of culture-specific symptomatology when making diagnosis. In addition, DSM-5 offers a section entitled "Cultural Formulation Interview (CFI)," which helps clinicians understand the values, experiences, and influences that have come to shape the client's worldview and provides an outline for how to interview clients from diverse backgrounds appropriately. Finally, DSM-5 offers definitions of some cross-cultural symptoms and identifies how cross-cultural issues affect a wide range of diagnoses. Clearly, when conducting a clinical assessment, counselors must be extra careful to eliminate cultural bias.

Ethical, Professional, and Legal Issues

Ethical Issues

Ethical Complaints and Ethical Concerns

One manner in which we can assess the kinds of ethical difficulties that mental health counselors may be facing is by examining the kinds of ethical complaints made against LPCs. Although many mental health counselors are not LPCs themselves, it is likely that most face similar ethical dilemmas. In surveying 45 licensing boards, Neukrug, Milliken, and Walden (2001) found that 24% of complaints were made about an inappropriate dual relationship; 17% for incompetence in the facilitation of a counseling relationship; 8% for practicing without a license or other misrepresentation of qualifications; 7% for having a sexual relationship with a client; 5% for breach of confidentiality; 4% for inappropriate fee assessment; 1% for failure to inform clients about goals, techniques, rules, and limitations of the counseling relationship; and 1% for failure to report abuse. Another 33% of the ethical complaints were listed in an "other" category, with many boards indicating that drug abuse and felony or misdemeanor conviction was the cause. Although ethical complaints do not necessarily translate into ethical violations, it is likely that trends in ethical violations can be deduced from these data.

Table 3.2 in Chapter 3 examines further research by Neukrug and Milliken (2011) that identifies behaviors about which counselors have little agreement regarding whether they are ethical (also see the further discussion in Chapter 3). To assess counselor responses, a random sample of ACA members (most of whom were mental health counselors) were pooled. The items in this table are grouped by logical categories. You may want to discuss these behaviors in class.

Ethics Codes: ACA or AMHCA?

Generally, one should abide by the ethics code of the professional association to which one belongs. However, what if you belong to two associations, both of which have an ethics code? Since AMHCA (2010) and ACA (2014a) both have ethics codes, this can be a real possibility, although, in point of fact, the ethics codes rarely conflict. However, if I was put in that position, I would examine the codes; consult with those who can give me good advice, such as the ethics committees of these organizations; and make a wise decision—not one that necessarily supports my leanings, but one that makes the most sense based on the situation that I'm facing.

Professional Issues

AMHCA

Because mental health counseling covers a wide spectrum of counselors who work in many different types of settings, there is no one "perfect" professional association to meet the needs of its entire constituency. However, probably the association that comes closest is the *American Mental Health Counselors Association (AMHCA)*. The mission of AMHCA is "to enhance the profession of mental health counseling through licensing, advocacy, education and professional development" (AMHCA, 2013d, para. 2), and its vision is "to be the national organization representing licensed mental health counselors and state chapters, with consistent standards of education, training, licensing, practice, advocacy and ethics" (AMHCA, 2013e, para. 3). A few of the many activities that AMHCA conducts include advocating for licensed counselors, providing workshops and conferences, offering malpractice insurance, providing a code of ethics, providing job links, helping clients find counselors, and publishing a journal.

As with ASCA, AMHCA felt that they could better address some of the unique needs of mental health counselors with their own separate association and has also moved to a semi-independent division status with ACA (Colangelo, 2009). Today, one can join AMHCA separately from ACA. If you want to join AMHCA, membership is rather inexpensive, especially considering the benefits. As you continue on your journey in the counseling profession, consider which organizations work best for you.

Credentialing

Many clinical mental health counselors are interested in becoming a National Certified Counselor (NCC) through the National Board for Certified Counselors (NBCC). In addition, many obtain additional certifications through NBCC as Certified Clinical Mental Health Counselors (CCMHCs) or Master Addiction Counselors (MACs) (NBCC, 2012b, 2012e). Of course, many clinical mental health counselors also want to become LPCs, as this will allow them to obtain third-party reimbursement. Most states require a master's degree and 60 credits in designated curriculum areas to become licensed, but check your state for the exact requirements. Usually, if your master's degree was fewer than 60 credits, you will need to pick up the additional credits. In addition, a minimum of two years of post-master's supervision and the passing of a licensing exam are generally required. While some states use the NCC or CCMHC for their licensure exam, other states have devised a separate licensing exam.

Of course, one can obtain other credentials depending on your area of specialization. For instance, on the national level, one can become a certified rehabilitation counselor, addiction counselor, art therapist, play therapist, or pastoral clinical supervisor. Increasingly, as other specialty areas become more popular, we will see additional certifications arise. Finally, you may want to find out if any specialty certifications exist in your state.

Salaries of Mental Health Counselors

As you can see, the settings in which you find the clinical mental health counselor vary dramatically. Generally, employment prospects for counselors are expected to be "much faster than average," as reported by the Occupational Outlook Handbook (U.S. Department of Labor, 2014–2015b). Although salaries might vary as a function of the setting or the region in which you live, the *Occupational Outlook Handbook* states that the median salary is 41,500. Because advancement in many of these agencies is possible, counselors can earn considerably more as they progress in their careers. Counselors in private practice who are well-networked and established can earn $100,000 or more (Ferguson's Careers in Focus, 2008).

Legal Issues

A number of legal issues that have a direct impact on clinical mental health counseling have been discussed throughout this book. The following discussion identifies a few of them that have been particularly important in recent years.

HIPAA

The passage of the *Health Insurance Portability and Accountability Act (HIPAA)* ensures the privacy of client records and adherence to rules concerning the sharing of such information (Zuckerman, 2008). In general, HIPAA restricts the amount of information that can be shared without client consent and allows for clients to have access to their records, except for process notes used in counseling (notes used to help a counselor remember salient points). In fact, HIPAA requires agencies to show how they have complied with this act. As a result of HIPAA, mental health professionals will generally have to do the following:

- ➤ Provide information to patients about their privacy rights and how that information can be used.
- ➤ Adopt clear privacy procedures for their practices.
- ➤ Train employees so that they understand the privacy procedures.
- ➤ Designate an individual to be responsible for seeing that privacy procedures are adopted and followed.
- ➤ Secure patient records. (APA, 2013c)

Confidentiality of Records

In addition to HIPAA, confidentiality of records continues to be a critical issue for clinical mental health counselors. As discussed throughout this book, a number of laws protect patients' rights to confidentiality. In terms of federal law, the *Freedom of Information Act of 1974* allows individuals access to any records maintained by a federal agency that contain personal information about the individual, and every state has followed along with similar laws governing state agencies (National Security Archive, 2009). Similarly, the *Family Education Rights and Privacy Act (FERPA)*, ensures parents the right to access their minor children's educational records, although this does not apply to process notes (U.S. Department of Education, 2014b). Also, clients probably have a legal right to view their counseling records, and they have been exercising that right increasingly in recent years (ACA, 2014a, Section B.6.e; Wheeler & Bertram, 2012). Relative to children, although ethical guidelines usually support a child's right to confidential counseling, it has generally been assumed that parents have the right to view records of their children. Of course, specific local and state laws may vary, and each counselor should become aware of how local laws apply.

Confidentiality and Privileged Communication

In Chapters 4 and 5, we distinguished between the ethical obligation that one holds toward *confidentiality* and the legal right that clients hold toward *privileged communication* (Remley & Herlihy, 2014; Wheeler & Bertram, 2012). As a reminder, privileged communication is a conversation conducted with someone that the law (state or federal statute) delineates as a person with whom conversations may be privileged (i.e., attorney–client, doctor–patient, therapist–patient, clergy–penitent, husband–wife, and the like). Because privileged communication is generally given only to clients of licensed practitioners, this raises issues for mental health counselors who are not licensed, as they cannot guarantee confidentiality to their clients should a court decide to subpoena the counselor.

Confinement Against One's Will

Earlier in this chapter and in Chapter 2, we discussed the case of Kenneth Donaldson, who had sued the state mental hospital in Florida for confining him against his will (see *Donaldson v. O'Connor*, 1975; and see Box 2.3). The Supreme Court unanimously upheld lower court decisions stating that the hospital could not hold him against his will if he was not in danger of harming himself or others (Swenson, 1997). As a result of this decision, every state in the country now prohibits long-term confinement of clients against their will unless there is a clear indication that they are a danger to self or others. Even in these cases, a court hearing to show cause is generally necessary. This law has had a dramatic effect on how clinical mental health counselors work with clients and the kinds of decisions they make concerning those clients who may not be quite ill enough to be committed but are also not well enough to adequately care for themselves. At times, clients such as these are cause for great concern among mental health counselors.

The Clinical Mental Health Counselor in Process: Growing, Changing, Accepting

The field of mental health counseling has undergone dramatic changes in recent years, and it is likely to continue to do so in the foreseeable future (Cannon & Cooper, 2010). The ever-increasing acceptance of diagnostic tools such as DSM, the dramatic shifts in the health care delivery system, the increase in the kinds of counseling services offered, the ever-expanding knowledge of multicultural issues and their effects on client treatment, and the development of new ways of treating individuals with various emotional problems are just a few of the many issues that currently face the clinical mental health counselor. Thus, the clinical mental health counselor must not hide his or her head in the sand and continue to operate as usual. He or she must change with the times, attend conferences and participate in continuing education opportunities, and be flexible enough to adapt to new ways of working with clients from all backgrounds.

Summary

In this chapter, we examined the unique characteristics of the clinical mental health counselor. We first began by describing clinical mental health counseling in light of the current CACREP standards and also noted that often, clinical mental health counselors go on to become LPCs. Then while exploring the history of mental health counseling, we noted that this counseling specialty area had its origins with the development of psychoanalysis, the testing movement, and vocational guidance at the turn of the century. Over the years, the field was greatly influenced by existentialists from Europe and the Western philosophy of taking charge of one's life. The profession was launched into modern-day America through a series of legislative acts in the 1940s, 1950s, and 1960s. As a result of this legislation, research uncovered innovative therapeutic treatment modalities and new psychotropic medications that were to vastly change the way that counseling was delivered. In addition, this legislation funded mental health centers and other counseling-related services, and soon counseling became more acceptable in the United States.

The growth of different types of agencies that offered various counseling services was rapid during the 1960s and 1970s. Very quickly, we began to see mental health centers emerge in almost every community in the United States. In addition, other agencies, such as substance abuse centers, family service agencies, and vocational rehabilitation agencies, became part of the American landscape. Today, we see counselors working in just about every agency where counseling services are offered.

Relative to recent events in the history of mental health counseling, we noted that all 50 states now have counselor licensure, that mental health counselors are now included as mental health providers (e.g., TRICARE), and that the Affordable Care Act has mandated that counseling and substance abuse services be offered by insurance companies and that this will likely increase the need for more mental health counselors. We noted that the increase in mental health counselors being accepted as providers by insurance companies has led to a need for mental health counselors to know about diagnosis and psychotropic medication. We discussed the pros and cons of diagnosis and noted that recent research seems to suggest there is a genetic link for some emotional disorders and that therapy and medication may sometimes be the best treatment path. As this section of the chapter concluded, we noted that whereas most students who entered counseling programs had specialized in school counseling, now it is evenly split between school and clinical mental health counseling.

Although we noted that the roles and functions of clinical mental health counselors vary dramatically based on the setting, we did highlight some of the more common ones. These include assessment and diagnosis; case manager; counseling and therapy;

consultant; cultural competence; crisis, disaster, and trauma work; ethical and legal issues; evaluation; maintaining records; psychoeducational activities; providing primary, secondary, and tertiary services; social justice advocate; supervisee/supervisor; and testing.

Because there are so many different settings, roles, and functions of a clinical mental health counselor, the theories used by such counselors vary dramatically. However, we were able to identify some broad principles that underlie the counseling process of mental health counselors. First, we highlighted some broad principles suggested by the AMHCA Standards of Practice, then we noted seven other principles. These included respect for the client, creating a facilitative environment for client growth, helping clients define goals, empowering clients and helping them view counseling as a process that involves client learning, focusing on the strengths of the client, understanding the client within his or her environment or context, and using up-to-date techniques.

Because counselors can be found in just about every setting where counseling takes place, it would be impossible to list every agency where we might find clinical mental health counselors today. However, some of the more common settings that we highlighted included career and employment agencies; community mental health centers; correctional facilities; family service agencies; gerontological settings; HMOs, PPOs, and EAPs; the military and government; pastoral, spiritual, and religious counseling agencies; private practice settings; rehabilitation agencies; residential treatment centers; substance abuse settings; and youth service programs.

During this discussion, we noted that when it comes to counseling clients from non-dominant groups, unfortunately they have often been negatively affected by racism, misdiagnosed, and misunderstood; feel uncomfortable working with a counselor who is not from their culture; are exposed to counseling theories that sometimes are not a good match for the client's culture; and sometimes are counseled by individuals who are incompetent in cross-cultural counseling and even discriminatory. We also stressed that the clinical mental health counselor needs to be aware of bias in testing and problems with diagnosing clients from diverse cultures.

Examining some of the more prevalent ethical, professional, and legal issues, we noted some ethical concerns that are likely to be impinging on clinical mental health counselors. Specifically, we reported that ethical complaints were more likely to be made about inappropriate dual relationships, incompetence in the facilitation of a counseling relationship, practicing without a license or other misrepresentation of qualifications, or having a sexual relationship with a client. Other complaints were made for breach of confidentiality; inappropriate fee assessment; failure to inform clients about goals, techniques, rules, and limitations of the counseling relationship; failure to report abuse; drug abuse; or having a misdemeanor or felony charge. We also highlighted a recent study that explored a number of behaviors that mental health counselors tend to struggle with in the ethical decision-making process. Finally, we discussed the dilemma of what to do if two separate ethical codes differ on how to respond to an ethical issue.

In regards to professional issues, we stated that many clinical mental health counselors belong to AMHCA, and those who work in rehabilitation settings usually join ARCA or NRCA. However, we also noted that because of the varied types of clinical mental health counselors, there are many professional associations that they can join. We stated that many clinical mental health counselors obtain an NCC, with some subsequently acquiring the CCMHC, licensure as professional counselors, or both. We also noted that there are other certifications for clinical mental health counselors, with two of the more popular ones being the Certified Rehabilitation Counselor (CRC) and the Master Addiction Counselor (MAC). Next, we highlighted some of the salaries that one might expect from employment in this specialty area.

Some select legal issues discussed included the passage of the Health Insurance Portability and Accountability Act (HIPAA), which addresses the privacy of clients; the Freedom of Information Act and FERPA, which assert the right of individuals to obtain their confidential records from state and federal agencies; the difference between confidentiality and privileged communication; and how the Supreme Court decision in *Donaldson v. O'Connor* asserted the rights of individuals to not be confined against their will unless they are in danger of harming themselves or others.

The chapter concluded by noting that clinical mental health counseling has undergone dramatic changes in recent years, and that the astute counselor must keep up with these changes if he or she is to work effectively with all clients.

Further Practice

Visit CengageBrain.com to respond to additional material that highlight the salient aspects of the chapter content. There, you can find ethical, professional, and legal vignettes, a number of experiential exercises, and study tools including a glossary, flashcards, and sample test items. Hopefully, these will enhance your learning and be fun and interesting.

18 Student Affairs and College Counseling (Postsecondary Counseling)

I was obtaining my master's degree in counseling, thinking that I would eventually work in a clinical mental health agency. However, I found myself in a program that stressed counseling in higher-education settings. Up until being admitted to that program, I had wrongly believed that the attainment of a counseling degree meant that you became a school counselor or a clinical mental health counselor. I had a lot to learn.

As I went through the program, it didn't take long for me to realize that the college experience was crucial in the development of the individual. In fact, I realized that I had gone through many changes in my own life as I had pursued my bachelor's degree. Suddenly, I was rather interested in learning about student affairs and the impact that a student affairs practitioner could have on the development of the college student. I began to see this as an option for my career.

Through my program, I learned that the history of student affairs practices is long and illustrious, and that student affairs practitioners (e.g., college counselors, career counselors, directors of multicultural centers, etc.) are critical to the development of college students. Today, it is common to find student affairs practitioners working in a variety of campus settings that focus on student development.

In this chapter, we will discuss the history of student affairs practice, including college counseling, and the various ways in which student affairs has affected the development of the emerging adult. We will explore models and theories of student development, the roles and functions of the student affairs practitioner, the settings in which student affairs counselors work, and the unique multicultural, ethical, professional, and legal issues that impinge on the work of the counselor in higher-education settings. But first let us look at what this specialty area is all about.

What Is Student Affairs?

There are a lot of names for this specialty area. It can be called *student affairs, student affairs practices, college student development, college counseling, student development in higher education*, and I've probably left out a few. So bear with me if throughout this chapter, I use all of these names at different times.

The label *student affairs* encompasses a broad range of services that includes, but is not limited to, recruitment activities, admissions, diversity and equity issues, registration, orientation, residence life, counseling, student development, and advising. Ideally, student affairs offices provide programs and services to enhance the college experience of all students, whether it is the 18-year-old first attending college, the 35-year-old married father of two returning to college, the 60-year-old grandmother attending college for the first time, the international student challenged by language and cultural differences, or the veteran pursing an education after returning from combat. Student affairs practitioners help to facilitate students' learning and knowledge of self by offering services directly to students, collaborating with faculty and administration, and being proactive in making changes in the institution.

Student affairs practitioners are found working in a wide variety of settings in higher education, including academic support services, career development centers, counseling centers, office of educational accessibility, health services, human resources, multicultural student services, residence life and housing services, student activities services, to name just a few. The most recent Council for Accreditation of Counseling and Related Educational Programs (CACREP) accreditation standards identify this specialty area as *student affairs and college counseling*, although college counseling is actually one of the many areas where the student affairs practitioner, with a degree in counseling, may work (CACREP, 2009). Tentatively, the latest draft of the 2016 CACREP standards has changed the name of this specialty area to *postsecondary counseling*. In either case, this category includes those counselors who are going to be working in any of a variety of postsecondary areas doing counseling-related activities.

The History of Student Affairs

The Beginning

Student affairs practices have a long history, dating to the 1700s and some of the earliest American colleges (Rentz & Howard-Hamilton, 2011). These colleges were almost exclusively religiously affiliated, and their major goal was the development of moral men for the clergy. Early college faculty believed that students were immature and in need of guidance if they were to develop morally. Not surprisingly, student affairs practices at this time were governed by the philosophy of *in loco parentis*, or the concept that college faculty takes on the role of parenting and guiding students (Thelin & Gasman, 2011). During these early years, the faculty took on most of the roles in which we find student development specialists today. For instance, it was common to find faculty doing informal counseling, being involved in the discipline of students, assisting with admissions and registration, and serving as moral and religious mentors for students. It was the educator who was charged with developing all facets of the student, including his (and, once in a while, her) intellectual, personal, physical, and spiritual parts.

The Expansion of Student Affairs Practices

During the early part of the nineteenth century, there was a movement away from faculty being involved with the moral and religious development of students and more toward an academically oriented relationship (Bowden, 2007; Gerda, 2006). In the latter part of the nineteenth century—perhaps as a backlash to a century in which there was little concern about the emotional and spiritual aspects of students—there was a shift back to an emphasis on the personal development of students. It was at this time that many colleges began to hire deans of students, who were charged with overseeing a broad range of student development concerns such as enrollment, admissions, and moral development (Gerda, 2006). In addition, this part of the century saw the first campus mental health services being organized, under the direction of psychiatrists, to address the emotional development of students and prevent personal concerns from affecting academic success (Kraft, 2009).

As with community agencies and schools, the emergence of *psychoanalysis, testing,* and the *vocational guidance* movement at the beginning of the twentieth century had an impact on the role that colleges played in the development of the student. Thus, the early part of the century saw a psychological and humanitarian focus toward students, a push toward the development of "mental hygiene" services, as well as the use of intelligence and aptitude testing for both vocational guidance and the provision of psychological services (Kraft, 2009; 2011). At this time some of the first student affairs associations were developed, including the *National Association of Women Deans and Counselors (NAWDAC),* the *National Association of Student Personnel Administrators (NASPA),* and the *American College Personnel Association (ACPA).*

The Great Depression of the late 1920s and 1930s brought cutbacks in counseling, guidance, and other support services. With declining college enrollment, administrators viewed student affairs as an unnecessary expense (Carpenter, 2011). However, as the country moved out of the Depression and into the 1940s, there was a resurgence of student affairs practices with what became known as the *student personnel point of view* (Rentz & Howard-Hamilton, 2011). This development was largely fueled by the *GI Bill* at the end of World War II, which gave financial assistance to veterans to attend college (Kraft, 2011). Thus, this era saw extremely large numbers of individuals going to college, many of whom needed academic guidance and personal support services. This trend continued well into the 1950s.

The 1960s brought with it civil rights rallies and antiwar protests on college campuses. As one might expect, it was during this period that the concept of in loco parentis changed, as students increasingly insisted that they were not to be controlled by individuals in positions of authority (Bowden, 2007). During the late 1960s, there was more federal aid for students and an increasingly diverse campus environment. *Theories of development* that focused on identity issues were introduced during the 1960s and increasingly applied during the 1970s, as student development specialists attempted to offer educationally oriented activities focused on supporting developmental changes. This decade also saw a rise in proactive interventions on campus, such as the establishment of crisis centers, women's centers, and substance abuse centers (Kraft, 2011). The 1960s and 1970s also saw growth in the popularity of counseling centers that offered a wide range of counseling-related services.

Next, the 1980s brought increased refinement and application of developmental theories, as well as the emergence of student services that offered assistance to individuals with disabilities, minorities, women, nontraditional students, and other students with special needs. This broadening of services was ironically happening during the same decade that funding cutbacks became more prevalent, thus forcing many student services offices to downsize. This decade also saw a number of legislative initiatives that affected the implementation of student services, such as affirmative action, laws concerning sexual harassment, and laws affecting the rights of students (e.g., freedom of speech).

Recent Trends

The early 1990s saw continued state and federal cutbacks to colleges, which often resulted in reduced services for students (Thelin & Gasman, 2011). Increasingly, colleges attempted to maintain academic programs while trying to reduce the cost of student services without eliminating them totally. It was also during this period that we saw a call within the profession to examine the effectiveness of student development theory. As the second half of the 1990s saw an economic upswing in the country, colleges and universities began to feel more solvent, and the place of student services was once again secure.

The late 1990s and the early years of the twenty-first century affected student affairs with advances in *technology* that changed how students and student affairs professionals interacted. In addition, campus violence became another issue of concern, as high-profile incidents changed the way that campuses regarded student safety and prevention.

Current Practices

Today, student affairs professionals have been challenged to respond to the impact of the economic downturn that began in 2007. These challenges include cutbacks in funding to higher education, tuition increases while families experience job loss, and decreased availability of student loans. In addition to helping students navigate these financial difficulties, student affairs practitioners must address other student needs (e.g., creating a multicultural environment, ensuring a safe and secure campus, and reducing the risk of drugs and alcohol) (Kraft, 2011). Also, with the spread of technology and the rise of distance learning, student affairs practitioners have needed to rethink how to address student needs when students may not be learning at the main campus. This has led to some creative ways of reaching out to the new nontraditional student. Amidst these challenges, student affairs continues to grow as an integral part of the college organizational structure, and the services offered have an impact on every college student.

The student affairs practitioner of today often has a degree in counseling, although some will have a degree in higher education or in student affairs administration. As you might expect, those with a degree in higher education or in student affairs administration are less likely to be found in settings where counseling or a more traditional helping role is needed. The settings that we will discuss later in the chapter generally hire individuals with a counseling degree, although there is no hard and fast rule for this. Of those who obtain degrees from a CACREP-accredited counseling program, approximately 8% specialize in student affairs or in college counseling, and approximately 13% of all who graduate from CACPREP-accredited programs find jobs in higher education (Schweiger, Henderson, McCaskill, & Clawson, 2012).

Roles and Functions of Student Affairs Specialists

Because the student affairs practitioner can be found in a wide variety of settings on the college campus, his or her roles and functions may vary considerably. However, most student affairs practitioners need to have expertise in a well-defined set of competencies. Thus, the following gives an abbreviated definition of the competencies needed by most student affairs practitioners as identified by College Student Educators International and the Student Affairs Administrators in Higher Education (known, respectively, by their former acronyms: ACPA and

NASPA) (see ACPA/NASPA, 2010). Each competency will be followed by a short description of how an individual with a master's degree in student affairs and counseling might use the specific competency in his or her work setting. The competencies include advising and helping; assessment, evaluation, and research; equity, diversity, and inclusion; ethical professional practice; history, philosophy, and values; human and organizational resources; law policy and governance; leadership; personal foundations; and student learning and development.

Advising and Helping

> *The Advising and Helping competency area addresses the knowledge, skills, and attitudes related to providing counseling and advising support, direction, feedback, critique, referral, and guidance to individuals and groups.*
>
> (ACPA/NASPA, 2010, p. 6)

Tamikia is a counselor at a community college counseling center. She uses her advising and helping skills when she sees students at the center for short-term counseling; and when she refers students with more serious concerns to counselors in the community, she provides a wide range of counseling services, including counseling students for personal concerns, issues relative to school, career counseling, substance abuse counseling, couples counseling, and more.

Assessment, Evaluation, and Research

> *The Assessment, Evaluation, and Research competency area (AER) focuses on the ability to use, design, conduct, and critique qualitative and quantitative AER analyses; to manage organizations using AER processes and the results obtained from them; and to shape the political and ethical climate surrounding AER processes and uses on campus.*
>
> (ACPA/NASPA, 2010, p. 8)

Joshua works for the Office of Assessment and Research at a small college. He is involved with helping the office conduct a wide range of evaluation services, such as conducting needs assessment of students and faculty, providing consultation for student services offices regarding assessment of their programs, and evaluating why some students do not complete college (retention services). Results of their assessment and research are used to develop programs for the college that will better serve students, staff, and faculty.

Equity, Diversity, and Inclusion

> *The Equity, Diversity, and Inclusion (EDI) competency area includes the knowledge, skills, and attitudes needed to create learning environments that are enriched with diverse views and people. It is also designed to create an institutional ethos that accepts and celebrates differences among people, helping to free them of any misconceptions and prejudices.*
>
> (ACPA/NASPA, 2010, p. 10)

Lanay works for the Office of Equity and Diversity at a mid-sized university. She is involved with helping the office provide training for faculty and staff regarding appropriate ways to conduct job searches; providing confidential consultation regarding sexual harassment, discrimination, and salary equity issues; and offering programs to assist faculty and staff in developing a culture at the college that embraces diverse individuals.

Ethical Professional Practice

> *The Ethical Professional Practice competency area pertains to the knowledge, skills, and attitudes needed to understand and apply ethical standards to one's work. While ethics is an integral component of all the competency areas, this competency area focuses specifically on the integration of ethics into all aspects of self and professional practice.*
>
> (ACPA/NASPA, 2010, p. 12)

Kendal works for the Dean of Students office at the local community college and is in charge of conducting hearings for honor code violations. It is his job to set up hearing dates, provide confidential hearings where all sides can be heard, provide guidelines for the hearings, and assemble a team of student and faculty judges to make decisions about possible cheating on exams and plagiarism. He is guided by a series of aspirational ethics, including making sure that he is fair, does not harm others, is doing good for the college, respects the rights of individuals, and is committed to ensuring a just process for all involved.

History, Philosophy, and Values

> *The History, Philosophy, and Values competency area involves knowledge, skills, and attitudes that connect the history, philosophy, and values of the profession to one's current professional practice. This competency area embodies the foundations of the profession from which current and future research and practice will grow. The commitment to demonstrating this competency area ensures that our present and future practices are informed by an understanding of our history, philosophy, and values.*
>
> (ACPA/NASPA, 2010, p. 14)

Brigit is an assistant to the president of a middle-sized university, providing a wide range of services as she works behind the scenes so that the president can work efficiently. One day, she might be ensuring that the university's board is notified of where and when they will be meeting; another time, she might be setting up a consultation with the president and the governor's chief of staff to ensure appropriate state funding for the university. She is acutely aware of the "ups and downs" of funding for student services over the last 100 years and is an advocate to the president and others for inclusion of a wide range of student services at the university.

Human and Organizational Resources

> *The Human and Organizational Resources competency area includes knowledge, skills, and attitudes used in the selection, supervision, motivation, and formal evaluation of staff; conflict resolution; management of the politics of organizational discourse; and the effective application of strategies and techniques associated with financial resources, facilities management, fundraising, technology use, crisis management, risk management, and sustainable resources.*
>
> (ACPA/NASPA, 2010, p. 16)

Jamal works for human resources at a small four-year college. It is his job to meet with all incoming staff and faculty to orient them to the university and help them choose benefit plans (including such elements as health insurance and retirement plans). He is also involved with conducting mediation when staff and faculty have interpersonal concerns and for assisting staff and faculty through a personal crisis in their lives that may affect their benefit package and well-being at the college. He is acutely aware of the sensitive nature of his job, the importance of using his helping skills, and of keeping concerns confidential.

Law Policy and Governance

> *The Law, Policy, and Governance area includes the knowledge, skills, attitudes relating to policy development processes used in various contexts, the application of legal constructs, and the understanding of governance structures and their effect on one's professional practice.*
>
> (ACPA/NASPA, 2010, p. 20)

Brett works for the Dean of Students and is the "go-to" person for legal issues that arise relative to students, parents, staff, and faculty. Although he is not a lawyer, while obtaining his master's degree in counseling, he learned about a number of important legal issues that often come up on a college campus, such as requests from students to see their personal records (see the discussion of the FERPA law later in this chapter), grievance complaints by faculty, privacy complaints made by students and parents (e.g., concerns about roommate behavior or cheating), and issues related to in loco parentis, especially as it relates to the duty of the college to ensure the safety of students. He is often given the role of consulting with parents, students, staff, and faculty on these issues and more.

Leadership

> *The Leadership competency area addresses the knowledge, skills, and attitudes required of a leader, whether it be a positional leader or a member of the staff in both an individual capacity and within a process of how individuals work together effectively to envision, plan, effect change in organizations, and respond to internal and external constituencies and issues.*
>
> (ACPA/NASPA, 2010, p. 22)

Jamie is Director of Counseling Services, which includes the Counseling Center, the Career Management Center, and the Student Crisis Center. She is charged with hiring staff, developing strategic plans, ensuring the smooth running of the centers, running staff meetings, periodically having "retreats" to discuss concerns and future directions of the center, and evaluating staff. She is a visionary who often needs to use both her organizational skills and her consulting and helping skills to ensure that all staff get along with one another and are satisfied at their work.

Personal Foundations

> *The Personal Foundations competency area involves the knowledge, skills, and attitudes to maintain emotional, physical, social, environmental, relational, spiritual, and intellectual wellness; be self-directed and self-reflective; maintain excellence and integrity in work; be comfortable with ambiguity; be aware of one's own areas of strength and growth; have a passion for work; and remain curious.*

(ACPA/NASPA, 2010, p. 24)

Braden has always wanted to work at a counseling center at a large, four-year university, and now that he has been there 15 years, he believes that he has made a difference in the lives of hundreds of students. However, he continues to consider ways that he can offer better services to students by providing a holistic approach to working with all aspects of the individual. He often attends workshops and trainings on new and more effective ways of working with students. He remains passionate about his work and believes he will work at this center for years to come.

Student Learning and Development

> *The Student Learning and Development competency area addresses the concepts and principles of student development and learning theory. This includes the ability to apply theory to improve and inform student affairs practice, as well as understanding teaching and training theory and practice.*

(ACPA/NASPA, 2010, p. 26)

Briana's lifelong dream was to work at the Intercultural Student Services office, and now that she is on staff, she wonders how she can best provide services for the diverse students who come to the office. She has learned about the many theories of student development, but more important, she knows how these theories may be applied to students from varying backgrounds. This information helps her relate to the students that come to the office in deeper and more profound ways and provide services that best meet their unique needs.

Conclusion

The above definitions and vignettes offer a glimpse into some of the unique roles of the student affairs practitioner. Although each practitioner may have particular knowledge and skills in the highlighted competency, most practitioners need to be versed in all the competencies to be effective. So a counselor who works in the counseling center not only needs advising and helping skills, but also needs to understand legal concerns, ethical issues, and have leadership qualities. And a student affairs practioner who works at the Intercultural Student Services office needs to know about resources in the community, understand how student services history and philosophy has been detrimental to minority students so that similar blocks to student success will not be repeated, and has to have passion for his or her job. You can easily see how all the competencies are important to each type of student services practitioner.

Theories of Student Development

Developmental Theory

The conceptual base behind student affairs work is that as students attend college and graduate school, they develop in predictable ways, and that student affairs practitioners can develop interventions that move students toward greater cognitive complexity (Pascarella & Terenzini, 2005). Many of the theories used by student practitioners to help us understand development and devise interventions have already been discussed in Chapter 9. For instance, they might rely on theories of moral development as noted by Kohlberg (1969) and Gilligan (1982); lifespan development as noted by Erikson (1963, 1968) and Levinson (1978, 1996); constructive/cognitive development as noted by Kegan (1982); psychosexual development (e.g., Freud, 1969/1940); and faith development (e.g., Fowler, 1995). In addition, recently student affairs practitioners have used racial/cultural and White identity development models (discussed in Chapter 14) to help understand an individual's development (e.g., McAuliffe, Goméz, & Grothaus, 2013; Helms, 1984, 1999, 2005; Sabnani, Ponterotto, & Borodovsky, 1991). Finally, person–environment models, or models that attempt to examine how the environment affects the behavior of the changing adult, have taken on some prominence lately (Pascarella & Terenzini, 2005).

Although a chapter such as this cannot touch on all of the developmental theories that may have an impact on students, two that have been consistently used to describe changes in students over time are Arthur Chickering's seven vectors model (Chickering, 1969; Chickering & Reisser, 1993) and William Perry's scheme of intellectual and ethical development (Pascarella & Terenzini, 2005; Perry, 1970).

Chickering's Seven Vectors of Student Development

In 1969, Chickering identified seven vectors that he believed were crucial in the development of college students (Evans, 2011; Evans, Forney, Guido, Paton, & Renn, 2010). These vectors have become the standard model used in understanding college student development, particularly the development of the traditional college student (i.e., 18–22 years old). Chickering postulated that students can mature along each vector, increasingly developing a more complex identity, and that, through knowledge of these vectors, student affairs specialists can foster student development. The vectors include the following:

1. *Achieving competence.* Chickering believed that each student's ability to successfully develop his or her intellectual, physical, and interpersonal competence is crucial during the college years, and that such growth ultimately leads one to a sense of self-worth.

2. *Managing emotions.* As students develop into adulthood, they increasingly struggle with finding ways of managing emotions, especially anger and emotions related to their sexuality, both of which become ever more salient in the college years. The task for students is to establish new, more mature ways of managing all of their emotions.

3. *Developing autonomy.* The developing college student is increasingly faced with issues of autonomy as he or she disengages from his or her family of origin and develops a separate sense of self.

4. *Establishing identity.* As students become autonomous, self-sufficient adults, they are better able to understand their intellectual, physical, and interpersonal competence and strive to more effectively manage their emotions. In this process, students begin to examine who they are within these domains and establish a sense of self—an identity.

5. *Forming interpersonal relationships.* As individuals increasingly become more aware of their own identity, they are better able to form relationships with others and ultimately become more tolerant of differences.

6. *Developing purpose.* Perhaps one of the most important vectors, developing purpose relates to how individuals make meaning out of their lives. Deciding what is worth striving for can only be accomplished if an individual has a clear sense of who he or she is.

7. *Developing integrity.* This last vector has to do with one's ability to develop a value system governed by a well-thought-out belief system. Such a value system is the basis for moral action in the developing adult.

The challenge for student affairs specialists is to find ways to stimulate and facilitate growth along each of these vectors and thus assist college students in the healthy development of identity.

Perry's Scheme of Intellectual and Ethical Development

Perry's cognitive development scheme asserts that there are developmental stages that reflect a logical and sequential manner in which students develop their cognitive processes (Evans et al., 2010; Hofer, 2002; Magolda & Porterfield, 1992; Moore, 2002). Thus, for the student affairs practitioner, it would be crucial to identify the probable stage of development from which most students operate in order to understand how they make meaning of the world. Equipped with such knowledge, interventions could be designed that would facilitate higher-level meaning-making. Although we have discussed Perry in previous chapters, below is a brief recap of his theory. Perry set forth a theory that identified nine positions interspersed through three stages. Below are descriptions of the three stages:

1. *Dualism.* Students who are dualists tend to view truth categorically as right or wrong and have little tolerance for ambiguity. Such students might see the professor, professional documents, texts, and the like as holding the truth to knowledge in their field. They believe that there is one right answer to questions and have difficulty with uncertainty and the unknown. These students want to be told "the truth" and will regurgitate such knowledge in class, on an exam, or in conversation. As students reach the latter position

in dualism, they approach what some call *multiplicity* or *transition,* in which a beginning recognition of the limits of authority occurs. These students are moving toward relativism.

2. *Relativism.* Relativists are able to think more abstractly and allow for differing opinions. In relativism, a student comes to understand that there may be many ways of constructing reality and of defining truth. They become more comfortable with ambiguity and realize that knowledge is relative and that there are limits to what we know. They are more comfortable sharing information and thoughts with one another and value not only the knowledge of experts, but also the knowledge of their peers.

3. *Commitment to relativism.* Generally, this stage is only reached by individuals who are older (have life experience) and who have a number of years of education. Individuals who have reached this stage have the capacity to maintain their relativistic outlook and are also able to commit themselves to specific behaviors and values. For example, the committed relativist may make a specific religious or job commitment while at the same time recognize the possibility that new information may modify that choice. Although most adults do not reach the higher levels of this development, these models suggest that if afforded the right opportunities, most can do so.

Although students develop intellectually, interpersonally, spiritually, and even physically in college, few would dispute that the most important aspect of the college experience is the development of one's cognitive processes. This is why Perry's scheme has attracted particular attention over the years.

Settings Where You Find Student Affairs Specialists

In their first year after graduating, most students who obtain their degrees in college counseling or in student affairs are able to find employment in higher education. Schweiger et al. (2008) found that 69% of those who obtained their degrees in college counseling and 75% of those who obtained their degree in student affairs worked in higher education during their first year after graduation. Other college counseling and student affairs graduates go on to attend an advanced graduate program or work in a variety of other settings, including managed care, private practice, agencies, or K-12 schools.

There are many career options in student affairs settings, as well as opportunities for progression within each division, all of which offer a positive employment outlook for students interested in this specialty area (Garner, 2008). Although the majority of counselors have the expectation of doing counseling once they obtain their degree, many settings within the postsecondary environment exist where the counselor can find work doing advising, consulting, supervising, and offering preventive educational workshops. The following discussion describes some of the many places where you might find the student affairs specialist.

Academic Support Services

The purpose of *academic support services* is to assist students in reaching their academic goals (Dungy, 2003; White & Lindhorst, 2011). A wide range of academic support services are offered at many colleges and universities these days, and it is common to find a counselor working in many of these settings. Some of them include academic advising, administering learning resource centers for students with special needs, and coordinating tutoring services. The kinds of services offered to students at these centers include assistance with scheduling, time management, study skills, stress reduction, and consulting with faculty concerning the special needs of these students. Student affairs practitioners at all levels (community colleges, four-year colleges, and in graduate education) can be found working in academic support services.

Career Development Services

Almost all colleges have an office that provides *career development services*. Although some of these offices are part of the counseling center, today they are more frequently separated from it. Career development services tend to include a wide range of activities (Dungy, 2003; Severy, 2011), including individual counseling related to career choice, testing and assessment for purposes of career decision making, access to career resource materials, computerized career development programs to assist in choice of major, and internship and job placement. In addition, most career development centers provide assistance with résumé writing, job interviewing skills, cooperative education programs (e.g., internships), finding employment, and obtaining graduate assistantships. Professionals in career services may be responsible for organizing job fairs, as well as developing and maintaining relationships with major employers.

Counseling Centers

Today, most colleges and universities have *counseling centers* staffed by counselors, psychologists, or both (see Box 18.1) (Dungy, 2003; Zhang, Brandel, & McCoy, 2011). Increasingly, counselors at large universities are required to have a doctorate in counseling or psychology, while smaller colleges and community colleges will often hire master's-level counselors. Less frequently, social workers may also be found at these centers. Counselors at counseling centers work with students who are experiencing adjustment problems and normal developmental concerns. In addition, staff often will provide remedial and preventive assistance by offering workshops, courses, or support groups on campus. Often, such centers offer testing as an adjunct to counseling. Some college counselors may work with students who are struggling with severe problems, while others are likely to refer such students to private practitioners or community agencies. Counselors work with students on a wide range of issues, such as concerns over academic success, self-esteem, relationship problems, test anxiety, stress, sexuality and sexual concerns, depression, suicidal thoughts, substance abuse, eating disorders, and career development concerns (Vespia, 2007; Zhang, Brandel, & McCoy, 2011). Increasingly, students are entering college with a history of mental health treatment, and many are on medication to help manage a range of mild to more severe mental health issues (Prescott, 2008; Vespia, 2007). In addition,

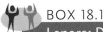

BOX 18.1

Lenora: Director of a University Counseling Service

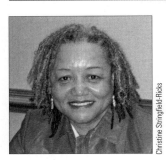

Christine Stringfield-Ricks

Helping others has always been a significant component of my life. As the oldest of five children, and the only daughter, I learned early in life how to help provide for others what they needed both physically and emotionally.

I was raised in Paterson, New Jersey, by parents who were determined to provide their children with a solid foundation of love, strength, support, and encouragement. As an African American child growing up in an urban environment and a society that did not embrace me, my gifts, or my abilities, it was my family who gave me their wisdom, determination, perseverance, and the knowledge that only I am in control of my destiny.

After surviving an urban miseducational system and being told by my White high school counselor that I should not attend college but pursue a job where I would work with my hands, I left Paterson to attend Shaw University in Raleigh, North Carolina. I knew I wanted to help make a difference in the lives of those I left behind, and I initially thought that teaching would be the best way to give back to the community. However, after gaining practical experience in elementary and junior high schools, I realized that teaching on those levels was not my calling. I therefore decided teacher training would be a better way to bring my goal to fruition, so I completed a graduate program in urban teacher education and obtained a position at the University of Massachusetts. This work was more fulfilling but not as satisfying as I expected.

Throughout this career exploration process, I realized that I was spending a great deal of time supporting my family, friends, and coworkers during their times of emotional upheaval. I would listen, ask critical questions, and help them develop a plan or strategy to ameliorate or change their particular life circumstance. These individuals would later call or write me to say how helpful our discussions had been in making changes in their lives.

From these experiences, my life's career path was established. I completed my doctoral degree in Humanistic Applications of the Behavioral Sciences (Counseling Psychology) with the goal of assisting adults with their mild to moderate mental health concerns.

The majority of my early clinical experiences were within a university environment, and these experiences, along with my life experiences and training, established a foundation for my current position as the director of a comprehensive urban university counseling service. In that capacity, I manage the daily functions of the office, manage the budget, recruit, hire, and supervise clinical staff and graduate students, facilitate seminars and psycho-educational workshops, provide consultation to the university community for mental health concerns, and of course, I carry a small clinical load. In addition, I sometimes find time to teach undergraduate and graduate courses. I find my career to be invigorating as I engage in a wide range of activities. Although my path has been a little circuitous in getting here, I'm glad I am where I am.

---

counselors may need to address posttraumatic stress disorder (PTSD) in veterans returning to college after combat, suicidal ideation as students face competitive programs and an unstable job market, or students suffering from the aftermath of sexual assault. Now, and in the coming years, counseling center staff will be challenged to find ways to respond to the increasing mental health needs of the college student population.

Office of Educational Accessibility (Disability Services)

Counselors who work for *disability services*, now sometimes called the *office of educational accessibility*, provide a wide range of services that support students with disabilities (Cory, 2011; Dungy, 2003). For instance, they can be found conducting short-term counseling, running support groups, ensuring compliance of the university with the *Americans with Disabilities Act* and other state and federal laws, assessing students for disabilities, assisting faculty in understanding how they can support individuals with disabilities in their academic pursuits, arranging transportation when appropriate, and assisting individuals with disabilities with campus housing. The range of disabilities with which the counselor works varies greatly. Some of the more common disabilities include the physically challenged, learning disabled, hearing impaired, and visually impaired.

Health Services

Many universities have their own *health services* that provide health care and preventive educational programs to students, faculty, staff, and administrators (Dungy, 2003; Keeling, Avery, Dickson, & Whipple, 2011). These health services are generally run by physicians, nurses, nurse practitioners, and physicians' assistants, and some may also offer counseling services, generally staffed by master's- or doctoral-level counselors. In addition, counselors will often be hired by health services to offer educational and preventive programs on such things as AIDS awareness, stress management, and living a healthy lifestyle. Some universities utilize student affairs professionals to organize student peer educator groups that work to promote such things as healthy lifestyles or safe sex practices on campus.

Human Resources

The *office of human resources* is involved with overseeing benefit packages for faculty, administrators, and staff and running preventive educational programs such as workshops on drug and alcohol abuse, stress management, communication skills, and financial management. Some human resource staff may be involved with hiring staff and assisting new faculty in their transition to the university, or helping faculty who are leaving the university find new jobs and/or move to a new area of the country. Some staff may also be involved in providing workshops and advice on sexual harassment issues and on affirmative action laws. In addition, human resource offices may house employee assistance programs that provide educational workshops, crisis intervention, short-term counseling, and referral to community agencies. Individuals who work for a human resource office may hold a degree in counseling or student affairs.

Intercultural Student Services

Today, most colleges and universities have an *office of intercultural student services*, sometimes called *multicultural or multiracial student services* that focuses on issues unique to ethnic minorities, women, men, religious groups, and sexual minority students (Dungy, 2003; Lopez-Mulnix & Mulnix, 2006; Shuford, 2011; Wong & Buckner, 2008). Staff who work in such offices will often have a degree in counseling or in student affairs and will provide a variety of services such as offering workshops for campus administrators, faculty, and staff to educate them on diversity issues; providing a supportive office where students from diverse backgrounds can feel welcome; assisting in providing a safe and accepting campuswide atmosphere; serving as advocates for individuals from diverse backgrounds; and educating the campus community on relevant laws (see Box 18.2). Some universities with high international student enrollment may have a separate office to support the needs of these students. This office may handle orientation, federal paperwork, and ongoing cultural exchange programs.

BOX 18.2
Carretta: Assistant to the Vice President, Student Affairs

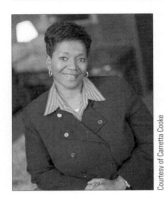

Courtesy of Carretta Cooke

I was always curious. I also wondered about people, and I grew up in a city where race, ethnicity, and class defined who you were. A wonderfully ethnic place, Detroit had kosher delis, Black Muslims, Polish bakeries, Italian and soul food restaurants, and world-famous museums.

Emigrating from the South, my father, a Korean War veteran, finished mortuary science school, married my mom, and settled in Detroit. I was lucky—my parents were able to afford me a life that was rare for an African American child growing up during the civil rights era. Ballet, voice, and piano lessons, dress-up social occasions, and private education were experiences that might have left me unaware of the fast-changing world around me. However, my parents helped educate me. At a time when Black history was a paragraph in history books about Lincoln freeing the slaves, I was being told about Denmark Vesey, Nat Turner, Harriet Tubman, and the contributions that African Americans made and were making in this country. I was a small child during the March on Washington but vividly remember the pride on my father's face as I sat on his lap and we watched it on television. I also remember not being able to use the bathroom in Tennessee, and looking at the signs that said "White Only" in Maryland as we drove to visit my relatives in the South. I guess that's why we always drove from Detroit to Sumter, South Carolina, in a day! I find it an honor to be part of a people who have endured and survived.

As an International Relations major in college, I was determined to be the first African American and female ambassador to China. I thought I would go on to law school. However, as an intern in the admissions office in college, I was fascinated by work in student services. Besides, my older sister was studying for the bar exam, and it scared the hell out of me! So, upon graduating, I began work as a financial aid counselor at a small Catholic college that had a diverse student body. I loved the college environment and decided China could wait—for a while anyway.

I came to multicultural student services still searching for my career in international relations. Accepting a position as Assistant Director for Minority Student Services at a large university near Washington, DC, I thought I could obtain a job at an international agency and move closer toward my goal of becoming a diplomat. However, I soon realized that I loved the work I was doing. After a racial incident on campus, I started pulling people together to have frank discussions about difference, "isms," to share perceptions. I found myself energized.

Now it is more than 30 years since my graduation, and I'm not the ambassador to China, but I have served more diverse groups than a career diplomat. I have served as executive director of a multicultural student affairs department that has more than four cultural units at a major selective university in the Midwest until recently. In my current position, I am still able to foment change as a senior level administrator and a campus expert on inclusion and diversity. I love working with the student community around issues of diversity. I love meeting people who have issues about race, ethnicity, and difference. I try to help them to better understand themselves and ultimately to heal.

I want to finish my doctorate and move into a position of greater authority and impact, possibly a vice president of student affairs. But, I will always be committed to diversity in the higher education setting. Whether it be speaking about the impact of diversity on college campuses, working with my faculty colleagues to infuse diversity issues into the curriculum, helping administrative staff deal with changing demographics, or helping people heal, I will never stop being that curious child—wanting to know the how and why of it all and, along the way, helping others and learning about myself.

Residence Life and Housing Services

The *office of residence life and housing services* generally provides a wide range of services related to student living (Akens & Novak, 2011; Dungy, 2003). Some residence life staff will live in student housing, oversee the day-to-day living of students, and assist with any housing-related problems that may arise. Other staff will assist students with their educational, social, and developmental concerns and may conduct preventive workshops on topics such as stress management, time management, communication skills, diversity

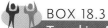

BOX 18.3
Tamekia: Area Coordinator for Residence Life

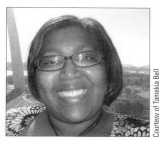

Courtesy of Tamekia Bell

In my opinion, there is no greater experience than working in residence life. I learned so much living with college students on a 24-hour basis for four years. From something as "simple" as roommate conflicts, to 3 a.m. fire alarms, to binge drinking, to students who have to go to the emergency room, to the many parent calls, residence life taught me how to manage and deal with difficult and complex issues. My journey to residence life was entirely coincidental. I was weeks away from graduating with my bachelor's in psychology and was planning to move to Tennessee to start my master's degree in counseling. I was moving to a new area where I had no family or friends, and I needed a job and a place to live. Thankfully, the person who interviewed me told me about a graduate assistantship in residence life. It seemed like a win-win situation. My out-of-state tuition would be waived and I would have a place to live. I applied, interviewed, and got the job.

I had no idea what I was getting myself into. I have worked in residence life for the past four years, spending three of those years as a resident director and a year as an area coordinator. In these roles, I learned so much about college student development and definitely put my counseling skills to good use. I also learned about crisis response and time management, how to be an effective supervisor, the importance of documentation, how to train staff, and many more transferable skills. There are aspects of residence life that I didn't like—like the numerous early morning calls I received—but, overall, I enjoyed my experience. The good definitely outweighed the bad.

College students are an amazing population of individuals to work with. It was amazing to see how they evolved throughout their college years. I was able to see my residents graduate and develop into successful, productive individuals. I recently resigned from my residence life position to pursue a doctorate in counseling. The reactions I received from residents upon my departure were just amazing. I had no idea that I impacted their lives so much. I enjoyed what I did and cared about them, which was reflected during every interaction I had with my residents. As I continue my doctoral studies, I bring each of my valuable learning experiences with me in the work that I do. My residence life experience was a worthwhile, valuable experience that I wouldn't take back for the world!

issues, and other concerns. In addition, staff will often be found assisting students who are having problems adjusting to college, struggling with personal problems, or dealing with interpersonal concerns with roommates and other students. Although staff who work in residence life may have a variety of degrees related to student affairs, clearly a master's in counseling is ideal, as many of the issues that face such staff are of a personal nature (see Box 18.3).

Student Activities Services

Often administered by the office of the dean of students, the *office of student activities services* is responsible for ensuring the smooth functioning of student organizations, advising student government, advising and coordinating sorority and fraternity chapters, scheduling campus activities, publishing student handbooks, enforcing student regulations, supervising student media (e.g., newspaper and radio), running intramural and recreational activities, and organizing social, cultural, and educational activities (Dungy, 2003; Whipple & O'Neil, 2011). As with many student affairs offices, a degree in counseling or student affairs is often needed to obtain a position with student services (see Box 18.4).

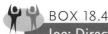

BOX 18.4
Joe: Director of Student Activities

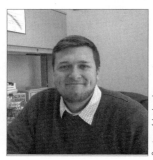

Courtesy of Joe Lowder

I often say that I did not grow up wanting to be a student affairs administrator. It is not a career that comes to mind until you are impacted by someone or something that shifts your perspective and direction. I grew up in a rural area of Mississippi, and my main goal was to push myself to graduate from college. My father dropped out of school in the eighth grade because of frequent moves. However, after a long road, he attained his GED and an associate's degree to better our family. My father's persistence helped me to truly understand the value of an education.

At first, I attended a small, residential community college in my hometown, where I was heavily involved on campus and thrived. Later, I transferred to a four-year college in Alabama where I lived and worked off campus. My grades dropped dramatically, and I found myself dissatisfied with the university. I decided to transfer back home to the large state land-grant university in Mississippi. There, I got involved in a campus organization and soon the organization's advisor suggested I examine a career in student affairs. Luckily, one of the master's degrees offered there was in counselor education. Although I took a number of common core classes with family and school counseling students, my emphasis was in student affairs in higher education. My master's degree helped me realize that I wasn't dissatisfied with the four-year university I had

been at, but rather with the experience that I had created for myself while there. This revelation is why I now have such a passion for student activities.

I consider myself lucky that I fell into a counseling degree, because counseling is the fundamental base of the work I do every day in student activities. My job is much more than planning events; it consists of mentoring, navigating conflict, team building, active listening, goal setting, informal career counseling, and asking students tough questions. I have learned that the one-on-one meetings are one of the most powerful tools I have to inspire and challenge students and staff to become well-rounded individuals.

Looking back, my educational journey has come full circle. I have my father and my student organization advisor to thank for shifting my perspective and helping me to find my direction. I did not realize until after I was in my current career that my father's path was also shifted by a college administrator at my small-hometown community college. It was the Dean of Students at this college who encouraged my father to attain his GED and gave him a small loan so he could work fewer hours and focus on the degree. For a long time, my father did not understand exactly what I did in student affairs, and always told his friends, "he teaches at the university or something." However, after hearing about his Dean of Students, I told my father that this type of guidance and nurturing is exactly what I strive to give my students. My dad now finally understands why I work in student affairs, and he has never been more proud of me!

Other Student Services Offices

The degree in counseling with a specialty in student services is versatile, and such individuals can be found in almost any setting on a college campus. Besides the ones listed above, some of the more prevalent offices include the *admissions office, office of assessment and evaluation, financial aid office, commuter services, distance learning site directors, women's/men's centers,* and *the office of the registrar* (Dungy, 2003; Zhang, 2011). Although traditional counseling is rarely offered at these offices, individuals with a background in counseling are often hired because of the heavy emphasis on advising, as counselors make excellent advisors. In addition, many graduates will obtain jobs in these offices as a stepping stone to other student services positions, positions that might have a more involved counseling role, more status, and better pay.

Multicultural/Social Justice Focus

Students who attend racially diverse institutions and are engaged in educationally purposeful activities that involve interactions with peers from different racial/ethnic backgrounds come to enjoy cognitive, psychosocial, and inter-personal gains that are useful during and after college.

(Harper & Hurtado, 2007, p.14)

With over one-third of all college students in the twenty-first century being identified as racial/cultural minorities (Fry & Lopez, 2012), multicultural issues are playing an increasingly important role in student affairs practices. Although offices of intercultural student services can be traced back to the 1960s, as more students of color and women attend colleges, addressing multicultural issues can no longer be the sole responsibility of this office. All student services offices and student affairs practitioners will need to learn how to effectively deliver services to this increasingly diverse population (Cuyjet, Howard-Hamilton, & Copper, 2011). The following discussion summarizes some of these approaches.

Applying Student Development Theory to Students from Diverse Backgrounds

Student affairs practitioners must ensure that the theories they apply with students are cross-culturally appropriate, as sometimes the "major" theories that have been applied have been based on the research from White students and can be misleading when applied to others (e.g., Chickering's and Perry's work) (MacKinnon, 2011).

Student affairs practitioners might do well in helping faculty and staff become educated on racial/cultural identity models (see Chapter 14). These theories can help faculty and staff understand students from diverse backgrounds, and when applied intentionally and appropriately, students from diverse backgrounds will feel an increased sense of being heard and understood. Such a deliberate focus, along with an ongoing commitment to improving the college experience of the students from nondominant groups, will help diverse students gain a positive experience on the college campus, increase retention rates, and develop leaders from non-dominant groups (Harper & Hurtado, 2007; Lopez-Mulnix & Mulnix, 2006; Pope, Reynolds, & Mueller, 2014).

Implementing a Cultural Environment Transitions Model

It is crucial that all student affairs practitioners jointly develop a model that will assist universities that operate mostly from a White Eurocentric perspective transition to one that embraces all cultures (Lopez-Mulnix & Mulnix, 2006). In making such a transition, a number of broad issues must be addressed (Cuyjet, 2011). For instance, a multicultural-friendly campus has diverse students and faculty, the social climate of the university is inviting, the physical environment is comfortable (e.g., it allows for places of worship yet feel comfortable for those who might be atheists), the interpersonal dynamics there are natural and respectful, the meaning that campus community members place on the campus environment is positive, and so forth.

"Hands-On" Changes That Encourage Cross-Cultural Sensitivity on Campus

Student affairs practitioners can actively assist all parts of the university in implementing specific changes that can move the university toward increased cultural sensitivity (Cooper, Howard-Hamilton, & Cuyjet, 2011; Pope et al., 2014). Just a few examples might include the following:

> ➤ Helping administrators see how the use of culture-specific terms such as "Christmas vacation" might be offensive to some non-Christians and to some cross-culturally sensitive Christians
> ➤ Helping orientation leaders assess the needs of minority students in order to better address their specific issues during orientation
> ➤ Assisting in the recruitment of staff who can better reflect the diversity on campus
> ➤ Encouraging the use of nonsexist and nonculturally biased language by the campuswide community
> ➤ Offering diversity workshops for students, staff, faculty, and administrators
> ➤ Providing assistance, such as scholarships, to encourage minority students to enroll
> ➤ Supporting the development of cultural student groups on campus
> ➤ Providing support for students from diverse backgrounds, especially those who have been disenfranchised and poor, and offering them a voice on campus
> ➤ Educating students about oppression and privilege and creating an environment that affirms other values and advocates for liberation of those who are oppressed
> ➤ Working to change policies and institutional structures that foster oppression

Removing the Barriers to Academic Excellence of Underrepresented Students

Rapidly increasing numbers of diverse college students have led to an artificial barrier between these new students and faculty members, the majority of which continue to be older White males (Gordon, 2007; Guthrie, Jones, Osteen, & Hu, 2013; Harper & Hurtado, 2007). Differences in language, ways of meaning-making, perceptions of racial and ethnic conflict, sexual orientation, and general cultural differences have made it difficult for underrepresented students to adjust to and achieve in college. One role of the student affairs practitioner is to lessen the gap between students and faculty so that all students will have an equal opportunity to achieve in all majors. This may mean working with faculty members to understand cultural or social barriers that may be impacting their students and helping faculty to devise strategies so that they can better relate to all students (Gordon, 2007; Harper & Hurtado, 2007).

Ethical, Professional, and Legal Issues

Ethical Issues

Ethical Guidelines

College Student Educators International (ACPA) offers ethical principles for student affairs practitioners (see ACPA, 2006). In addition, the *American College Counseling Association (ACCA)*, a division of the *American Counseling Association (ACA)*, applies the ACA ethical code to student affairs practitioners (see ACA, 2014a). Although the ACPA ethical principles are more specific to higher education settings, both guidelines are important for addressing ethical issues.

Confidentiality and Foreseeable Harm

Although confidentiality is an issue that all counselors must face, it has been particularly focused on in college settings following a landmark case that resulted in what has become known as the *Tarasoff rule* (Corey, Corey, Corey, & Callanan, 2015; Wheeler & Bertram, 2012; also see Chapter 4 of this book). This case, which examined the liability the university holds when an individual is in danger of harming another, has far-reaching implications for counselors who work in a college setting. Confidentiality is an important professional standard. However, in light of acts of campus violence, student affairs professionals may be called to take potential safety risks more seriously, thus limiting the extent of confidentiality offered to each student (Fisher, 2007).

Confidentiality, Informed Consent, and the Breaking of Rules

Because student affairs specialists are working for both students and the institution, they are sometimes faced with the dilemma of deciding to whom they owe their allegiance (Winston, 2003). Thus, students will sometimes come to student affairs practitioners with confidential information that the practitioner may be obligated to pass on to the institution. An example of this might be a student revealing to an advisor that he or she has cheated on an examination or knows of someone who has cheated. Thus, the student affairs practitioner must be clear on the limits of confidentiality when working with students and must obtain informed consent from the student for any advising or counseling that will take place under these limitations.

Professional Issues

Professional Associations

The sheer number of professional associations reflects the broad diversity in the field of student affairs today. Today, the *American College Counseling Association* (ACCA; www.collegecounseling.org), which is a division of ACA, and the *College Student Educators International* (ACPA; www.myacpa.org) are the two associations joined most frequently by counselors who work in student affairs. ACPA typically attracts those who identify with student affairs in general, while individuals who work in a counseling capacity in higher education generally join ACCA. Another important association is the *Student Affairs Administrators in Higher Education* (NASPA, www.naspa.org), which focuses on concerns of administrators in higher education. Also, many who work in student development offices will join associations specific to their field of interest. For instance, we often find those working in career services joining the *National Career Development Association* (NCDA, www.ncda.org) and those working in counseling centers joining the *American Mental Health Counselors Association* (AMHCA, www.amhca.org).

Technology and Student Affairs

Technology has greatly affected how some students learn, and it has increasingly become commonplace to find students learning via live TV or audio transmission, live online courses, or prepackaged online courses (Pullan, 2010). As accreditation bodies have increasingly accepted this new way of teaching (see CACREP, 2009), student affairs practitioners have had to devise new ways of meeting the needs of these new nontraditional students. Today, colleges and universities have placed student affairs practitioners at distant sites and have found creative ways to reach students who are not located on the main campus, such as offering online counseling, online remediation of writing, and intensive short-term institutes on campus where students can have their college needs addressed.

Even on campus, advances in technology have made it necessary for student affairs professionals to be proficient in the technologies available to students. Professionals may need to engage in online communication, create online social communities, and provide constant access to up-to-date information (Alemán, 2014; Alemán & Wartman, 2010). Additionally, many professionals may struggle with ensuring confidentiality across various media. Student affairs professionals unfamiliar with current technology will need to receive regular training to keep up with students' ever-changing online habits. The need to be constantly available in a time of instant communication, as well as the need for continuous access to information, will likely remain a challenge for the field of student affairs.

Salaries of Student Affairs Practitioners

Because of the diversity of student affairs practitioners on college campuses, salaries vary considerably within any one institution. In addition, colleges and universities vary dramatically on how much they pay student affairs practitioners. This tends to be a function of the geographical location of the college, whether it is a private or public institution, the financial stability of the institution, and the value that the institution places on the specific student affairs job. For instance, the median salary for a career counselor is $43,672 (Higheredjobs, 2013–2014a), for college counselors is $51,144 (salary.com, 2014), for directors of multicultural student services is $60,205 (Higheredjobs, 2013–2014b), and for postsecondary education administrators is $87,410 (U.S. Department of Labor, 2014–2015b). Please note, however, that salaries at some institutions can be quite a bit higher.

Legal Issues

Campus Safety

With the tragedy of thirty-two students and faculty being murdered at Virginia Tech, as well as violence on campus at numerous other universities, ensuring campus safety has become a major concern for student services. Indeed, nearly every student affairs office has been affected by the creation of policies and procedures to minimize risks and identify threats while protecting individual rights. Among these policies are methods to alert students to potential dangers, as well as identify worrisome student behaviors to prevent future violence. Many universities have adopted crisis alerts that can instantly notify students via text or email if there is a situation on or near campus. Heightened security in campus buildings has also been widely adopted following recent acts of violence (Rasmussen & Johnson, 2008). Additionally, student affairs professionals in various offices have the added responsibility of gatekeeping and referral.

Most colleges and universities now have threat assessment teams that work to identify potentially problematic students. Student affairs professionals and faculty members contact the team with any evidence that a student is exhibiting any abnormal or threatening behaviors. These students are then frequently referred to the counseling center for assessment and may be referred again to an outside agency if the concerns are severe (McBain, 2008). Counseling center staff may also be asked to disclose information on students to the threat assessment team, thus complicating the practice of confidentiality. Whatever the individual school's policy, staff from across all departments of student affairs must work together to protect campus safety, while also maintaining an environment that is supportive of students with mental health needs.

Liability Concerns

Student affairs practitioners face liability concerns that many other counselors do not. Some of the more common liability concerns are described below.

In loco parentis: In recent years, a number of student-initiated lawsuits have suggested that colleges may have a duty to protect students from physical harm that might occur through such things as sexual attacks, psychological problems such as suicidal ideation, sports-related injuries, and substance abuse (Bowden, 2007; LaCroix, 2008; Sloan & Fisher, 2011; White, 2007). Whereas in loco parentis was formerly seen as protecting student moral development, this new interpretation suggests that there is a duty of colleges to protect students from harm. Student affairs practitioners will need to pay special attention to these and other issues in the decades to come.

Alcohol abuse: When a university has condoned the use of alcohol, which subsequently becomes the reason for an accident or death, the university may be found to be at fault (Dowdall, 2013). For example, not being vigilant about addressing underage drinking or allowing alcohol at events, both of which could result in a car accident, could lead to legal action. Campuses have responded to this threat very differently. Some campuses are designated as "dry," meaning that alcohol is not allowed anywhere on school grounds and students may be penalized for being caught under the influence. Other campuses are "wet," which allow students to drink in designated locations and under certain guidelines. Regardless of the approach, colleges and universities must continually balance student safety and legal considerations when making and enforcing alcohol-related policies (Scribner et al., 2009).

Defamation and libel: When written or oral materials are used with the intention of defaming a person, a university may be held liable (Barr, 2003; Foundation for Individual Rights, 2009; Monaghan, 2012). However, universities have a history of upholding the right of students and others to freedom of expression. Thus, all universities must find the appropriate balance between the right to free speech and the right that an individual has to not be harmed by someone else's free speech. Thus, student affairs specialists who work with students, faculty, student organizations, the media (such as student newspapers,

Facebook, or Twitter) must be knowledgeable about the appropriate and legal balance between the right to free speech and the right of freedom from harm.

Civil rights liability: A number of civil rights laws have been passed over the years that prohibit discrimination of protected classes of individuals (e.g., minorities). In addition, universities today are increasingly being challenged to protect the civil rights of all people (Barr, 2003; Fagin, 2005; Safransky, 2010). Thus, when rights are in some way violated, the university may be held liable.

Contract liability: Numerous publications are initiated by a university, many of which are viewed as a contract (e.g., the university catalog) (Beckham, 2011; Palfreyman, 2003). Thus, student affairs specialists who are involved in the development of such publications must be keenly aware of potential liability concerns.

The right to records: The Family Educational Rights and Privacy Act (FERPA) ensures that all individuals have the right to inspect their educational records and to request a formal hearing if they believe the record to be false (Wheeler & Bertram, 2012; White, 2007). Parents do not have rights to student records at postsecondary institutions unless their child is a dependent according to the tax code, or if the student signs a release of information. Thus, student affairs practitioners need to know when and how to disperse requested records to students. It should be noted that if certain conditions are followed, FERPA excludes counseling process notes from the category of educational records.

The Counselor in Process: The Student Affairs Practitioner

Colleges and universities have historically been on the cutting edge; they are our nation's laboratories, where we experiment for the future. They exist to provide and expand our knowledge base. Any individual who wants to work at such an institution must be a forward thinker who is willing to take risks, test new paradigms, and provide new ways of offering services. The student affairs practitioner must be willing to move forward with the changes that will inevitably take place at our universities and later be reflected in society. Whether it is women's centers, multiculturalism, political correctness, or new student development models to be tested, the realm of the student affairs practitioner is ever-moving and ever-changing. As Rentz (2004) succinctly stated:

> *The role, mission, and goals of student affairs have never been, and hopefully never will be, static. For it is in the dynamic tension that resides within and between the field and higher education's changing institutions that the seeds of our power and value can be found.*

(p. 54)

Summary

This chapter began by highlighting the fact that the main purpose of the student affairs practitioner is to help facilitate the learning and self-knowledge of all students by offering services directly to students, collaborating with faculty and administration, and by being proactive in making changes in the institution.

The history of student services, we noted, dates to the early American colleges in the 1700s, which were mostly religiously oriented, had as their purpose the development of moral persons, and stressed the concept of in loco parentis, in which faculty took on the parental role of ensuring the safety and growth of students—roles that today, are loosely filled by student affairs practitioners. We noted that as the nineteenth century began, faculty were more concerned with the academic relationship they had with students than their personal lives, but by the end of the century, they became involved with the personal development of students.

With the rise of psychoanalysis and vocational guidance at the beginning of the twentieth century, there was an increased push toward mental hygiene services in higher education. It was also at this time that the first professional associations were formed: the National Association of Women Deans and Counselors (NAWDAC), the National Association of Student Personnel Administrators (NASPA), and the American College Personnel Association (ACPA). During the early years of the twentieth century, student services became firmly established, and except during the Depression, the focus generally remained on the whole person. The end of World War II saw extremely large increases in the number of college students and a concomitant rise in student affairs practices, fueled by the GI bill. This trend continued well into the 1950s. The 1960s saw a movement away from the traditional concept of in loco parentis as students demanded more independence and saw an increased emphasis on the application of developmental theories. The 1970s saw an expansion of student affairs practices, especially in the area of proactive interventions like crisis centers, women's centers, substance abuse centers, and counseling centers. With the 1980s came a greater refinement and application of development theories and an increased focus on nontraditional and minority students, while the beginning part of the 1990s saw an increased emphasis on promoting academic success and an attempt to find ways of reducing the cost of student services.

The latter part of the 1990s brought increased economic solvency on the part of student services, and in the early part of the twenty-first century, we saw a focus on the importance of creating a multicultural environment on campus, having a safe and secure campus, reducing the use of drugs and alcohol, and dealing with the spread of technology, including the rise of distance learning. In recent years, we saw student affairs professionals challenged to respond to the impact of the economic downturn that started around 2007, the continued spread of technology, and the increased professionalization of student affairs practices. We noted that the student affairs practitioner of today often have their master's degree in counseling, may work in a number of student affairs positions, and often obtain their degree from a CACREP-accredited institution.

We noted that the development of the student affairs profession was reflected in the establishment of a number of professional associations over the years, including the American College Counseling Association (ACCA), which is a division of ACA; the College Students Educators International (formerly the American College Personnel Association, but keeping the ACPA acronym); and Student Affairs Administrators in Higher Education (formerly, the National Association of Student Personnel Administrators, but keeping the NASPA acronym).

As the chapter continued, we noted that despite the fact that there is great variability in the roles and functions of student affairs practitioner, a number of competencies have been identified that most student practitioners should know. They include advising and helping; assessment, evaluation, and research; equity, diversity, and inclusion; ethical professional practice; history, philosophy, and values; human and organizational resources; law policy and governance; leadership; personal foundations; and student learning and development.

As the chapter continued, we noted that developmental theories offer a conceptual basis for student affairs practice. We pointed out that many of the developmental theories discussed in Chapter 9 guide student affairs practice, and that two theories in particular, Chickering's seven vectors model and Perry's scheme of intellectual and ethical development, have been relied upon by practitioners in this area. We noted that Chickering believed that students mature along seven vectors, which include achieving competence, managing emotions, developing autonomy, establishing identity, forming mature interpersonal relationships, developing purpose, and developing integrity. Perry, on the other hand, examined changes in cognitive development as a function of college experience, noting that individuals tend to move from a dualistic, rigid way of viewing the world to a relativistic, more open mode of understanding.

As the chapter continued, we identified some of the student affairs offices where one is likely to find individuals who hold a degree in counseling. These include academic support services, career development centers, counseling centers, office of educational accessibility, health services, human resources, intercultural student services, residence life and housing services, and student activities services. We also noted that many other student services offices are staffed by individuals with counseling degrees.

Relative to multicultural and social justice issues, we noted that college campuses are becoming increasingly diverse, and we highlighted a few issues that student affairs practitioners should address. They included the importance of ensuring that developmental theory is not biased and are applied accurately to students from diverse backgrounds, ways to implement a cultural environment transitions model, "hands-on" changes that encourage cross-cultural sensitivity on campus, and ways to remove the barriers to academic excellence of underrepresented students.

Relative to ethical concerns, we noted that ACPA and ACA both provide ethical codes, although ACPA's code is more focused on student services and less focused on counseling. Two major ethical issues that we identified included concerns over confidentiality, especially in reference to the responsibility toward an individual who may be in danger of harming oneself or another (e.g., the Tarasoff rule), and the conflict that sometimes exists between confidential information that we receive from students (e.g., a student who has cheated on an exam) and the responsibility to report such information to supervisors or the institution at large.

Relative to professional issues, we highlighted four associations in this field: the American College Counseling Association (ACCA), which tends to focus on counseling issues; the College Student Educators International (ACPA), which generally attracts those who identify with student affairs in general; the Student Affairs Administrators in Higher Education (NASPA), which focuses on concerns of administrators, and the National Career Development Association (NCDA). Also relative to professional issues, we pointed out that technology and distance learning have greatly affected how student affairs practitioners reach students, and we discussed the importance of finding creative ways of addressing the needs of these new nontraditional students and some of the struggles that professionals may have with confidentiality with constantly changing technology. We noted that because there are so many types of student affairs practitioners, the salaries of such staff can vary dramatically. However, we were able to identify some median salaries of career counselors, college counselors, directors of multicultural student services, and postsecondary educational administrators.

As the chapter neared its conclusion, we discussed a number of legal issues that affect the student affairs practitioner. First, we highlighted how policies and procedures have changed to better ensure campus safety. Then, we examined a number of liability issues, including in loco parentis to ensure that students are protected from harm; keeping students safe from the effects of alcohol abuse; ensuring that students aren't defamed or libeled; ensuring the civil rights of students; contract liability, or ensuring that publications are accurate (e.g., the catalog); and the rights of students to their records as stated by FERPA. Finally, we concluded the chapter by noting that the student affairs practitioner of today must be willing to move forward in response to the changes that will inevitably take place in our universities and later be reflected in society.

Further Practice

Visit CengageBrain.com to respond to additional material that highlight the salient aspects of the chapter content. There, you can find ethical, professional, and legal vignettes, a number of experiential exercises, and study tools including a glossary, flashcards, and sample test items. Hopefully, these will enhance your learning and be fun and interesting.

Afterword

A Look Toward Your Future:
Applying for Graduate Programs and Finding a Job

My path toward the attainment of master's and doctoral degrees in counselor education was by no means direct. At first, since I had majored in biology, counseling hardly seemed like the career that I would end up choosing. For one thing, when I went to school, career counselors were not as aware of degrees in counseling as they are now. Thus, when I went to my career counseling center to seek help in deciding my future, it was not the best experience for me. In addition, source books with information about the field of counseling or specifics about where to apply for a graduate degree were not readily available. And, of course, there was no Internet. Today, the degree is often sought after, and it is much easier to find out about various programs.

I've had many jobs over the years. How I learned about these jobs and each of their application processes differed. I've also been on the other end of the application process, where I reviewed materials and assisted in making decisions about whether an applicant should be admitted to a graduate program or recommended for a job. As an interviewee, I've made some mistakes. And as a reviewer of applicants' materials, I've seen mistakes made.

With my experience over the years, I humbly believe that I might be able to help others by identifying resources and by offering some helpful "tips" for those considering a master's or doctorate in counseling and for those applying for a job. This afterword is intended to help you in that process.

Select Items to Consider When Choosing a Program or Finding a Job

Although there are dozens of items to consider when selecting a graduate program or finding a job, the following pinpoint some critical elements. For instance, when making an informed decision about going on to graduate school, one should probably consider the following:

➤ Whether the program is accredited
➤ The kinds of counseling specialties and degrees offered
➤ The philosophical orientation of the program
➤ Entry requirements
➤ The size of the program and university

- Faculty-student ratios
- Diversity of the student body and of the faculty
- The cost and number of available scholarships
- Location
- Job placement possibilities

Similarly, the job seeker should know the following:

- The minimum credentials needed for the job
- Specific requirements necessary to fulfill the job
- The philosophical orientation of the setting
- The number and type of clients that one is expected to see
- Other job roles and functions
- Salary
- Diversity of coworkers
- Possibilities for job advancement

The Application Process

Having sat on selection committees for graduate schools and for counseling jobs in the public and private sector, I have been amazed at the number of applicants who miss the basics in their application process. The following represent some items that one should address when completing such applications:

- Complete all necessary forms and meet all application deadlines.
- Make sure that you address each item asked of you in the graduate application or job advertisement.
- Do not submit cookie-cutter applications to different jobs or different graduate schools. Make sure that your application "speaks to" the particular school or job for which you are applying.
- Be prepared for and take any necessary tests (e.g., GREs for graduate schools, or personality tests that are required for some jobs).
- Write a great essay or statement of philosophy.
- Find out if an interview is required, and if so, prepare for it.
- Find out about faculty members' research or be knowledgeable about your employer's background and find an opportunity to ask questions about what they have accomplished.
- Provide a well-written résumé.
- Consider submitting a portfolio.
- Use spell-check, check your grammar, and have someone else check your materials for errors and flow, too.
- Be positive, focused, and prepared.
- Don't be negative or cynical.

The Résumé

Some programs and most potential employers will ask you to submit a résumé. Good résumés present a well-rounded picture of who you are, so it's usually a good idea to submit one even if it is not requested. Some general guidelines when developing your résumé include:

➤ Make it readable, attractive, grammatically correct, and to the point.
➤ Do not use gender biased words or phrases.
➤ Do not be overly concerned about length. There has been a tendency in recent years to keep résumés under two pages. I don't agree. Whatever you decide the length of your résumé needs to be, make sure that major points stand out and it is easy for the reader to understand who you are and what you have accomplished.
➤ Do not make the résumé too wordy or too chaotic.
➤ Tailor your résumé to the requirements of the program or job being pursued.
➤ Do not add detail that could eliminate you from the selection process. For instance, sometimes individuals include a career goal that is at odds with the goals of the program or the job at hand.
➤ Do not sell yourself short. For example, I have seen many individuals not list jobs they have had because they were not in the counseling field. Don't forget that all experience is good experience and that jobs have transferrable skills.
➤ Brag about yourself, but don't sound narcissistic.

For a more detailed look at résumés, get a good book on résumé writing, such as *The Perfect Resume* (Quinlen, 2014) or *Best Résumés for College Students and New Grads* (Kursmark, 2012). In addition, there are some great websites to help you build a terrific résumé (e.g., Microsoft's website templates can be found at http://office .microsoft.com/en-us/templates/results.aspx?qu=resumes).

The Portfolio

In addition to a résumé, a portfolio may increase your chance of being admitted to graduate school or obtaining a job (Cobia et al., 2005). Portfolios include materials that demonstrate the ability of the student or counselor and can be used when applying for graduate school or for jobs. Competencies highlighted through accreditation processes [e.g., by the Council for the Accreditation of Counseling and Related Educational Programs (CACREP)] or goals highlighted in job advertisements will often drive what is included in the portfolio.

As an example of what may be placed in a portfolio, students who have completed a degree in school counseling may have developed a portfolio that could be used for potential employment purposes and includes a résumé (as discussed previously), transcripts or videos of the student's work with clients (with the clients' identities hidden), supervisor's assessment of the student's work, a paper that highlights the student's view of human nature, examples of how to build a multicultural school environment, ways that the student shows a commitment to the school counseling profession, a test report written by the student, letters of recommendation, and a project that shows how the student would build a comprehensive school counseling program. Although in the past, portfolios have consisted of only hard-copy materials, today's portfolios are often placed on a CD or online (Andrade, 2013; Barnes, Clark, & Thull, 2003).

Locating a Graduate Program/Finding a Job

You're ready to apply to a program or find a job. So where do you look? There are some specific places to contact to find the graduate program of your choice, and there are ways to increase your chances of obtaining your dream job. The following section provides some resources for your school or job selection process.

Finding a Graduate Program

A number of resources are available to assist students in locating a graduate school. Some of these include the following:

Master's and doctoral programs in counseling:

addiction counseling
career counseling
clinical mental health counseling
couples, family, and marriage counseling
school counseling
student affairs and college counseling

Council for Accreditation of Counseling and Related Educational Programs
1001 North Fairfax St., Suite 510
Alexandria, VA 22314
Phone: 703.535.5990
Web site: www.cacrep.org
Related association: American Counseling Association

Counselor Preparation: Programs, Faculty, Trends (13th ed.) (2013)
Authors: Schweiger, W. K., Henderson, D. A., McCaskill, K., Clawson, T., & Collins, D. R.
7625 Empire Dr.
Florence, KY 41042-2919
Phone: 800.634.7064
Web site: http://www.routledge.com/
Email: orders@taylorandfrancis.com

Doctoral programs in counseling and clinical psychology:

American Psychological Association (APA)
Graduate and Postdoctoral Education
750 First St. NE
Washington, DC 20002
Phone: 800-374-2721
Web site: www.apa.org/education/grad/index.aspx
Related association: American Psychological Association (www.apa.org)

Master's programs in rehabilitation counseling:

Council on Rehabilitation Education
1699 Woodfield Rd., Suite 300
Schauburg, IL 60173
Phone: 847.944.1345
Email: sdenys@cpcredentialing.com
Web site: www.core-rehab.org
Related associations: American Rehabilitation Counseling Association (www.ar-caweb.org), National Rehabilitation Counseling Association (http://nrca-net.org)

Master's programs in marriage and family therapy:

Commission on Accreditation for Marriage and Family Therapy Education
112 South Alfred St.
Alexandria, VA 22314-3061
Phone: 703.838.9808
Web site: http://www.aamft.org/imis15/content/coamfte/coamfte.aspx
Related association: American Association for Marriage and Family Therapy
(www.aamft.org)

Clinical pastoral programs:

Association for Clinical Pastoral Education, Inc.
1549 Clairmont Rd., Suite 103
Decatur, GA 30033
Phone: 404.320.1472
Web site: www.acpe.edu

Master's programs in social work:

Council on Social Work Education
1725 Duke St., Suite 200
Alexandria, VA 22314

Phone: 703.683.8080
Web site: http://www.cswe.org/Accreditation.aspx
Related associations: Council on Social Work Education (www.cswe.org)
National Association of Social Workers (www.naswdc.org)

Master's programs in art therapy:

American Art Therapy Association
4875 Eisenhower Ave., Suite 240
Alexandria, VA 22304
Phone: 888.290.0878
Web site: http://www.arttherapy.org/aata-educational-programs.html
Related association: American Art Therapy Association (www.arttherapy.org)

Finding a Job

There are a number of things you can do to increase your chances of finding a job. Some of these include networking, going on informational interviews, responding to ads in professional publications, interviewing at national conferences, using college and university job-placement services, and more.

Networking. You've finished your training, and now are ready to find a job. What do you do? Well, if you wanted to get a head start on the process, you would have joined your local, state, and national professional associations prior to finishing your training. Networking in this manner is one of the most widely used and best methods of obtaining a job. When people see you and are impressed with you, you have put one foot in the door. Sometimes you might even get a job on the spot (see Afterword, Box 1)!

Going on Informational Interviews. So you have written your résumé and developed a portfolio, you're networked, and you look and sound good—now what do you do? Well, you've probably identified a few different types of jobs in the counseling field.

AFTERWORD, BOX 1
Networking

Randy was a former student of mine who was enthusiastic about the counseling field. He joined his professional associations, he worked with me on research, and he participated in professional activities whenever possible. Because Randy was so involved, he had the opportunity to co-present a workshop with me at a state professional association conference. His enthusiasm and knowledge so impressed one of the participants that at the end of one workshop, she offered him a job—right then and there.

Now it's time to find some people who have these jobs and go on some informational interviews. These interviews will allow you to get a closer look at exactly what people do and will help you make a decision regarding whether you really want to pursue a particular job. In fact, sometimes people will let you shadow them on the job—and sometimes informational interviews can lead you to a specific job opening.

Responding to Ads in Professional Publications.   Today, there are a number of professional publications that list jobs locally, statewide, and nationally. An active counseling association in your community or state may have a job bank and list jobs in its newsletter. *Counseling Today*, the monthly American Counseling Association (ACA) periodical, lists a variety of counseling-related jobs throughout the country. So does the APA newspaper, *The Monitor*. Similarly, the *Chronicle of Higher Education* lists jobs nationally, although most of these jobs are confined to the area of student affairs or are at the doctoral level.

Interviewing at National Conferences.   Often, the large national conferences, such as the annual counselor conference sponsored by ACA, will offer a process whereby individuals who are looking for jobs can interview with a prospective employer at the conference. Although this is generally focused on doctoral-level counselor educator jobs, some master's-level jobs are also available.

College and University Job Placement Services.   Job-placement services and career-management centers at colleges and universities will often have information about local community agencies that can be helpful when conducting a job search. Sometimes these placement services will have job listings and offer job fairs that are relevant for graduate students in counseling.

Other Job-Finding Methods.   Remember the tried-and-true methods for finding jobs—such as applying directly to an employer, responding to a newspaper ad, contacting a private or state employment agency, and placing an ad in a professional journal. These methods sometimes do work!

Being Chosen, Being Denied

Counselor educators avoid saying that a person is "rejected" from a program or a job, suggesting instead that the individual was denied admission or given other opportunities. Nevertheless, most people who are not admitted to their first-choice school or not offered their dream job generally feel rejected. If you are denied admission or not offered a desired job, ask for feedback about your application and the interview process. Although it is sometimes hard *not* to take a denial personally, this can be a great opportunity to discover what you can do to improve your application process. Once you know what was amiss, you can increase the chances of obtaining your chosen graduate program or job.

In Process and Moving Forward

Change can be painful. It requires giving up a former way of living in the world and accommodating to a new way. Even when the past way is not working, it is our security blanket. It is what we know, and often it feels safer to stick with the familiar than take the risk of moving into unknown territory. After all, if people weren't afraid of change, they would hardly need counselors.

There is something to be said for sticking with what has worked. It's like our favorite old armchair. We can rely on it to be comfortable and faithful to us. We can always fall back on it. On the other hand, there is something exhilarating about taking risks. Like rollerblading for the first time, it's exciting and you may fall down (and even get hurt), but generally you end up on your feet.

As you move into your career as a counselor, are you feeling comfy in your armchair, or are you going rollerblading? Consider your choices and think about your future. If you get too comfortable, then move on for a doctorate or get a new job—but whatever you do, get up on those rollerblades and keep moving.

Appendix

2014 ACA Code of Ethics
As approved by the ACA Governing Council

Mission

The mission of the American Counseling Association is to enhance the quality of life in society by promoting the development of professional counselors, advancing the counseling profession, and using the profession and practice of counseling to promote respect for human dignity and diversity.

Contents

ACA Code of Ethics Preamble

The American Counseling Association (ACA) is an educational, scientific, and professional organization whose members work in a variety of settings and serve in multiple capacities. Counseling is a professional relationship that empowers diverse individuals, families, and groups to accomplish mental health, wellness, education, and career goals.

Professional values are an important way of living out an ethical commitment. The following are core professional values of the counseling profession:

1. enhancing human development throughout the life span;
2. honoring diversity and embracing a multicultural approach in support of the worth, dignity, potential, and uniqueness of people within their social and cultural contexts;
3. promoting social justice;
4. safeguarding the integrity of the counselor–client relationship; and
5. practicing in a competent and ethical manner.

These professional values provide a conceptual basis for the ethical principles enumerated below. These principles are the foundation for ethical behavior and decision making. The fundamental principles of professional ethical behavior are

- *autonomy*, or fostering the right to control the direction of one's life;
- *nonmaleficence*, or avoiding actions that cause harm;
- *beneficence*, or working for the good of the individual and society by promoting mental health and well-being;
- *justice*, or treating individuals equitably and fostering fairness and equality;
- *fidelity*, or honoring commitments and keeping promises, including fulfilling one's responsibilities of trust in professional relationships; and
- *veracity*, or dealing truthfully with individuals with whom counselors come into professional contact.

ACA Code of Ethics Purpose

The *ACA Code of Ethics* serves six main purposes:

1. The *Code* sets forth the ethical obligations of ACA members and provides guidance intended to inform the ethical practice of professional counselors.
2. The *Code* identifies ethical considerations relevant to professional counselors and counselors-in-training.
3. The *Code* enables the association to clarify for current and prospective members, and for those served by members, the nature of the ethical responsibilities held in common by its members.

4. The *Code* serves as an ethical guide designed to assist members in constructing a course of action that best serves those utilizing counseling services and establishes expectations of conduct with a primary emphasis on the role of the professional counselor.
5. The *Code* helps to support the mission of ACA.
6. The standards contained in this *Code* serve as the basis for processing inquiries and ethics complaints concerning ACA members.

The *ACA Code of Ethics* contains nine main sections that address the following areas:

Section A:	The Counseling Relationship
Section B:	Confidentiality and Privacy
Section C:	Professional Responsibility
Section D:	Relationships With Other Professionals
Section E:	Evaluation, Assessment, and Interpretation
Section F:	Supervision, Training, and Teaching
Section G:	Research and Publication
Section H:	Distance Counseling, Technology, and Social Media
Section I:	Resolving Ethical Issues

Each section of the *ACA Code of Ethics* begins with an introduction. The introduction to each section describes the ethical behavior and responsibility to which counselors aspire. The introductions help set the tone for each particular section and provide a starting point that invites reflection on the ethical standards contained in each part of the *ACA Code of Ethics*. The standards outline professional responsibilities and provide direction for fulfilling those ethical responsibilities.

When counselors are faced with ethical dilemmas that are difficult to resolve, they are expected to engage in a carefully considered ethical decision-making process, consulting available resources as needed. Counselors acknowledge that resolving ethical issues is a process; ethical reasoning includes consideration of professional values, professional ethical principles, and ethical standards.

Counselors' actions should be consistent with the spirit as well as the letter of these ethical standards. No specific ethical decision-making model is always most effective, so counselors are expected to use a credible model of decision making that can bear public scrutiny of its application. Through a chosen ethical decision-making process and evaluation of the context of the situation, counselors work collaboratively with clients to make decisions that promote clients' growth and development. A breach of the standards and principles provided herein does not necessarily constitute legal liability or violation of the law; such action is established in legal and judicial proceedings.

The glossary at the end of the *Code* provides a concise description of some of the terms used in the *ACA Code of Ethics*.

Section A

The Counseling Relationship

. . . .

Introduction

Counselors facilitate client growth and development in ways that foster the interest and welfare of clients and promote formation of healthy relationships. Trust is the cornerstone of the counseling relationship, and counselors have the responsibility to respect and safeguard the client's right to privacy and confidentiality. Counselors actively attempt to understand the diverse cultural backgrounds of the clients they serve. Counselors also explore their own cultural identities and how these affect their values and beliefs about the counseling process. Additionally, counselors are encouraged to contribute to society by devoting a portion of their professional activities for little or no financial return (*pro bono publico*).

A.1.   Client Welfare

A.1.a.   Primary Responsibility

The primary responsibility of counselors is to respect the dignity and promote the welfare of clients.

A.1.b.   Records and Documentation

Counselors create, safeguard, and maintain documentation necessary for rendering professional services. Regardless of the medium, counselors include sufficient and timely documentation to facilitate the delivery and continuity of services. Counselors take reasonable steps to ensure that documentation accurately reflects client progress and services provided. If amendments are made to records and documentation, counselors take steps to properly note the amendments according to agency or institutional policies.

A.1.c.   Counseling Plans

Counselors and their clients work jointly in devising counseling plans that offer reasonable promise of success and are consistent with the abilities, temperament, developmental level, and circumstances of clients. Counselors and clients regularly review and revise counseling plans to assess their continued viability and effectiveness, respecting clients' freedom of choice.

A.1.d.   Support Network Involvement

Counselors recognize that support networks hold various meanings in the lives of clients and consider enlisting the support, understanding, and involvement of others (e.g., religious/spiritual/community leaders, family members, friends) as positive resources, when appropriate, with client consent.

A.2.   Informed Consent in the Counseling Relationship

A.2.a.   Informed Consent

Clients have the freedom to choose whether to enter into or remain in a counseling relationship and need adequate information about the counseling process and the counselor. Counselors have an obligation to review in writing and verbally with clients the rights and responsibilities of both counselors and clients. Informed consent is an ongoing part of the counseling process, and counselors appropriately document discussions of informed consent throughout the counseling relationship.

A.2.b.   Types of Information Needed

Counselors explicitly explain to clients the nature of all services provided. They inform clients about issues such as, but not limited to, the following: the purposes, goals, techniques, procedures, limitations, potential risks, and benefits of services; the counselor's qualifications, credentials, relevant experience, and approach to counseling; continuation of services upon the incapacitation or death of the counselor; the role of technology; and other pertinent information. Counselors take steps to ensure that clients understand the implications of diagnosis and the intended use of tests and reports. Additionally, counselors inform clients about fees and billing arrangements, including procedures for nonpayment of fees. Clients have the right to confidentiality and to be provided with an explanation of its limits (including how supervisors and/or treatment or interdisciplinary team professionals are involved), to obtain clear information about their records, to participate in the ongoing counseling plans, and to refuse any services or modality changes and to be advised of the consequences of such refusal.

A.2.c.   Developmental and Cultural Sensitivity

Counselors communicate information in ways that are both developmentally and culturally appropriate. Counselors use clear and understandable language when discussing issues related to informed consent. When clients have difficulty understanding the language that counselors use, counselors provide necessary services (e.g., arranging for a qualified interpreter or translator) to ensure comprehension by clients. In collaboration with clients, counselors consider cultural implications of informed consent procedures and, where possible, counselors adjust their practices accordingly.

A.2.d.   Inability to Give Consent

When counseling minors, incapacitated adults, or other persons unable to give voluntary consent, counselors seek the assent of clients to services and include them in decision making as appropriate. Counselors recognize the need to balance the ethical rights of clients to make choices, their capacity to give consent or assent to receive services, and parental or familial legal rights and responsibilities to protect these clients and make decisions on their behalf.

A.2.e.   Mandated Clients

Counselors discuss the required limitations to confidentiality when working with clients who have been mandated for counseling services. Counselors also explain what type of information and with whom that information is shared prior to the beginning of counseling. The client may choose to refuse services. In this case, counselors will, to the best of their ability, discuss with the client the potential consequences of refusing counseling services.

A.3.   Clients Served by Others

When counselors learn that their clients are in a professional relationship with other mental health professionals, they request release from clients to inform the other professionals and strive to establish positive and collaborative professional relationships.

A.4.   Avoiding Harm and Imposing Values

A.4.a.   Avoiding Harm

Counselors act to avoid harming their clients, trainees, and research participants and to minimize or to remedy unavoidable or unanticipated harm.

A.4.b.   Personal Values

Counselors are aware of—and avoid imposing—their own values, attitudes, beliefs, and behaviors. Counselors respect the diversity of clients, trainees, and research participants and seek training in areas in which they are at risk of imposing their values onto clients, especially when the counselor's values are inconsistent with the client's goals or are discriminatory in nature.

A.5.   Prohibited Noncounseling Roles and Relationships

A.5.a.   Sexual and/or Romantic Relationships Prohibited

Sexual and/or romantic counselor client interactions or relationships with current clients, their romantic partners, or their family members are prohibited. This prohibition applies to both in-person and electronic interactions or relationships.

A.5.b.   Previous Sexual and/or Romantic Relationships

Counselors are prohibited from engaging in counseling relationships with persons with whom they have had a previous sexual and/or romantic relationship.

A.5.c.   Sexual and/or Romantic Relationships With Former Clients

Sexual and/or romantic counselor client interactions or relationships with former clients, their romantic partners, or their family members are prohibited for a period of 5 years following the last professional contact. This prohibition applies to both in-person and electronic interactions or relationships. Counselors, before engaging in sexual and/or romantic interactions or relationships with former clients, their romantic partners, or their family members, demonstrate forethought and document (in written form) whether the interaction or relationship can be viewed as exploitive in any way and/or whether there is still potential to harm the former client; in cases of potential exploitation and/or harm, the counselor avoids entering into such an interaction or relationship.

A.5.d.   Friends or Family Members
Counselors are prohibited from engaging in counseling relationships with friends or family members with whom they have an inability to remain objective.

A.5.e.   Personal Virtual Relationships With Current Clients
Counselors are prohibited from engaging in a personal virtual relationship with individuals with whom they have a current counseling relationship (e.g., through social and other media).

A.6.   Managing and Maintaining Boundaries and Professional Relationships

A.6.a.   Previous Relationships
Counselors consider the risks and benefits of accepting as clients those with whom they have had a previous relationship. These potential clients may include individuals with whom the counselor has had a casual, distant, or past relationship. Examples include mutual or past membership in a professional association, organization, or community. When counselors accept these clients, they take appropriate professional precautions such as informed consent, consultation, supervision, and documentation to ensure that judgment is not impaired and no exploitation occurs.

A.6.b.   Extending Counseling Boundaries
Counselors consider the risks and benefits of extending current counseling relationships beyond conventional parameters. Examples include attending a client's formal ceremony (e.g., a wedding/commitment ceremony or graduation), purchasing a service or product provided by a client (excepting unrestricted bartering), and visiting a client's ill family member in the hospital. In extending these boundaries, counselors take appropriate professional precautions such as informed consent, consultation, supervision, and documentation to ensure that judgment is not impaired and no harm occurs.

A.6.c.   Documenting Boundary Extensions
If counselors extend boundaries as described in A.6.a. and A.6.b., they must officially document, prior to the interaction (when feasible), the rationale for such an interaction, the potential benefit, and anticipated consequences for the client or former client and other individuals significantly involved with the client or former client. When unintentional harm occurs to the client or former client, or to an individual significantly involved with the client or former client, the counselor must show evidence of an attempt to remedy such harm.

A.6.d.   Role Changes in the Professional Relationship
When counselors change a role from the original or most recent contracted relationship, they obtain informed consent from the client and explain the client's right to refuse services related to the change. Examples of role changes include, but are not limited to

1. changing from individual to relationship or family counseling, or vice versa;
2. changing from an evaluative role to a therapeutic role, or vice versa; and
3. changing from a counselor to a mediator role, or vice versa.

Clients must be fully informed of any anticipated consequences (e.g., financial, legal, personal, therapeutic) of counselor role changes.

A.6.e.   Nonprofessional Interactions or Relationships (Other Than Sexual or Romantic Interactions or Relationships)
Counselors avoid entering into nonprofessional relationships with former clients, their romantic partners, or their family members when the interaction is potentially harmful to the client. This applies to both in-person and electronic interactions or relationships.

A.7. Roles and Relationships at Individual, Group, Institutional, and Societal Levels

A.7.a. Advocacy
When appropriate, counselors advocate at individual, group, institutional, and societal levels to address potential barriers and obstacles that inhibit access and/or the growth and development of clients.

A.7.b. Confidentiality and Advocacy
Counselors obtain client consent prior to engaging in advocacy efforts on behalf of an identifiable client to improve the provision of services and to work toward removal of systemic barriers or obstacles that inhibit client access, growth, and development.

A.8. Multiple Clients
When a counselor agrees to provide counseling services to two or more persons who have a relationship, the counselor clarifies at the outset which person or persons are clients and the nature of the relationships the counselor will have with each involved person. If it becomes apparent that the counselor may be called upon to perform potentially conflicting roles, the counselor will clarify, adjust, or withdraw from roles appropriately.

A.9. Group Work

A.9.a. Screening
Counselors screen prospective group counseling/therapy participants. To the extent possible, counselors select members whose needs and goals are compatible with the goals of the group, who will not impede the group process, and whose well-being will not be jeopardized by the group experience.

A.9.b. Protecting Clients
In a group setting, counselors take reasonable precautions to protect clients from physical, emotional, or psychological trauma.

A.10. Fees and Business Practices

A.10.a. Self-Referral
Counselors working in an organization (e.g., school, agency, institution) that provides counseling services do not refer clients to their private practice unless the policies of a particular organization make explicit provisions for self-referrals. In such instances, the clients must be informed of other options open to them should they seek private counseling services.

A.10.b. Unacceptable Business Practices
Counselors do not participate in fee splitting, nor do they give or receive commissions, rebates, or any other form of remuneration when referring clients for professional services.

A.10.c. Establishing Fees
In establishing fees for professional counseling services, counselors consider the financial status of clients and locality. If a counselor's usual fees create undue hardship for the client, the counselor may adjust fees, when legally permissible, or assist the client in locating comparable, affordable services.

A.10.d. Nonpayment of Fees
If counselors intend to use collection agencies or take legal measures to collect fees from clients who do not pay for services as agreed upon, they include such information in their informed consent documents and also inform clients in a timely fashion of intended actions and offer clients the opportunity to make payment.

A.10.e. Bartering
Counselors may barter only if the bartering does not result in exploitation or harm, if the client requests it, and if such arrangements are an accepted practice among professionals in the community. Counselors consider the cultural implications of bartering and discuss relevant concerns with clients and document such agreements in a clear written contract.

A.10.f. Receiving Gifts
Counselors understand the challenges of accepting gifts from clients and recognize that in some cultures, small gifts are a token of respect and gratitude. When determining whether to accept a gift from clients, counselors take into account the therapeutic relationship, the monetary value of the gift, the client's motivation for giving the gift, and

the counselor's motivation for wanting to accept or decline the gift.

A.11.   Termination and Referral

A.11.a.   Competence Within Termination and Referral

If counselors lack the competence to be of professional assistance to clients, they avoid entering or continuing counseling relationships. Counselors are knowledgeable about culturally and clinically appropriate referral resources and suggest these alternatives. If clients decline the suggested referrals, counselors discontinue the relationship.

A.11.b.   Values Within Termination and Referral

Counselors refrain from referring prospective and current clients based solely on the counselor's personally held values, attitudes, beliefs, and behaviors. Counselors respect the diversity of clients and seek training in areas in which they are at risk of imposing their values onto clients, especially when the counselor's values are inconsistent with the client's goals or are discriminatory in nature.

A.11.c.   Appropriate Termination

Counselors terminate a counseling relationship when it becomes reasonably apparent that the client no longer needs assistance, is not likely to benefit, or is being harmed by continued counseling. Counselors may terminate counseling when in jeopardy of harm by the client or by another person with whom the client has a relationship, or when clients do not pay fees as agreed upon. Counselors provide pretermination counseling and recommend other service providers when necessary.

A.11.d.   Appropriate Transfer of Services

When counselors transfer or refer clients to other practitioners, they ensure that appropriate clinical and administrative processes are completed and open communication is maintained with both clients and practitioners.

A.12.   Abandonment and Client Neglect

Counselors do not abandon or neglect clients in counseling. Counselors assist in making appropriate arrangements for the continuation of treatment, when necessary, during interruptions such as vacations, illness, and following termination.

Section B

Confidentiality and Privacy

. . . .

Introduction

Counselors recognize that trust is a cornerstone of the counseling relationship. Counselors aspire to earn the trust of clients by creating an ongoing partnership, establishing and upholding appropriate boundaries, and maintaining confidentiality. Counselors communicate the parameters of confidentiality in a culturally competent manner.

B.1.   Respecting Client Rights

B.1.a.   Multicultural/Diversity Considerations

Counselors maintain awareness and sensitivity regarding cultural meanings of confidentiality and privacy. Counselors respect differing views toward disclosure of information. Counselors hold ongoing discussions with clients as to how, when, and with whom information is to be shared.

B.1.b.   Respect for Privacy

Counselors respect the privacy of prospective and current clients. Counselors request private information from clients only when it is beneficial to the counseling process.

B.1.c.   Respect for Confidentiality

Counselors protect the confidential information of prospective and current clients. Counselors disclose information only with appropriate consent or with sound legal or ethical justification.

B.1.d.   Explanation of Limitations

At initiation and throughout the counseling process, counselors inform clients of the limitations of confidentiality and seek to identify situations in which confidentiality must be breached.

B.2. Exceptions

B.2.a. Serious and Foreseeable Harm and Legal Requirements

The general requirement that counselors keep information confidential does not apply when disclosure is required to protect clients or identified others from serious and foreseeable harm or when legal requirements demand that confidential information must be revealed. Counselors consult with other professionals when in doubt as to the validity of an exception. Additional considerations apply when addressing end-of-life issues.

B.2.b. Confidentiality Regarding End-of-Life Decisions

Counselors who provide services to terminally ill individuals who are considering hastening their own deaths have the option to maintain confidentiality, depending on applicable laws and the specific circumstances of the situation and after seeking consultation or supervision from appropriate professional and legal parties.

B.2.c. Contagious, Life-Threatening Diseases

When clients disclose that they have a disease commonly known to be both communicable and life threatening, counselors may be justified in disclosing information to identifiable third parties, if the parties are known to be at serious and foreseeable risk of contracting the disease. Prior to making a disclosure, counselors assess the intent of clients to inform the third parties about their disease or to engage in any behaviors that may be harmful to an identifiable third party. Counselors adhere to relevant state laws concerning disclosure about disease status.

B.2.d. Court-Ordered Disclosure

When ordered by a court to release confidential or privileged information without a client's permission, counselors seek to obtain written, informed consent from the client or take steps to prohibit the disclosure or have it limited as narrowly as possible because of potential harm to the client or counseling relationship.

B.2.e. Minimal Disclosure

To the extent possible, clients are informed before confidential information is disclosed and are involved in the disclosure decision-making process. When circumstances require the disclosure of confidential information, only essential information is revealed.

B.3. Information Shared With Others

B.3.a. Subordinates

Counselors make every effort to ensure that privacy and confidentiality of clients are maintained by subordinates, including employees, supervisees, students, clerical assistants, and volunteers.

B.3.b. Interdisciplinary Teams

When services provided to the client involve participation by an interdisciplinary or treatment team, the client will be informed of the team's existence and composition, information being shared, and the purposes of sharing such information.

B.3.c. Confidential Settings

Counselors discuss confidential information only in settings in which they can reasonably ensure client privacy.

B.3.d. Third-Party Payers

Counselors disclose information to third-party payers only when clients have authorized such disclosure.

B.3.e. Transmitting Confidential Information

Counselors take precautions to ensure the confidentiality of all information transmitted through the use of any medium.

B.3.f. Deceased Clients

Counselors protect the confidentiality of deceased clients, consistent with legal requirements and the documented preferences of the client.

B.4. Groups and Families

B.4.a. Group Work

In group work, counselors clearly explain the importance and parameters of confidentiality for the specific group.

B.4.b. Couples and Family Counseling

In couples and family counseling, counselors clearly define who is considered "the client" and discuss expectations and limitations of confidentiality.

Counselors seek agreement and document in writing such agreement among all involved parties regarding the confidentiality of information. In the absence of an agreement to the contrary, the couple or family is considered to be the client.

B.5.   Clients Lacking Capacity to Give Informed Consent

B.5.a.   Responsibility to Clients

When counseling minor clients or adult clients who lack the capacity to give voluntary, informed consent, counselors protect the confidentiality of information received—in any medium—in the counseling relationship as specified by federal and state laws, written policies, and applicable ethical standards.

B.5.b.   Responsibility to Parents and Legal Guardians

Counselors inform parents and legal guardians about the role of counselors and the confidential nature of the counseling relationship, consistent with current legal and custodial arrangements. Counselors are sensitive to the cultural diversity of families and respect the inherent rights and responsibilities of parents/guardians regarding the welfare of their children/charges according to law. Counselors work to establish, as appropriate, collaborative relationships with parents/guardians to best serve clients.

B.5.c.   Release of Confidential Information

When counseling minor clients or adult clients who lack the capacity to give voluntary consent to release confidential information, counselors seek permission from an appropriate third party to disclose information. In such instances, counselors inform clients consistent with their level of understanding and take appropriate measures to safeguard client confidentiality.

B.6.   Records and Documentation

B.6.a.   Creating and Maintaining Records and Documentation

Counselors create and maintain records and documentation necessary for rendering professional services.

B.6.b.   Confidentiality of Records and Documentation

Counselors ensure that records and documentation kept in any medium are secure and that only authorized persons have access to them.

B.6.c.   Permission to Record

Counselors obtain permission from clients prior to recording sessions through electronic or other means.

B.6.d.   Permission to Observe

Counselors obtain permission from clients prior to allowing any person to observe counseling sessions, review session transcripts, or view recordings of sessions with supervisors, faculty, peers, or others within the training environment.

B.6.e.   Client Access

Counselors provide reasonable access to records and copies of records when requested by competent clients. Counselors limit the access of clients to their records, or portions of their records, only when there is compelling evidence that such access would cause harm to the client. Counselors document the request of clients and the rationale for withholding some or all of the records in the files of clients. In situations involving multiple clients, counselors provide individual clients with only those parts of records that relate directly to them and do not include confidential information related to any other client.

B.6.f.   Assistance With Records

When clients request access to their records, counselors provide assistance and consultation in interpreting counseling records.

B.6.g.   Disclosure or Transfer

Unless exceptions to confidentiality exist, counselors obtain written permission from clients to disclose or transfer records to legitimate third parties. Steps are taken to ensure that receivers of counseling records are sensitive to their confidential nature.

B.6.h.   Storage and Disposal After Termination

Counselors store records following termination of services to ensure reasonable future access, maintain records in accordance with federal and state laws and statutes such as licensure laws and policies governing records, and dispose of client records and other sensitive materials in a manner that protects client confidentiality. Counselors apply careful discretion and deliberation before destroying records that may be needed by a court of law, such as notes on child abuse, suicide, sexual harassment, or violence.

B.6.i. Reasonable Precautions

Counselors take reasonable precautions to protect client confidentiality in the event of the counselor's termination of practice, incapacity, or death and appoint a records custodian when identified as appropriate.

B.7.   Case Consultation

B.7.a.   Respect for Privacy

Information shared in a consulting relationship is discussed for professional purposes only. Written and oral reports present only data germane to the purposes of the consultation, and every effort is made to protect client identity and to avoid undue invasion of privacy.

B.7.b.   Disclosure of Confidential Information

When consulting with colleagues, counselors do not disclose confidential information that reasonably could lead to the identification of a client or other person or organization with whom they have a confidential relationship unless they have obtained the prior consent of the person or organization or the disclosure cannot be avoided. They disclose information only to the extent necessary to achieve the purposes of the consultation.

Section C

Professional Responsibility

. . . .

Introduction

Counselors aspire to open, honest, and accurate communication in dealing with the public and other professionals. Counselors facilitate access to counseling services, and they practice in a nondiscriminatory manner within the boundaries of professional and personal competence; they also have a responsibility to abide by the *ACA Code of Ethics*. Counselors actively participate in local, state, and national associations that foster the development and improvement of counseling. Counselors are expected to advocate to promote changes at the individual, group, institutional, and societal levels that improve the quality of life for individuals and groups and remove potential barriers to the provision or access of appropriate services being offered. Counselors have a responsibility to the public to engage in counseling practices that are based on rigorous research methodologies. Counselors are encouraged to contribute to society by devoting a portion of their professional activity to services for which there is little or no financial return (*pro bono publico*). In addition, counselors engage in self-care activities to maintain and promote their own emotional, physical, mental, and spiritual well-being to best meet their professional responsibilities.

C.1.   Knowledge of and Compliance With Standards

Counselors have a responsibility to read, understand, and follow the *ACA Code of Ethics* and adhere to applicable laws and regulations.

C.2.   Professional Competence

C.2.a.   Boundaries of Competence

Counselors practice only within the boundaries of their competence, based on their education, training, supervised experience, state and national professional credentials, and appropriate professional experience. Whereas multicultural counseling competency is required across all counseling specialties, counselors gain knowledge, personal awareness, sensitivity, dispositions, and skills pertinent to being a culturally competent counselor in working with a diverse client population.

C.2.b.   New Specialty Areas of Practice

Counselors practice in specialty areas new to them only after appropriate education, training, and supervised experience. While developing skills in new specialty areas, counselors take steps to ensure the competence of their work and protect others from possible harm.

C.2.c.   Qualified for Employment

Counselors accept employment only for positions for which they are qualified given their education, training, supervised experience, state and national professional credentials, and appropriate professional experience. Counselors hire for professional counseling positions only individuals who are qualified and competent for those positions.

C.2.d.   Monitor Effectiveness

Counselors continually monitor their effectiveness as professionals and take steps to improve when necessary. Counselors take reasonable steps to seek peer supervision to evaluate their efficacy as counselors.

C.2.e.   Consultations on Ethical Obligations

Counselors take reasonable steps to consult with other counselors, the ACA Ethics and Professional Standards Department, or related professionals when they have questions regarding their ethical obligations or professional practice.

C.2.f.   Continuing Education

Counselors recognize the need for continuing education to acquire and maintain a reasonable level of awareness of current scientific and professional information in their fields of activity. Counselors maintain their competence in the skills they use, are open to new procedures, and remain informed regarding best practices for working with diverse populations.

C.2.g.   Impairment

Counselors monitor themselves for signs of impairment from their own physical, mental, or emotional problems and refrain from offering or providing professional services when impaired. They seek assistance for problems that reach the level of professional impairment, and, if necessary, they limit, suspend, or terminate their professional responsibilities until it is determined that they may safely resume their work. Counselors assist colleagues or supervisors in recognizing their own professional impairment and provide consultation and assistance when warranted with colleagues or supervisors showing signs of impairment and intervene as appropriate to prevent imminent harm to clients.

C.2.h.   Counselor Incapacitation, Death, Retirement, or Termination of Practice

Counselors prepare a plan for the transfer of clients and the dissemination of records to an identified colleague or records custodian in the case of the counselor's incapacitation, death, retirement, or termination of practice.

C.3.   Advertising and Soliciting Clients

C.3.a.   Accurate Advertising

When advertising or otherwise representing their services to the public, counselors identify their credentials in an accurate manner that is not false, misleading, deceptive, or fraudulent.

C.3.b.   Testimonials

Counselors who use testimonials do not solicit them from current clients, former clients, or any other persons who may be vulnerable to undue influence. Counselors discuss with clients the implications of and obtain permission for the use of any testimonial.

C.3.c.   Statements by Others

When feasible, counselors make reasonable efforts to ensure that statements made by others about them or about the counseling profession are accurate.

C.3.d.   Recruiting Through Employment

Counselors do not use their places of employment or institutional affiliation to recruit clients, supervisors, or consultees for their private practices.

C.3.e.   Products and Training Advertisements

Counselors who develop products related to their profession or conduct workshops or training events ensure that the advertisements concerning these products or events are accurate and disclose adequate information for consumers to make informed choices.

C.3.f.   Promoting to Those Served

Counselors do not use counseling, teaching, training, or supervisory relationships to promote their products or training events in a manner that is deceptive or would exert undue influence on individuals who may be vulnerable. However, counselor educators may adopt textbooks they have authored for instructional purposes.

C.4. Professional Qualifications

C.4.a. Accurate Representation

Counselors claim or imply only professional qualifications actually completed and correct any known misrepresentations of their qualifications by others. Counselors truthfully represent the qualifications of their professional colleagues. Counselors clearly distinguish between paid and volunteer work experience and accurately describe their continuing education and specialized training.

C.4.b. Credentials

Counselors claim only licenses or certifications that are current and in good standing.

C.4.c. Educational Degrees

Counselors clearly differentiate between earned and honorary degrees.

C.4.d. Implying Doctoral-Level Competence

Counselors clearly state their highest earned degree in counseling or a closely related field. Counselors do not imply doctoral-level competence when possessing a master's degree in counseling or a related field by referring to themselves as "Dr." in a counseling context when their doctorate is not in counseling or a related field. Counselors do not use "ABD" (all but dissertation) or other such terms to imply competency.

C.4.e. Accreditation Status

Counselors accurately represent the accreditation status of their degree program and college/university.

C.4.f. Professional Membership

Counselors clearly differentiate between current, active memberships and former memberships in associations. Members of ACA must clearly differentiate between professional membership, which implies the possession of at least a master's degree in counseling, and regular membership, which is open to individuals whose interests and activities are consistent with those of ACA but are not qualified for professional membership.

C.5. Nondiscrimination

Counselors do not condone or engage in discrimination against prospective or current clients, students, employees, supervisees, or research participants based on age, culture, disability, ethnicity, race, religion/spirituality, gender, gender identity, sexual orientation, marital/partnership status, language preference, socioeconomic status, immigration status, or any basis proscribed by law.

C.6. Public Responsibility

C.6.a. Sexual Harassment

Counselors do not engage in or condone sexual harassment. Sexual harassment can consist of a single intense or severe act, or multiple persistent or pervasive acts.

C.6.b. Reports to Third Parties

Counselors are accurate, honest, and objective in reporting their professional activities and judgments to appropriate third parties, including courts, health insurance companies, those who are the recipients of evaluation reports, and others.

C.6.c. Media Presentations

When counselors provide advice or comment by means of public lectures, demonstrations, radio or television programs, recordings, technology-based applications, printed articles, mailed material, or other media, they take reasonable precautions to ensure that

1. the statements are based on appropriate professional counseling literature and practice,
2. the statements are otherwise consistent with the *ACA Code of Ethics*, and
3. the recipients of the information are not encouraged to infer that a professional counseling relationship has been established.

C.6.d. Exploitation of Others

Counselors do not exploit others in their professional relationships.

C.6.e. Contributing to the Public Good
(Pro Bono Publico)

Counselors make a reasonable effort to provide services to the public for which there is little or no financial return (e.g., speaking to groups, sharing professional information, offering reduced fees).

C.7.   Treatment Modalities

C.7.a.   Scientific Basis for Treatment

When providing services, counselors use techniques/procedures/modalities that are grounded in theory and/or have an empirical or scientific foundation.

C.7.b.   Development and Innovation

When counselors use developing or innovative techniques/procedures/ modalities, they explain the potential risks, benefits, and ethical considerations of using such techniques/procedures/ modalities. Counselors work to minimize any potential risks or harm when using these techniques/procedures/modalities.

C.7.c.   Harmful Practices

Counselors do not use techniques/procedures/modalities when substantial evidence suggests harm, even if such services are requested.

C.8.   Responsibility to Other Professionals

C.8.a.   Personal Public Statements

When making personal statements in a public context, counselors clarify that they are speaking from their personal perspectives and that they are not speaking on behalf of all counselors or the profession.

Section D

Relationships With Other Professionals

. . . .

Introduction

Professional counselors recognize that the quality of their interactions with colleagues can influence the quality of services provided to clients. They work to become knowledgeable about colleagues within and outside the field of counseling. Counselors develop positive working relationships and systems of communication with colleagues to enhance services to clients.

D.1.   Relationships With Colleagues, Employers, and Employees

D.1.a.   Different Approaches

Counselors are respectful of approaches that are grounded in theory and/or have an empirical or scientific foundation but may differ from their own. Counselors acknowledge the expertise of other professional groups and are respectful of their practices.

D.1.b.   Forming Relationships

Counselors work to develop and strengthen relationships with colleagues from other disciplines to best serve clients.

D.1.c.   Interdisciplinary Teamwork

Counselors who are members of interdisciplinary teams delivering multifaceted services to clients remain focused on how to best serve clients. They participate in and contribute to decisions that affect the well-being of clients by drawing on the perspectives, values, and experiences of the counseling profession and those of colleagues from other disciplines.

D.1.d.   Establishing Professional and Ethical Obligations

Counselors who are members of interdisciplinary teams work together with team members to clarify professional and ethical obligations of the team as a whole and of its individual members. When a team decision raises ethical concerns, counselors first attempt to resolve the concern within the team. If they cannot reach resolution among team members, counselors pursue other avenues to address their concerns consistent with client well-being.

D.1.e.   Confidentiality

When counselors are required by law, institutional policy, or extraordinary circumstances to serve in more than one role in judicial or administrative proceedings, they clarify role expectations and the parameters of confidentiality with their colleagues.

D.1.f.   Personnel Selection and Assignment

When counselors are in a position requiring personnel selection and/or assigning of responsibilities to others, they select competent staff and assign responsibilities compatible with their skills and experiences.

D.1.g. Employer Policies

The acceptance of employment in an agency or institution implies that counselors are in agreement with its general policies and principles. Counselors strive to reach agreement with employers regarding acceptable standards of client care and professional conduct that allow for changes in institutional policy conducive to the growth and development of clients.

D.1.h. Negative Conditions

Counselors alert their employers of inappropriate policies and practices. They attempt to effect changes in such policies or procedures through constructive action within the organization. When such policies are potentially disruptive or damaging to clients or may limit the effectiveness of services provided and change cannot be affected, counselors take appropriate further action. Such action may include referral to appropriate certification, accreditation, or state licensure organizations, or voluntary termination of employment.

D.1.i. Protection From Punitive Action

Counselors do not harass a colleague or employee or dismiss an employee who has acted in a responsible and ethical manner to expose inappropriate employer policies or practices.

D.2. Provision of Consultation Services

D.2.a. Consultant Competency

Counselors take reasonable steps to ensure that they have the appropriate resources and competencies when providing consultation services. Counselors provide appropriate referral resources when requested or needed.

D.2.b. Informed Consent in Formal Consultation

When providing formal consultation services, counselors have an obligation to review, in writing and verbally, the rights and responsibilities of both counselors and consultees. Counselors use clear and understandable language to inform all parties involved about the purpose of the services to be provided, relevant costs, potential risks and benefits, and the limits of confidentiality.

Section E

Evaluation, Assessment, and Interpretation

. . . .

Introduction

Counselors use assessment as one component of the counseling process, taking into account the clients' personal and cultural context. Counselors promote the well-being of individual clients or groups of clients by developing and using appropriate educational, mental health, psychological, and career assessments.

E.1. General

E.1.a. Assessment

The primary purpose of educational, mental health, psychological, and career assessment is to gather information regarding the client for a variety of purposes, including, but not limited to, client decision making, treatment planning, and forensic proceedings. Assessment may include both qualitative and quantitative methodologies.

E.1.b. Client Welfare

Counselors do not misuse assessment results and interpretations, and they take reasonable steps to prevent others from misusing the information provided. They respect the client's right to know the results, the interpretations made, and the bases for counselors' conclusions and recommendations.

E.2. Competence to Use and Interpret Assessment Instruments

E.2.a. Limits of Competence

Counselors use only those testing and assessment services for which they have been trained and are competent. Counselors using technology-assisted test interpretations are trained in the construct being measured and the specific instrument being used prior to using its technology-based application. Counselors take reasonable measures to ensure the proper use of assessment techniques by persons under their supervision.

E.2.b.   Appropriate Use
Counselors are responsible for the appropriate application, scoring, interpretation, and use of assessment instruments relevant to the needs of the client, whether they score and interpret such assessments themselves or use technology or other services.

E.2.c.   Decisions Based on Results
Counselors responsible for decisions involving individuals or policies that are based on assessment results have a thorough understanding of psychometrics.

E.3.   Informed Consent in Assessment

E.3.a.   Explanation to Clients
Prior to assessment, counselors explain the nature and purposes of assessment and the specific use of results by potential recipients. The explanation will be given in terms and language that the client (or other legally authorized person on behalf of the client) can understand.

E.3.b.   Recipients of Results
Counselors consider the client's and/ or examinee's welfare, explicit understandings, and prior agreements in determining who receives the assessment results. Counselors include accurate and appropriate interpretations with any release of individual or group assessment results.

E.4.   Release of Data to Qualified Personnel
Counselors release assessment data in which the client is identified only with the consent of the client or the client's legal representative. Such data are released only to persons recognized by counselors as qualified to interpret the data.

E.5.   Diagnosis of Mental Disorders

E.5.a.   Proper Diagnosis
Counselors take special care to provide proper diagnosis of mental disorders. Assessment techniques

(including personal interviews) used to determine client care (e.g., locus of treatment, type of treatment, recommended follow-up) are carefully selected and appropriately used.

E.5.b.   Cultural Sensitivity
Counselors recognize that culture affects the manner in which clients' problems are defined and experienced. Clients' socioeconomic and cultural experiences are considered when diagnosing mental disorders.

E.5.c.   Historical and Social Prejudices in the Diagnosis of Pathology
Counselors recognize historical and social prejudices in the misdiagnosis and pathologizing of certain individuals and groups and strive to become aware of and address such biases in themselves or others.

E.5.d.   Refraining From Diagnosis
Counselors may refrain from making and/or reporting a diagnosis if they believe that it would cause harm to the client or others. Counselors carefully consider both the positive and negative implications of a diagnosis.

E.6.   Instrument Selection

E.6.a.   Appropriateness of Instruments
Counselors carefully consider the validity, reliability, psychometric limitations, and appropriateness of instruments when selecting assessments and, when possible, use multiple forms of assessment, data, and/or instruments in forming conclusions, diagnoses, or recommendations.

E.6.b.   Referral Information
If a client is referred to a third party for assessment, the counselor provides specific referral questions and sufficient objective data about the client to ensure that appropriate assessment instruments are utilized.

E.7.   Conditions of Assessment Administration

E.7.a.   Administration Conditions
Counselors administer assessments under the same conditions that were established in their standardization. When assessments are not administered under standard

conditions, as may be necessary to accommodate clients with disabilities, or when unusual behavior or irregularities occur during the administration, those conditions are noted in interpretation, and the results may be designated as invalid or of questionable validity.

E.7.b. Provision of Favorable Conditions

Counselors provide an appropriate environment for the administration of assessments (e.g., privacy, comfort, freedom from distraction).

E.7.c. Technological Administration

Counselors ensure that technologically administered assessments function properly and provide clients with accurate results.

E.7.d. Unsupervised Assessments

Unless the assessment instrument is designed, intended, and validated for self-administration and/or scoring, counselors do not permit unsupervised use.

E.8. Multicultural Issues/Diversity in Assessment

Counselors select and use with caution assessment techniques normed on populations other than that of the client. Counselors recognize the effects of age, color, culture, disability, ethnic group, gender, race, language preference, religion, spirituality, sexual orientation, and socioeconomic status on test administration and interpretation, and they place test results in proper perspective with other relevant factors.

E.9. Scoring and Interpretation of Assessments

E.9.a. Reporting

When counselors report assessment results, they consider the client's personal and cultural background, the level of the client's understanding of the results, and the impact of the results on the client. In reporting assessment results, counselors indicate reservations that exist regarding validity or reliability due to circumstances of the assessment or inappropriateness of the norms for the person tested.

E.9.b. Instruments With Insufficient Empirical Data

Counselors exercise caution when interpreting the results of instruments not having sufficient empirical data to support respondent results. The specific purposes for the use of such instruments are stated explicitly to the examinee. Counselors qualify any conclusions, diagnoses, or recommendations made that are based on assessments or instruments with questionable validity or reliability.

E.9.c. Assessment Services

Counselors who provide assessment, scoring, and interpretation services to support the assessment process confirm the validity of such interpretations. They accurately describe the purpose, norms, validity, reliability, and applications of the procedures and any special qualifications applicable to their use. At all times, counselors maintain their ethical responsibility to those being assessed.

E.10. Assessment Security

Counselors maintain the integrity and security of tests and assessments consistent with legal and contractual obligations. Counselors do not appropriate, reproduce, or modify published assessments or parts thereof without acknowledgment and permission from the publisher.

E.11. Obsolete Assessment and Outdated Results

Counselors do not use data or results from assessments that are obsolete or outdated for the current purpose (e.g., noncurrent versions of assessments/ instruments). Counselors make every effort to prevent the misuse of obsolete measures and assessment data by others.

E.12. Assessment Construction

Counselors use established scientific procedures, relevant standards, and current professional knowledge for assessment design in the development, publication, and utilization of assessment techniques.

E.13. Forensic Evaluation: Evaluation for Legal Proceedings

E.13.a. Primary Obligations

When providing forensic evaluations, the primary obligation of counselors is to produce objective findings that can be substantiated based on information and techniques appropriate to the evaluation, which may include examination of the individual and/or review of records. Counselors form professional opinions based on their professional knowledge and expertise that can be supported by the data gathered in evaluations. Counselors define the limits of their reports or testimony, especially when an examination of the individual has not been conducted.

E.13.b.   Consent for Evaluation

Individuals being evaluated are informed in writing that the relationship is for the purposes of an evaluation and is not therapeutic in nature, and entities or individuals who will receive the evaluation report are identified. Counselors who perform forensic evaluations obtain written consent from those being evaluated or from their legal representative unless a court orders evaluations to be conducted without the written consent of the individuals being evaluated. When children or adults who lack the capacity to give voluntary consent are being evaluated, informed written consent is obtained from a parent or guardian.

E.13.c.   Client Evaluation Prohibited

Counselors do not evaluate current or former clients, clients' romantic partners, or clients' family members for forensic purposes. Counselors do not counsel individuals they are evaluating.

E.13.d.   Avoid Potentially Harmful Relationships

Counselors who provide forensic evaluations avoid potentially harmful professional or personal relationships with family members, romantic partners, and close friends of individuals they are evaluating or have evaluated in the past.

Section F

Supervision, Training, and Teaching

. . . .

Introduction

Counselor supervisors, trainers, and educators aspire to foster meaningful and respectful professional relationships and to maintain appropriate boundaries with supervisees and students in both face-to-face and electronic formats. They have theoretical and pedagogical foundations for their work; have knowledge of supervision models; and aim to be fair, accurate, and honest in their assessments of counselors, students, and supervisees.

F.1.   Counselor Supervision and Client Welfare

F.1.a.   Client Welfare

A primary obligation of counseling supervisors is to monitor the services provided by supervisees. Counseling supervisors monitor client welfare and supervisee performance and professional development. To fulfill these obligations, supervisors meet regularly with supervisees to review the supervisees' work and help them become prepared to serve a range of diverse clients. Supervisees have a responsibility to understand and follow the *ACA Code of Ethics*.

F.1.b.   Counselor Credentials

Counseling supervisors work to ensure that supervisees communicate their qualifications to render services to their clients.

F.1.c.   Informed Consent and Client Rights

Supervisors make supervisees aware of client rights, including the protection of client privacy and confidentiality in the counseling relationship. Supervisees provide clients with professional disclosure information and inform them of how the supervision process influences the limits of confidentiality. Supervisees make clients aware of who will have access to records of the counseling relationship and how these records will be stored, transmitted, or otherwise reviewed.

F.2.   Counselor Supervision Competence

F.2.a.   Supervisor Preparation

Prior to offering supervision services, counselors are trained in supervision methods and techniques. Counselors who offer supervision services regularly pursue continuing education activities, including both counseling and supervision topics and skills.

F.2.b. Multicultural Issues/Diversity in Supervision

Counseling supervisors are aware of and address the role of multiculturalism/diversity in the supervisory relationship.

F.2.c. Online Supervision

When using technology in supervision, counselor supervisors are competent in the use of those technologies. Supervisors take the necessary precautions to protect the confidentiality of all information transmitted through any electronic means.

F.3. Supervisory Relationship

F.3.a. Extending Conventional Supervisory Relationships

Counseling supervisors clearly define and maintain ethical professional, personal, and social relationships with their supervisees. Supervisors consider the risks and benefits of extending current supervisory relationships in any form beyond conventional parameters. In extending these boundaries, supervisors take appropriate professional precautions to ensure that judgment is not impaired and that no harm occurs.

F.3.b. Sexual Relationships

Sexual or romantic interactions or relationships with current supervisees are prohibited. This prohibition applies to both in person and electronic interactions or relationships.

F.3.c. Sexual Harassment

Counseling supervisors do not condone or subject supervisees to sexual harassment.

F.3.d. Friends or Family Members

Supervisors are prohibited from engaging in supervisory relationships with individuals with whom they have an inability to remain objective.

F.4. Supervisor Responsibilities

F.4.a. Informed Consent for Supervision

Supervisors are responsible for incorporating into their supervision the principles of informed consent and participation. Supervisors inform supervisees of the policies and procedures to which supervisors are to adhere and the mechanisms for due process appeal of individual supervisor actions. The issues unique to the use of distance supervision are to be included in the documentation as necessary.

F.4.b. Emergencies and Absences

Supervisors establish and communicate to supervisees procedures for contacting supervisors or, in their absence, alternative on-call supervisors to assist in handling crises.

F.4.c. Standards for Supervisees

Supervisors make their supervisees aware of professional and ethical standards and legal responsibilities.

F.4.d. Termination of the Supervisory Relationship

Supervisors or supervisees have the right to terminate the supervisory relationship with adequate notice. Reasons for considering termination are discussed, and both parties work to resolve differences. When termination is warranted, supervisors make appropriate referrals to possible alternative supervisors.

F.5. Student and Supervisee Responsibilities

F.5.a. Ethical Responsibilities

Students and supervisees have a responsibility to understand and follow the *ACA Code of Ethics*. Students and supervisees have the same obligation to clients as those required of professional counselors.

F.5.b. Impairment

Students and supervisees monitor themselves for signs of impairment from their own physical, mental, or emotional problems and refrain from offering or providing professional services when such impairment is likely to harm a client or others. They notify their faculty and/or supervisors and seek assistance for problems that reach the level of professional impairment, and, if necessary, they limit, suspend, or terminate their professional responsibilities until it is determined that they may safely resume their work.

F.5.c. Professional Disclosure

Before providing counseling services, students and supervisees disclose their status as supervisees and explain how this status affects the limits of confidentiality. Supervisors ensure that clients are aware of the services rendered and the qualifications of the students and supervisees rendering those services. Students and super-visees obtain client permission before they use any information concerning the counseling relationship in the training process.

F.6. Counseling Supervision Evaluation, Remediation, and Endorsement

F.6.a. Evaluation

Supervisors document and provide supervisees with ongoing feedback regarding their performance and schedule periodic formal evaluative sessions throughout the supervisory relationship.

F.6.b. Gatekeeping and Remediation

Through initial and ongoing evaluation, supervisors are aware of supervisee limitations that might impede performance. Supervisors assist supervisees in securing remedial assistance when needed. They recommend dismissal from training programs, applied counseling settings, and state or voluntary professional credentialing processes when those supervisees are unable to demonstrate that they can provide competent professional services to a range of diverse clients. Supervisors seek consultation and document their decisions to dismiss or refer supervisees for assistance. They ensure that supervisees are aware of options available to them to address such decisions.

F.6.c. Counseling for Supervisees

If supervisees request counseling, the supervisor assists the supervisee in identifying appropriate services. Supervisors do not provide counseling services to supervisees. Supervisors address interpersonal competencies in terms of the impact of these issues on clients, the supervisory relationship, and professional functioning.

F.6.d. Endorsements

Supervisors endorse supervisees for certification, licensure, employment, or completion of an academic or training program only when they believe that supervisees are qualified for the endorsement. Regardless of qualifications, supervisors do not endorse supervisees whom they believe to be impaired in any way that would interfere with the performance of the duties associated with the endorsement.

F.7. Responsibilities of Counselor Educators

F.7.a. Counselor Educators

Counselor educators who are responsible for developing, implementing, and supervising educational programs are skilled as teachers and practitioners. They are knowledgeable regarding the ethical, legal, and regulatory aspects of the profession; are skilled in applying that knowledge; and make students and supervisees aware of their responsibilities. Whether in traditional, hybrid, and/or online formats, counselor educators conduct counselor education and training programs in an ethical manner and serve as role models for professional behavior.

F.7.b. Counselor Educator Competence

Counselors who function as counselor educators or supervisors provide instruction within their areas of knowledge and competence and provide instruction based on current information and knowledge available in the profession. When using technology to deliver instruction, counselor educators develop competence in the use of the technology.

F.7.c. Infusing Multicultural Issues/Diversity

Counselor educators infuse material related to multiculturalism/diversity into all courses and workshops for the development of professional counselors.

F.7.d. Integration of Study and Practice

In traditional, hybrid, and/or online formats, counselor educators establish education and training programs that integrate academic study and supervised practice.

F.7.e. Teaching Ethics

Throughout the program, counselor educators ensure that students are aware of the ethical responsibilities and standards of the profession and the ethical responsibilities of students to the profession. Counselor educators infuse ethical considerations throughout the curriculum.

F.7.f. Use of Case Examples

The use of client, student, or supervisee information for the purposes of case examples in a lecture or classroom setting is permissible only when (a) the client, student, or supervisee has reviewed the material and agreed to its presentation or (b) the information has been sufficiently modified to obscure identity.

F.7.g. Student-to-Student Supervision and Instruction

When students function in the role of counselor educators or supervisors, they understand that they have the same ethical obligations as counselor educators, trainers, and supervisors. Counselor educators make every effort to ensure that the rights of students are not compromised when their peers lead experiential counseling activities in traditional, hybrid, and/or online formats (e.g., counseling groups, skills classes, clinical supervision).

F.7.h. Innovative Theories and Techniques

Counselor educators promote the use of techniques/procedures/modalities that are grounded in theory and/or have an empirical or scientific foundation. When counselor educators discuss developing or innovative techniques/procedures/modalities, they explain the potential risks, benefits, and ethical considerations of using such techniques/procedures/modalities.

F.7.i. Field Placements

Counselor educators develop clear policies and provide direct assistance within their training programs regarding appropriate field placement and other clinical experiences. Counselor educators provide clearly stated roles and responsibilities for the student or supervisee, the site supervisor, and the program supervisor. They confirm that site supervisors are qualified to provide supervision in the formats in which services are provided and inform site supervisors of their professional and ethical responsibilities in this role.

F.8. Student Welfare

F.8.a. Program Information and Orientation

Counselor educators recognize that program orientation is a developmental process that begins upon students' initial contact with the counselor education program and continues throughout the educational and clinical training of students. Counselor education faculty provide prospective and current students with information about the counselor education program's expectations, including

1. the values and ethical principles of the profession;
2. the type and level of skill and knowledge acquisition required for successful completion of the training;
3. technology requirements;
4. program training goals, objectives, and mission, and subject matter to be covered;
5. bases for evaluation;
6. training components that encourage self-growth or self-disclosure as part of the training process;
7. the type of supervision settings and requirements of the sites for required clinical field experiences;
8. student and supervisor evaluation and dismissal policies and procedures; and
9. up-to-date employment prospects for graduates.

F.8.b. Student Career Advising

Counselor educators provide career advisement for their students and make them aware of opportunities in the field.

F.8.c. Self-Growth Experiences

Self-growth is an expected component of counselor education. Counselor educators are mindful of ethical principles when they require students to engage in self-growth experiences. Counselor educators and supervisors inform students that they have a right to decide what information will be shared or withheld in class.

F.8.d.   Addressing Personal Concerns

Counselor educators may require students to address any personal concerns that have the potential to affect professional competency.

F.9.   Evaluation and Remediation

F.9.a.   Evaluation of Students

Counselor educators clearly state to students, prior to and throughout the training program, the levels of competency expected, appraisal methods, and timing of evaluations for both didactic and clinical competencies. Counselor educators provide students with ongoing feedback regarding their performance throughout the training program.

F.9.b.   Limitations

Counselor educators, through ongoing evaluation, are aware of and address the inability of some students to achieve counseling competencies. Counselor educators do the following:

1. assist students in securing remedial assistance when needed,
2. seek professional consultation and document their decision to dismiss or refer students for assistance, and
3. ensure that students have recourse in a timely manner to address decisions requiring them to seek assistance or to dismiss them and provide students with due process according to institutional policies and procedures.

F.9.c.   Counseling for Students

If students request counseling, or if counseling services are suggested as part of a remediation process, counselor educators assist students in identifying appropriate services.

F.10.   Roles and Relationships Between Counselor Educators and Students

F.10.a.   Sexual or Romantic Relationships

Counselor educators are prohibited from sexual or romantic interactions or relationships with students currently enrolled in a counseling or related program and over whom they have power and authority. This prohibition applies to both in-person and electronic interactions or relationships.

F.10.b.   Sexual Harassment

Counselor educators do not condone or subject students to sexual harassment.

F.10.c.   Relationships With Former Students

Counselor educators are aware of the power differential in the relationship between faculty and students. Faculty members discuss with former students potential risks when they consider engaging in social, sexual, or other intimate relationships.

F.10.d.   Nonacademic Relationships

Counselor educators avoid nonacademic relationships with students in which there is a risk of potential harm to the student or which may compromise the training experience or grades assigned. In addition, counselor educators do not accept any form of professional services, fees, commissions, reimbursement, or remuneration from a site for student or supervisor placement.

F.10.e.   Counseling Services

Counselor educators do not serve as counselors to students currently enrolled in a counseling or related program and over whom they have power and authority.

F.10.f.   Extending Educator–Student Boundaries

Counselor educators are aware of the power differential in the relationship between faculty and students. If they believe that a nonprofessional relationship with a student may be potentially beneficial to the student, they take precautions similar to those taken by counselors when working with clients. Examples of potentially beneficial interactions or relationships include, but are not limited to, attending a formal ceremony; conducting hospital visits; providing support during a stressful event; or maintaining mutual membership in a professional association, organization, or community. Counselor educators discuss with students the rationale for such interactions, the potential benefits and drawbacks, and the anticipated consequences for the student. Educators clarify the specific nature and limitations of the additional role(s) they will have with the student prior to engaging in a nonprofessional relationship. Nonprofessional relationships with students should be time limited and/or context specific and initiated with student consent.

F.11. Multicultural/Diversity Competence in Counselor Education and Training Programs

F.11.a. Faculty Diversity
Counselor educators are committed to recruiting and retaining a diverse faculty.

F.11.b. Student Diversity
Counselor educators actively attempt to recruit and retain a diverse student body. Counselor educators demonstrate commitment to multicultural/diversity competence by recognizing and valuing the diverse cultures and types of abilities that students bring to the training experience. Counselor educators provide appropriate accommodations that enhance and support diverse student well-being and academic performance.

F.11.c. Multicultural/Diversity Competence
Counselor educators actively infuse multicultural/diversity competency in their training and supervision practices. They actively train students to gain awareness, knowledge, and skills in the competencies of multicultural practice.

Section G

Research and Publication
. . . .

Introduction
Counselors who conduct research are encouraged to contribute to the knowledge base of the profession and promote a clearer understanding of the conditions that lead to a healthy and more just society.

Counselors support the efforts of researchers by participating fully and willingly whenever possible. Counselors minimize bias and respect diversity in designing and implementing research.

G.1. Research Responsibilities

G.1.a. Conducting Research
Counselors plan, design, conduct, and report research in a manner that is consistent with pertinent ethical principles, federal and state laws, host institutional regulations, and scientific standards governing research.

G.1.b. Confidentiality in Research
Counselors are responsible for understanding and adhering to state, federal, agency, or institutional policies or applicable guidelines regarding confidentiality in their research practices.

G.1.c. Independent Researchers
When counselors conduct independent research and do not have access to an institutional review board, they are bound to the same ethical principles and federal and state laws pertaining to the review of their plan, design, conduct, and reporting of research.

G.1.d. Deviation From Standard Practice
Counselors seek consultation and observe stringent safeguards to protect the rights of research participants when research indicates that a deviation from standard or acceptable practices may be necessary.

G.1.e. Precautions to Avoid Injury
Counselors who conduct research are responsible for their participants' welfare throughout the research process and should take reasonable precautions to avoid causing emotional, physical, or social harm to participants.

G.1.f. Principal Researcher Responsibility
The ultimate responsibility for ethical research practice lies with the principal researcher. All others involved in the research activities share ethical obligations and responsibility for their own actions.

G.2.   Rights of Research Participants

G.2.a.   Informed Consent in Research

Individuals have the right to decline requests to become research participants. In seeking consent, counselors use language that

1. accurately explains the purpose and procedures to be followed;
2. identifies any procedures that are experimental or relatively untried;
3. describes any attendant discomforts, risks, and potential power differentials between researchers and participants;
4. describes any benefits or changes in individuals or organizations that might reasonably be expected;
5. discloses appropriate alternative procedures that would be advantageous for participants;
6. offers to answer any inquiries concerning the procedures;
7. describes any limitations on confidentiality;
8. describes the format and potential target audiences for the dissemination of research findings; and
9. instructs participants that they are free to withdraw their consent and discontinue participation in the project at any time, without penalty.

G.2.b.   Student/Supervisee Participation

Researchers who involve students or supervisees in research make clear to them that the decision regarding participation in research activities does not affect their academic standing or supervisory relationship. Students or supervisees who choose not to participate in research are provided with an appropriate alternative to fulfill their academic or clinical requirements.

G.2.c.   Client Participation

Counselors conducting research involving clients make clear in the informed consent process that clients are free to choose whether to participate in research activities. Counselors take necessary precautions to protect clients from adverse consequences of declining or withdrawing from participation.

G.2.d.   Confidentiality of Information

Information obtained about research participants during the course of research is confidential. Procedures are implemented to protect confidentiality.

G.2.e.   Persons Not Capable of Giving Informed Consent

When a research participant is not capable of giving informed consent, counselors provide an appropriate explanation to, obtain agreement for participation from, and obtain the appropriate consent of a legally authorized person.

G.2.f.   Commitments to Participants

Counselors take reasonable measures to honor all commitments to research participants.

G.2.g.   Explanations After Data Collection

After data are collected, counselors provide participants with full clarification of the nature of the study to remove any misconceptions participants might have regarding the research. Where scientific or human values justify delaying or withholding information, counselors take reasonable measures to avoid causing harm.

G.2.h.   Informing Sponsors

Counselors inform sponsors, institutions, and publication channels regarding research procedures and outcomes. Counselors ensure that appropriate bodies and authorities are given pertinent information and acknowledgment.

G.2.i.   Research Records Custodian

As appropriate, researchers prepare and disseminate to an identified colleague or records custodian a plan for the transfer of research data in the case of their incapacitation, retirement, or death.

G.3.   Managing and Maintaining Boundaries

G.3.a.   Extending Researcher–Participant Boundaries

Researchers consider the risks and benefits of extending current research relationships beyond conventional parameters. When a nonresearch interaction between the researcher and the research participant may be potentially beneficial, the researcher must document, prior to the interaction (when feasible), the rationale for such an interaction, the potential benefit, and anticipated consequences for the research participant. Such interactions should be initiated with appropriate consent of the research participant. Where unintentional harm occurs to the research participant, the researcher must show evidence of an attempt to remedy such harm.

G.3.b. Relationships With Research Participants

Sexual or romantic counselor–research participant interactions or relationships with current research participants are prohibited. This prohibition applies to both in-person and electronic interactions or relationships.

G.3.c. Sexual Harassment and Research Participants

Researchers do not condone or subject research participants to sexual harassment.

G.4. Reporting Results

G.4.a. Accurate Results

Counselors plan, conduct, and report research accurately. Counselors do not engage in misleading or fraudulent research, distort data, misrepresent data, or deliberately bias their results. They describe the extent to which results are applicable for diverse populations.

G.4.b. Obligation to Report Unfavorable Results

Counselors report the results of any research of professional value. Results that reflect unfavorably on institutions, programs, services, prevailing opinions, or vested interests are not withheld.

G.4.c. Reporting Errors

If counselors discover significant errors in their published research, they take reasonable steps to correct such errors in a correction erratum or through other appropriate publication means.

G.4.d. Identity of Participants

Counselors who supply data, aid in the research of another person, report research results, or make original data available take due care to disguise the identity of respective participants in the absence of

specific authorization from the participants to do otherwise. In situations where participants selfidentify their involvement in research studies, researchers take active steps to ensure that data are adapted/changed to protect the identity and welfare of all parties and that discussion of results does not cause harm to participants.

G.4.e. Replication Studies

Counselors are obligated to make available sufficient original research information to qualified professionals who may wish to replicate or extend the study.

G.5. Publications and Presentations

G.5.a. Use of Case Examples

The use of participants', clients', students', or supervisees' information for the purpose of case examples in a presentation or publication is permissible only when (a) participants, clients, students, or supervisees have reviewed the material and agreed to its presentation or publication or (b) the information has been sufficiently modified to obscure identity.

G.5.b. Plagiarism

Counselors do not plagiarize; that is, they do not present another person's work as their own.

G.5.c. Acknowledging Previous Work

In publications and presentations, counselors acknowledge and give recognition to previous work on the topic by others or self.

G.5.d. Contributors

Counselors give credit through joint authorship, acknowledgment, footnote statements, or other appropriate means to those who have contributed significantly to research or concept development in accordance with such contributions. The principal contributor is listed first, and minor technical or professional contributions are acknowledged in notes or introductory statements.

G.5.e. Agreement of Contributors

Counselors who conduct joint research with colleagues or students/supervisors establish agreements in advance regarding allocation of tasks, publication credit, and types of acknowledgment that will be received.

G.5.f.   Student Research

Manuscripts or professional presentations in any medium that are substantially based on a student's course papers, projects, dissertations, or theses are used only with the student's permission and list the student as lead author.

G.5.g.   Duplicate Submissions

Counselors submit manuscripts for consideration to only one journal at a time. Manuscripts that are published in whole or in substantial part in one journal or published work are not submitted for publication to another publisher without acknowledgment and permission from the original publisher.

G.5.h.   Professional Review

Counselors who review material submitted for publication, research, or other scholarly purposes respect the confidentiality and proprietary rights of those who submitted it. Counselors make publication decisions based on valid and defensible standards. Counselors review article submissions in a timely manner and based on their scope and competency in research methodologies. Counselors who serve as reviewers at the request of editors or publishers make every effort to only review materials that are within their scope of competency and avoid personal biases.

Section H

Distance Counseling, Technology, and Social Media

. . . .

Introduction

Counselors understand that the profession of counseling may no longer be limited to in-person, face-to-face interactions. Counselors actively attempt to understand the evolving nature of the profession with regard to distance counseling, technology, and social media

and how such resources may be used to better serve their clients. Counselors strive to become knowledgeable about these resources. Counselors understand the additional concerns related to the use of distance counseling, technology, and social media and make every attempt to protect confidentiality and meet any legal and ethical requirements for the use of such resources.

H.1.   Knowledge and Legal Considerations

H.1.a.   Knowledge and Competency

Counselors who engage in the use of distance counseling, technology, and / or social media develop knowledge and skills regarding related technical, ethical, and legal considerations (e.g., special certifications, additional course work).

H.1.b.   Laws and Statutes

Counselors who engage in the use of distance counseling, technology, and social media within their counseling practice understand that they may be subject to laws and regulations of both the counselor's practicing location and the client's place of residence. Counselors ensure that their clients are aware of pertinent legal rights and limitations governing the practice of counseling across state lines or international boundaries.

H.2.   Informed Consent and Security

H.2.a.   Informed Consent and Disclosure

Clients have the freedom to choose whether to use distance counseling, social media, and/or technology within the counseling process. In addition to the usual and customary protocol of informed consent between counselor and client for face-to-face counseling, the following issues, unique to the use of distance counseling, technology, and / or social media, are addressed in the informed consent process:

> ➤ distance counseling credentials, physical location of practice, and contact information;
> ➤ risks and benefits of engaging in the use of distance counseling, technology, and/or social media;
> ➤ possibility of technology failure and alternate methods of service delivery;

➤ anticipated response time;
➤ emergency procedures to follow when the counselor is not available;
➤ time zone differences;
➤ cultural and/or language differences that may affect delivery of services;
➤ possible denial of insurance benefits; and
➤ social media policy.

H.2.b. Confidentiality Maintained by the Counselor
Counselors acknowledge the limitations of maintaining the confidentiality of electronic records and transmissions. They inform clients that individuals might have authorized or unauthorized access to such records or transmissions (e.g., colleagues, supervisors, employees, information technologists).

H.2.c. Acknowledgment of Limitations
Counselors inform clients about the inherent limits of confidentiality when using technology. Counselors urge clients to be aware of authorized and/or unauthorized access to information disclosed using this medium in the counseling process.

H.2.d. Security
Counselors use current encryption standards within their websites and/or technology-based communications that meet applicable legal requirements. Counselors take reasonable precautions to ensure the confidentiality of information transmitted through any electronic means.

H.3. Client Verification

Counselors who engage in the use of distance counseling, technology, and/or social media to interact with clients take steps to verify the client's identity at the beginning and throughout the therapeutic process. Verification can include, but is not limited to, using code words, numbers, graphics, or other nondescript identifiers.

H.4. Distance Counseling Relationship

H.4.a. Benefits and Limitations
Counselors inform clients of the benefits and limitations of using technology applications in the provision of counseling services. Such technologies include, but are not limited to, computer hardware and/or software, telephones and applications, social media and Internet-based applications and other audio and/or video communication, or data storage devices or media.

H.4.b. Professional Boundaries in Distance Counseling
Counselors understand the necessity of maintaining a professional relationship with their clients. Counselors discuss and establish professional boundaries with clients regarding the appropriate use and/or application of technology and the limitations of its use within the counseling relationship (e.g., lack of confidentiality, times when not appropriate to use).

H.4.c. Technology-Assisted Services
When providing technology-assisted services, counselors make reasonable efforts to determine that clients are intellectually, emotionally, physically, linguistically, and functionally capable of using the application and that the application is appropriate for the needs of the client. Counselors verify that clients understand the purpose and operation of technology applications and follow up with clients to correct possible misconceptions, discover appropriate use, and assess subsequent steps.

H.4.d. Effectiveness of Services
When distance counseling services are deemed ineffective by the counselor or client, counselors consider delivering services face-to-face. If the counselor is not able to provide face-to-face services (e.g., lives in another state), the counselor assists the client in identifying appropriate services.

H.4.e. Access
Counselors provide information to clients regarding reasonable access to pertinent applications when providing technology-assisted services.

H.4.f. Communication Differences in Electronic Media
Counselors consider the differences between face-to-face and electronic communication (nonverbal and verbal cues) and how these may affect the counseling process. Counselors educate clients on how to

prevent and address potential misunderstandings arising from the lack of visual cues and voice intonations when communicating electronically.

H.5.   Records and Web Maintenance

H.5.a.   Records

Counselors maintain electronic records in accordance with relevant laws and statutes. Counselors inform clients on how records are maintained electronically. This includes, but is not limited to, the type of encryption and security assigned to the records, and if/for how long archival storage of transaction records is maintained.

H.5.b.   Client Rights

Counselors who offer distance counseling services and/or maintain a professional website provide electronic links to relevant licensure and professional certification boards to protect consumer and client rights and address ethical concerns.

H.5.c.   Electronic Links

Counselors regularly ensure that electronic links are working and are professionally appropriate.

H.5.d.   Multicultural and Disability Considerations

Counselors who maintain websites provide accessibility to persons with disabilities. They provide translation capabilities for clients who have a different primary language, when feasible. Counselors acknowledge the imperfect nature of such translations and accessibilities.

H.6.   Social Media

H.6.a.   Virtual Professional Presence

In cases where counselors wish to maintain a professional and personal presence for social media use, separate professional and personal web pages and profiles are created to clearly distinguish between the two kinds of virtual presence.

H.6.b.   Social Media as Part of Informed Consent

Counselors clearly explain to their clients, as part of the informed consent procedure, the benefits, limitations, and boundaries of the use of social media.

H.6.c.   Client Virtual Presence

Counselors respect the privacy of their clients' presence on social media unless given consent to view such information.

H.6.d.   Use of Public Social Media

Counselors take precautions to avoid disclosing confidential information through public social media.

Section I

Resolving Ethical Issues

. . . .

Introduction

Professional counselors behave in an ethical and legal manner. They are aware that client welfare and trust in the profession depend on a high level of professional conduct. They hold other counselors to the same standards and are willing to take appropriate action to ensure that standards are upheld. Counselors strive to resolve ethical dilemmas with direct and open communication among all parties involved and seek consultation with colleagues and supervisors when necessary. Counselors incorporate ethical practice into their daily professional work and engage in ongoing professional development regarding current topics in ethical and legal issues in counseling. Counselors become familiar with the ACA Policy and Procedures for Processing Complaints of Ethical Violations[1] and use it as a reference for assisting in the enforcement of the *ACA Code of Ethics*.

I.1.   Standards and the Law

I.1.a.   Knowledge

Counselors know and understand the *ACA Code of Ethics* and other applicable ethics codes from professional organizations or certification and licensure bodies of which they are members. Lack of knowledge or misunderstanding of an ethical responsibility is not a defense against a charge of unethical conduct.

I.1.b. Ethical Decision Making

When counselors are faced with an ethical dilemma, they use and document, as appropriate, an ethical decision-making model that may include, but is not limited to, consultation; consideration of relevant ethical standards, principles, and laws; generation of potential courses of action; deliberation of risks and benefits; and selection of an objective decision based on the circumstances and welfare of all involved.

I.1.c. Conflicts Between Ethics and Laws

If ethical responsibilities conflict with the law, regulations, and/or other governing legal authority, counselors make known their commitment to the *ACA Code of Ethics* and take steps to resolve the conflict. If the conflict cannot be resolved using this approach, counselors, acting in the best interest of the client, may adhere to the requirements of the law, regulations, and/or other governing legal authority.

I.2. Suspected Violations

I.2.a. Informal Resolution

When counselors have reason to believe that another counselor is violating or has violated an ethical standard and substantial harm has not occurred, they attempt to first resolve the issue informally with the other counselor if feasible, provided such action does not violate confidentiality rights that may be involved.

I.2.b. Reporting Ethical Violations

If an apparent violation has substantially harmed or is likely to substantially harm a person or organization and is not appropriate for informal resolution or is not resolved properly, counselors take further action depending on the situation. Such action may include referral to state or national committees on professional ethics, voluntary national certification bodies, state licensing boards, or appropriate institutional authorities. The confidentiality rights of clients should be considered in all actions. This standard does not apply when counselors have been retained to review the work of another counselor whose professional conduct is in question (e.g., consultation, expert testimony).

I.2.c. Consultation

When uncertain about whether a particular situation or course of action may be in violation of the *ACA Code of Ethics*, counselors consult with other counselors who are knowledgeable about ethics and the *ACA Code of Ethics*, with colleagues, or with appropriate authorities, such as the ACA Ethics and Professional Standards Department.

I.2.d. Organizational Conflicts

If the demands of an organization with which counselors are affiliated pose a conflict with the *ACA Code of Ethics*, counselors specify the nature of such conflicts and express to their supervisors or other responsible officials their commitment to the *ACA Code of Ethics* and, when possible, work through the appropriate channels to address the situation.

I.2.e. Unwarranted Complaints

Counselors do not initiate, participate in, or encourage the filing of ethics complaints that are retaliatory in nature or are made with reckless disregard or willful ignorance of facts that would disprove the allegation.

I.2.f. Unfair Discrimination Against Complainants and Respondents

Counselors do not deny individuals employment, advancement, admission to academic or other programs, tenure, or promotion based solely on their having made or their being the subject of an ethics complaint. This does not preclude taking action based on the outcome of such proceedings or considering other appropriate information.

I.3. Cooperation With Ethics Committees

Counselors assist in the process of enforcing the *ACA Code of Ethics*. Counselors cooperate with investigations, proceedings, and requirements of the ACA Ethics Committee or ethics committees of other duly constituted associations or boards having jurisdiction over those charged with a violation.

---

[1]See the American Counseling Association web site at http://www.counseling.org/knowledge-center/ethics

Glossary of Terms

Abandonment – the inappropriate ending or arbitrary termination of a counseling relationship that puts the client at risk.

Advocacy – promotion of the well-being of individuals, groups, and the counseling profession within systems and organizations. Advocacy seeks to remove barriers and obstacles that inhibit access, growth, and development.

Assent – to demonstrate agreement when a person is otherwise not capable or competent to give formal consent (e.g., informed consent) to a counseling service or plan.

Assessment – the process of collecting in-depth information about a person in order to develop a comprehensive plan that will guide the collaborative counseling and service provision process.

Bartering – accepting goods or services from clients in exchange for counseling services.

Client – an individual seeking or referred to the professional services of a counselor.

Confidentiality – the ethical duty of counselors to protect a client's identity, identifying characteristics, and private communications.

Consultation – a professional relationship that may include, but is not limited to, seeking advice, information, and/or testimony.

Counseling – a professional relationship that empowers diverse individuals, families, and groups to accomplish mental health, wellness, education, and career goals.

Counselor Educator – a professional counselor engaged primarily in developing, implementing, and supervising the educational preparation of professional counselors.

Counselor Supervisor – a professional counselor who engages in a formal relationship with a practicing counselor or counselor-in-training for the purpose of overseeing that individual's counseling work or clinical skill development.

Culture – membership in a socially constructed way of living, which incorporates collective values, beliefs, norms, boundaries, and lifestyles that are cocreated with others who share similar worldviews comprising biological, psychosocial, historical, psychological, and other factors.

Discrimination – the prejudicial treatment of an individual or group based on their actual or perceived membership in a particular group, class, or category.

Distance Counseling – The provision of counseling services by means other than face-to-face meetings, usually with the aid of technology.

Diversity – the similarities and differences that occur within and across cultures, and the intersection of cultural and social identities.

Documents – any written, digital, audio, visual, or artistic recording of the work within the counseling relationship between counselor and client.

Encryption – process of encoding information in such a way that limits access to authorized users.

Examinee – a recipient of any professional counseling service that includes educational, psychological, and career appraisal, using qualitative or quantitative techniques.

Exploitation – actions and/or behaviors that take advantage of another for one's own benefit or gain.

Fee Splitting – the payment or acceptance of fees for client referrals (e.g., percentage of fee paid for rent, referral fees).

Forensic Evaluation – the process of forming professional opinions for court or other legal proceedings, based on professional knowledge and expertise, and supported by appropriate data.

Gatekeeping – the initial and ongoing academic, skill, and dispositional assessment of students' competency for professional practice, including remediation and termination as appropriate.

Impairment – a significantly diminished capacity to perform professional functions.

Incapacitation – an inability to perform professional functions.

Informed Consent – a process of information sharing associated with possible actions clients may choose to take, aimed at assisting clients in acquiring a full appreciation and understanding of the facts and implications of a given action or actions.

Instrument – a tool, developed using accepted research practices, that measures the presence and strength of a specified construct or constructs.

Interdisciplinary Teams – teams of professionals serving clients that may include individuals who may not share counselors' responsibilities regarding confidentiality.

Minors – generally, persons under the age of 18 years, unless otherwise designated by statute or regulation. In some jurisdictions, minors may have the right to consent to counseling without consent of the parent or guardian.

Multicultural/Diversity Competence – counselors' cultural and diversity awareness and knowledge about self and others, and how this awareness and knowledge are applied effectively in practice with clients and client groups.

Multicultural/Diversity Counseling – counseling that recognizes diversity and embraces approaches that support the worth, dignity, potential, and uniqueness of individuals within their historical, cultural, economic, political, and psychosocial contexts.

Personal Virtual Relationship – engaging in a relationship via technology and/or social media that blurs the professional boundary (e.g., friending on social networking sites); using personal accounts as the connection point for the virtual relationship.

Privacy – the right of an individual to keep oneself and one's personal information free from unauthorized disclosure.

Privilege – a legal term denoting the protection of confidential information in a legal proceeding (e.g., subpoena, deposition, testimony).

Pro bono publico – contributing to society by devoting a portion of professional activities for little or no financial return (e.g., speaking to groups, sharing professional information, offering reduced fees).

Professional Virtual Relationship – using technology and/ or social media in a professional manner and maintaining appropriate professional boundaries; using business accounts that cannot be linked back to personal accounts as the connection point for the virtual relationship (e.g., a business page versus a personal profile).

Records – all information or documents, in any medium, that the counselor keeps about the client, excluding personal and psychotherapy notes.

Records of an Artistic Nature – products created by the client as part of the counseling process.

Records Custodian – a professional colleague who agrees to serve as the caretaker of client records for another mental health professional.

Self-Growth – a process of self-examination and challenging of a counselor's assumptions to enhance professional effectiveness.

Serious and Foreseeable – when a reasonable counselor can anticipate significant and harmful possible consequences.

Sexual Harassment – sexual solicitation, physical advances, or verbal/nonverbal conduct that is sexual in nature; occurs in connection with professional activities or roles; is unwelcome, offensive, or creates a hostile workplace or learning environment; and/ or is sufficiently severe or intense to be perceived as harassment by a reasonable person.

Social Justice – the promotion of equity for all people and groups for the purpose of ending oppression and injustice affecting clients, students, counselors, families, communities, schools, workplaces, governments, and other social and institutional systems.

Social Media – technology-based forms of communication of ideas, beliefs, personal histories, etc. (e.g., social networking sites, blogs).

Student – an individual engaged in formal graduate-level counselor education.

Supervisee – a professional counselor or counselor-in-training whose counseling work or clinical skill development is being overseen in a formal supervisory relationship by a qualified trained professional.

Supervision – a process in which one individual, usually a senior member of a given profession designated as the supervisor, engages in a collaborative relationship with another individual or group, usually a junior member(s) of a given profession designated as the supervisee(s) in order to (a) promote the growth and development of the supervisee(s), (b) protect the welfare of the clients seen by the supervisee(s), and (c) evaluate the performance of the supervisee(s).

Supervisor – counselors who are trained to oversee the professional clinical work of counselors and counselors-in-training.

Teaching – all activities engaged in as part of a formal educational program that is designed to lead to a graduate degree in counseling.

Training – the instruction and practice of skills related to the counseling profession. Training contributes to the ongoing proficiency of students and professional counselors.

Virtual Relationship – a non–face-to-face relationship (e.g., through social media).

Index

Ethics Related Resources from ACA!

➤ Free consultation on ethics for ACA Members
➤ Bestselling publications revised in accordance with the 2014 *Code of Ethics*, including *ACA Ethical Standards Casebook*, *Boundary Issues in Counseling*, *Ethics Desk Reference for Counselors*, and *The Counselor and the Law*
➤ Podcast and six-part webinar series on the 2014 *Code*
➤ The latest information on ethics at *counseling.org/ethics*

References

Aasheim, L. L. (2010). Guidance/psychoeducational groups. In D. Capuzzi, D. R. Gross, & M. D. Stauffer (Eds.), *Group work* (5th ed., pp. 281–307). Denver, CO: Love Publishing.

Ackerman, N. W. (1958). *The psychodynamics of family life.* New York, NY: Basic Books.

Ackerman, N. W. (1966). *Treating the troubled family.* New York, NY: Basic Books.

ACT (2014). *Discover.* Retrieved from http://www.act.org/discover/

Adam, B. D. (2007). Homophobia and heterosexism. In R. George (Ed.), *Blackwell encyclopedia of sociology.* Retrieved from http://www.sociologyencyclopedia.com/

Addams, J. (2012). *Twenty years at Hull House.* Charleston, SC: Nabu Press. (Original work published 1910)

Agazarian, Y. M. (2008). Introduction to a theory of living human systems and systems-centered practice. In G. M. Saiger, S. Rubenfeld, & M. D. Dluhy (Eds.), *Windows into today's group therapy* (pp. 23–31). New York, NY: Routledge.

Agresta, J. (2004). Professional role perceptions of school social workers, psychologists, and counselors. *Children and Schools, 26*(3), 151–163. doi: org/10.1093/cs/26.3.151

Aiken, L. R., & Groth-Marnat, G. (2006). *Psychological testing and assessment* (12th ed.). Upper Saddle River, NJ: Pearson.

Akens, C., & Novak, J. (2011). Residence halls. In N. Zhang (Ed.), *Rentz's student affairs practice in higher education* (4th ed., pp. 315–358). Springfield, IL: Charles C. Thomas.

Alarcon, R. D. (2009). Culture, cultural factors, and psychiatric diagnosis: Review and projections. *World Psychiatry, 8*(3), 131–139.

Albert, K. A., & Luzzo, D. A. (1999). The role of perceived barriers in career development: A social cognitive perspective. *Journal of Counseling and Development, 77*(4), 431–436.

Alberto, P., & Troutman, A. C. (2012). *Applied behavior analysis for teachers* (9th ed.). Upper Saddle River, NJ: Merrill Prentice Hall.

Alemán, A. M. (2014, January/February). Social media go to college. *Change: The Magazine of Higher Learning,* 13–20. doi: 10.1080/00091383.2014.867203

Alemán, A. M., & Wartman, K. L. (2010). Using technology in student affairs practice. In J. H. Schuh, S. R. Jones, & S. R. Harper (Eds.), *Student services: A handbook for the profession* (5th ed., pp. 515–533). San Francisco, CA: Jossey Bass.

Allen, J. P., & Turner, E. J. (1988). *We the people: An atlas of America's ethnic diversity.* New York, NY: Macmillan.

Altekruse, M. K., & Wittmer, J. (1991). Accreditation in counselor education. In F. O. Bradley (Ed.), *Credentialing in counseling* (pp. 81–85). Alexandria, VA: Association for Counselor Education and Supervision.

Alvarez, A., & Piper, R. (2005). Integrating theory and practice: A racial-cultural counseling model. In R. T. Carter (Ed.), *Handbook of racial-cultural psychology and counseling, Vol. 2: Training and practice* (pp. 235–248). Hoboken, NJ: John Wiley & Sons.

American Art Therapy Association (2013). *The American Art Therapy Association's mission.* Retrieved from http://www.arttherapy.org/aata-aboutus.html

American Association of Marriage and Family Therapists (AAMFT) (2002–2013a). *About AAMFT.* Retrieved from http://www.aamft.org/imis15/content/about_aamft/AAMFT.aspx

American Association of Marriage and Family Therapists (AAMFT) (2002–2013c). *Home page.* Retrieved from http://www.aamft.org/iMIS15/AAMFT/

American Association of Marriage and Family Therapists (AAMFT) (2002–2013d). *Commission on Accreditation for Marital and Family Therapy Education.* Retrieved from http://www.aamft.org/imis15/content/coamfte/About_COAMFTE.aspx

American Association of Marriage and Family Therapists (AAMFT) (2012). *Code of ethics.* Retrieved from http://www.aamft.org/imis15/Content/Legal_Ethics/Code_of_Ethics.aspx

American Association of Marriage and Family Therapy (2002–2013b). *MFT licensing boards.* Retrieved from http://www.aamft.org/imis15/Content/Directories/MFT_Licensing_Boards.aspx

American Association of Pastoral Counselors (2005–2012). *Approved service centers.* Retrieved from http://www.aapc.org/links-resources/centers/service-centers.aspx?

American Association of State Counseling Boards (2009). *Listserv survey-licensing art therapist in your state.* Retrieved from http://www.aascb.org/aws/AASCB/asset_manager/get_file/37355/licsening_art_therapist_in_your_state-0809.pdf

American Counseling Association (ACA) (1995a). *ACA history: 1995.* Alexandria, VA: Author.

American Counseling Association (ACA) (1995b). *Code of ethics and standards of practice* (rev. ed.). Alexandria, VA: Author.

American Counseling Association (ACA) (2003). *Standards for qualifications of test users*. Alexandria, VA: Author.

American Counseling Association (ACA) (2005). *Code of ethics* (rev. ed.). Alexandria, VA: Author.

American Counseling Association (ACA) (2009, August 1). *Membership report*. Alexandria, VA: Author.

American Counseling Association (ACA) (2011). 2011 statistics on mental health professions. Retrieved from http://www.counseling.org/docs/public-policy-resources-reports/mental_health_professions-_statistics_2011-(1).pdf?sfvrsn=2

American Counseling Association (ACA) (2012a). *Licensure requirements for professional counselors: A state-by-state report*. Alexandria, VA: Author.

American Counseling Association (ACA) (2012b). *The Affordable Care Act: What counselors should know*. Retrieved from http://www.counseling.org/PublicPolicy/PDF/What_counselors_should_know-the_Affordable_Care_Act_12-12.pdf

American Counseling Association (ACA) (2013a). 20/20: Consensus definition of counseling. Retrieved from http://www.counseling.org/knowledge-center/20-20-a-vision-for-the-future-of-counseling/consensus-definition-of-counseling

American Counseling Association (ACA) (2013b). *Our mission*. Retrieved from http://www.counseling.org/about-us/about-aca/our-mission

American Counseling Association (ACA) (2013c). Knowledge center—20/20: A vision for the future of counseling. Retrieved from http://www.counseling.org/knowledge-center/20-20-a-vision-for-the-future-of-counseling/statement-of-principles

American Counseling Association (ACA) (2013d). Common Core State Standards: Essential information for school counselors. Retrieved from http://www.counseling.org/docs/resources—school-counselors/common-core-state-standards.pdf?sfvrsn=2

American Counseling Association (ACA) (2014a). *Code of ethics*. Retrieved from http://www.counseling.org/resources/aca-code-of-ethics.pdf

American Counseling Association (ACA) (2014b). *Membership benefits: Professional liability insurance*. Retrieved from http://www.counseling.org/membership/aca—membership-benefits

American Counseling Association (ACA) (2014c). *Licensure and certification*. Retrieved from http://www.counseling.org/knowledge-center/licensure-requirements

American Counseling Association (ACA) (2014d). *Government affairs*. Retrieved from http://www.counseling.org/PublicPolicy

American Counseling Association (ACA) (2014e). *Public policy news view: More details on Tricare*. Retrieved from http://www.counseling.org/government-affairs/public-policy/public-policy-news-view/legislative-news/2014/03/10/More-details-on-Tricare

American Educational Research Association (AERA) (1999). *Standards for educational and psychological testing*. Washington, DC: AERA.

American Group Psychotherapy Association (AGPA) (n.d.). *Practice guidelines for group psychotherapy: Group process*. Retrieved from http://agpa.org/home/practice-resources/practice-guidelines-for-group-psychotherapy

American Mental Health Counselors Association (AMHCA) (2010). AMHCA Code of Ethics. Retrieved from https://www.amhca.org/about/codetoc.aspx

American Mental Health Counselors Association (AMHCA) (2011). *Standards for the practice of clinical mental health counseling*. Retrieved from http://www.amhca.org/assets/content/AMHCA_Standards_1-26-2012.pdf

American Mental Health Counselors Association (AMHCA) (2013a). *Facts about mental health counselors*. Retrieved from http://www.amhca.org/about/facts.aspx

American Mental Health Counselors Association (AMHCA) (2013b). *Obamacare mental health benefits extended to 62 million Americans*. Retrieved from http://www.amhca.org/news/detail.aspx?ArticleId=615

American Mental Health Counselors Association (AMHCA) (2013c). *Facts about clinical mental health counselors*. Retrieved from http://www.amhca.org/about/facts.aspx

American Mental Health Counselors Association (AMHCA) (2013d). *Our mission*. Retrieved from https://www.amhca.org/about/default.aspx

American Mental Health Counselors Association (AMHCA) (2013e). *Our vision*. Retrieved from https://www.amhca.org/about/default.aspx

American Psychiatric Association (1994). *Diagnostic and statistical manual of mental disorders* (4th ed.). Washington, DC, Author.

American Psychiatric Association (2000). *Diagnostic and statistical manual of mental disorders,* (4th ed., text rev.). Washington, DC, Author.

American Psychiatric Association (2012). *About APA and Psychiatry*. Retrieved from http://www.psychiatry.org/about-apa–psychiatry

American Psychiatric Association (2013a). *Diagnostic and statistical manual of mental disorders* (5th ed.). Arlington, VA: American Psychiatric Association.

American Psychiatric Association (2013b). *The principles of medical ethics: With annotations especially applicable to psychiatry*. Retrieved from http://www.psych.org/practice/ethics

American Psychiatric Association (2013c). *Cultural concepts in DSM-5*. Retrieved from file:///C:/Users/Edward/Downloads/cultural-concepts-in-dsm-5.pdf

American Psychiatric Association (2014a). *DSM-5 field trials.* Retrieved from http://www.dsm5.org/Research/Pages/DSM-5FieldTrials.aspx

American Psychiatric Association (2014b). *African Americans.* Retrieved from http://www.psychiatry.org/african-americans

American Psychiatric Nurses Association (APNA) (n.d.a). *Home page.* Retrieved from http://www.apna.org/

American Psychiatric Nurses Association (APNA) (n.d.b). *About the American Psychiatric Nurses Association: An introduction.* Retrieved from http://www.apna.org/i4a/pages/index.cfm?pageid=3277

American Psychoanalytic Association (APsaA) (2012). *Standards in education and training in psychoanalysis.* Retrieved from http://apsa.org/Portals/1/docs/Training/Standards.pdf

American Psychological Association (APA) (1954). *Technological recommendations for psychological tests and diagnostic techniques.* Washington, DC: Author.

American Psychological Association (APA) (1973). Guidelines for psychologists conducting growth groups. *American Psychologist, 28,* 933. doi: 10.1037/h0035596

American Psychological Association (APA) (2007). *Guidelines for psychological practice with girls and women.* Washington, DC: Author.

American Psychological Association (APA) (2010a). *Ethical principles of psychologists and code of conduct: 2010 amendments.* Retrieved from http://www.apa.org/ethics/code/index.aspx

American Psychological Association (APA) (2010b). *Publication manual of the American Psychological Association* (6th ed.). Washington, DC: Author.

American Psychological Association (APA) (2013a). *Careers in psychology.* Retrieved from http://www.apa.org/careers/resources/guides/careers.aspx?item=1

American Psychological Association (APA) (2013b). *About APA.* Retrieved from http://www.apa.org/about/index.aspx

American Psychological Association (APA) (2013c). *HIPAA: What you need to know: The privacy rule—A primer for psychologists.* Retrieved from http://apapracticecentral.org/business/hipaa/hippa-privacy-primer.pdf

American Psychological Association (APA) (2014a). *Accreditation.* Retrieved from http://www.apa.org/ed/accreditation/

American Psychological Association (APA) (2014b). *Health and homelessness.* Retrieved from http://www.apa.org/pi/ses/resources/publications/homelessness-health.aspx

American School Counselor Association (ASCA) (2005a). *The ASCA National Model: A framework for school counseling programs* (2nd ed.). Arlington, VA: Author.

American School Counselor Association (ASCA) (2005b). *NBCC and NBPTS: Comparison of costs and benefits.* Retrieved from http://www.schoolcounselor.org/asca/media/asca/home/SC_MA05_NBCC_NBPTS_CertChart.pdf

American School Counselor Association (ASCA) (2008). *The professional school counselor and response to intervention.* Retrieved from http://www.schoolcounselor.org/asca/media/asca/PositionStatements/PS_Intervention.pdf

American School Counselor Association (ASCA) (2010). *Ethical standards for school counselors.* Retrieved from http://www.schoolcounselor.org/asca/media/asca/Resource%20Center/Legal%20and%20Ethical%20Issues/Sample%20Documents/EthicalStandards2010.pdf

American School Counselor Association (ASCA) (2010). *Ethical standards for school counselors.* Retrieved from http://www.schoolcounselor.org/asca/media/asca/Resource%20Center/Legal%20and%20Ethical%20Issues/Sample%20Documents/EthicalStandards2010.pdf

American School Counselor Association (ASCA) (2012). *The ASCA National Model: A framework for school counseling programs* (3rd ed.). Alexandria, VA: Author.

American School Counselor Association (ASCA) (2013). *ASCA announces 2013 RAMP schools.* Retrieved from http://www.schoolcounselor.org/asca/media/asca/Press%20releases/RAMP2013.pdf

American School Counselor Association (ASCA) (2014). *ASCA mindsets and behaviors for student success: K-12 college- and career-readiness standards for every student.* Alexandria, VA: Author.

American School Counselor Association (ASCA) (n.d.). *The role of the professional school counselor.* Retrieved from http://www.schoolcounselor.org/asca/media/asca/home/RoleStatement.pdf

Ancis, J. R., & Marshall, D. S. (2010). Using a multicultural framework to assess supervisees' perceptions of culturally competent supervision. *Journal of Counseling and Development, 88,* 277–284. doi: 10.1002/j.1556-6678.2010.tb00023.x

Anderson, E. (2009). *Inclusive masculinity: The changing nature of masculinities.* New York, NY: Routledge.

Anderson, M. L. Goodman, J., & Schlossberg, N. K. (2012). *Counseling adults in transition: Linking practice with theory* (4th ed.). New York, NY: Springer Publishing Company.

Anderson, T., Lunnen, K. M., & Ogles, B. M. (2010). Putting models and techniques in context. In B. L. Duncan, S. D. Miller, B. E. Wampold, & M A. Hubble (Eds.), *The heart and soul of change* (2nd ed., pp. 143–166). Washington, DC: American Psychological Association.

Andrade, M. S. (2013). Launching e-portfolios: An organic process. *Assessment Update: Progress, Trends, and Practices in Higher Education, 25*(3), 1–2, 14–15.

Ansbacher, H. L. (1964). The increasing recognition of Adler. In H. L. Ansbacher & R. R. Ansbacher (Eds.), *Superiority and social interest: A collection of later writings* (pp. 3–19). Evanston, IL: Northwestern University Press.

Anthony, E. J. (1972). The history of group psychotherapy. In H. I. Kaplan & B. J. Sadock (Eds.), *The origins of group psychoanalysis* (pp. 1–26). New York, NY: Jason Aronson.

Arredondo, P. (1999). Multicultural counseling competencies as tools to address oppression and racism. *Journal of Counseling and Development, 77,* 102–108. doi: 10.1002/j.1556-6676.1999.tb02427.x

Arredondo, P., Rosen, D., Rice, T., Perez, P., & Tovar-Gamero, Z. (2005). Multicultural counseling: A 10-year content analysis of the *Journal of Counseling and Development. Journal of Counseling and Development, 83*(2), 155–161.

Arredondo, P., Toporek, R., Brown, S. P., Jones, J., Locke, D. C., Sanchez, J., & Stadler, H. (1996). Operationalization of the multicultural counseling competencies. *Journal of Multicultural Counseling and Development, 24*(1), 42–78. doi: 10.1002/j.2161-1912.1996.tb00288.x

Arredondo, P., Tovar-Blank, Z., & Parham, T. A. (2008). Challenges and promises of becoming a culturally competent counselor in a sociopolitical era of change and empowerment. *Journal of Counseling and Development, 86,* 261–268.

Art Therapy Credentials Board. (2012). *Welcome to the Art Therapy Credentials Board, Inc.!* Retrieved from http://www.atcb.org/

Arthur, M. M. L. (2007). Race. In G. Ritzer (Ed.), *Blackwell encyclopedia of sociology.* Retrieved from http://www.blackwellreference.com/subscriber/tocnode?id=g9781405124331_chunk_g978140512433124_ss1-1

Arthur, N., & Achenbach, K. (2002). Developing multicultural counseling competencies through experiential learning. *Counselor Education and Supervision, 42*(1), 2–14.

Arthur, N., & Collins, S. (2011). Infusing culture in career counseling. *Journal of Employment Counseling, 48*(4), 147–149.

Arthur, N., & McMahon, M. (2005). Multicultural career counseling: Theoretical applications of the systems theory framework. *Career Development Quarterly, 53*(3), 208–222.

Association for Assessment and Research in Counseling (AARC) (2003). *Responsibilities of users of standardized tests (RUST)* (3rd ed.). Alexandria, VA: Author.

Association for Assessment and Research in Counseling (AARC) (2012). *Standards for multicultural assessment* (4th revision). Retrieved from http://aarc-counseling.org/assets/cms/uploads/files/AACE-AMCD.pdf

Association for Assessment and Research in Counseling (AARC) (2014a). *Resources.* Retrieved from http://aarc-counseling.org/resources

Association for Assessment and Research in Counseling (AARC) (2014b). *About us: Vision.* Retrieved from http://aarc-counseling.org/about-us

Association for Counselor Education and Supervision (1990). Standards for counseling supervisors. *Journal of Counseling and Development, 69,* 30–36.

Association for Counselors and Educators in Government (AECG) (2014). *About us.* Retrieved from http://acegonline.org/

Association for Specialists in Group Work (2000). *Professional standards for the training of group workers.* Retrieved from http://www.asgw.org/PDF/training_standards.pdf

Association for Specialists in Group Work (2007). *ASGW best practices guidelines.* Retrieved from http://www.asgw.org/PDF/Best_Practices.pdf

Association for Specialists in Group Work (2012a). *Multicultural and social justice competence principles for group workers.* Retrieved from http://www.asgw.org/pdf/ASGW_MC_SJ_Principles_Final_ASGW.pdf

Association for Specialists in Group Work (2012b). *Purpose of ASGW.* Retrieved from http://www.asgw.org/purpose.htm

Association for Spiritual, Ethical, and Religious Values in Counseling (2009). *Spiritual competencies.* Retrieved from http://aservic.org/?page_id=133

Association of Marital and Family Therapy Regulatory Boards (2014). *Home page.* Retrieved from http://www.amftrb.org/

Association of Social Work Boards (2013). *Licenses.* Retrieved from http://www.aswb.org/licensees/

Ata, R., Ludden, A., & Lally, M. (2007). The effects of gender and family, friend, and media influences on eating behaviors and body image during adolescence. *Journal of Youth and Adolescence, 36*(8), 1024–1037. doi: 10.1007/s10964-006-9159-x

Atkinson, D. R. (2004a). Defining populations and terms. In D. R. Atkinson (Ed.), *Counseling American minorities* (6th ed., pp. 3–26). Boston, MA: McGraw-Hill.

Atkinson, D. R. (2004b). Within-group differences among ethnic minorities. In D. R. Atkinson (Ed.), *Counseling American minorities* (6th ed., pp. 27–56). New York, NY: McGraw-Hill.

Atkinson, D., & Israel, T. (2003). The future of multicultural counseling competence. In D. B. Pope-Davis, H. L. K. Coleman, W. M. Lieu, & R. Toporek (Eds.), *Handbook of multicultural competencies: In counseling and psychology* (pp. 591–606). Thousand Oaks, CA: Sage.

Attridge, W. C. (2000). *Ethical considerations for internet counseling*. Retrieved from ERIC database (ED 448369)

Aubrey, R. F. (1977). Historical development of guidance and counseling and implications for the future. *Personnel and Guidance Journal, 55,* 288–295. doi: 10.1002/j.2164-4918.1977.tb04991.x

Aubrey, R. F. (1982). A house divided: Guidance and counseling in twentieth-century America. *Personnel and Guidance Journal, 61,* 198–204. doi: 10.1002/j.2164-4918.1982.tb00312.x

Auwarter, A. E., & Aruguete, M. S. (2008). Counselor perceptions of students who vary in gender and socioeconomic status. *Social Psychology of Education, 11,* 389–395. doi: 10.1007/ s11218-008-9056-0

Aviv, R. (2005, August 16). The interpretation of reams: Talking with Albert Ellis, world- renowned anti-Freud therapist. *Village Voice.* Retrieved from http://www.villagevoice.com/2005-08-16/people/the-interpretation-of-reams/full/

Axelson, J. A. (1999). *Counseling and development in a multicultural society* (3rd ed.). Pacific Grove, CA: Brooks/Cole.

Axthelm, P. (1978, December 4). The emperor Jones. *Newsweek,* pp. 54–60.

Baditoi, B. E., & Brott, P. B. (2011). *What school counselors need to know about special education and students with disabilities.* Arlington, VA: Council for Exceptional Children.

Bagalman, R., & Napili, A. (2014). *Prevalence of mental illness in the United States: Data sources and estimates.* Retrieved from http://www.fas.org/sgp/crs/misc/R43047.pdf

Baker, C. (2004). *Behavioral genetics: An introduction to how genes and environments interact through development to shape differences in mood, personality, and intelligence.* New York, NY: American Association for the Advancement of Science.

Baker, S., & Gerler, E. (2008). *School counseling for the twenty-first century* (5th ed.). Upper Saddle River, NJ: Merrill.

Baker, S. B., & Gerler Jr., E. R. (2008). *School counseling for the twenty-first century* (5th ed.). Upper Saddle River, NJ: Pearson.

Baker, S. B., Robichaud, T. A., Dietrich, V., Wells, S. C., & Schreck, R. E. (2009). School counselor consultation: A pathway to advocacy, collaboration, and leadership. *Professional School Counseling, 12*(3), 200–206. doi: 10.5330/PSC.n.2010-12.200

Baker, S. R., Robinson, J. E., Danner, M. J. E., & Neukrug, E. (2001). *Community social disorganization theory applied to adolescent academic achievement.* Retrieved from ERIC database (ED453301)

Ballas, C. A., Evans, D. L., & Dinges, D. F. (2009). Psychostimulants in psychiatry: Amphetamine, methylphenidate, and modafinil. In A. F. Schatzberg & C. B. Nemeroff (Eds.), *Textbook of psychopharmacology* (4th ed., pp. 843–861). Washington, DC: American Psychiatric Press.

Bandura, A. T. (1969). *Principles of behavior modification.* New York, NY: Holt, Rinehart, & Winston.

Bandura, A. T. (1977). *Social learning theory.* Englewood Cliffs, NJ: Prentice Hall.

Bandura, A. T. (1997). *Self-efficacy: The exercise of control.* New York, NY: W. H. Freeman.

Bandura, A. T., Ross, D., & Ross, S. A. (1963). Imitation of film-mediated aggressive models. *Journal of Abnormal and Social Psychology, 67,* 3–11. doi: 10.1037/h0048687

Banmen, J. (2015). Virginia Satir. In E. Neukrug (Ed.), *The Sage encyclopedia of theory in counseling and psychotherapy* (Vol. 2, pp. 905–907). Thousand Oaks, CA: Sage.

Banning, N. (2013). Talking business. *Therapy Today, 24*(8), 1–4.

Bannink, F. (2010). *1001 solution-focused questions* (I. De Taye, Trans.). New York, NY: W. W. Norton & Company. (Original work published 2006)

Barber, P. (2012). *Facilitating change in groups and teams: A gestalt approach to mindfulness.* Farringdon, UK: Libri Publishing.

Barker, P., & Chang, J. (2013). *Basic family therapy* (6th ed.). Hoboken, NJ: John Wiley & Sons.

Barlow, S. H. (2014). The history of group counseling and psychotherapy. In J. DeLucia-Waack, C. R. Kalodner, & M. Riva (Eds.), *Handbook of group counseling and psychotherapy* (pp. 3–34). Thousand Oaks, CA: Sage.

Barlow, S. H., Burlingame, G., & Fuhriman, A. (2000). Therapeutic applications of groups: From Pratt's "thought control classes" to modern group psychotherapy. *Group Dynamics: Theory, Research, and Practice, 4*(1), 115–134. doi: 10.1037/1089-2699.4.1.115

Barnes, P., Clark, P., & Thull, B. (2003). Web-based digital portfolios and counselor supervision. *Journal of Technology in Counseling, 3*(1). Retrieved from http://jtc.colstate.edu/vol3_1/Barnes/Barnes.htm

Barr, M. J. (2003). Legal foundations of student affairs practice. In S. R. Komives & D. B. Woodward (Eds.), *Student services: A handbook for the profession* (4th ed., pp. 128–150). San Francisco, CA: Jossey-Bass.

Barstow, S., & Lum, C. (2011). *Federal information resources for professional counselors.* Alexandria, VA: American Counseling Association.

Basseches, M. (1984). *Dialectical thinking and adult development.* Norwood, NJ: Ablex.

Baxter, W. E. (1994). American psychiatry celebrates 150 years of caring. *Psychiatric Clinics of North America, 17,* 683–693.

Beck, A. T. (1967). *Depression: Clinical, experimental, and theoretical aspects.* New York, NY: Harper and Row. Republished in 1972 as *Depression: Causes and treatment.* Philadelphia, PA: University of Pennsylvania Press.

Beck, A. T. (1976). *Cognitive therapy and the emotional disorders.* New York, NY: International Universities Press.

Beck, A. T. (1991). Cognitive therapy: A 30-year retrospective. *American Psychologist, 46*(4), 368–375. doi: 10.1037/0003-066X.46.4.368

Beck, A. T. (1999). *Prisoners of hate: The cognitive basis of anger, hostility, and violence.* New York, NY: HarperCollins.

Beck, A. T. (2005). The current state of cognitive therapy: A 40-year retrospective. *Archives of General Psychiatry, 62,* 953–959. doi: 10.1001/archpsyc.62.9.953

Beck, J. (1995). *Cognitive therapy: Basics and beyond.* New York, NY: Guilford Press.

Beck, J. (2005). *Cognitive therapy for challenging problems.* New York, NY: Guilford Press.

Beckham, J. C. (2011). Negligent liability involving colleges and students: An evolving duty to care. In R. Fossey, K. B. Melear, & J. Beckham, J. (Eds.). *Contemporary issues in higher education law* (pp. 207–234). Dayton, OH: Education Law Association.

Becvar, D. S., & Becvar, R. J. (2013). *Family therapy: A systemic integration* (8th ed.). Boston, MA: Allyn & Bacon.

Bedi, R. P. (2006). Concept mapping the client's perspective on counseling alliance formation. *Journal of Counseling Psychology, 53*(1), 26–35.

Beers, C. W. (1948). *A mind that found itself* (7th ed.) Garden City, NY: Doubleday.

Behuniak, P. (2003). Educational assessment in an era of accountability. In J. Wall & G. Waltz (Eds.), *Measuring up: Assessment issues for teachers, counselors, and administrators* (pp. 335–348). Retrieved from ERIC database (ED 380066)

Belenky, M. F., Clinchy, B. M., Goldberger, N. R., & Tarule, J. M. (1997). *Women's ways of knowing.* New York, NY: Basic Books. (Original work published 1986)

Belgium, D. (1992). Guilt. In M. T. Burker & J. G. Miranti (Eds.), *Ethical and spiritual values in counseling.* (pp. 53–66). Alexandria, VA: American Association for Counseling and Development.

Belkin, G. S. (1988). *Introduction to counseling* (3rd ed.). Dubuque, IA: William C. Brown.

Bemak, F., & Chung, R. C. (2004). Teaching multicultural group counseling: Perspectives for a new era. *Journal for Specialists in Group Work, 29,* 31–42. doi: 10.1080/01933920490275349

Bemak, F., & Chung, R. C. (2008). New professional roles and advocacy strategies for school counselors: A multicultural/social justice perspective to move beyond the nice counselor syndrome. *Journal of Counseling and Development, 86,* 372–382.

Benack, S. (1984). Post-formal epistemologies and the growth of empathy. In M. Commons, F. A. Richards, & C. Armon (Eds.), *Beyond formal operations* (pp. 340–356). New York, NY: Praeger.

Benack, S. (1988). Relativistic thought: A cognitive basis for empathy in counseling. *Counselor Education and Supervision, 27*(3), 216–232. doi: 10.1002/j.1556-6978.1988.tb00760.x

Benjamin, A. (2001). *The helping interview, with case illustrations.* Boston, MA: Houghton Mifflin.

Berg, I. K. (1994). *Family-based services: A solution-focused approach.* New York, NY: W. W. Norton.

Berger, J. M., Levant, R. F., McMillan, K. K., Kelleher, W., & Sellers, A. (2005). Impact of gender role conflict, traditional masculinity ideology, alexithymia, and age on men's attitudes toward psychological help-seeking. *Psychology of Men and Masculinity, 6*(1), 73–78. doi: 10.1037/1524-9220.6.1.73

Berger, M. (2006). Computer assisted clinical assessment. *Child and Adolescent Mental Health, 11*(2), 64–75. doi: 10.1111/j.1475-3588.2006.00394.x

Bernard, J. M., & Goodyear, R. K. (2013). *Fundamentals of clinical supervision* (5th ed.). Upper Saddle River, NJ: Pearson.

Berne, E. (1964). *Games people play.* New York, NY: Simon & Schuster.

Best, J. W., & Kahn, J. V. (2006). *Research in education* (10th ed.). Boston, MA: Allyn & Bacon.

Beutler, L. E., & Malik, M. L. (Eds.). (2002). *Rethinking the DSM: A psychological perspective.* Washington, DC: American Psychological Association.

Biancoviso, A. N., Bishop-Towle, W., & Fuertes, J. N. (2004). *Planned group counseling: An alternative group method for reluctant chemically dependent and psychiatric patients.* New York, NY: Springer Publishing.

Bidwell, D. R. (2007). Miraculous knowing: Epistemology and solution-focused therapy. In T. S. Nelson & F. N. Thomas (Eds.), *Handbook of solution-focused brief therapy: Clinical applications* (pp. 65–87). New York, NY: Haworth Press.

Binswanger, L. (1963). *Being-in-the-world: Selected papers.* New York, NY: Basic Books.

Bishop, A. (2015). Freudian psychoanalysis. In E. Neukrug (Ed.), *The Sage encyclopedia of theory in counseling and psychotherapy* (Vol. 1, pp. 437–441). Thousand Oaks, CA: Sage.

Bitter, J. R. (2014). *Theory and practice of family therapy and counseling* (2nd ed.). Belmont, CA: Brooks/Cole.

Bjork, D. (2015). B. F. Skinner. In E. Neukrug (Ed.), *The Sage encyclopedia of theory in counseling and psychotherapy* (Vol. 2, pp. 935–937). Thousand Oaks, CA: Sage.

Blackburne, L. D. (2011). We are family. *Crisis, 118*(3), 3.

Blau, G. M., Caldwell, B., & Lieberman, R. E. (2014). *Residential interventions for children, adolescents, and families.* New York, NY: Routledge.

Blocher, D. (1988). Developmental counseling revisited. In R. Hayes & R. Aubrey (Eds.), *New directions for counseling and human development* (pp. 13–21). Denver, CO: Love Publishing Company.

Bloom, J. (1996). *Credentialing professional counselors for the 21st century.* Retrieved from ERIC database (ED399498)

Bloomgarden, A., & Mennuti, R. B. (2009). Therapist self-disclosure: Beyond the taboo. In A. Bloomgarden & R. B. Mennuit (Eds.), *Psychotherapist revealed: Therapists speak about self-disclosure in psychotherapy* (pp. 3–16). New York, NY: Taylor and Francis Group.

Blustein, D. L. (2006). *The psychology of work: A new perspective for career development counseling and public policy.* Mahwah, NJ: Lawrence Erlbaum Associates.

Bobby, C. L. (2013). The evolution of specialties in the CACREP standards: CACREP's role in unifying the profession. *Journal of Counseling & Development, 91,* 35–43. doi: 10.1002/j.1556-6676.2013.00068.x

Bolles, R. N. (2014). *What color is your parachute? 2014: A practical manual for job-hunters and career changes.* New York, NY: Ten Speed Press.

Bonitz, V. (2008). Use of physical touch in the "talking cure": A journey to the outskirts of psychotherapy. *Psychotherapy: Theory, Research, Practice, Training, 45,* 391–404. doi: 10.1037/a0013311

Borders, L. D., & Brown, L. L. (2005). *The new handbook of counseling supervision.* Mahwah, NJ: Erlbaum.

Borders, L. D., Welfare, E., Greason, P. B., Paladino, D. A., Mobley, A. K., Villalba, J. A., & Wester, K. L. (2012). Individual and triadic and group: Supervisee and supervisor perceptions of each modality. *Counselor Education & Supervision, 51*(4), 281–295. doi.org/10.1002/j.1556-6978.2012.00021.x

Boszormenyi-Nagy, I. (1973). *Invisible loyalties: Reciprocity in intergenerational family therapy.* New York, NY: Harper & Row.

Boszormenyi-Nagy, I. (1987). *Foundations of contextual therapy.* New York, NY: Brunner/Mazel.

Bottome, P. (1957). *Alfred Adler: A portrait from life.* New York, NY: Vanguard Press.

Bowden, R. (2007). Evolution of responsibility: from "in loco parentis" to "ad meliora vertamur." *Education, 127,* 480–489.

Bowen, M. (1976). Theory in the practice of psychotherapy. In P. J. Guerin (Ed.), *Family therapy: Theory and practice* (pp. 42–90). New York, NY: Gardner Press.

Bowen, M. (1978). *Family therapy in clinical practice.* New York, NY: Jason Aronson.

Bowen, M. (1985). *Family therapy in clinical practice.* Lanham, MD: Rowman & Littlefield Publishers.

Bowman, S. L., & Roysircar, G. (2011). Training and practice in trauma, catastrophes, and disaster counseling. *Counseling Psychologist, 39,* 1160–1181. doi: 101177/0011000010397934

Brabender, V., & Fallon, A. (2009). *Group development in practice: Guidance for clinicians and researchers on stages and dynamics of change.* Washington, DC: American Psychological Association.

Brack, G., Jones, E. S., Smith, R. M., White, J., & Brack, C. J. (1993). A primer on consultation theory: Building a flexible worldview. *Journal of Counseling and Development, 71,* 619–628. doi: 10.1002/j.1556-6676.1993.tb02251.x

Bradley, L. J. (1995). Certification and licensure. *Journal of Counseling and Development, 74,* 185–186.

Brammer, L. M., & MacDonald, G. (2003). *The helping relationship: Process and skills* (8th ed.). Boston, MA: Allyn & Bacon.

Brault, M. W. (2012). *United States Census Bureau: Americans with disabilities: 2010.* Retrieved from http://www.census.gov/prod/2012pubs/p70-131.pdf

Braun, S., & Cox, J. (2005). Managed mental health care: Intentional misdiagnosis of mental disorders. *Journal of Counseling and Development, 83,* 425–433. doi: 10.1002/j.1556-6678.2005.tb00364.x

Breasted, J. H. (1930). *The Edwin Smith surgical papyrus.* Chicago, IL: University of Chicago Press.

Breasted, J. H. (1934). *The dawn of conscience.* New York, NY: Scribner's.

Brennan, C. (2013). Ensuring ethical practice: Guidelines for mental health counselors in private practice. *Journal of Mental Health Counseling, 35,* 245–261.

Brewer, J. M. (1932). *Education as guidance.* New York, NY: Macmillan.

Brickell, J. (2007, February). Reality therapy: Helping people take more effective control of their lives. *Counseling at Work,* 6–9.

Briddick, W. (2009a). Frank findings: Frank Parsons and the Parson family. *Career Development Quarterly, 57*(3), 207–214. doi: 0.1002/j.2161-0045.2009.tb00106.x

Briddick, W. C. (2009b). Frank Parsons on interests. *Journal of Vocational Behavior, 24*(2), 230–233. doi: 10.1016/j.jvb.2008.12.003

Bridge, J. A., Iyengar, S., Salary, C. B., Barbe, R. P., Birmaher, B., Pincus, H. A., & Brent, D. A. (2007). Clinical response and risk for reported suicidal ideation and suicide attempts in pediatric antidepressant treatment: A meta-analysis of randomized controlled trials. *JAMA, 297,* 1683–1696. doi: 10.1001/jama.297.15.1683

Bridgeman, B., Burton, N., & Cline, F. (2009). A note on presenting what predictive validity numbers mean. *Applied Measurement in Education, 22,* 109–119.

Bridges, J. (2007). *Respectable sins.* Colorado Springs, CO: NavPress.

Brill, A. (2010). *Basic principles of psychoanalysis.* London, UK: Kessinger Publishing. (Original work published 1921)

Brooks-Gunn, J. (2004). Intervention and policy as change agents for young children. In P. L. Chase-Lansdale, K. Kiernan, & R. J. Friedman (Eds.), *Human development across lives and generations: The potential for change* (pp. 293–342). New York, NY: Cambridge University Press.

Brown, C. G., Weber, S., & Ali, S. (2008). Women's body talk: A feminist narrative approach. *Journal of Systemic Therapies, 27*(2), 92–104.

Brown, D. (2012). *Career information, career counseling, and career development* (10th ed.). Boston, MA: Pearson.

Brown, K. J., Johnson, R. J., Bender, J. A., & Roberts, M. C. (2009). Positive psychology for children: Development, prevention, and promotion. In C. R. Snyder & S. J. Lopez (Eds.), *Handbook of positive psychology* (2nd ed., pp. 133–146). New York, NY: Oxford University Press.

Brown, L. S., & Bryan, T. C. (2007). Feminist therapy with people who self-inflict violence. *Journal of Clinical Psychology: In Session, 63*(11), 1121–1133. doi: 10.1521/jsyt.2008.27.2.92

Brown, M., Lum, J., & Voyle, K. (1997). Roe revisited: A call for the reappraisal of the theory of personality development and career choice. *Journal of Vocational Behavior, 51*, 283–94.

Brown, N. (2015a). Group counseling and psychotherapy theories: Overview. In E. Neukrug (Ed.), *The Sage encyclopedia of theory in counseling and psychotherapy* (Vol. 1, pp. 471–477). Thousand Oaks, CA: Sage.

Brown, N. (2015b). Psychoeducational groups. In E. Neukrug (Ed.), *The Sage encyclopedia of theory in counseling and psychotherapy* (Vol. 2, pp. 825–830). Thousand Oaks, CA: Sage.

Bryan, J., & Henry, L. (2008). Strengths-based partnerships: A school-family-community partnership approach to empowering students. *Professional School Counseling, 12*, 149–156.

Bryant, J., & Milsom, A. (2005). Child abuse reporting by school counselors. *Professional School Counseling, 9*, 63–71.

Brymer, M., Jacobs, A., Layne, C., Pynoos, R., Ruzek, J., Steinberg, A., . . ., & Watson, P. (2009). *Psychological first aid: Field operations guide* (2nd ed.). Durham, N.C.: National Child Traumatic Stress Network and National Center for PTSD.

Buckley, M. R. (2010). Grounded theory methodology. In C. J. Sheperis, J. C. Young, & M. H. Daniels (Eds.), *Counseling research: Quantitative, qualitative, and mixed methods* (pp. 115–150). Upper Saddle River, NJ: Pearson.

Buckley, T. R., & Franklin-Jackson, C. F. (2005). Diagnosis in racial-cultural practice. In R. T. Carter (Ed.), *Handbook of racial-cultural psychology and counseling: Theory and research* (Vol. 2, pp. 286–296). Hoboken, NJ: John Wiley.

Budman, S. H., & Gurman, A. S. (1988). *Theory and practice of brief therapy.* New York, NY: Guilford Press.

Bugental, J. F. T. (1976). *The search for existential identity: Patient–therapist dialogues in humanistic psychotherapy.* San Francisco, CA: Jossey-Bass.

Bujold, C. (2002). Constructing career through narrative. *Journal of Vocational Behavior, 64*, 470–484.

Bureau of Justice Statistics (2013). *Total U.S. correctional population declined in 2012 for fourth year.* Retrieved from http://www.bjs.gov/content/pub/press/cpus12pr.cfm.

Bureau of Justice Statistics (2014). *Prison inmate characteristics.* Retrieved from http://www.bjs.gov/index.cfm?ty=tp&tid=132

Bureau of Labor Statistics (2014). Occupational outlook handbook: School and career counselors. Retrieved from http://www.bls.gov/ooh/community-and-social-service/school-and-career-counselors.htm

Burger, W. R. (2014). *Human services in contemporary America* (9th ed.). Belmont, CA: Brooks/Cole.

Burkard, A. W., Gillen, M., Martinez, M. J., & Skytte, S. (2012). Implementation challenges and training need for comprehensive school counseling programs in Wisconsin high schools. *Professional School Counseling, 16*, 136–145. doi: 10.5330/PSC.n.2012-16.136

Burlingame, G. M., MacKenzie, K. R., & Strauss, B. (2004). Small group treatment: Evidence for effectiveness and mechanism of change. In M. J. Lambert (Ed.), *Bergin and Garfield's handbook of psychotherapy and behavior change* (5th ed., pp. 647–696). New York, NY: Wiley.

Burlingame, G., & Krogel, J. (2005). Relative efficacy of individual versus group psychotherapy. *International Journal of Group Psychotherapy, 55*(4), 607–611. doi: 10.1521/ijgp.2005.55.4.607

Burnham, J. J., & Jackson, C. M. (2000). School counselor roles: Discrepancies between actual practice and existing models. *Professional School Counseling, 4*, 41–49.

BUROS Center for Testing. (2014). *Tests reviews online.* Retrieved from http://buros.org/test-reviews-information

Burton, N. W., & Wang, M. (2005). *Predicting long-term success in graduate school: A collaborative validity study.* Princeton, NJ: Educational Testing Service.

Byars-Winston, A., & Fouad, N. (2006). Metacognition and multicultural competence: expanding the culturally appropriate career counseling model. *Career Development Quarterly, 54*(3), 187–201.

Cade, B. (2005). *Obituary: Steve de Shazer: 1940–2005.* Retrieved from http://www.ebta.nu/page28/page32/page32.html

Cade, B. (2007). Springs, streams, and tributaries: A history of the brief, solution-focused approach. In T. S. Nelson & F. N. Thomas (Eds.), *Handbook of solution-focused brief therapy: Clinical applications* (pp. 25–64). New York, NY: Haworth Press.

Caetano, R. (2011). There is potential for cultural and social bias in DSM-V. *Addiction, 106*(5), 885–887. doi:10.1002/da.20753

Cain, D. J. (2002). Defining characteristics, history, and evolution of humanistic psychotherapies. In D. J. Cain (Ed.), *Humanistic psychotherapies: Handbook of research and practice* (pp. 3–54). Washington, DC: American Psychological Association.

Calmes, S. A., Piazza, N. J., & Laux, J. M. (2013). The use of touch in counseling: An ethical decision-making model. *Counseling and Values, 58*(1), 59–68. doi: 10.1002 /j.2161–007X.2013.00025.x

Camargo-Borges, C., & Rasera, E. (2013, April–June). Social constructionism in the context of organization development: Dialogue, imagination, and co-creation as resources of change. *SAGE Open,* 1–7. doi: 10.1177 /2158244013487540

Cameron, S., & turtle-song, i. (2002). Learning to write case notes using the SOAP format. *Journal of Counseling and Development, 80,* 286–92.

Campbell, C. A., & Dahir, C. A. (1997). *Sharing the vision: The national standards for school counseling programs.* Alexandria, VA: American School Counselor Association.

Campbell, D. P. (1968). The Strong vocational interest blank: 1927–1967. In P. McReynolds (Ed.), *Advances in psychological assessment* (Vol. 1, pp. 105–130). Palo Alto, CA: Science and Behavior Books.

Campbell, D. T., & Stanley, J. C. (1963). *Experimental and quasi-experimental designs for research.* Chicago, IL: Rand McNally.

Cannon, E., & Cooper, J. (2010). Clinical mental health counseling: A national survey of counselor educators. *Journal of Mental Health Counseling, 32,* 236–246.

Caplan, G. (1970). *The theory and practice of mental health consultation.* New York, NY: Basic Books.

Caplan, G., & Caplan-Moskovich, R. B. (2004). Recent advances in mental health consultation and mental health collaboration. In N. M. Lambert, I. Hylander, & J. H. Sandoval (Eds.), *Consultee-centered consultation: Improving the quality of professional services in schools and community organizations* (pp. 21–35). Mahwah, NJ: Lawrence Erlbaum.

Capshew, J. H. (1992). Psychologists on site: A reconnaissance of the historiography of the laboratory. *American Psychologist, 47,* 132–142. doi: 10.1037/0003-066X.47.2.132

Capuzzi, D., & Gross, D. R. (2010). Group work: An introduction. In D. Capuzzi, D. R. Gross, & M. D. Stauffer, (Eds.), *Introduction to group work* (5th ed., pp. 3–38). Denver, CO: Love Publishing.

Carey, J., Harrington, K., Martin, I., & Stevenson, D. (2012). A statewide evaluation of the outcomes of the implementation of ASCA national model school counseling programs in Utah high schools. *Professional School Counseling, 16,* 89–99. doi: 10.5330/PSC.n.2012-16.89

Carkhuff, R. R. (1969). *Helping and human relations* (Vol. 2). New York, NY: Holt, Rinehart, & Winston.

Carkhuff, R. R. (2009). *The art of helping in the twenty-first century* (9th ed.). Amherst, MA: Human Resource Development Press.

Carlisle, R. M., Carlisle, K. L., Hill, T., Kirk-Jenkins, A. J., & Polychronopoulos, G. B. (2013). Distance supervision in human services. *Journal of Human Services, 33,* 17–28.

Carlson, J. C. (2002). Strategic family therapy. In J. Carlson & D. Kjos (Eds.), *Theories and strategies of family therapy* (pp. 80–97). Boston, MA: Allyn & Bacon.

Carlson, J., Watts, R. E., & Maniacci, M. (2006). *Adlerian therapy: Theory and practice.* Washington, DC: American Psychological Association.

Carpenter, S. (2011). The philosophical heritage of student affairs. In N. Zhang (Ed.), *Rentz's student affairs practice in higher education* (4th ed., pp. 3–29). Springfield, IL: Charles C. Thomas.

Carson, A. D., & Altai, N. M. (1994). 1000 years before Parsons: Vocational psychology in classical Islam. *The Career Development Quarterly, 43,* 197–206. doi: 10.1002/ j.2161-0045.1994.tb00858.x

Casas, J. M., Raley, J. D., & Vasquez, M. J. T. (2015). ¡Adelante! Counseling the Latina/o from guiding theory to practice. In P. B. Pedersen, J. G. Draguns, W. J. Lonner, & J. E. Trimble (Eds.), *Counseling across cultures* (6th ed., pp. 113–128). Thousand Oaks, CA: Sage.

Cashwell, C. S. (1994). *Interpersonal process recall.* Retrieved from ERIC database (ED 372342)

Cashwell, C. S., Young, J. S., Fulton, C. L., Willis, B. T., Giordano, A., Daniel, L. W., . . .Welch, M. L. (2013). Clinical behaviors for addressing religious/spiritual issues: Do we practice what we preach? *Counseling |and values, 58*(1), 45–58. doi: 10.1002 /j.2161-007X.2013.00024.x

Cautin, R. L. (2011). A century of psychotherapy, 1860–1960. In J. C. Norcross, G. R. VandenBos, & D. K. Freedheim (Eds.), *History of psychotherapy: Continuity and change* (2nd ed., pp. 3–38). Washington, DC: American Psychological Association.

Cazzaniga, E., & Schinco, M. (2015). Systemic family therapy. In E. Neukrug (Ed.), *The Sage encyclopedia of theory in counseling and psychotherapy* (Vol. 2, pp. 986–991). Thousand Oaks, CA: Sage.

Centers for Disease Control. (2013, December 3). *HIV and AIDS in the United States: At a glance.* Retrieved from http://www.cdc.gov/hiv/resources/factsheets/us.htm

Centers for Medicare and Medicaid Services (2013). *Community mental health centers.* Retrieved from http:// www.cms.gov/Medicare/Provider-Enrollment-and-Certification/CertificationandComplianc /CommunityHealthCenters.html

Champe, J., & Kleist, D. M. (2003). Live supervision: A review of the research. *Family Journal, 11*, 268–275. doi: 10.1177/1066480703252755

Chang, C. Y., Hays, D. G., & Gray, G. (2010). Multicultural issues in research. In C. J. Sheperis, J. C. Young, & M. H. Daniels (Eds.), *Counseling research: Quantitative, qualitative, and mixed methods* (pp. 262–273). Upper Saddle River, NJ: Pearson.

Chang, C., Chrethar, H. C., & Ratts, M. J. (2010). A national imperative for counselor education and supervision. *Counselor Education and Supervision, 50*, 82–87. doi: 10.1002/j.1556-6978.2010.tb00110.x

Chao, R., & Nath, S. R. (2011). The role of ethnic identity, gender roles, and multicultural training in college counselors' multicultural counseling competence: A mediation model. *Journal of College Counseling, 14*(1), 50–64. doi: 10.1002/j.2161-1882.2011.tb00063.x

Chapa, T. (2004). *Mental health services in primary care settings for racial and ethnic minority populations.* Rockville, MD: U.S. Department of Health and Human Services, Office of Minority Health.

Chaplin, J. P. (1975). *Dictionary of psychology* (2nd ed.). New York, NY: Dell.

Chapman, R. R., Baker, S. B., Nassar-McMillan, S. C., & Gerler, E. R. (2011). Cybersupervision: Further examination of synchronous and asynchronous modalities in counseling practicum supervision. *Counselor Education & Supervision, 50*(5), 298–313. doi: 10.1002/j.1556-6978.2011.tb01917.x

Chase, R. (2012). *The physical basis of mental illness.* Piscataway, NJ: Transaction Publishers.

Chickering, A. W., & Reisser, L. (1993). *Education and identity* (2nd ed.). San Francisco, CA: Jossey-Bass.

Choate, L., & Granello, D. (2006). *Counselor Education and Supervision, 46*(2), 116–130. doi: 10.1002/j.1556-6978.2006.tb00017.x

Cholewa, V., & West-Olatunji, C. (2008). Exploring the relationship among cultural discontinuity, psychological distress, and academic achievement outcomes for low-income, culturally diverse students. *Professional School Counseling, 12*, 54–61.

Chou, T., Asnaani, A., & Hofmann, S. G. (2012). Perception of racial discrimination and psychopathology across three U.S. ethnic minority groups. *Cultural Diversity and Ethnic Minority Psychology, 18*(1), 74–81. doi: 10.1037/a0025432

Christensen, T. M., & Brumfield, K. A. (2010). Phenomenological designs: The philosophy of phenomenological research. In C. J. Sheperis, J. C. Young, & M. H. Daniels (Eds.), *Counseling research: Quantitative, qualitative, and mixed methods* (pp. 135–149). Upper Saddle River, NJ: Pearson.

Cincotta, N. F. (2008). The journey of middle childhood: Who are "latency-age children?" In S. G. Austrian (Ed.), *Developmental theories through the life cycle* (2nd ed., pp. 79–122). New York, NY: Columbia University Press.

Cipriani, R. (2007). Religion. In R. George, (Ed.), *Blackwell encyclopedia of sociology.* Retrieved from http://www.blackwellreference.com/subscriber/tocnode?id=g9781405124331_chunk_ g978140512433124_ss1-48

Claiborn, C. D. (Ed.). (1991). *Multiculturalism as a fourth force in counseling* [Special issue]. *Journal of Counseling and Development, 70*(1).

Clare, M. (2009). Decolonizing consultation: Advocacy as the strategy, diversity as the context. *Journal of Educational and Psychological Consultation, 19*(1), 8–25. doi.org/10.1080/10474410802494929

Clark, A. J. (2002). Scapegoating: Dynamics and interventions in group counseling. *Journal of Counseling and Development, 80*, 271–276.

Clark, L. A., & Watson, D. (2008). Temperament: An organizing paradigm for trait psychology. In O. P. John, R. W., Robins, & L. A. Pervin (Eds.), *Handbook of personality: Theory and research* (3rd ed., pp. 265–287). New York, NY: Guilford Press.

Clemens, E. V., Milsom, A., & Cashwell, C. C. (2009). Using leader-member exchange theory to examine principal-school counselor relationship, school counselors' roles, job satisfaction, and turnover intentions. *Professional School Counseling, 13*, 75–85. doi: 10.5330/PSC.n.2010-13.75

Cobia, C. D., Carney, J. S., Buckhalt, J. A., Middleton, R. A., Shannon, D. M., Trippany, R., & Kunkel, E. (2005). The doctoral portfolio: Centerpiece of a comprehensive system of evaluation. *Counselor Education and Supervision, 44*(4), 242–254.

Cobia, D. C., & Pipes, R. B. (2002). Mandated supervision: An intervention for disciplined professionals. *Journal of Counseling and Development, 80*, 140–144. doi: 10.1002/j.1556-6678.2002.tb00176.x

Cochrane, W. S., & Salyers, K. M. (2006). Collaborative consultation training: The missing link to the enhancement of collaborative relationships among education and mental health professionals. *Improving Schools, 9*, 131–140. doi: 10.1177/1365480206064737

Coe, D. M., & Zimpfer, D. G. (1996). Infusing solution-oriented theory and techniques into group work. *The Journal for Specialists in Group Work, 21*, 49–57. doi: 10.1080/01933929608411358.

Colangelo, J. J. (2009). The American Mental Health Counselors Association: Reflection on 30 historic years. *Journal of Counseling & Development, 87*, 234–240. doi: 10.1002/j.1556-6678.2009.tb00572.x

Colapinto, J. (2015). Structural family therapy. In E. Neukrug (Ed.), *The Sage encyclopedia of theory in counseling and psychotherapy* (Vol. 2, pp. 966–971). Thousand Oaks, CA: Sage.

Cole, W., Gorman, C., Barrett, L. I., & Thompson, D. (1993, April 26). The shrinking 10 percent. *Time*, 27–29.

College Student Educators International (2006). *Statement of ethical principles and standards.* Retrieved from http://www.acpa.nche.edu/ethics

College Student Educators International/Student Affairs Administrators in Higher Education (ACPA /NASPA). (2010). *Professional competency areas for student affairs practitioners.* Retrieved from https://www.naspa.org/images/uploads/main/Professional_Competencies.pdf

Colley, L. (2009). *The power of groups: Solution-focused group counseling in the schools.* Thousand Oaks, CA: Corwin.

Commission on Accreditation for Marital and Family Therapy Education (COAMFTE) (2002–2013). *Accreditation.* Retrieved from http://www.aamft.org/iMIS15/AAMFT /Education_and_Training/Accreditation/Content /COAMFTE/Accreditation_Resources.aspx?hkey =5cb74a42-815a-4b75-9c29-64e5e70f02d5

Commission on Rehabilitation Counselor Certification (CRCC) (2010). *Code of professional ethics for rehabilitation counselors.* Retrieved from https://www.crccertification .com/filebin/pdf/CRCC_COE_1-1-10_Rev12-09.pdf

Commission on Rehabilitation Counselor Certification (CRCC) (2014). *Home page.* Retrieved from http://www .crccertification.com/

Connors, J., & Caple, R. (2005). A review of group systems theory. *Journal for Specialists in Group Work, 30*(2), 93–110. doi: 10.1080/01933920590925940

Constantine, M. G., & Sue, D. W. (2005). *Strategies for building multicultural competence in mental health and educational settings.* Hoboken, NJ: John Wiley & Sons.

Cook, J. M., Biyanova, T., & Coyne, J. C. (2009). Influential psychotherapy figures, authors, and books: An Internet survey of over 2,000 psychotherapists. *Psychotherapy: Theory, Research, Practice, Training, 46*(1), 42–51. doi: 10.1037/a0015152

Cook, T. D., & Campbell, D. T. (1979). *Quasi-experimentation: Design and analysis issues for field settings.* Chicago, IL: Rand McNally.

Cooper, D. L., Howard-Hamilton, M. F., & Cuyjet, M. J. (2011). Achieving cultural competence as a student practitioner, student, or faculty member. In M. J. Cuyjet, Howard-M. F. Hamilton, & D. L. Cooper, D. L. (Eds.) (2011). *Multiculturalism on campus: Theory, models, and practices for understanding diversity and creating inclusion* (pp. 401–420). Sterling, VA: Stylus Publishing.

Cooper, J. O., Heron, T. E., & Heward, W. L. (2007). *Applied behavior analysis* (2nd ed.). Columbus, OH: Merrill.

Cooper, M. (2011). Meeting the demand for evidence-based practice. *Therapy Today, 22*(4), 10–16.

Cooper, S. (2003). College counseling centers as internal organizational consultants to universities. *Consulting Psychology Journal: Practice and Research, 55*(4), 230–238. doi: 10.1037/1061-4087.55.4.230

Corey, G. (2012). *Theory and practice of group counseling* (8th ed.). Belmont, CA: Cengage.

Corey, G. (2013). *Theory and practice of counseling and psychotherapy* (9th ed.). Belmont, CA: Brooks/Cole.

Corey, G. (2015). Eclecticism. In E. Neukrug (Ed.), *The Sage encyclopedia of theory in counseling and psychotherapy* (Vol. 1, pp. 307–310). Thousand Oaks, CA: Sage.

Corey, G., Corey, M. S., Corey, C., & Callanan, P. (2015). *Issues and ethics in the helping professions* (9th ed.). Belmont, CA: Cengage.

Corey, G., Haynes, R., & Moulton, P., & Muratori, M. (2010). *Clinical supervision in the helping professions: A practical guide* (2nd ed.). Alexandria, VA: American Counseling Association.

Corey, M. S., Corey, G., & Corey, C. (2014). *Groups: Process and practice* (9th ed.). Belmont, CA: Brooks/Cole.

Cormier, S., Nurius, P. S., & Osborn, C. J. (2012). *Interviewing and change strategies for helpers* (7th ed.). Belmont, CA: Cengage.

Cory, R. C. (2011). Disability services offices for students with disabilities: A campus resource. *New Directions for Higher Education, 2011*(154), 27–36. doi: 10.1002/he

Cottone, R. R. (2001). A social constructivism model of ethical decision making in counseling. *Journal of Counseling And Development, 79*, 39–45. doi: 10.1002/j.1556-6676 .2001.tb01941.x

Cottone, R. R., & Claus, R. E. (2000). Ethical decision-making models: A review of the literature. *Journal of Counseling and Development, 78*, 275–283. doi: 10.1002 /j.1556-6676.2000.tb01908.x

Couch, R. D. (1995). Four steps for conducting a pregroup screening interview. *Journal for Specialists in Group Work, 20*(1), 10–25. doi: 10.1080/01933929508411321

Council for the Accreditation of Counseling and Related Educational Programs (CACREP) (2009). *2009 standards.* Retrieved from http://www.cacrep.org/wp-content /uploads/2013/12/2009-Standards.pdf

Council for the Accreditation of Counseling and Related Educational Programs (CACREP) (2014a). *CACREP /Core Updates.* Retrieved from http://www.cacrep.org /news-and-events/cacrepcore-updates/

Council for the Accreditation of Counseling and Related Educational Programs (CACREP) (2014b). About

CACREP. Retrieved from http://www.cacrep.org/index.cfm/about-cacrep

Council for the Accreditation of Counseling and Related Educational Programs (CACREP) (2014c). *IRCEP: Welcome and history.* Retrieved from http://www.ircep.org/ircep/template/index.cfm

Council for the Accreditation of Counseling and Related Educational Programs (CACREP) (2014d). *IRCEP: Vision, mission, and core values.* Retrieved from http://www.ircep.org/ircep/template/page.cfm?id=93

Council for the Accreditation of Counseling and Related Educational Programs (CACREP) (2014e). *Home page.* Retrieved from http://www.cacrep.org

Council on Rehabilitation Education. (2014a). *CORE-CACREP affiliation.* Retrieved from http://www.core-rehab.org/CORE-CACREP

Council on Rehabilitation Education. (2014b). *Home page.* Retrieved from http://www.core-rehab.org/

Council on Social Work Education. (2014). *Accreditation.* Retrieved from http://www.cswe.org/

Coursol, D. (2004). *Cybersupervision: Conducting supervision on the information superhighway.* Retrieved from ERIC database (ED 478213)

CPP. (2004). *Technical brief for the newly revised Strong Interest Inventory assessment: Content, reliability, and validity.* Retrieved from http://www.cpp.com/products/strong/StrongTechnicalBrief.pdf

CPP. (2009a). *Strong Interest Inventory.* Retrieved from https://www.cpp.com/products/strong/index.aspx

CPP. (2009b). *Myers-Briggs Type Indicator.* Retrieved from https://www.cpp.com/products/mbti/index.aspx

CPP. (2009c). *The CPI Assessments.* Retrieved from https://www.cpp.com/products/cpi/index.aspx

Craigen, L. M., Cole, R. F., & Cowan, R. G. (2013). Online relationships and the role of the human service practitioner. *Journal of Human Services, 33,* 29–43.

Crandell, T. L, Crandell, C. H., & Vander Zanden, J. M. (2012). *Human development* (10th ed.). New York, NY: McGraw-Hill.

Creswell, J. W. (2012a). *Educational research: Planning, conducting and evaluating quantitative and qualitative research* (4th ed.). Boston, MA: Pearson.

Creswell, J. W. (2012b). *Qualitative inquiry and research design: Choosing among the five approaches* (3rd ed.). Thousand Oaks, CA: Sage Publications.

Crethar, H., Rivera, E., & Nash, S. (2008). In search of common threads: Linking multicultural, feminist, and social justice counseling paradigms. *Journal of Counseling and Development, 86*(3), 269–278.

Crews, J. A., & Hill, N. R. (2005a). Diagnosis in marriage and family counseling: An ethical double bind. *Family Journal: Counseling and Therapy for Couples and Families, 13,* 63–66.

Crews, J. A., & Hill, N. R. (2005b). The application of an ethical lens to the issue of diagnosis in marriage and family counseling. *Family Journal: Counseling and Therapy for Couples and Families, 13,* 176–180.

Crighton, D. A., & Towl, G. J. (2008). *Psychology in prisons* (2nd ed.). Malden, MA: Blackwell.

Cross-disorder Group of the Psychiatric Genomics Consortium. (2013). Genetic relationships between five psychiatric disorders estimated from genome-wide SNPs. *Nature Genetics, 45,* 984–994. doi: 10.1038/ng.2711

Crothers, L., Hughes, T., & Morine, K. (2008). *Theory and cases in school-based consultation: A resource for school psychologists, school counselors, special educators, and other mental health professionals.* New York, NY: Routledge/Taylor & Francis Group.

Cummings, N. A. (1990). The credentialing of professional psychologists and its implications for the other mental health disciplines. *Journal of Counseling and Development, 68,* 490. doi: 10.1002/j.1556-6676.1990.tb01395.x

Cuyjet, M. J. (2011). Environmental influences on college culture. In M. J. Cuyjet, Howard-M. F. Hamilton, & D. L. Cooper, D. L. (Eds.) (2011). *Multiculturalism on campus: Theory, models, and practices for understanding diversity and creating inclusion* (pp. 37–64). Sterling, VA: Stylus Publishing.

Cuyjet, M. J., Howard-Hamilton, M. F., & Cooper, D. L. (Eds.) (2011). *Multiculturalism on campus: Theory, models, and practices for understanding diversity and creating inclusion.* Sterling, VA: Stylus Publishing.

Czander, W., & Eisold, K. (2003). Psychoanalytic perspectives on organizational consulting: Transference and counter-transference. *Human Relations, 56,* 475–491.

D'Andrea, M., & Daniels, J. (1991). Exploring the different levels of multicultural counseling training in counselor education. *Journal of Counseling and Development, 70,* 78–85.

D'Andrea, M., & Daniels, J. (1999). Exploring the psychology of White racism through naturalistic inquiry. *Journal of Counseling and Development, 77*(1), 93–101. doi: 10.1002/j.1556-6676.1999.tb02426.x

D'Andrea, M., & Heckman, E. (2008a). A 40-year review of multicultural counseling outcome research: Outlining a future research agenda for the multicultural counseling movement. *Journal of Counseling & Development, 86,* 356–363. doi: 10.1002/j.1556-6678.2008.tb00520.x

D'Andrea, M., & Heckman, E. F. (2008b). Contributing to the ongoing evolution of the multicultural counseling movement: An introduction to the special issue. *Journal of Counseling and Development, 86,* 259–260. doi: 10.1002/j.1556-6678.2008.tb00507.x

Dahir, C. A., & Stone, C. B. (2012). *The transformed school counselor* (2nd ed.). Belmont, CA: Cengage.

Dahlbeck, D. T., & Lease, S. H. (2010). Career issues and concerns for persons living with HIV/AIDS. *Career Development Quarterly, 58,* 359–368. doi: 10.1002/j.2161-0045.2010.tb00184.x

Dana, R., Gamst, G., Der-Karabetian, A., & Kramer, T. (2001). Asian American mental health clients: Effects of ethnic match and age on global assessment and visitation. *Journal of Mental Health Counseling, 23*(1), 57–71.

Daniel-Burke, R. (Host). (2014). The new 2014 code of ethics: An overview [Audio podcast]. Retrieved from http://www.counseling.org/knowledge-center/ethics

Dasenbrook, N. C. (2014). *The complete guide to private practice.* Rockford, IL: Dasenbrook Consulting.

Day, S. X. (2007). *Groups in practice.* Boston, MA: Houghton Mifflin.

Day-Vines, N. L., & Day-Hairston, B. O. (2005). Culturally congruent strategies for addressing the behavioral needs of urban, African American male adolescents. *Professional School Counseling, 8,* 236–243.

Day-Vines, N. L., & Terriquez, V. (2008). A strength-based approach to promoting prosocial behavior among African-American and Latino students. *Professional School Counseling, 12,* 170–175.

De Jong, P., & Berg, I. K. (2002). *Interviewing for solutions* (2nd ed.). Pacific Grove, CA: Brooks/Cole.

de Shazer, S. (1982). *Patterns of brief family therapy: An ecosystemic approach.* New York, NY: Guilford Press.

de Shazer, S. (1988). *Clues: Investigating solutions in brief therapy.* New York, NY: W. W. Norton & Company.

de Shazer, S., & Dolan, Y. V. (2007). *More than miracles: The state of the art of solution-focused therapy.* Binghamton, NY: Haworth Press.

Deaver, S. (2015). Creative and expressive therapies: Overview. In E. Neukrug (Ed.), *The Sage encyclopedia of theory in counseling and psychotherapy* (Vol. 1, pp. 253–256). Thousand Oaks, CA: Sage.

Debunking the concept of race. (2005, July 30). Editorial Page Editor, *New York Times,* A28.

Del Corso, J., & Rehfuss, M. C. (2011). The role of narrative in career construction theory. *Journal of Vocational Behavior, 79*(2), 334–339.

Delgado-Romero, E. A., Nevels, B. J., & Capielo, C. (2013). Culturally alert counseling with Latino/Latina Americans. In G. J. McAuliffe (Ed.), *Culturally alert counseling: A comprehensive introduction* (2nd ed., pp. 293–314). Thousand Oaks, CA: Sage Publications.

DeLucia-Waack, J. L., & Nitza, A. (2014). *Effective planning for groups.* Thousand Oaks, CA: Sage Publications.

DeRicco, J. N., & Sciarra, D. T. (2005). The immersion experience in multicultural counselor training: Confronting covert racism. *Journal of Multicultural Counseling and Development, 33*(1), 2–16.

Desjarlais, R.R. (1997). *Shelter blues: Sanity and selfhood among the homeless.* Philadelphia, PA: University of Pennsylvania Press.

DeVoss, J. A., & Andrews, M. F. (2006). *School counselors as educational leaders.* Boston, MA: Lahaska Press.

Dewey, J. (1956). *School and society.* Chicago, IL: University of Chicago Press. (Original work published 1900)

Di Leo, J. H. (2012). *Child development: Analysis and synthesis.* New York, NY: Routledge. (Original work published 1977)

Dimmitt, C., Carey, J.C., & Hatch, T (2007). *Evidence-based school counseling: Making a difference with data-driven practices.* Thousand Oaks, CA: Corwin Press.

Dimmock, C., & Walker, A. (2005). *Educational leadership: Culture and diversity.* Thousand Oaks, CA: Sage.

Dinkmeyer, D., & Dreikurs, R. (1963). *Encouraging children to learn: The encouragement process.* Englewood Cliffs, NJ: Prentice Hall.

Dolgoff, R., Loewenberg, F. M., & Harrington, D. (2009). *Ethical decisions for social work practice* (8th ed.). Belmont, CA: Brooks/Cole.

Dollarhide, C., & Miller, G. (2006). Supervision for preparation and practice of school counselors: Pathways to excellence. *Counselor Education and Supervision, 45*(4), 242–252.

Donaldson v. O'Connor, 422 U.S. 563 (U.S. Supreme Ct., 1975).

Dougherty, A. M. (2014). *Psychological consultation and collaboration in school and community settings* (6th ed.). Belmont, CA: Cengage.

Dowdall, G. W. (2013). *College drinking: Reframing a social problem/changing the culture.* Sterling, VA: Stylus Publishing.

Dressel, J. L., Consoli, A. J., Kim, B. S. K., & Atkinson, D. (2007). Successful and unsuccessful multicultural supervisory behaviors: A Delphi poll. *Journal of Multicultural Counseling & Development, 35*(1), 51–64. doi: 10.1002/j.2161-1912.2007.tb00049.x

Drummond, R. J., & Jones, K. D. (2010). *Appraisal procedures for counselors and helping professionals* (7th ed.). Upper Saddle River, NJ: Merrill.

DuBois, P. (1970). *A history of psychological testing.* Boston, MA: Allyn & Bacon.

Ducommun-Nagy, C. (2015). Ivan Boszormenyi-Nagy. In E. Neukrug (Ed.), *The Sage encyclopedia of theory in counseling and psychotherapy* (Vol. 1, pp. 131–133). Thousand Oaks, CA: Sage.

Duffy, M. & Chenail, R. J. (2008). Values in qualitative and quantitative research. *Counseling and Values, 53,* 22–38.

Duffy, R. D., Bott, E. M., Allan, B. A., Torrey, C. L., & Dik, B. J. (2012). Perceiving a calling, living a calling, and job satisfaction: Testing a moderated, multiple mediator model. *Journal of Counseling Psychology, 59*(1), 50–59. doi: 10.1037/a0026129

Duncan, E. (2005, October). Genes are not destiny. *Discover,* 62–63.

Dungy, G. J. (2003). Organization and functions of student affairs. In S. R. Komives & D. B. Woodward (Eds.), *Student services: A handbook for the profession* (4th ed., pp. 339–357). San Francisco, CA: Jossey-Bass.

Dykeman, B. F. (2011). Intervention strategies with the homeless population. *Journal of Instructional Psychology, 38*(1), 32–39.

Dykhuizen, G. (1973). *The life and mind of John Dewey.* Carbondale, IL: Southern Illinois University Press.

Eaves, S. H. (2010). Methodological issues. In C. J. Sheperis, J. C. Young, & M. H. Daniels (Eds.), *Counseling research: Quantitative, qualitative, and mixed methods* (pp. 32–45). Upper Saddle River, NJ: Pearson.

Education Trust. (2006). *Yes we can: Telling truths and dispelling myths about race and education in America.* Washington, DC: Author.

Egan, G. (1975). *The skilled helper: A model for systematic helping and interpersonal relating.* Pacific Grove, CA: Brooks /Cole.

Egan, G. (2014). *The skilled helper: A problem management and opportunity-development approach to helping* (10th ed.). Belmont, CA: Cengage.

Ellis, A., & Harper, R. A. (1961). *A guide to rational living.* Englewood Cliffs, NJ: Prentice Hall.

Ellis, A., & Harper, R. A. (1997). *A guide to rational living* (3rd ed.). North Hollywood, CA: Wilshire Book Company.

Ellis, A., & Maclaren, C. (2005). *Rational emotive behavior therapy: A therapist's guide* (2nd ed.). Atascadero, CA: Impact publishers.

Ellis, R. A. (2009). *Best practices in residential treatment.* New York, NY: Routledge.

Ellwood, R. S., & McGraw, B. A. (2014). *Many peoples, many faiths: Women and men in the world religions* (10th ed.). Upper Saddle River, NJ: Pearson.

Elmore, P., & Elkstrom, R. B. (2003). Assessment competencies for school counselors. In J. Wall & G. Waltz (Eds.), *Measuring up: Assessment issues for teachers, counselors, and administrators* (pp. 343–352). Retrieved from ERIC database (ED 380066)

Else-Quest, N., Hyde, J., & Linn, M. (2010). Cross-national patterns of gender differences in mathematics: A meta-analysis. *Psychological Bulletin, 136*(1), 103–127. doi: 10.1037/a0018053

Encyclopedia of Black America (1981). New York, NY: McGraw-Hill.

Englar-Carlson, M., & Kiselica, M. S. (2013). Affirming the strengths in men: A positive masculinity approach to assisting male clients. *Journal of Counseling & Development, 91*, 399–409. doi: 10.1002/j.1556-6676.2013.00111.x

Epstein, M. (2013). *The trauma of everyday life.* New York, NY: Penguin Press.

Erchul, W. (2009). Gerald Caplan: A tribute to the originator of mental health consultation. *Journal of Educational and Psychological Consultation, 19*(2), 95–105. doi: 10.1080 /10474410902888418

Erford, B. T. (2015). Becoming a professional school counselor: Current perspectives, historical roots, and future challenges. In B. T. Erford (Ed.), *Transforming the school counseling profession* (4th ed., pp. 1–28). Boston, MA: Pearson.

Erford, B. T., House, R. M., & Martin, P. J. (2007). Transforming the school counseling profession. In B. T. Erford (Ed.), *Transforming the school counseling profession* (2nd ed., pp. 1–12). Upper Saddle River, NJ: Pearson.

Erford, B. T., Lee, V. V., & Rock, E. (2015). Systemic approaches to counseling students experiencing complex and specialized problems. In B. T. Erford (Ed.), *Transforming the school counseling profession* (4th ed., pp. 325–349). Boston, MA: Pearson.

Eriksen, K., & Kress, V. (2005). *Beyond the DSM story: Ethical quandaries, challenges, and best practices.* Thousand Oaks, CA: Sage.

Eriksen, K., & Kress, V. (2006). The *DSM* and the professional counseling identity: Bridging the gap. *Journal of Mental Health Counseling, 28*, 202–217.

Eriksen, K., & Kress, V. (2008). Gender and diagnosis: Struggles and suggestions for counselors. *Journal of Counseling and Development, 86*, 152–162. doi: 10.1002/ j.1556-6678.2008.tb00492.x

Eriksen, K., & McAuliffe, G. J. (2006). Constructive development and counselor competence. *Counselor Education and Supervision, 45*(3), 180–192. doi: 10.1002 /j.1556-6978.2006.tb00141.x

Eriksen, K., Jackson, S. A., & Weld, C., & Lester, S. (2013). Religion and spirituality. In G. J. McAuliffe (Ed.), *Culturally alert counseling: A comprehensive introduction* (2nd ed., pp. 453–504). Thousand Oaks, CA: Sage Publications.

Erikson, E. H. (1950). *Childhood and society.* New York, NY: Norton.

Erikson, E. H. (1963). *Childhood and society* (2nd ed.). New York, NY: Norton.

Erikson, E. H. (1968). *Identity: Youth and crisis.* New York, NY: Norton.

Erikson, E. H. (1980). *Identity and the life cycle.* New York, NY: Norton.

Erikson, E. H. (1982). The *life cycle completed.* New York, NY: Norton.

Essandoh, P. K. (1996). Multicultural counseling as the "fourth force": A call to arms. *Counseling Psychologist, 24*, 126–138. doi: 10.1177/0011000096241008

Ethridge, G., Burnshill, D., & Dong, S. (2009). Career counseling across the life span. In I. Marini & M. A. Stebnicki (Eds.), *The professional counselor's desk reference* (pp. 443–465). New York, NY: Springer Publishing Company.

Evans, A. C., Delphin, M., Simmons, R., Omar, G., & Tebes, J. (2005). Developing a framework for culturally competent systems care. In R. T. Carter (Ed.), *Handbook of racial-cultural psychology and counseling: Theory and research* (Vol. 2, pp 492–513). Hoboken, NJ: John Wiley.

Evans, K. M. (2013). Culturally alert counseling with African Americans. In G. J. McAuliffe (Ed.), *Culturally alert counseling: A comprehensive introduction* (2nd ed., pp. 125–156). Thousand Oaks, CA: Sage Publications.

Evans, K. M., & Larrabee, M. J. (2002). Teaching the multicultural counseling competencies and revised career counseling competencies simultaneously. *Journal of Multicultural Counseling and Development, 30*(1), 21–39. doi: 10.1002/j.2161-1912.2002.tb00475.x

Evans, M. P., Duffey, T., & Englar-Carlson, M. (2013). Introduction to the special issue: Men in counseling. *Journal of Counseling & Development, 91*, 387–389. doi: 10.1002/j.1556-6676.2013.00108.x

Evans, N. J. (2011). Psychosocial and cognitive-structural perspectives on student development. In J. H. Schuh, S. R. Jones, & S. R. Harper (Eds.), *Student services: A handbook for the profession* (5th ed., pp. 168–186). San Francisco, CA: John Wiley & Sons.

Evans, N. J., Forney, D. S., Guido, F. M., Patton, L.D., & Renn, K. A. (2010). Student development in college: Theory, research, and practice (2nd ed.). New York, NY: John Wiley & Sons.

Eysenck, H. J. (1952). The effects of psychotherapy: An evaluation. *Journal of Consulting Psychology, 16*, 319–324.

Fagin, J. A. (2005). *Academic Leader, 21*(12), 4–8.

Fall, M. (1995). Planning for consultation: An aid for the elementary school counselor. *The School Counselor, 43*, 151–157.

Fall, M., & Sutton, J. M. (2004). *Clinical supervision: A handbook for practitioners*. Boston, MA: Pearson.

Farber, B. A. (2006). *Self-disclosure in psychotherapy.* New York, NY: Guilford Press.

Farr, J. M., & Shatkin, L. (2006). *Guide for occupational exploration* (4th ed.). St. Paul, MN: JIST Publishing.

Farrell, R. (2009). Developing a diverse counseling posture. In C. M Ellis & J. Carlson (Eds.), (pp. 45–60). New York, NY: Routledge/Taylor & Francis Group.

Faust, H. S., & Menzel, P. T. (2011). *Prevention vs. treatment.* New York, NY: Oxford University Press.

Fava, G. A. (2012). The clinical role of psychological well-being. *World Psychiatry, 11*(2), 102–103. doi: 10.1016/j.wpsyc.2012.05.018

Fawcett, J., & Busch, K. A. (1998). Stimulants in psychiatry. In A. F. Schatzberg & C. B. Nemeroff (Eds.), *Textbook of psychopharmacology* (2nd ed., pp. 503–522). Washington, DC: American Psychiatric Press.

Fenell, D. L. (2012). *Counseling families: An introduction to marriage, couple, and family therapy* (4th ed.). Denver, CO: Love.

Ferguson, E. (2010). Adler's innovative contributions regarding the need to belong. *Journal of Individual Psychology, 66*(1), 1–7.

Ferguson's Careers in Focus. (2008). *Careers in focus: Therapists* (2nd ed). New York, NY: Ferguson.

Fernando, D. M. (2007). Existential theory and solution-focused strategies: Integration and application. *Journal of Mental Health Counseling, 29*, 226–241.

Fisher, G. L., & Harrison, T. C. (2009). *Substance abuse: Information for school counselors, social workers, therapists, and counselors* (5th ed.). Boston, MA: Pearson.

Fisher, K. (2007). Report on Virginia Tech shootings urges clarification of privacy laws. *Chronicle of Higher Education, 53*(42), A30.

Fitzpatrick, J. L., Sanders, J. R., & Worthen, B. R. (2011). *Program evaluation: Alternative approaches and practical guidelines* (4th ed.). Boston, MA: Pearson.

Flavell, J. H. (1963). *The developmental psychology of Jean Piaget.* New York, NY: Van Nostrand.

Ford, D. Y., Moore, J. L. III, & Whiting, G. W. (2006). Eliminating deficit orientations: Creating classrooms and curricula for gifted students from diverse cultural backgrounds. In M. G. Constantine & D. W. Sue (Eds.), *Addressing racism: Facilitating cultural competence in mental health and educational settings* (pp. 173–193). Hoboken, NJ: John Wiley & Sons.

Fossey, R., Melear, K. B., Beckham, J. (Eds.) (2011). *Contemporary issues in higher education law.* Dayton, OH: Education Law Association.

Foster, L. H. (2010). A best kept secret: Single-subject research design in counseling. *Counseling Outcome Research and Evaluation, 1*(2), 30–39.

Foster, V., & McAdams, C. (2009). A framework for creating a climate of transparency for professional performance assessment: Fostering student investment in gatekeeping. *Counselor Education and Supervision, 48*, 271–284. doi: 10.1002/j.1556-6978.2009.tb00080.x

Foundation for Individual Rights in Education. (2009). Spotlight on speech codes, 2009. The state of free speech on our nation's campuses. Foundation for individual rights in education. Available from Educational Resources Information Center (ERIC), Ipswich, MA.

Fowler, J. W. (1976). Stages in faith: The structural-developmental approach. In T. C. Hennessy (Ed.),

Values and Moral Development (pp. 173–211). New York, NY: Paulist Press.

Fowler, J. W. (1991). The vocation of faith developmental theory. In J. W. Fowler, K. E. Nipkow, & F. Schweitzer (Eds.), *Stages of faith and religious development: Implications for church, education, and society* (pp. 19–37). New York, NY: Crossroad Publishing.

Fowler, J. W. (1995). *Stages of faith: The psychology of human development and the quest for meaning.* New York, NY: Harper & Row. (Original work published 1981)

Fowler, J. W. (2000). *Becoming adult, becoming Christian: Adult development and Christian faith* (rev. ed.). San Francisco, CA: Jossey-Bass.

Fox, T. (1987). *The essential Moreno: Writings on psychodrama, group method, and spontaneity.* New York, NY: Springer.

Fraenkel, J. R., Wallen, N. E. & Hyun, H. H. (2015). *How to design and evaluate research in education* (9th ed.). New York, NY: McGraw-Hill.

Frances, A. (2013). *Essentials of psychiatric diagnosis: Responding to the challenge of DSM-5* (rev. ed.). New York, NY: Guilford Press.

Frankl, V. E. (1963). *Man's search for meaning.* Boston, MA: Beacon.

Frankl, V. E. (1968). *Psychotherapy and existentialism.* New York, NY: Simon & Schuster.

Frankl, V. E. (2004). *The doctor and the soul: From psychotherapy to logotherapy.* London, UK: Souvenir. (Original work published 1946)

Frankl, V. E. (2006). *Man's search for meaning.* Boston, MA: Beacon Press. (Original work published 1946)

Freedman, J., & Combs, G. (1996). *Narrative therapy: The social construction of preferred realities.* New York, NY: W. W. Norton and Company.

Freeman, M. P., Wiegand, C., Gelenberg, A. J. (2009). Lithium. In A. F. Schatzberg & C. B. Nemeroff (Eds.), *Textbook of psychopharmacology* (4th ed., pp. 697–718). Washington, DC: American McElroy & Keck.

Freud, A. (1966). *The ego and the mechanisms of defense.* New York, NY: International Universities Press. (Original work published 1936)

Freud, S. (1961). *Beyond the pleasure principle* (J. Strachey, Trans.). New York, NY: W. W. Norton. (Original work published 1920)

Freud, S. (1975). *Group psychology and the analysis of the ego* (J. Strachey, Trans.). New York, NY: Norton. (Original work published 1922)

Freud, S. (1976a). *The interpretation of dreams.* (J. Strachey, Trans.). New York, NY: Penguin Books. (Original work published 1899)

Freud, S. (1976b). *Jokes and their relation to the unconscious.* (J. Strachey, Trans.). New York, NY: Penguin Books. (Original work published 1905)

Freud, S. (2003). *An outline of psychoanalysis* (rev. ed.) (J. H. Ragg-Kirby, Trans.). New York, NY: Penguin Group. (Original work published 1940)

Freud, S., & Breuer, J. (1974). *Studies in hysteria.* (J. Strachey, Trans.). New York, NY: Penguin Books. (Original work published 1895)

Friedman, M. (1989). Martin Buber and Ivan Boszormenyi-Nagy: The role of dialogue in contextual therapy. *Psychotherapy, 26,* 402–409.

Fry, R., & Lopez, M. H. (2012). *Pew Research Center: Hispanic student enrollments reach new highs in 2011.* Retrieved from http://www.pewhispanic.org/2012/08/20/iv-college-graduation-and-hispanics/

Gale, A. U., & Austin, B. D. (2003). Professionalism's challenges to professional counselors' collective identity. *Journal of Counseling and Development, 81,* 3–10. doi: 10.1002/j.1556-6678.2003.tb00219.x

Gall, M. D. Gall, J. P., & Borg, W. R. (2007). *Educational research: An introduction* (8th ed.). Boston, MA: Allyn & Bacon.

Gall, M. D. Gall, J. P., & Borg, W. R. (2010). *Applying educational research: How to read, do, and use research to solve problems* (6th ed.). Boston, MA: Pearson.

Gallagher, B. J., & Streeter, J. (2012). *The sociology of mental illness* (5th ed., revised). Cornwall-on-Hudson, NY: Sloan Educational Publishing.

Gallup. (2014). *Gay and lesbian rights.* Retrieved from http://www.gallup.com/poll/1651/gay-lesbian-rights.aspx

Gamst, G., Dana, R., Der-Karabetian, A., & Kramer, T. (2004). Ethnic match and treatment outcomes for child and adolescent mental health center clients. *Journal of Counseling and Development, 82,* 457–465. doi: 10.1002/j.1556-6678.2004.tb00334.x

Garcia, A. (1990). An examination of the social work profession's efforts to achieve legal regulation. *Journal of Counseling and Development, 68,* 491–497. doi: 10.1002/j.1556-6676.1990.tb01396.x

Garner, G. O. (2008). *Careers in social and rehabilitation services* (3rd ed.). New York, NY: Wiley.

Garrett, M. T. (2004). Profile of Native Americans. In D. R. Atkinson (Ed.), *Counseling American minorities* (6th ed., pp. 147–170). Boston, MA: McGraw-Hill.

Garrett, M. T., Garrett, J. T., Grayshield, L., Williams, C., Portman, T. A. A., Rivera, E. T., . . . Kawulich, B. (2013). Culturally alert counseling with Native Americans. In G. J. McAuliffe (Ed.), *Culturally alert counseling: A comprehensive introduction* (2nd ed., pp. 185–222). Thousand Oaks, CA: Sage Publications.

Garske, G. G. (2009). Psychiatric disability: A biopsychosocial challenge. In I. Marini, & M. A. Stebnicki (Eds.), *The professional counselor's desk reference* (pp. 647–654). New York, NY: Springer.

Gates, G. J. (2011). How many people are lesbian, gay, bisexual, and transgender? Retrieved from http://williamsinstitute.law.ucla.edu/wp-content/uploads/Gates-How-Many-People-LGBT-Apr-2011.pdf

Gay, L. R., Mills, G. E., & Airasian, P. (2012). *Educational research: Competencies for analysis and application* (10th ed.). Upper Saddle River, NJ: Pearson.

Geller, J. L. (2000). The last half-century of psychiatric services as reflected in *Psychiatric Services. Psychiatric Services, 51*, 41–67.

Gelso, C. (2009). The real relationship in a postmodern world: Theoretical and empirical explorations. *Psychotherapy Research, 19*, 253–264. doi: 10.1080/10503300802389242

Gelso, C. J., Kelley, F. A., Fuertes, J. N., Marmarosh, C., Holmes, S. E., Costa, C., & Hancock, G. R. (2005). Measuring the real relationship in psychotherapy: Initial validation of the therapist form. *Journal of Counseling Psychology, 52*, 640–649. doi: 10.1037/0022-0167.52.4.640

Gerda, J. (2006). Gathering together: A view of the earliest student affairs professional organizations. *NASPA Journal, 43*(4), 147–163. doi.org/10.2202/1949-6605.1727

Gergen, K. J. (1985). The social constructionist movement in modern psychology. *American Psychologist, 40*, 266–275. doi: 10.1037/0003-066X.40.3.266

Gergen, K. M. (2009). *An invitation to social construction* (2nd ed.). Thousand Oaks, CA: Sage.

Gerrig, R. (2014). *Psychology and life* (20th ed.). Upper Saddle River, NJ: Pearson.

Gerson, M. (2009). *The embedded self: An integrative psychodynamic and systemic perspective on couples and family therapy.* New York, NY: Routledge.

Gerstein, L. H., Heppner, P. P., Aegisdóttir, S., Leung, S. A. & Norsworthy, K. L. (Eds.) (2009). *International handbook of cross-cultural counseling: Cultural assumptions and practices worldwide.* Thousand Oaks, CA: Sage.

Gert, B. (2005). *Morality* (rev. ed.). New York, NY: Oxford University Press.

Gibson, R., & Mitchell, M. (2008). *Introduction to counseling and guidance* (7th ed.). Upper Saddle River, NJ: Merrill.

Gibson, W. T., & Pope, K. S. (1993). The ethics of counseling: A national survey of certified counselors. *Journal of Counseling & Development, 71*, 330–336.

Gillham, N. (2001). *A life of Sir Francis Galton: From African exploration to the birth of eugenics.* New York, NY: Oxford University Press.

Gilligan, C. (1982). *In a different voice: Psychological theory and women's development.* Cambridge, MA: Harvard University Press.

Gilligan, C. (2008). *Kyra.* New York, NY: Random House.

Gingerich, W. (2006). Obituary: Steve de Shazer. *Research on Social Work Practice, 16*, 549–550. doi: 10.1177/1049731506289129

Ginzberg, E. (1972). Toward a theory of occupational choice: A restatement. *Vocational Guidance Quarterly, 20*, 169–176.

Ginzberg, E., Ginsburg, S. W., Axelrad, S., & Herma, J. (1951). *Occupational choice: An approach to a general theory.* New York, NY: Columbia University Press.

Girl can sue for telling mom she's gay: Federal judge allows violation of privacy case to proceed to California (2005, December 4). Retrieved from http://msnbc.msn.com/id/10299356/from/ET/

Gladding, S. T. (2006). *The counseling dictionary: Concise definitions of frequently used terms* (2nd ed.). Upper Saddle River, NJ: Pearson.

Gladding, S. T. (2011). *Family therapy: History, theory, and practice* (5th ed.). Boston, MA: Prentice Hall.

Gladding, S. T. (2012). *Groups: A counseling specialty* (6th ed.). New York, NY: Merrill.

Gladding, S., & Newsome. D. W. (2014). *Clinical mental health counseling in community and agency settings* (4th ed.). Upper Saddle River, NJ: Pearson Education.

Glasser, W. (1961). *Mental health or mental illness?* New York, NY: Harper & Row.

Glasser, W. (1965). *Reality therapy: A new approach to psychiatry.* New York, NY: Harper & Row.

Glasser, W. (1998). *Choice theory: A new psychology of personal freedom.* New York, NY: HarperCollins.

Glasser, W. (2001). *Counseling with choice theory: The new reality therapy.* New York, NY: HarperCollins.

Glasser, W., & Glasser, C. (1999). *The language of choice theory.* New York, NY: HarperCollins.

Glosoff, H. L., & Matrone, K. F. (2010). Ethical issues in rehabilitation counselor supervision and the New 2010 code of ethics. *Rehabilitation Counseling Bulletin, 53*, 249–254. doi: 10.1177/0034355210368729

Godby, D. D., Hopper, E., & Sharpe, M. (2015). Group analysis. In E. Neukrug (Ed.), *The Sage encyclopedia of theory in counseling and psychotherapy* (Vol. 1, pp. 466–471). Thousand Oaks, CA: Sage.

Goldberg, J. F., & Ernst, C. L. (2102). *Managing the side effects of psychotropic medications.* Arlington, VA: American Psychiatric Publishing.

Goldenberg, H., & Goldenberg, I. (2013). *Family therapy: An overview* (8th ed.). Belmont, CA: Brooks/Cole.

Goldenberg, M. J. (2006). Evidence and evidence-based medicine: Lessons from the philosophy of science. *Social Science & Medicine, 62*, 2621–2632.

Goldfinger, K., & Pomerantz, A. M. (2014). *Psychological assessment and report writing.* Thousand Oaks, CA: Sage Publications.

Gompertz, K. (1960). The relation of empathy to effective communication. *Journalism Quarterly, 37*, 535–546.

Good, E. M. (2012). Personality disorders in the DSM-5: Proposed revisions and critiques. *Journal of Mental Health Counseling, 34*, 1–13.

Good, G. E., & Brooks, G. R. (2005). *The new handbook of psychotherapy and counseling with men: A comprehensive guide to settings, problems, and treatment approaches* (rev. ed.). New York, NY: Wiley.

Goodman, J., Schlossberg, N. K., & Anderson, M. L. (2006). *Counseling adults in transition: Linking practice with theory* (3rd ed.). New York, NY: Springer Publications.

Goodman-Scott, E. (2011, Fall). School counselors and principals: Creating a powerful partnership. *VSCA Voices*, 7–8.

Goodman-Scott, E. (in press). School counselors' perceptions of their academic preparedness and job activities. *Counselor Education and Supervision.*

Goodrich, K. M. (2015). Sexual orientation change efforts. In E. Neukrug (Ed.), *The Sage encyclopedia of theory in counseling and psychotherapy* (Vol. 2, 931–933). Thousand Oaks, CA: Sage.

Goodspeed-Grant, P., & Mackie, K. L. (2013). Social class. In G. McAuliffe (Ed.), *Culturally alert counseling: A comprehensive introduction* (2nd ed., pp. 347–382). Los Angeles, CA: Sage Publications.

Goodwin, L. (2002). The meaning of validity. *Journal of Pediatric Gastroenterology and Nutrition, 35*, 6–7. doi: 10.1097/00005176-200207000-00003

Goodyear, R. K. (1984). On our journal's evolution: Historical developments, transitions, and future directions. *Journal of Counseling and Development, 63*, 3–9. doi: 10.1002/j.1556-6676.1984.tb02669.x

Gordon, E. W. (2006). Establishing a system of public education in which all children achieve at high levels and reach their full potential. In T. Smiley (Ed.), *The covenant with Black America* (pp. 23–45). Chicago, IL: Third World Press.

Gordon, J. (2007). What can White faculty do? *Teaching in Higher Education, 12*(3), 337–347. doi: 10.1080/13562510701278682

Gorton, R., & Alston, J. A. (2012). School leadership and administration: Important concepts, case studies, and simulations. New York, NY: McGraw-Hill.

Gottfredson, G. D., Holland, J. L., & Ogawa, D. K. (1996). *Dictionary of Holland occupational codes*. Odessa, FL: Psychological Assessment Resources.

Graham. L. B. (2010). Implementing CACREP disasters/crisis standards for counseling students. Retrieved from http://counselingoutfitters.com/vistas/vistas10/Article_90.pdf

Granello, D. H. (2002). Assessing the cognitive development of counseling students: Changes in epistemological assumptions. *Counselor Education and Supervision, 41*, 279–293. doi: 10.1002/j.1556-6978.2002.tb01291.x

Granello, D., Kindsvatter, A., Granello, P., Underfer-Babalis, J., & Moorhead, H. (2008). Multiple perspectives in supervision: Using a peer consultation model to enhance supervisor development. *Counselor Education and Supervision, 48*(1), 32–47. doi: 10.1002/j.1556-6978.2008.tb00060.x

Grant, J., Schofield, M. J., & Crawford, S. (2012). Managing difficulties in supervision: Supervisors' perspectives. *Journal of Counseling Psychology, 59*, 528–541. doi: 10.1037/a0030000

Green, C. D. (2009). Darwinian theory, functionalism, and the first American psychological revolution. *American Psychologist, 64*(2), 75–83. doi: 10.1037/a0013338

Greenfield, S. F., Cummings, A. M., Kuper, L., Wigderson, S. B., & Koro-Ljungberg, M. (2013). A qualitative analysis of women's experiences in single-gender versus mixed-gender substance abuse group therapy. *Substance Use & Misuse, 48*, 750–760.

Greenhaus, J. H., & Callanan, G. A. (Eds.). (2006). *Encyclopedia of career development*. Thousand Oaks, CA: Sage.

Greer, M. (2005, June). Keeping them hooked in. *APA Monitor, 36*(6), p. 60.

Griffin, D., & Farris, A. (2010). School counselors and collaboration: Finding resources through community mapping. *Professional School Counseling, 13*, 248–256.

Griffiths, P., & Stotz, K. (2013). *Genetics and philosophy: An introduction*. New York, NY: Cambridge University Press.

Griggs v. Duke Power Company, 401 U. S. 424 (1971).

Grothaus, T., & Cole, R. (2010). Meeting the challenges together: School counselors collaborating with students and families with low income. *Journal of School Counseling, 8*. Retrieved from http://files.eric.ed.gov/fulltext/EJ895909.pdf

Grothaus, T., & Johnson, K. F. (2012). *Making diversity work: Creating culturally competent school counseling programs*. Alexandria, VA: American School Counselor Association.

Grothaus, T., Crum, K.S., & James, A.B. (2010). Effective leadership in a culturally diverse learning environment. *International Journal of Urban Educational Leadership, 4*, 111–125.

Guerrero, L. K., & Floyd, K. (2006). *Nonverbal communication in close relationships*. Mahwah, NJ: Lawrence Erlbaum Associates.

Guest, C. L., & Dooley, K. (1999). Supervisor malpractice: Liability to the supervisee in clinical supervision. *Counselor Education and Supervision, 38*, 269–279. doi: 10.1002/j.1556-6978.1999.tb00577.x

Guidelines for psychotherapy with lesbian, gay, and bisexual clients (2000). *American Psychologist, 55*(12), 1440–1451. doi:10.1037/0003-066X.55.12.1440

Guterman, J. T. (2006). *Solution-focused counseling.* Alexandria, VA: American Counseling Association.

Guterman, J. T., & Rudes, J. (2008). Social constructionism and ethics: Implications for counseling. *Journal of Counseling and Development, 52,* 136–144. doi:10.1002/j.2161–007X.2008.tb00097.x

Guthrie, K. L., Jones, T. B., Osteen, L., & Hu, S. (2013). Cultivating leader identity and capacity in students from diverse backgrounds, *ASHE Higher Education Report, 39*(4). New York, NY: John Wiley & Sons.

Guthrie, R. V. (2003). *Even the rat was white: A historical view of psychology* (2nd ed.). Boston, MA: Pearson.

Gysbers, N. C., & Henderson, P. (2012). *Developing and managing your school guidance and counseling program* (5th ed.). Alexandria, VA: American Counseling Association.

Gysbers, N. C., Heppner, M. J., & Johnston, J. A. (2009). *Career counseling: Contexts, processes, and techniques* (3rd ed.). Alexandria, VA: American Counseling Association.

Hackney, H., & Cormier, L. S. (2012). *The professional counselor: A process guide to helping* (6th ed.). Upper Saddle River, NJ: Pearson.

Hackney, H., & Cormier, L. S. (2013). *The professional counselor: A process guide to helping* (7th ed.). Columbus, OH: Merrill.

Haley, A. (2001). *The autobiography of Malcolm X.* London, UK: Penguin.

Haley, J. (1973). *Uncommon therapy.* New York, NY: Norton.

Haley, J. (1976). *Problem-solving therapy.* San Francisco, CA: Jossey-Bass.

Haley, J. (1986). *The power tactics of Jesus Christ and other essays* (2nd ed.). Rockville, MD: Triangle.

Haley, J. (1997–2014). *Jay Haley: The family therapist.* Retrieved from http://www.jay-haley-on-therapy.com/html/family_therapy.html

Hall, C. S. (1999). *A primer of Freudian psychology.* New York, NY: Meridian. (Original work published 1954)

Halstead, R. W. (2007). *Assessment of client core issues.* Alexandria, VA: American Counseling Association.

Hansen, J. (2003). Including diagnostic training in counseling curricula: Implications for professional identity development. *Counselor Education and Supervision, 43,* 96–107. doi:10.1002/j.1556-6978.2003.tb01834.x

Harkins, A. K., Hansen, S. S., & Gama, E. M. P. (2008). Updating gender issues in multicultural counseling. In P. B. Pedersen, J. G. Draguns, W. J. Lonner, & J. E. Trimble (Eds.), *Counseling across cultures* (6th ed., pp. 185–200). Thousand Oaks, CA: Sage.

Harper, D. (2014). *Online etymology dictionary: Diagnosis.* Retrieved from http://www.etymonline.com/index.php?term=diagnosis

Harper, S., & Hurtado, S. (2007). Nine themes in campus racial climates and implications for institutional transformation. *New Directions for Student Services, 120,* 7–24. doi: 10.1002/ss.254

Harrington, J. A. (2013). Contemporary issues in private practice: Spotlight on the self-employed mental health counselor. *Journal of Mental Health Counseling, 35,* 189–197.

Hart, J., Corriere, R., & Binder, J. (1975). *Going sane: An introduction to feeling therapy.* New York, NY: Jason Aronson.

Hatch, T. (2014). *The use of data in school counseling: Hatching results for students, programs, and the profession.* Thousand Oaks, CA: Corwin Press.

Haverkamp, B. E., Morrow, S. L., & Ponterotto, G. E. (Eds). (2005). Knowledge in context: Qualitative methods in counseling psychology research *[Special issue]. Journal of Counseling Psychology, 52*(2).

Havighurst, R. J. (1972). *Developmental tasks and education* (3rd ed.). New York, NY: David McKay.

Hays, D. (2010). Introduction to counseling outcome research and evaluation. *Counseling Outcome Research and Evaluation, 1*(1), 1–7.

Hays, D., Chang, C. Y., & Havic, P. (2005) White racial identity statuses as predictors of white privilege awareness. *Journal of Humanistic Counseling, Education, & Development, 47*(2): 234–246.

Helms, J. E. (1984). Toward a theoretical model of the effects of race on counseling: A black and white model. *The Counseling Psychologist, 12,* 153–165. doi: 10.1177/0011000084124013

Helms, J. E. (1999). Another meta-analysis of the White Racial Identity Attitude Scale's Cronbach alphas: Implications for validity. *Measurement and Evaluation in Counseling and Development, 32,* 122–137.

Helms, J. E. (2005). Challenging some misuses of reliability as reflected in evaluations of the White Racial Identity Attitude Scale (WRIAS). (2005). In R. T. Carter (Ed.), *Handbook of racial-cultural psychology and counseling, theory, and research* (Vol. 1, pp. 360–390). Hoboken, NJ: John Wiley & Sons.

Helms, J. E., & Cook, D. A. (1999). Using race and culture in counseling and psychotherapy: theory and process. Needham Heights, MA: Allyn & Bacon.

Hendricks, B. E., Bradley, L. J., Southern, S., Oliver, M., & Birdsall, B. (2011). Ethical code for the International Association of Marriage and Family Counselors. *The Family Journal, 19,* 217–224. doi: 10.1177/1066480711400814

Hendrix, L. R. (2001). Health and health care of American Indian and Alaska Native Elders. In U. S. Department of Human Services, *Curriculum ethnogeriatics: Core curriculum and ethnic specific modules.* Retrieved from http://web.stanford.edu/group/ethnoger/

Heppner, P. P., Wampold, B. E., & Kivlighan, D. M. (2008). *Research design in counseling* (3rd ed.). Belmont, CA: Wadsworth.

Herek, G. M. (2000). The psychology of sexual prejudice. *Current Directions in Psychological Science, 9*(1), 19–22. doi: 10.1111/1467-8721.00051

Herlihy, B., & Dufrene, R. L. (2011). Current and emerging ethical issues in counseling: A Delphi study of expert opinions. *Counseling and Values, 56,* 10–25. doi: 10.1002/j.2161-007X.2011.tb01028.x

Hermann, M. A., Legget, D. G. & Remley, T. P. (2008). A study of counselors' legal challenges and their perceptions of their ability to respond. *International Journal of Education Policy & Leadership, 3*(5), 1–11.

Hermann, M. A., Remley, T. P., Jr., & Huey, W. C. (Eds.). (2010). *Ethical and legal issues in school counseling* (3rd Ed.). Alexandria, VA: American School Counselor Association.

Hernández-Wolfe, P. (2010). Family counseling supervision. In N. Ladany & L. J. Bradley (Eds.), *Counselor supervision* (4th ed., pp. 287–308). New York, NY: Routledge.

Herr, E. L. (1985). *Why counseling?* (2nd ed.). Alexandria, VA: American Association for Counseling and Development.

Herr, E. L., Cramer, S. H., & Niles, S. G. (2004). *Career guidance and counseling through the life span: Systematic approaches* (6th ed.). Boston, MA: Pearson/Allyn & Bacon.

Herring, R. D. (2004). Physical and mental health needs of Native American Indian and Alaska Native populations. In D. R. Atkinson (Ed.), *Counseling American minorities* (6th ed., pp. 171–192). Boston, MA: McGraw-Hill.

Hershenson, D. B. (2008). A head of its time: Career counseling's roots in phrenology. *Career Development Quarterly, 57*(2), 181–190.

Hershenson, D. B. (2009). Historical perspectives in career development theory. In I. Marini & M. A. Stebnicki (Eds.), *The professional counselor's desk reference* (pp. 411–420). New York, NY: Springer Publishing Company.

Hershenson, D. B., & Berger, G. P. (2001). The state of community counseling: A survey of directors of CACREP-accredited programs. *Journal of Counseling and Development, 79,* 188–193. doi: 10.1002/j.1556-6676.2001.tb01959.x

Hershenson, D. B., Power, P.W., & Waldo, M. (2003). *Community counseling: Contemporary theory and practice.* Long Grove, IL: Waveland Press.

Higgins, L. T., & Sun, C. H. (2002). The development of psychological testing in China. *International Journal of Psychology, 37*(4), 246–254. doi: 10.1080/00207590244000025

Higheredjobs. (2013–2014a). Professionals in higher education salaries: Career counselor. Retrieved July 5, 2014, from http://www.higheredjobs.com/salary/salaryDisplay.cfm?SurveyID=23

Higheredjobs. (2013–2014b). Professionals in higher education salaries: Director of multicultural student services. Retrieved July 5, 2014, from http://www.higheredjobs.com/salary/salaryDisplay.cfm?SurveyID=23

Hill, A. L. (2004). Ethical analysis in counseling: A case for narrative ethics, moral visions, and virtue ethics. *Counseling & Values, 48*(2), 131–148. doi: 10.1002/j.2161-007X.2004.tb00240.x

Hill, C. E. (2014). *Helping skills: Facilitating exploration, insight, and action* (4th ed.). Washington, DC: American Psychological Association.

Hill, C. E., & Knox, S. (2002). Self-disclosure. In J. C. Norcross (Ed.), *Psychotherapy relationships that work: Therapist contributions and responsiveness to patients* (pp. 255–266). New York, NY: Oxford University Press.

Hill, C. E., Thompson, B. J. & Williams, E. N. (1997). A guide to conducting consensual qualitative research. *The Counseling Psychologist, 25,* 517–572.

Hines, P., & Fields, T. H. (2002). Pregroup screening issues for school counselors. *Journal for Specialists in Group Work, 27,* 358–376.

Hinkle, J. S., & O'Brien, S. (2010). The human services-board certified practitioners: An overview of a new national credential. *Journal of Human Services, 30*(1), 23–28.

Hinson, G. (2011). *Fire in my bones: Transcendence and the holy spirit in African American gospel.* Philadelphia, PA: University of Pennsylvania Press.

Hipolito-Delgado, C. P., Cook, J. M., Avrus, E. M., & Boham, E. J. (2011). Developing counseling students' multicultural competence through the multicultural action project. *Counselor Education & Supervision, 50,* 402–421. doi: 10.1002/j.1556-6978.2011.tb01924.x

History of the McKinney Act. (2014). *William and Mary School of Education Project Hope—Virginia.* Retrieved from http://education.wm.edu/centers/hope/resources/mckinneyact/

Ho, M. K., Rasheed, J. M., & Rasheed, M. N. (2004). *Family therapy with ethnic minorities* (2nd ed.). Thousand Oaks, CA: Sage.

Hoare, C. (2006). *Handbook of adult development and learning.* New York, NY: Oxford University Press.

Hodges, S. (2012). *101 careers in counseling.* New York, NY: Springer.

Hoekstra, R., Bartels, M., & Boomsma, D. (2007). Longitudinal genetic study of verbal and nonverbal IQ from early childhood to young adulthood. *Learning and Individual Differences, 17*(2), 97–114. doi: 10.1016/j.lindif.2007.05.005

Hofer, B. K. (2002). Personal epistemology as a psychological and educational construct: An Introduction. In B. Hofer & P. Pintrich, P. (Eds.), *Personal epistemology: The psychology of beliefs about knowledge and knowing* (pp. 3–14). Mahwah, NJ: Lawrence Erlbaum Associates Publishers.

Hoffman, E. (1994). *The drive for self: Alfred Adler and the founding of individual psychology.* New York, NY: Addison-Wesley.

Hoffman, M., Phillips, E., Noumair, D., Shullman, S., Geisler, C., Gray, J., . . . Ziegler, D. (2006). Toward a feminist and multicultural model of consultation and advocacy. *Journal of Multicultural Counseling and Development, 34*(2), 116. doi: 10.1002/j.2161-1912.2006.tb00032.x

Høglend, P., Bøgwald, K., Amlo, S., Marble, A., Ulberg, R., Sjaastad, M., & Johansson, P. (2008). Transference interpretations in dynamic psychotherapy: Do they really yield sustained effects? *American Journal of Psychiatry, 165,* 763–771. doi: 10.1176/appi.ajp.2008.07061028

Holcomb-McCoy, C. (2007). *School counseling to close the achievement gap: A social justice framework for success.* Thousand Oaks, CA: Corwin.

Holcomb-McCoy, C. (2008). A response to "social privilege, social justice, and group counseling: An inquiry." *Journal for Specialists in Group Work, 33*(4), 367–369. doi: 10.1080/01933920802424423

Holland, J. L. (1973). *Making vocational choices: A theory of career.* Englewood Cliffs, NJ: Prentice Hall.

Holland, J. L., & Gottfredson, G. D. (1976). Using a topology of persons and environments to explain careers: Some extensions and clarifications. *Counseling Psychologist, 6,* 20–29.

Hollis, J. W., & Dodson, T. A. (2000). *Counselor preparation 1999–2001: Programs, faculty, trends* (10th ed.). Philadelphia, PA: Taylor & Francis.

Homan, M. S. (2011). *Promoting community change: Making it happen in the real world* (5th ed.) Pacific Grove, CA: Brooks/Cole.

Hopkins, G. (2005). School counselors reflective on what makes them effective. *Education World.* Retrieved from http://www.educationworld.com/a_curr/curr198.shtml

Hosie, T. (1991). Historical antecedents and current status of counselor licensure. In F. O. Bradley (Ed.), *Credentialing in counseling* (pp. 23–52). Alexandria, VA: Association for Counselor Education and Supervision.

Houser, R. (2015). *Counseling and educational research: Evaluation and application* (3rd ed.). Thousand Oaks, CA: Sage.

Howard, K. A. S., & Solberg, V. S. H. (2006). School-based social justice: The achieving success identity pathways program. *Professional School Counseling, 9,* 278–287.

Hoyt, M. F. (1994). *Introduction: Competency-based future-oriented therapy.* In M. F. Hoyt (Ed.). *Constructive therapies* (pp. 1–11). New York, NY: Guilford Press.

Hoyt, M. F. (1996). Solution building and language games: A conversation with Steve de Shazer. In M. F. Hoyt (Ed.), *Constructive therapies* (Vol. 2, pp. 60–86). New York, NY: Guilford Press.

Hubert, M. (1995, December). Disaffiliation: An ethical consideration. *The ASCA Counselor.* Alexandria, VA: Author.

Hull, G. H., & Mather, J. (2006). *Understanding generalist practice with families.* Belmont, CA: Brooks/Cole.

Hulse-Killacky, D., Killacky, J., & Donigian, J. (2001). *Making task groups work in your world.* Upper Saddle River, NJ: Merrill.

Humphreys, K. (2011). *Circles of recovery: Self-help organizations for addictions.* New York, NY: Cambridge University Press.

Hurston, Z. N. (1942/2006). *Dust tracks on a road: An autobiography.* New York, NY: Harper Perennial.

Hutchison, B., & Niles, S. G. (2009). Career development theories. In I. Marini & M. A. Stebnicki (Eds.), *The professional counselor's desk reference* (pp. 467–476). New York, NY: Springer Publishing Company.

Hyde, J. S. (2005). The gender similarities hypothesis. *American Psychologist, 60,* 581–592. doi: 10.1037/0003-066X.60.6.581

Idol, L., Nevin, A., & Paolucci-Whitcomb, P. (2000). *Collaborative consultation* (3rd ed.). Austin, TX: Pro-Ed.

Ingersoll, R. (2000). Teaching a psychopharmacology course to counselors: Justification, structure, and methods. *Counselor Education and Supervision, 40,* 58–69. doi: 10.1002/j.1556-6978.2000.tb01799.x

Inhelder, B., & Piaget, J. (1958). *The growth of logical thinking: From childhood to adolescence.* New York, NY: Basic Books.

International Association of Counseling Services (2010). *Standards for university and college counseling services.* Retrieved from http://www.iacsinc.org/IACS%20STANDARDS%20rev%2010-3-11.pdf

International Association of Marriage and Family Counselors (IAMFC) (n.d.). *Welcome to IAMFC.* Retrieved from http://www.provisionsconsultingcms.com/~iamfc/

International Association of Marriage and Family Counselors (IAMFC) (2011). *Ethical code.* Retrieved from http://www.iamfconline.org/public/department3.cfm

International Association of Marriage and Family Counselors (IAMFC) (2014). *Home page.* Retrieved from http://www.iamfconline.org/public/main.cfm

International Registry of Counselor Education Programs. (2014). *Welcome.* Retrieved from http://www.ircep.org/ircep/template/index.cfm

Irving, B. A. (2010). (Re)constructing career education as a socially just practice: An antipodean reflection. *International Journal for Educational and Vocational Guidance, 10,* 49–63. doi: 10.1007/s10775-009-9172-1

Isaacson, W. (2007). *Einstein: His life and universe.* New York, NY: Simon & Schuster.

Ivey, A., E. & Ivey, M. (1998). Reframing *DSM-IV:* Positive strategies from developmental counseling and therapy. *Journal of Counseling and Development, 76*(3), 334–350.

Ivey, A., E., & Gluckstein, N. (1974). *Basic attending skills: An introduction to microcounseling and helping.* N. Amherst, MA: Microtraining Associates.

Ivey, A., E., Ivey, M., & Zalaquett, C. P. (2014). *Intentional interviewing and counseling: Facilitating client development in a multicultural society* (8th ed.). Belmont, CA: Brooks /Cole.

Ivey, A., E., Pedersen, P. B., & Ivey, M. B. (2001). *Intentional group counseling: A microskills approach.* Belmont, CA: Brooks/Cole.

Jackson, C. (2012). Diagnostic disarray. *Therapy Today, 23*(3), 4–8.

Jackson, M., & Grant, G. (2004). Equity, access, and career development: Contextual conflicts. In R. Perusse & G. E. Goodnough (Eds.), *Leadership, advocacy, and direct service strategies for professional school counselors* (pp. 125–153). Belmont, CA: Brooks/Cole.

Jacobs, E. E., Masson, R. L., & Harvill, R. L. (2012). *Group counseling: Strategies and skills* (7th ed.). Belmont, CA: Cengage.

Jayakar, P. (2003). *J. Krishnamurti: A biography.* New York, NY: Penguin Books. (Original work published 1986)

Jenkins, R. (2007). Ethnicity. In R. George (Ed.), *Blackwell encyclopedia of sociology.* Retrieved from http://www .blackwellreference.com/subscriber/tocnode?id =g9781405124331_chunk_g978140512433111 _ss1-68

Jennings, L. (2007). Prejudice. In R. George (Ed.), *Blackwell encyclopedia of sociology.* Retrieved from http://www .blackwellreference.com.proxy.lib.odu.edu/subscriber /uid=2165/tocnode?id=g9781405124331_chunk _g978140512433122_ss1-97

Jensen, M. (2011, January 1). The relationship of cognitive development level, supervision, and counselor skills in preparing counselors. Proquest dissertations and theses. Retrieved from http://www.proquest.com

Johnson, K. F. (2013). Preparing ex-offenders for work: Applying the self-determination theory to social cognitive career counseling. *Journal of Employment Counseling, 50*(2), 83–93.

Joint Committee on Testing Practices. (2000). *Rights and responsibilities of test takers: Guidelines and expectations.* Washington, DC: American Psychological Association.

Joint Committee on Testing Practices (JCTP) (2004). *Code of fair testing practices in education.* Washington, DC: American Psychological Association.

Jones, J., & Wilson, W. (2006). An incomplete education (3rd ed.). New York, NY: Ballantine Books.

Jones, L. K. (1994). Frank Parsons' contribution to career counseling. *Journal of Career Development, 20*(4), 287–294. doi.org/10.1177/089484539402000403

Jozefowiez, J., & Staddon, J. E. R. (2015). Operant conditioning. In E. Neukrug (Ed.). *The Sage encyclopedia of theory in counseling and psychotherapy* (Vol. 2, pp. 738–742). Thousand Oaks, CA: Sage.

Jung, C. G. (1968). *Analytical psychology, its theory and practice: The Tavistock lectures.* New York, NY: Pantheon Books. (Original work published 1935)

Jung, C. G. (1975). *Critique of psychoanalysis* (R. F. C. Hull, Trans.). Princeton, NJ: Princeton University Press. (Original work published 1929)

Juntunen, C. L., & Morin, P. M. (2004). Treatment issues for Native Americans: An overview of individual, family, and group strategies. In D. R. Atkinson (Ed.), *Counseling American minorities* (6th ed., pp. 193–213). Boston, MA: McGraw-Hill.

Juve, J. (2008). Testing and assessment. In S. F. Davis & W. Buskit (Eds.), *21st-century psychology: A reference handbook* (Vol. 1, pp. 383–391). Thousand Oaks, CA: Sage Publications.

Kaffenberger, C., & Young, A. (2013). *Making DATA work.* Alexandria, VA: American School Counselor Association.

Kagan, N. (1980). Influencing human interaction: Eighteen years with IPR. In A. I. Hess (Ed.), *Psychotherapy supervision: Theory, research, and practice* (pp. 262–283). New York, NY: Wiley.

Kagan, N., & Kagan, N. I. (*1997*). Interpersonal process recall: Influencing human interaction. In C. E. Watkins (Ed.), *Handbook of psychotherapy supervision* (pp. 296–309). New York, NY: Wiley.

Kahn, M. (2001). *Between therapist and client: The new relationship* (rev. ed.). New York, NY: W. H. Freeman/Owl.

Kail, R. V., & Cavanaugh, J. C. (2013). *Human development: A life-span view* (6th ed.). Belmont, CA: Cengage.

Kalichman, S. C., Klein, S. J., Kalichman, M. O., O'Connell, D. A., Freedman, J. A., Eaton, L. C. & Cain, D. (2007). HIV/AIDS case managers and client HIV status disclosure: Perceived client needs, practices, and services. *Health and Social Work, 32*(4), 259–267.

Kampwirth, T. J., & Powers, K. M. (2012). *Collaborative consultation in the schools: Effective practices for students with learning and behavior problems* (4th ed.). Upper Saddle River, NJ: Pearson.

Kaplan, D. M., & Gladding, S. T. (2011). A vision for the future of counseling: The 20/20 principles for unifying and strengthening the profession. *Journal of Counseling and Development, 89,* 367–372. doi: 10.1002/j.1556-6678 .2011.tb00101.x

Kaplan, D. M., Tarvydas, V. M., Gladding, S. T. (2014). 20/20: A vision for the future of counseling: The new consensus definition of counseling. *Journal of Counseling & Development, 92,* 366–372. doi: 10.1002 /j.1556-6676.2014.00164.x

Kaplan, M., & Cuciti, P. L. (Eds.) (1986). *The Great Society and its legacy: Twenty years of U.S. social policy.* Durham, NC: Duke University Press.

Kaplan, R. M., & Saccuzzo, D. P. (2013). *Psychological testing: Principles, applications, and issues* (8th ed). Belmont, CA: Brooks/Cole.

Kapur, S., Phillips, A. G., & Insel, T. R. (2012). Why has it taken so long for biological psychiatry to develop clinical tests and what to do about it? *Mol Psychiatry, 12,* 1174–1179. doi: 10.1038/mp.2012.105

Kaslow, N. J., Rubin, N. J., Forrest, L., Elman, N. S., Van Horne, B. A., Jacobs, S. C., . . . Thorn, B. E. (2007). Recognizing, assessing, and intervening with problems of professional competence. *Professional Psychology: Research and Practice, 38,* 479–492. doi: 10.1037 /0735-7028.38.5.479

Keeling, R. P., Avery, T., Dickson, J. S. M., & Whipple, E. G. (2011). Student health. In N. Zhang (Ed.), *Rentz's student affairs practice in higher education* (4th ed., pp. 430–459). Springfield, IL: Charles C. Thomas.

Kees, N. L. (Ed.). (2005). Special issue on women and counseling. *Journal of Counseling and Development, 83*(3).

Kees, N. L., Carlson, L. A., Parmley, R., Dahlen, P., Evans, K., Marbley, A. R., . . .& Snyder, B. (2005). Women and counseling: A vision for the future. *Journal of Counseling and Development, 83,* 381–383. doi: 10.1002 /j.1556-6678.2005.tb00359.x

Kegan, R. (1982). *The evolving self.* Cambridge, MA: Harvard University Press.

Kegan, R. (1994). *In over our heads.* Cambridge, MA: Harvard University Press.

Keith, D. V. (2015). Carl Whitaker. In E. Neukrug (Ed.), *The Sage encyclopedia of theory in counseling and psychotherapy* (Vol. 2, 1048–1049). Thousand Oaks, CA: Sage.

Keith-Spiegel, P., & Wiederman, M. W. (2000). *The complete guide to graduate school admission: Psychology, counseling and related professions* (2nd ed.). Mahwah, NJ: Erlbaum.

Kelsey, D., & Smart, J. F. (2012). Social justice, disability, and rehabilitation education. *Rehabilitation Research, Policy, and Education, 26*(2–3), 229–239. doi: 10.1891 /216866612X664970

Kemeny, J. (1970, producer). *The hidden nature of man.* Columbus, OH: Learning Corporation of America.

Kenneally, C. (2014). *The invisible history of the human race: How DNA and history shape our identities and our futures.* New York: Random House.

Kerr, M. S. (2008). Psychometrics. In S. F. Davis & W. Buskit (Eds.), *21st-century psychology: A reference handbook* (Vol. 1, pp. 374–382). Thousand Oaks, CA: Sage Publications.

Kerzner, S. (2009). Psychoanalytic school consultation: A collaborative approach. *Schools: Studies in Education, 6,* 117–128. doi: 10.1086/597661

Kim, B. S. K., Ng, G. F., & Ahn, A. J. (2009). Client adherence to Asian cultural values, common factors in counseling, and session outcome with Asian American clients at a university counseling center. *Journal of Counseling & Development, 87,* 131–142. doi: 10.1002 /j.1556-6678.2009.tb00560.x

Kim, B. S., & Park, Y. S. (2013). Culturally alert counseling with East and Southeast Asian Americans. In G. J. McAuliffe (Ed.), *Culturally alert counseling: A comprehensive introduction* (2nd ed., pp. 157–184). Thousand Oaks, CA: Sage Publications.

Kimbel, T. M., & Goodman-Scott, E. (2011). Major matters in crafting master school counselors. *Counseling Today 54,* 56–57.

King, P. M. (1978). William Perry's theory of intellectual and ethical development. In L. Knefelkamp, C. Widick, & C. L. Parker (Eds.), *Applying new developmental findings* (pp. 34–51). San Francisco, CA: Jossey-Bass.

Kinnier, R. T.; Hofsess, C; Pongratz, R.; Lambert, C. (2009). Attributions and affirmations for overcoming anxiety and depression. *Psychology & Psychotherapy: Theory, Research, & Practice, 82*(2), 153–169. doi: 10.1348 /147608308X389418

Kinsey, A. C., Pomeroy, W. B., & Martin, C. E. (1948). *Sexual behavior in the human male.* Philadelphia, PA: Saunders.

Kinsey, A. C., Pomeroy, W. B., Martin, C. E., & Gebhard, P. H. (1953). *Sexual behavior in the human female.* Philadelphia, PA: Saunders.

Kirkpatrick, D. L., & Kirkpatrick, J. D. (2006). *Evaluating training programs: The four levels.* San Francisco, CA: Berrett-Koehler Publishers Inc.

Kirschenbaum, H. (2009). *The life and work of Carl Rogers.* Alexandria, VA: American Counseling Association.

Kirschenbaum, H., & Henderson, V. L. (Eds.) (1989). *The Carl Rogers reader.* Boston, MA: Houghton Mifflin.

Kirst-Ashman, K. K., & Hull, G. H. (2015). *Understanding generalist practice.* Belmont, CA: Cengage.

Kitchener, K. S. (1984). Intuition, critical evaluation and ethical principles: The foundation for ethical decisions in counseling psychology. *The Counseling Psychologist, 12*(3), 43–45. doi: 10.1177/0011000084123005

Kitchener, K. S. (1986). Teaching applied ethics in counselor education: An integration of psychological processes and philosophical analysis. *Journal of Counseling and Development, 64*(5), 306–311. doi: 10.1177 /0011000084123005

Kleinke, C. L. (1994). *Common principles of psychotherapy.* Pacific Grove, CA: Brooks/Cole.

Kleist, D., & Bitter, J. R. (2009). In J. Bitter (Ed.), *Theory and practice of family therapy and counseling* (pp. 43–65). Belmont, CA: Brooks/Cole.

Klever, P. (2004). The multigenerational transmission of nuclear family processes and symptoms. *The American Journal of Family Therapy, 32,* 337–351.

Kliewer, S. P., McNally, M., & Trippany, R. L. (2009). Deinstitutionalization: Its impact on community mental health centers and the seriously mentally ill. *Alabama Counseling Association Journal, 35*(1), 40–45.

Kline, R. B. (2009). *Becoming a behavioral science researcher: Producing research that matters.* New York, NY: Guilford Press.

Kline, W. B. (Ed.) (2006). Supervision in schools [special section]. *Counselor Education and Supervision, 45*(4), 242–303. doi: 10.1002/j.1556-6978.2006.tb00001.x

Kluckhohn, C., & Murray, H. A. (Eds.) (1948). *Personality in nature, society, and culture.* New York, NY: Alfred A. Knopf.

Knapp, M. L., & Hall, J. A. (2010). *Nonverbal communication in human interaction* (7th ed.). Belmont, CA: Cengage.

Kohlberg, L. (1969). *Stages in the development of moral thought and action.* New York, NY: Holt, Rinehart, & Winston.

Kohlberg, L. (1981). *The philosophy of moral development: Moral stages and the idea of justice.* San Francisco, CA: Harper and Row.

Kohlberg, L. (1984). *The psychology of moral development: The nature and validity of moral stages.* San Francisco, CA: Harper & Row.

Kolb, B. & Whishaw, I. (2009). *Fundamentals of human neuro-psychology* (6th ed.) New York, NY: Worth Publishers.

Kongstvedt, P. R. (2013). *Essentials of managed health care* (6th ed.). Burlington, MA: Jones and Bartlett.

Konopik, D. & Cheung, M. (2013). Psychodrama as a social work modality. *Social Work, 58*(1), 9–20.

Kosciw, J. G., Greytak, E. A., Bartkiewicz, M. J., Boesen, M. J., & Palmer, N. A. (2012). The 2011 national school climate survey: The experiences of lesbian, gay, bisexual and transgender youth in our nation's schools. New York, NY: GLSEN.

Kottler, J. A. (1994). *Advanced group leadership.* Pacific Grove, CA: Brooks/Cole.

Kottler, J. A., & Shepard, D. S. (2015). *Introduction to counseling: Voices from the field* (8th ed.). Belmont, CA: Cengage.

Kraft, D. P. (2009). *Mens sana:* The growth of mental health in the American College Health Association. *Journal of American College Health, 58,* 267–275. doi: 10.1080/ 07448480903297546

Kraft, D. P. (2011). One hundred years of college mental health. *Journal of American College Health, 59,* 477–482. doi: org/10.1080/07448481.2011.569964

Kress, V., Eriksen, K., Rayle, A., & Ford, S. (2005). The DSM-IV-TR and culture: Considerations for counselors. *Journal of Counseling and Development, 83,* 97–104. doi: 10.1002/j.1556-6678.2005.tb00584.x

Kring, A. M., Davison, G. C., & Neale, J. M., & Johnson, S. L. (2007). *Abnormal psychology* (10th ed.). New York, NY: Wiley.

Kring, A. M., Johnson, S. L., Davison, G. C., & Neale, J. M. (2012). *Abnormal psychology* (12th ed.). New York, NY: John Wiley & Sons.

Krishnan, K. R. R. (2009). Monoamine oxidase inhibitors. In A. F. Schatzberg & C. B. Nemeroff (Eds.), *Textbook of psychopharmacology* (4th ed., pp. 389–403). Washington, DC: American Psychiatric Press.

Krueger, R. F., & Eaton, N. R. (2010). Personality traits and the classification of mental disorders: Toward a more complete integration in DSM-5 and an empirical model of psychopathology. *Personality Disorders: Theory, Research, and Treatment, 1,* 97–118. doi: 10.1037/a0018990

Krumboltz, J. D. (1966a). Promoting adaptive behavior. In J. D. Krumboltz (Ed.), *Revolution in counseling* (pp. 3–26). Boston, MA: Houghton Mifflin.

Krumboltz, J. D. (Ed.). (1966b). *Revolution in counseling.* Boston, MA: Houghton Mifflin.

Kubler-Ross, E., & Kessler, D. (2005). *On grief and grieving.* New York, NY: Scribner.

Kuhn, T. S. (1962). *The structure of scientific revolutions.* Chicago, IL: University of Chicago Press.

Kuriansky, J. (2008). A clinical toolbox for cross-cultural counseling and training. In U. P. Gielen, J. G. Draguns, & J. M. Fish (Eds.), *Principles of multicultural counseling and therapy.* New York, NY: Routledge.

Kurpius, D. J., & Robinson, S. E. (1978). An overview of consultation. *Personnel and Guidance Journal, 56,* 321–323.

Kursmark, L. M. (2012). *Best resumes for college students and new grads: Jump-start your career* (3rd ed.). Indianapolis, IN: JIST Works.

LaCroix, T. (2008). Student drug testing: The blinding appeal of in loco parentis and the importance of state protection of student privacy. *Brigham Young University Education and Law Journal, 2,* 251–279.

Laing, R. D. (1967). *The politics of experience.* New York, NY: Ballantine.

Lam, T., Kolomitro, K., & Alamparambil, F. C. (2011). Empathy training: Methods, evaluation practices, and validity. *Journal of Multidisciplinary Evaluation, 7,* 162–200.

Lambert, M. J., & Barley, D. E. (2001). Research summary on the therapeutic relationship and psychotherapy outcome. *Psychotherapy, 38,* 357–361. doi: 10.1037/ 0033-3204.38.4.357

Lambert, N., Hylander, I., & Sandoval, J. H. (Eds.). (2004). *Consultee-centered consultation. Improving the quality of professional services in schools and community organizations.* Mahwah, NJ: Lawrence Erlbaum Associates.

Lambie, G., & Williamson, L. L. (2004). The challenge to change from guidance counseling to professional school counseling: A historical proposition. *Professional School Counseling, 8*(2), 124–131.

Lambie, G. W., Hagedor, W. B., & Ieva, K. P. (2010). Social-cognitive development, ethical and legal knowledge, and ethical decision making of counselor education students. *Counselor Education and Supervision, 49,* 228–246. doi: 10.1002/j.1556-6978.2010.tb00100.x

Lambie, G. W., Smith, H. L., & Ieva. K. P. (2009). Graduate counseling students' levels of ego development, wellness, and psychological disturbance: An exploratory investigation. *Adultspan Journal, 8,* 114–127. doi: 10.1002/j.2161-0029.2009.tb00064.x

Langer, J. (1969). *Theories of development.* New York, NY: Holt, Rinehart, & Winston.

Langewitz, W., Nübling, M., & Weber, H. (2003). A theory-based approach to analysing conversation sequences. *Epidemiologia e Psichiatria Sociale, 12*(2), 103–108.

Lapan, R. T., Gysbers, N. C., & Kayson, M. A. (2007). *Missouri school counselors benefit all students.* Jefferson City, MO: Missouri Department of Elementary and Secondary Education.

Lapan, R. T., Gysbers, N. C., & Petroski, G. (2001). Helping 7th graders be safe and academically successful: A statewide study of the impact of comprehensive guidance programs. *Journal of Counseling & Development, 79,* 320–330. doi: 10.1002/j.1556-6676.2001.tb01977.x

Lapan, R. T., Gysbers, N. C., Stanley, B., & Pierce, M. E. (2012). Missouri professional school counselors: Ratios matter, especially in high-poverty schools. *Professional School Counselors, 16,* 108–116. doi: 10.5330/PSC.n.2012-16.108

Lapan, R. T., Gysbers, N. C., & Sun, Y. (1997). The impact of more fully implemented guidance programs on the school experiences of high school students: A statewide evaluation study. *Journal of Counseling & Development, 75,* 292–302. doi: 10.1002/j.1556-6676.1997.tb02344.x

Lapan, R. T., Whitcomb, S. A., & Aleman, N. M. (2012). Connecticut professional school counselors: College and career counseling services and smaller ratios benefit students. *Professional School Counseling, 16,* 117–124. doi: 10.5330/PSC.n.2012-16.124

Lassiter, P., Napolitano, L., Culbreth, J. R., & Ng, K. (2008). Developing multicultural competence using the structured peer group supervision model. *Counselor Education & Supervision, 47*(3), 164–178.

Law, I. (2007). *Discrimination.* In R. George (Ed.), *Blackwell encyclopedia of sociology.* Retrieved from http://www .blackwellreference.com/subscriber/tocnode?id =g9781405124331_ chunk_g98140512433110_ss2-27

Lawson, G. (2007). Counselor wellness and impairment: A national survey. *Journal of Humanistic Counseling, Education, and Development, 46*(1), 20–34.

Lawson, G., Hein, S., & Getz, H. (2009). A model for using triadic supervision in counselor preparation programs. *Counselor Education and Supervision, 48*(4), 257–270. doi: 10.1002/j.1556-6978.2009.tb00079.x

Leahy, M., Muenzen, P., Saunders, J., & Strauser, D. (2009). Essential knowledge domains underlying effective rehabilitation counseling practice. *Rehabilitation Counseling Bulletin, 2*(2), 95–106. doi: 10.1177/ 0034355208323646

Leahy, R. L. (2003). *Cognitive therapy techniques: A practitioner's guide.* New York, NY: Guilford Publications.

Leary, D. (1992). William James and the art of human understanding. *American Psychologist, 47,* 152–160. doi: 10.1037/0003-066X.47.2.152

Leary, M. R. (2012). *Introduction to behavioral research methods* (6th ed.). Upper Saddle River, NJ: Pearson Education Inc.

Lee, C. (2001). Culturally responsive school counselors and programs: Addressing the needs of all students. *Professional School Counseling, 4,* 163–171.

Lee, R. E., Nichols, D. P., Nichols, W. C., & Odom, T. (2004). Trends in family therapy supervision: The past 25 years and into the future. *Journal of Marital and Family Therapy, 30,* 61–69. doi: 10.1111/j.1752-0606.2004.tb01222.x

Lee, V. V, & Goodnough, G. E. (2015). Systemic, data-driven school counseling practice and programming for equity. In B. T. Erford (Ed.), *Transforming the school counseling profession* (4th ed., pp. 66–91). Boston, MA: Pearson.

Leiby, J. (1978). *A history of social welfare and social work in the United States.* New York, NY: Columbia University Press.

Lent, R. W. (2013). Social cognitive career theory. In S. D. Brown & R. W. Lent (Eds.), *Career development and counseling: Putting theory and research to work* (2nd ed., pp. 115–146). New York, NY: John Wiley & Sons.

Lent, R. W., & Brown, S. D. (2013). Promoting work satisfaction and performance. In S. D. Brown & R. W. Lent (Eds.), *Career development and counseling: Putting theory and research to work* (2nd ed., pp. 621–652). New York, NY: John Wiley & Sons.

Lent, R. W., & Brown, S. D. (2013a). Understanding and facilitating career development in the 21st century. In S. D. Brown & R. W. Lent (Eds.), *Career development and counseling: Putting theory and research to work* (2nd ed.). Hoboken, NY: John Wiley & Sons.

Lent, R. W., Brown, S. D., & Hackett, G. (2002). Social cognitive career theory. In D. Brown et al., *Career choice and development* (4th ed., pp. 255–311). San Francisco, CA: Jossey-Bass.

Leong, F. T. L., & Flores, L. Y. (2013). Multicultural perspectives in vocational psychology. In W. B. Walsh, M. L. Savickas, & P. J. Hartung (Eds.), *Handbook of vocational psychology: Theory, research, and practice* (4th ed., pp. 51–80). New York, NY: Taylor and Francis.

Leucht, S., Hierl, S., Kissling, W., Dold, M., & Davis, J. M. (2012). Putting the efficacy of psychiatric and general medication into perspective: Review of meta-analyses. *British Journal of Psychiatry, 200,* 97–106. doi: 10.1192/bjp.bp.111.096594

Levenkron, H. (2009). Engaging the implicit: Meeting points between the Boston Change Process Study Group and relational psychoanalysis. *Contemporary Psychoanalysis, 45*(2), 179–217.

Levinson, D. L. (1978). *The seasons of a man's life.* New York, NY: Alfred A. Knopf.

Levinson, D. L. (1996). *The seasons of a woman's life.* New York, NY: Alfred A. Knopf.

Levinson, H. (2009). Assessing organizations. *Consulting psychology: Selected articles by Harry Levinson* (pp. 137–166). Washington, DC: American Psychological Association. doi: 10.1037/11848-008

Levitt, H. M. (2001). Sounds of silence in psychotherapy: The categorization of client's pauses. *Psychotherapy Research, 11,* 295–309. doi: 10.1080/713663985

Lewis, J. A., Lewis, M. D., Daniels, J. A., & D'Andrea, M. J. (2011). *Community counseling: A multicultural-social justice perspective* (4th ed.). Belmont, CA: Cengage.

Lezak, M., Howieson, D., & Bigler, E. D., Tranel, D. (2012). *Neuropsychological assessment* (5th ed.). New York, NY: Oxford University Press.

Lieberman, M. A., & Keith, H. (2002). Self-help groups and substance abuse: An examination of Alcoholics Anonymous. In. D. W. Brook & H. Spitz (Eds.), *The group therapy of substance abuse* (pp. 203–221). New York, NY: Haworth Press.

Lincoln, Y. S., & Guba, E. G. (1985). *Naturalistic inquiry.* Beverly Hills, CA: Sage.

Linnell, S., Bansel, P., Ellwood, C., & Gannon, S. (2008). Precarious listening. *Qualitative Inquiry, 14,* 285–306. doi: 10.1177/1077800407312041

Linstrum, K. S. (2005). The effects of training on ethical decision-making skills as a function of moral development and context in master-level counseling students. Commerce, TX: Texas A & M University–Commerce.

Lipps, T. (1960). Empathy, inner-imitation, and sense feelings. In M. M. Rader (Ed.), *A modern book of esthetics: An anthology* (3rd ed., pp. 374–381). New York, NY: Holt, Rinehart, and Winston. (Original work published 1903)

Livingston, R. (1979). The history of rehabilitation counselor certification. *Journal of Applied Rehabilitation Counseling, 10,* 111–118.

Loevinger, J. (1976). *Ego development.* San Francisco, CA: Jossey-Bass.

Lonergan, E. C. (1994). Using theories of group therapy. In H. S. Bernard & K. R. MacKenzie (Eds.), *Basics of group psychotherapy* (pp. 191–216). New York, NY: Guilford.

Lopez-Mulnix, E., & Mulnix, M. (2006). Models of excellence in multicultural colleges and universities. *Journal of Hispanic Higher Education, 5*(1), 4–21. doi: 10.1177/1538192705282566

Love, P., & Maxam, S. (2011). Advising and consultation. In J. H. Schuh, S. R. Jones, & S. R. Harper (2011). *Student services: A handbook for the profession* (5th ed., pp. 413–432). San Francisco, CA: Jossey-Bass.

Lovell, C. (1999) Empathic-cognitive development in students of counseling. *Journal of Adult Development, 6*(4), 195–203.

Luke, M. D., Goodrich, K. M., Gilbride, D. D. (2013). Testing the intercultural model of ethical decision making with counselor trainees. *Counselor Education & Supervision, 52,* 222–234. doi: 10.1002/j.1556-6978.2013.00039.x

Lum, C. (2003). *A guide to state laws and regulations on professional school counseling.* Retrieved from ERIC database (ED 474113)

Lum, D. (2004). *Social work practice and people of color: A process-stage approach* (5th ed.). Pacific Grove, CA: Brooks /Cole.

Lyon, R. E., & Potkar, K. A. (2010). The supervisory relationship. In N. Ladany & L. J. Bradley (Eds.), *Counselor supervision* (4th ed., pp. 15–52). New York, NY: Routledge.

Maccartney, S., Bishaw, A., & Fontenot, K. (2013). *U.S. Census Bureau: Poverty rates for select detailed race and Hispanic groups by state and place, 2007–2011.* Retrieved from http://www.census.gov/prod/2013pubs/acsbr11-17.pdf

Macionis. J. J. (2014). *Sociology.* (15th ed.). Upper Saddle River, NJ: Pearson.

MacKinnon, F. J. D. (2011). Afterward. In N. Zhang (Ed.), *Rentz's student affairs practice in higher education* (4th ed., pp. 460–470). Springfield, IL: Charles C. Thomas.

Madanes, C. (1981). *Strategic family therapy.* San Francisco, CA: Jossey-Bass.

Madanes, C. (2015a). Cloe Madanes. In E. Neukrug (Ed.), *The Sage encyclopedia of theory in counseling and psychotherapy* (Vol. 2, pp. 623–624). Thousand Oaks, CA: Sage.

Madanes, C. (2015b). Strategic family therapy. In E. Neukrug (Ed.), *The Sage encyclopedia of theory in counseling and psychotherapy* (Vo. 2, pp. 957–962). Thousand Oaks, CA: Sage.

Madigan, S. P. (2015). Michael White. In E. Neukrug (Ed.), *The Sage encyclopedia of theory in counseling and psychotherapy* (Vol 2., pp. 1050–1052). Thousand Oaks, CA: Sage.

Madsen, K., & Leech, P. (2007). *The ethics of labeling in mental health.* Jefferson, NC: MacFarland & Company.

Magolda, M. B., & Porterfield, W. D. (1992). *Assessing intellectual development: The link between theory and practice.* Alexandria, VA: American College Personnel Association.

Maia, S., & Jozefowiez, J. (2015). Classical conditioning. In E. Neukrug (Ed.), *The Sage encyclopedia of theory in counseling and psychotherapy* (Vol. 1, pp. 163–167). Thousand Oaks, CA: Sage.

Male, R. A. (1996). Careers in public and private agencies. In B. B. Collison & N. J. Garfield (Eds.), *Careers in counseling and human services* (2nd ed., pp. 81–89). Washington, DC: Taylor & Francis.

Maples, M., & Abney, P. (2006). Baby boomers mature and gerontological counseling comes of age. *Journal of Counseling and Development, 84*(1), 3–9. doi: 10.1002 /j.1556-6678.2006.tb00374.x

Marchand, M. M. (2010). Application of Paulo Freire's *Pedagogy of the Oppressed* to human services education. *Journal of Human Services, 30*(1), 43–53.

Markus, H. E., & King, D. A. (2003). A survey of group psychotherapy training during predoctoral psychology internship. *Professional Psychology: Research and Practice, 34*(2), 203–209. doi: 10.1037/0735-7028.34.2.203

Maroda, K. J. (2009). Less is more: An argument for the judicious use of self-disclosure. In A. Bloomgarden & R. B. Mennuit (Eds.), *Psychotherapist revealed: Therapists speak about self-disclosure in psychotherapy* (pp. 17–29). New York, NY: Taylor and Francis Group.

Marquis, A. (2015). Integrative approaches: Overview. In E. Neukrug (Ed.), *The Sage encyclopedia of theory in counseling and psychotherapy* (Vol. 1, pp. 546–551). Thousand Oaks, CA: Sage.

Martin, E. D. (Ed.) (2007). *Principles and practices of case management in rehabilitation counseling.* Springfield, IL: Charles C. Thomas.

Martin, I., Carey, J., & DeCoster, K. (2009). A national study of the current status of state school counseling models. *Professional School Counseling, 12*, 378–386. doi: 10.5330 /PSC.n.2010-12.378

Martin, P. J. (2015). Transformational thinking in today's schools. In B. T. Erford (Ed.), *Transforming the school counseling profession* (4th ed., pp. 45–65). Boston, MA: Pearson.

Martin, W. E., Easton, C., Wilson, S., Takemoto, M., & Sullivan, S. (2004). Salience of emotional intelligence as a core characteristic of being a counselor. *Counselor Education and Supervision, 44*(1), 17–30.

Maslow, A. (1943). A theory of human motivation. *Psychological Review, 50*(4), 370–396. doi: 10.1037 /h0054346

Maslow, A. (1970). *Motivation and personality* (rev. ed.). New York, NY: Harper & Row.

Maslow, A. H. (1968). *Toward a psychology of being.* Princeton, NJ: Van Nostrand.

Matsumoto, D. (2006). Culture and nonverbal behavior. In V. Manusov & M. L. Patterson (Eds.), *The Sage handbook of nonverbal communication* (pp. 219–236). Thousand Oaks, CA: Sage Publishing.

Mattern, K. D., & Patterson, B. F. (2012). *2012–3).* New York, NY: The College Board.

Matthews, C. H. (2015). Gender-aware therapy. In E. Neukrug (Ed.), *The Sage encyclopedia of theory in counseling and psychotherapy* (Vol. 1, pp. 449–452). Thousand Oaks, CA: Sage Publishing.

Matthews, C. O. (1992). An application of general system theory (GST) to group therapy. *Journal for Specialists in Group Work, 17*(3), 161–169. doi: 10.1080 /01933929208413725

Matsumoto, D., Frank, M. G., & Hwang, H. S. (Eds.). (2013). *Nonverbal communication: Science and applications.* Thousand Oaks, CA: Sage.

May, R. (1950). *The meaning of anxiety.* New York, NY: Ronald Press.

May, R., Angel, E., & Ellenberg, H. F. (Eds.) (1958). *Existence: A new dimension in psychiatry and psychology.* New York, NY: Basic Books.

Mayotte-Blum, J., Slavin-Mulford, J., Lehmann, M., Pesale, F., Becker-Matero, N., & Hilsenroth, M. (2012). Therapeutic immediacy across long-term psychodynamic psychotherapy: An evidence-based case study. *Journal of Counseling Psychology, 59*(1), 27–40. doi: 10.1037/a0026087.

McAdams, R. (2015). Couples, family, and relational models: Overview. In E. Neukrug (Ed.) *The Sage encyclopedia of theory in counseling and psychotherapy* (Vol. 1, pp. 247–253). Thousand Oaks, CA: Sage.

McAuliffe, G. (2013a). Culture and diversity defined. In G. McAuliffe (Ed.), *Culturally alert counseling: A comprehensive introduction* (2nd ed., pp. 3–23). Los Angeles, CA: Sage Publications.

McAuliffe, G. (2013b). The practice of culturally alert counseling: Part 1. In G. McAuliffe (Ed.), *Culturally alert counseling: A comprehensive introduction* (2nd ed., pp. 543–548). Los Angeles, CA: Sage Publications.

McAuliffe, G., & Eriksen, K. (Eds.) (2010). *Handbook of counselor preparation.* Thousand Oaks, CA: Sage, and Alexandria, VA: Association for Counselor Education and Supervision.

McAuliffe, G., Goméz, E., & Grothaus, T. (2013). Conceptualizing race and racism. In G. McAuliffe (Ed.), *Culturally alert counseling: A comprehensive introduction* (2nd ed., pp. 89–124).Thousand Oaks, CA: Sage Publications.

McAuliffe, G., Grothaus, T., Paré, D., & Wolf, A. K. (2013). The practice of culturally alert counseling: Part 2. In G. McAuliffe (Ed.), *Culturally alert counseling: A comprehensive introduction* (pp. 559–586). Thousand Oaks, CA: Sage.

McBain, L. (2008, Winter). Balancing student privacy, campus security, and public safety: Issues for campus leaders. *Perspectives*, 1–22.

McBride, R. G. (2012). Survival on the streets: Experiences of the homeless population and constructive suggestions for assistance. *Journal of Multicultural Counseling and Development, 40*(1), 49–61. doi: 10.1111 /j.2161-1912.2012.00005.x

McCarthy, J., & Holliday, E. L. (2004). Help-seeking and counseling within a traditional male gender role: An examination from a multicultural perspective. *Journal of Counseling and Development, 82*, 25–30. doi: 10.1002 /j.1556-6678.2004.tb00282.x

McDaniels, C., & Watts, G. A. (Eds.) (1994). Frank Parsons: Light, information, inspiration, cooperation [Special issue]. *Journal of Career Development, 20*(4). doi: 10.1007 /BF02106306

McDonald, J. D., & Chaney, J. M. (2003). Resistance to multiculturalism: The "Indian problem." In J. S. Mio & G. Y. Iwamasa (Eds.), *Culturally diverse mental health: The challenges of research and resistance* (pp. 39–54). New York, NY: Brunner-Routledge.

McElroy, S. L., & Keck, P. E. (2009). Topirmate. In A. F. Schatzberg & C. B. Nemeroff (Eds.), *Textbook of psychopharmacology* (4th ed., pp. 795–810). Washington, DC: American Psychiatric Press.

McGoldrick, M. (2005). History, genograms, and the family life cycle: Freud in context. In B. Carter & M. McGoldrick (Eds.), *The expanded family life cycle: Individual, family, and social perspectives* (3rd ed., pp. 47–68). Boston, MA: Allyn & Bacon.

McGoldrick, M., Carter, B., & Garcia-Preto, N. G. (Eds.). (2011). *The expanded family life cycle: Individual, family, and social perspectives* (4th ed.). Boston, MA: Allyn & Bacon.

McGoldrick, M., Gerson, R., & Petry, S. (2008). *Genograms: Assessment and intervention* (3rd ed.). New York, NY: W.W. Norton & Company.

McGoldrick, M., Giordano, J., & Garcia-Petro, N. (2005). *Ethnicity and family therapy* (3rd ed.). New York, NY: Guilford Press.

McKnight, A. (2015). Murray Bowen. In E. Neukrug (Ed.), *The Sage encyclopedia of theory in counseling and psychotherapy* (Vol. 1, pp. 133–136). Thousand Oaks, CA: Sage.

McMahon, M., Arthur, N., & Collins, S. (2008). Social justice and career development: Looking back, looking forward. *Australian Journal of Career Development, 17*(2), 21–29.

McMillan, J. H., & Schumacher, S. (2010). *Research in education: Evidence-based inquiry* (7th ed.). Boston, MA: Allyn & Bacon.

McWhirter, J. J., McWhirter, B. T., McWhirter, E. H., & McWhirter, R. J. (2013). *At-risk youth: A comprehensive response for counselors, teachers, psychologists, and human service professionals* (5th ed.). Belmont, CA: Cengage.

Mead, M. (1961). *Coming of age in Samoa: A psychological study of primitive youth for western civilization.* New York, NY: Morrow.

Meara, N. M., Schmidt, L. D., & Day, J. D. (1996) Principles and virtues: A foundation for ethical decisions, policies, and character. *The Counseling Psychologist, 24*(9), 4–77. doi: 10.1177/0011000096241002

Mehrens, W. A. (1992). Leadership to researchers and practitioners. *Journal of Counseling and Development, 70,* 439–440.

Meichenbaum, D. (1977). *Cognitive behavior modification: An integrative approach.* New York, NY: Basic Books.

Mejia, X. (2005). Gender matters: Working with adult male survivors of trauma. *Journal of Counseling and Development, 83,* 29–40. doi: 10.1002/j.1556-6678.2005 .tb00577.x

Mellin, E. (2009). Responding to the crisis in children's mental health: Potential roles for the counseling profession. *Journal of Counseling and Development, 87*(4), 501–506. doi: 10.1002/j.1556-6678.2009.tb00136.x

Mendoza, D. W. (1993). A review of Gerald Caplan's theory and practice of mental health consultation. *Journal of Counseling and Development, 71,* 629–635. doi: 10.1002 /j.1556-6676.1993.tb02252.x

Mental Research Institute. (2008). *About us.* Retrieved from http://www.mri.org/about_us.html

Merlone, L. (2005). Record keeping and the school counselor. *Professional School Counseling, 8,* 372–376.

Merrel, K. W., Ervin, R. A., & Peacock, G. G. (2012). *School psychology for the 21st century: Foundations and practices* (2nd ed.). New York, NY: Guilford Press.

Mertler, C. A., & Charles, C. M. (2011). *Introduction to educational research* (7th ed.). Boston, MA: Pearson.

Meyers, L. (2014). A living document of ethical guidance. *Counseling Today.* Retrieved from http://ct.counseling .org/2014/05/a-living-document-of-ethical-guidance/

Mezzich, J. E., & Caracci, G. (Eds.) (2008). *Cultural formation: A reader for psychiatric diagnosis.* Lanham, MD: Jason Aronson.

Michaels, M. H. (2006). Ethical considerations in writing psychological assessment reports. *Journal of Clinical Psychology, 62*(1), 47–58. doi.org/10.1002/jclp.20199

Middleton, R., Stadler, H., Simpson, C., Guo, Y., Brown, M., Crow, G., . . . Lazarte, A. A. (2005). Mental health practitioners: The relationship between White racial identity attitudes and self-reported multicultural counseling competencies. *Journal of Counseling and Development*, *83*(4), 444–456.

Migration Policy Institute. (2014). *Frequently requested statistics on immigrants and immigration in the United States*. Retrieved from http://www.migrationpolicy.org/article/frequently-requested-statistics-immigrants-and-immigration-united-states

Military OneSource. (2014). Counseling options for service members and their families. Retrieved from http://www.militaryonesource.mil/non-medical-counseling?content_id=268934

Miller, G. (2012). Criticism continues to dog psychiatric manual as deadline approaches. *Science*, *336*, 1088–1089. doi: 10.1177/0004867413518825

Miller, J. G. (1956). General behavior systems theory and summary. *Journal of Counseling Psychology*. *3*(2), 120–124. doi: 10.1037/h0048504

Miller, W. R., & Rollnick, S. (2013). *Motivational interviewing: Helping people change* (3rd ed.). New York, NY: Guilford Press.

Milsom, A., & Akos, P. (2003). Preparing school counselors to work with students with disabilities. *Counselor Education and Supervision, 43*, 86–95.

Minuchin, S. (1974). *Families and family therapy*. Cambridge, MA: Harvard University Press.

Minuchin, S. (1981). *Family therapy techniques*. Cambridge, MA: Harvard University Press.

Mislevy, R. J. (2004). Can there be reliability without "reliability"? *Journal of Educational and Behavioral Statistics, 29*(2), 241–244. doi: 10.3102/10769986029002241

Monaghan, P. (2012). Sticks, stones—and words too? *Chronicle of Higher Education*. Retrieved from http://chronicle.com/article/Sticks-Stones-and-Words/132045/

Moore, W. S. (2002). Understanding learning in a postmodern world: Reconsidering the Perry scheme of intellectual and ethical development. In B. Hofer & P. Pintrich (Eds.), *Personal epistemology: The psychology of beliefs about knowledge and knowing* (pp. 17–36). Mahwah, NJ: Lawrence Erlbaum Associates Publishers.

Morales, A. T., Sheafor, B. W., & Scott, M. E. (2012). *Social work: A profession of many faces* (12th ed.). Boston, MA: Allyn & Bacon.

Morrow, S. L. (2004). Finding the "yes" within ourselves: Counseling lesbian and bisexual women. In D. R. Atkinson & G. Hackett (Eds.), *Counseling diverse populations* (3rd ed., pp. 366–387). Boston, MA: McGraw-Hill.

Mortola, P., & Carlson, J. (2003). "Collecting an anecdote": The role of narrative in school consultation. *Family Journal: Counseling and Therapy for Couples and Families*, *11*(1), 7–12. doi: 10.1080/87568220903400138

Moss, P. (2004). The meaning and consequences of reliability. *Journal of Educational and Behavioral Statistics, 29*(2), 245–249. doi:10.3102/10769986029002245

Much, K., Wagener, A., & Hellenbrand, M. (2010). Practicing in the 21st century college counseling center. *Journal of College Student Psychotherapy*, *24*(1), 32–38. doi: 10.1080/87568220903400138

Murdach, A. D. (2007). Situational approaches to direct practice: Origin, decline, and re-emergence. *Social Work, 52*, 211–218.

Murdin, L. (2000). *How much is enough? Endings in psychotherapy and counseling*. New York, NY: Routledge.

Muro, J. J., & Dinkmeyer, D. C. (1977). *Counseling in the elementary and middle schools: A pragmatic approach*. Dubuque, IA: William C. Brown.

Murphy, J. J. (2008). *Solution-focused counseling in schools* (2nd ed.). Alexandria, VA: American Counseling Association.

Murray, T. (2006). The other side of psychopharmacology: A review of the literature. *Journal of Mental Health Counseling, 28*(4), 309–317.

Myers, J. E., & Harper, M. C. (2004). Evidence-based effective practice with older adults. *Journal of Counseling and Development, 82*, 207–218. doi: 10.1002/j.1556-6678.2004.tb00304.x

Myers, J. E., & Sweeney, T. J. (2004). *Counselors for wellness: Theory, research, and practice*. Alexandria, VA: American Counseling Association.

Myers, J. E., & Sweeney, T. J. (2005). The indivisible self: An evidence-based model of wellness. *Journal of Individual Psychology, 61*(3), 269–278.

Myers, J. E., & Sweeney, T. J. (2008). Wellness counseling: The evidence base for practice. *Journal of Counseling and Development, 86*, 482–493. doi: 10.1002/j.1556-6678.2008.tb00536.x

Nadal, K. L. (2011). The Racial and Ethnic Microaggressions Scale (REMS): Construction, reliability, and validity. *Journal of Counseling Psychology, 58*(4), 470–480. doi: 10.1037/a0025193

Napier, A., & Whitaker, C. (1972). A conversation about co-therapy. In A. Ferber, M. Mendelsohn, & A. Napier (Eds.), *The book of family therapy* (pp. 480–506). New York, NY: Jason Aronson.

Napier, A., & Whitaker, C. (1978). *The family crucible*. New York, NY: Harper & Row.

Napier, G. (2002). Experiential family therapy. In J. Carlson & D. Kjos, *Theories and strategies of family therapy* (pp. 296–316). Boston, MA: Allyn & Bacon.

Napier, R. W., & Gershenfeld, M. K. (2004). *Groups: Theory and experience* (7th ed.). New York, NY: Houghton Mifflin.

Nasrallah, H. A., & Tandon, F. (2009). Classic antipsychotic medications. In A. F. Schatzberg and C. B.

Nemeroff (Eds.), *Textbook of psychopharmacology* (4th ed., pp. 533–554). Washington, DC: American Psychiatric Press.

Nassar, J. L., & Devlin, A. (2011). Impressions of psychotherapists' offices. *Journal of Counseling Psychology, 58,* 310–320. doi: 10.1037/a0023887

National Association of School Psychologists (NASP) (n.d.). *What is a school psychologist?* Retrieved from http://www.nasponline.org/about_sp/whatis.aspx

National Association of Social Workers (NASW) (2008). *Code of ethics.* Retrieved from http://www.socialworkers.org/pubs/code/code.asp

National Association of Social Workers (NASW) (2013). *About NASW.* Retrieved from http://www.naswdc.org/nasw/default.asp

National Association of Social Workers (NASW) (2014). *Credentialing center home.* Retrieved from http://www.socialworkers.org/credentials/default.asp

National Board for Certified Counselors (NBCC) (2012). *Code of ethics.* Retrieved from http://www.nbcc.org/Assets/Ethics/NBCCCodeofEthics.pdf

National Board for Certified Counselors (NBCC) (2014a). *Understanding national certification and state licensure.* Retrieved from http://www.nbcc.org/Certification/CertificationorLicensure

National Board for Certified Counselors (NBCC) (2014b). *About NBCC.* Retrieved from http://www.nbcc.org/Footer/AboutNBCC

National Board for Certified Counselors (NBCC) (2014c). *More information on TRICARE.* Retrieved from http://www.nbcc.org/InnerPageLinks/MoreInformationOnTRICARE

National Career Development Association (2007). *Code of ethics.* Retrieved from http://www.ncda.org/aws/NCDA/asset_manager/get_file/3395

National Career Development Association (2008). *Career development: A policy statement of the National Career Development Association board of directors.* Retrieved from http://lifeworkps.com/HPH/NCDA/NCDA-Policy-Statement-on-Seven-Stages-of-CD.html

National Career Development Association (2009a). *Minimum competencies of multicultural career counseling and development.* Retrieved from http://www.associationdatabase.com/aws/NCDA/asset_manager/get_file/9914/minimum_competencies_for_multi-cultural_career_counseling.pdf

National Career Development Association (2009b). *Career counseling competencies.* Retrieved from http://association-database.com/aws/NCDA/pt/sd/news_article/37798/_self/layout_ccmsearch/true

National Center for Children in Poverty (2014). *Child poverty.* Retrieved from http://nccp.org/topics/childpoverty.html

National Center for Transgender Equality (2014). *Transgender terminology.* http://transequality.org/Resources/TransTerminology_2014.pdf

National Coalition for the Homeless (2009). *How many people experience homelessness?* Retrieved from http://www.nationalhomeless.org/factsheets/How_Many.html

National Council for Behavioral Health (2014). *Community Mental Health Act.* Retrieved from http://www.thenationalcouncil.org/about/national-mental-health-association/overview/community-mental-health-act/

National Credentialing Academy (n.d.). *Overview and general information.* Retrieved from http://www.natlacad.4t.com/overview.html

National Human Genome Research Project (2012). *From blueprint to you.* Retrieved from https://www.genome.gov/12511466

National Institute of Drug Abuse (2014). *DrugFacts: Nationwide trends.* Retrieved from http://www.drugabuse.gov/publications/drugfacts/nationwide-trends

National Institute of Mental Health (2001). *NIH policy and guidelines on the inclusion of women and minorities as subjects in clinical research.* Retrieved from http://grants1.nih.gov/grants/funding/women_min/guidelines_amended_10_2001.htm

National Institute of Mental Health (2010). *Mental health medications.* Retrieved from http://www.nimh.nih.gov/health/publications/mental-health-medications/nimh-mental-health-medications.pdf

National Institute of Mental Health (n.d.). *The numbers count: Mental disorders in America.* Retrieved from http://www.nimh.nih.gov/health/publications/the-numbers-count-mental-disorders-in-america/index.shtml

National Organization for Human Services (n.d.). *About us.* Retrieved from http://www.nationalhumanservices.org/about-us-page

National Organization of Human Services (NOHS) (1996). *Ethics of human services.* Retrieved from http://www.nationalhumanservices.org/mc/page.do?sitePageId=89927&orgId=nohs

National Organization of Human Services (NOHS) (2013). *Home page.* Retrieved from http://www.nationalhumanservices.org/

National Public Health Partnership (2006). The language of prevention. Retrieved from http://www.nphp.gov.au/publications/language_of_prevention.pdf

National Security Archive (2009). *FOIA Basics.* Retrieved from http://www.gwu.edu/~nsarchiv/nsa/foia/guide.html

National Training Laboratory (2014). *About NTL.* Retrieved from http://www.ntl.org/inner.asp?id=177&category=2

Naugle, A. E., & Maher, S. (2003). Modeling and behavioral rehearsal. In W. O'Donohue, U. J. Fisher, & S. C. Hayes (Eds.), *Cognitive behavior therapy: Applying empirically supported techniques in your practice* (pp. 238–246). Hoboken, NJ: John Wiley & Sons.

Naugle, K. A. (2010). Counseling and testing: What counselors need to know about state laws on assessment and testing. *Measurement and Evaluation in Counseling and Development, 42*(1), 31–45. doi: 10.1177/0748175609333561

Nelson, J. C. (2009). Tricyclic and tetracyclic drugs. In A. F. Schatzberg & C. B. Nemeroff (Eds.), *Textbook of psychopharmacology* (4th ed., pp. 263–288). Washington, DC: American Psychiatric Press.

Neuer, C. A. A. (2013). Endless possibilities: Diversifying service options in private practice. *Journal of Mental Health Counseling, 35*, 198–210.

Neukrug, E. (1980). The effects of supervisory style and type of praise upon counselor trainees' level of empathy and perception of supervisor. (Doctoral dissertation, University of Cincinnati, 1980.) *Dissertation Abstracts International, 41*(04A), 1496.

Neukrug, E. (1998). Support and challenge: Use of metaphor as a higher-level empathic response. In H. Rosenthal (Ed.), *Favorite counseling and therapy techniques* (pp. 139–141). Bristol, PA: Accelerated Development.

Neukrug, E. (2002). *Skills and techniques for human service professionals: Counseling environment, helping skills, treatment issues.* Pacific Grove, CA: Brooks/Cole.

Neukrug, E. (2011). *Counseling theory and practice.* Belmont, CA: Brooks/Cole.

Neukrug, E. (2013). *Theory, practice, and trends in human services: An introduction* (5th ed.). Belmont, CA: Brooks/Cole.

Neukrug, E. (2014). A brief orientation to counseling. Belmont, CA: Cengage.

Neukrug, E. (Ed.) (2015a). *The Sage encyclopedia of theory in counseling and psychotherapy* (Vols. 1 and 2). Thousand Oaks, CA: Sage.

Neukrug, E. (2015b). Existential-humanistic therapies: Overview. In E. Neukrug (Ed.), *The Sage encyclopedia of theory in counseling and psychotherapy* (Vol. 1, pp. 374–378). Thousand Oaks, CA: Sage Publishing.

Neukrug, E. (2015c). Person-centered counseling. In E. Neukrug (Ed.), *The Sage encyclopedia of theory in counseling and psychotherapy* (Vol. 2, pp. 767–772). Thousand Oaks, CA: Sage.

Neukrug, E. S., & Fawcett, R. C. (2015). *Essentials of testing and assessment: A practical guide for counselors, social workers, and psychologists* (3rd ed.). Belmont, CA: Brooks/Cole.

Neukrug, E., & McAuliffe, G. (1993). Cognitive development and human service education. *Human Service Education, 13*, 13–26.

Neukrug, E., & Milliken, T. (2011). Counselors' perceptions of ethical behaviors. *Journal of Counseling and Development, 89*, 206–217. doi: 10.1002/j.1556-6678.2011.tb00079.x

Neukrug, E., & Schwitzer, A. M. (2006). *Skills and tools for today's counselors and psychotherapists: From natural helping to professional counseling.* Pacific Grove, CA: Brooks/Cole.

Neukrug, E., Bayne, H., Dean-Nganga, L., & Pusateri, C. (2012). Creative and novel approaches to empathy: A neo-Rogerian perspective. *Journal of Mental Health Counseling, 35*(1), 29–42.

Neukrug, E., Lovell, C., & Parker, R. (1996). Employing ethical codes and decision-making models: A developmental process. *Counseling and Values, 40*, 98–106.

Neukrug, E., Milliken, T., & Walden, S. (2001). Ethical practices of credentialed counselors: An updated survey of state licensing boards. *Counselor Education and Supervision, 41*(1), 57–70.

Neukrug, E., Peterson, C., Bonner, M., & Lomas, G. (2013). A national survey of assessment instruments taught by counselor educators. *Counselor Education and Supervision, 52*, 207–221. doi: 10.1002/j.1556-6978.2013.00038.x

Newport, F. (2011, December 23). *Gallup: Christianity remains dominant religion in the United States: Majority still says religion is very important in their lives.* Retrieved from http://www.gallup.com/poll/151760/Christianity-Remains-Dominant-Religion-United-States.aspx

Newton, P. (1994). Daniel Levinson and his theory of adult development: A reminiscence and some clarifications. *Journal of Adult Development, 1*(3), 135–137. doi: 10.1007/BF02260089

Nicholi, A. M. (2002). *The question of God: C. S. Lewis and Sigmund Freud debate God, love, sex, and the meaning of life.* New York, NY: Free Press.

Nichols, M. P., & Schwartz, R. C. (2008). *Family therapy: Concepts and methods* (8th ed.). Boston, MA: Allyn & Bacon.

Nichols, M. P., & Schwartz, R. C. (2014). *The essentials of family therapy* (6th ed.). Boston, MA: Allyn & Bacon.

Niles, S. (Ed.). (2009). Special section: Advocacy competencies. *Journal of Counseling and Development, 87*(3).

Niles, S. G., & Harris-Bowlsbey, J. (2013). *Career development interventions in the 21st century* (4th ed.). New York, NY: Pearson.

Ninnemann, K. (2012). Variability in the efficacy of psychopharmaceuticals: Contributions from pharmacogenomics, ethnopsychopharmacology, and psychological and psychiatric anthropologies. *Culture, Medicine & Psychiatry, 36*(1), 10–25. doi: 10.1007/s11013-011-9242-y

Nishino, S., Mishima, K., Mignot, E., & Dement, W. C. (2009). Sedative-hypnotics. In A. F. Schatzberg & C. B. Nemeroff (Eds.), *Textbook of psychopharmacology* (4th ed., pp. 821–842). Washington, DC: American Psychiatric Press.

Norcross, J. C. (2010). The therapeutic relationship. In B. L. Duncan, S. D. Miller, B. E. Wampold, & M A. Hubble (Eds.), *The heart and soul of change* (2nd ed., pp. 113–142). Washington, DC: American Psychological Association.

Norcross, J. C. (Ed.). (2011). *Psychotherapy relationships that work: Evidence-based responsiveness.* New York, NY: Oxford University Press.

Norcross, J. C., Bike, D. H., Evans, K. L., & Schatz, D. M. (2008). Psychotherapists who abstain from personal therapy: Do they practice what they preach? *Journal of Clinical Psychology, 64*(12), 1368–1376. doi: 10.1002/jclp.20523

Norcross, J. C., Bike, H., & Evans, K. L. (2009). The therapist's therapist: A replication and extension 20 years later. *Psychotherapy Theory, Research, Practice, Training, 46*(1), 32–41. doi: 10.1037/a0015140

Nugent, F. A., & Jones, K. D. (2009). *An introduction to the profession of counseling* (5th ed.). Upper Saddle River, NJ: Merrill.

Nye, R. D. (2000). *Three psychologies: Perspectives from Freud, Skinner, and Rogers* (6th ed.). Belmont, CA: Brooks/Cole.

O*NET Online (2010). *Summary report for: 21-1011.00— Substance abuse and behavioral disorder counselors.* Retrieved from http://www.onetonline.org/link/summary/21-1011.00#Skills

O*NET Online (2012). *Marriage and family therapists.* Retrieved from http://www.onetonline.org/link/summary/21-1013.00

O*NET Online (2013). *Summary report for 21-1014.00— Mental health counselors.* Retrieved from http://www.onetonline.org/link/summary/21-1014.00

O'Connell, B. (2003). Introduction to the solution-focused approach. In B. O'Connell & S. Palmer (Eds.), *Handbook of solution-focused therapy* (pp. 1–11). Thousand Oaks, CA: Sage.

O'Hanlon, B., & Weiner-Davis, M. (2003). *In search of solutions: A new direction in psychotherapy* (rev. ed.). New York, NY: Norton.

Ober, A., Granello, D., & Henfield, M. (2009). A synergistic model to enhance multicultural competence in supervision. *Counselor Education and Supervision, 48*(3), 204–221. doi: 10.1002/j.1556-6978.2009.tb00075.x

Office of Minority Health (n.d.). Publications. Retrieved from http://minorityhealth.hhs.gov/templates/browse.aspx?lvl=3&lvlid=83

Ohler, D. L., & Levinson, E. M. (2012). Using Holland's theory in employment counseling: Focus on service occupations. *Journal of Employment Counseling, 49*(4), 148–159. doi: 10.1002/j.2161-1920.2012.00016.x

Orcher, L. T. (2014). *Conducting research: Social and behavioral science methods.* Glendale, CA: Pyrczak Publishing.

Orlinsky, D. E., Ronnestad, M. H., & Willutzki, U. (2004). Fifty years of psychotherapy process-outcome research: Continuity and change. In M. J. Lambert (Ed.), *Bergin and Garfield's handbook of psychotherapy and behavior change* (5th ed., pp. 307–389). New York, NY: Wiley.

Orlinsky, D. E., Schofield, M. J., Schroder, & T., Kazantzis, N. (2011). Utilization of personal therapy by psychotherapists: A practice-friendly review and a new study. *Journal Of Clinical Psychology, 67,* 828–842. doi: org/10.1002/jclp.20821

Osborn, D., Street, S., & Bradham-Cousar, M. (2012). Spiritual needs and practices of counselor education students. *ADULTSPAN Journal, 11*(1), 27–38. doi: 10.1002/j.2161-0029.2012.00003.x

Osherson, S. (2001). *Finding our fathers: How a man's life is shaped by his relationship with his father.* New York, NY: McGraw-Hill. (Original work published 1986)

Paisley, P. O., & Borders, L. (1995). School counseling: An evolving specialty. *Journal of Counseling and Development, 74,* 150–153.

Palazzoli, S. M., Boscolo, L., Cecchin, G., & Prata, G. (1978). *Paradox and counter-paradox.* New York, NY: Jason Aronson.

Palfreyman, D. (2003). Phelps . . . Clark . . . and now Rycotewood? Disappointment damages for breach of contract to educate. *Education and the Law, 15,* 237–247.

Parham, T. A. (1993). White researchers conducting multicultural counseling research: Can their efforts be "Mo Betta"? *The Counseling Psychologist, 21*(2), 250–256.

Parker, R. M., & Patterson, J. B. (Eds.) (2012). *Rehabilitation counseling: Basics and beyond* (5th ed.). Austin, TX: PRO-ED.

Parker, S. (2009). Faith development theory as a context for supervision of spiritual and religious issues. *Counselor Education and Supervision, 49*(1), 39–53. doi: 10.1002/j.1556-6978.2009.tb00085.x

Parks-Savage, A. (2015). Self-help groups. In E. Neukrug (Ed.), *The Sage encyclopedia of theory in counseling and psychotherapy* (Vol. 2, pp. 914–917). Thousand Oaks, CA: Sage.

Parsons, F. (2009). *Choosing a vocation.* Charleston, SC: Biblioboard. (Original work published 1909)

Parsons, R. D., & Kahn, W. J. (2005). *The school counselor as consultant: An integrated model for school-based consultation.* Belmont, CA: Cengage.

Pascarella, E. T., & Terenzini, P. T. (2005). *How college affects students: A third decade of research* (Vol. 2). San Francisco, CA: Jossey-Bass.

Patterson, C. H. (1986). *Theories of counseling and psychotherapy* (4th ed.). New York, NY: HarperCollins.

Patterson, J., Albala, A. A., McCahill, M. E., & Edwards, T. M. (2010). *The therapist's guide to psychopharmacology: Working with patients, families, and physicians to optimize care* (rev. ed.). New York, NY: Guilford Press.

Patton, W., & McIlveen, P. (2009). *Practice and research in career counseling and development—2008. Career Development Quarterly*, 58(2), 118–161.

Patureau-Hatchett, M. (2009). Counselors' perceptions of training, theoretical orientation, cultural and gender bias, and use of the "Diagnostic and Statistical Manual of Mental Disorders-IV-Text Revision." *Dissertation Abstracts International*, 69, 10A.

Pearson, Q. M. (2001). A case in clinical supervision: A framework for putting theory into practice. *Journal of Mental Health Counseling, 23*, 174–183.

Pearson, Q. M. (2006). Psychotherapy-driven supervision: Integrating counseling theories into role-based supervision. *Journal of Mental Health Counseling, 28*(3), 241–252.

Pearson. (2014). *Differential aptitude tests* (5th ed.). Retrieved from http://www.pearsonassessments. com/learningassessments/products/100000564 /differential-aptitude-tests-fifth-edition-dat-dat.html

Pedersen, P. (2008). Ethics, competence, and professional issues in cross-cultural counseling. In Pedersen, P., Lonner, W., Draguns, J. G., & Trimble, J. E. (Eds.), *Counseling across cultures* (6th ed., pp. 5–20). Thousand Oaks, CA: Sage Publications.

Pedersen, P. B. (2001). Triad counseling. In R. Corsini (Ed.), *Handbook of innovative psychotherapies* (2nd ed., pp. 704–714). New York, NY: Wiley.

Pedersen, P. B., Crethar, H., & Carlson, J. (2008). *Inclusive cultural empathy: Making relationships central in counseling and psychotherapy*. Washington, DC: American Psychological Association.

Pepinsky, H. B. (2001). Counseling psychology: History. In W. E. Crawford & C. B. Nemeroff (Eds.), *The Corsini encyclopedia of psychology and behavioral science* (Vol. 1, pp. 375–379). New York, NY: Wiley.

Perera-Diltz, D. M., & Mason, K. L. (2012). A national survey of school counselor supervision practices: Administrative, clinical, peer, and technology mediated supervision. *Journal of School Counseling, 10*(4), 1–34.

Perls, F. (1969). *Gestalt therapy verbatim*. Moab, UT: Real People Press.

Perls, F. (1970). Four lectures. In J. Fagan & I. L. Shepherd (Eds.), *Gestalt therapy now* (pp. 14–46). New York, NY: Harper & Row.

Perls, F. (1973). *The gestalt approach and eyewitness to therapy*. Palo Alto: Science and Behavior Books.

Perls, F. (1978). Finding self through Gestalt therapy. *Gestalt Journal, 1*(1), 54–73.

Perls, F., Hefferline, R., & Goodman, P. (1951). *Gestalt therapy: Excitement and growth in human personality*. New York, NY: Julian Press.

Perry, W. G. (1970). *Forms of intellectual and ethical development in the college years: A scheme*. New York, NY: Holt, Rinehart, & Winston.

Perusse, R., Goodnough, G., & Lee, V. V. (2009). Group counseling in the schools. *Psychology in the Schools, 46*(3), 225–231. doi: 10.1002/pits.20369

Peters, T. (1989). *Thriving on chaos*. New York, NY: Park Avenue Press.

Petersen, J. (2008). The intersection of oral history and the role of white researchers in cross-cultural contexts. *Educational Foundations, 22*(3–4), 33–52.

Petersen, J., & Hyde, J. (2010). A meta-analytic review of research on gender differences in sexuality, 1993–2007. *Psychological Bulletin, 136*(1), 21–38. doi: 10.1037 /a0017504

Peterson, C., Lomas, G., Neukrug, E., & Bonner, M. (2014). Assessment use by counselors in the United States: Implications for policy and practice. *Journal of Counseling and Development. 92*, 90–98. doi: 10.1002 /j.1556-6676.2013.00134.x

Pew Forum on Religion and Public Life (2009). *Results from the 2009 annual religion and public life survey*. Retrieved from http://people-press.org/reports/pdf/542.pdf

Pew Research (2013). *Religion and public life project: Religious landscape survey*. Retrieved from http://religions .pewforum.org/reports.

Piaget, J. (1954). *The construction of reality in the child*. New York, NY: Basic Books.

Pichot, T. (2015). de Shazer, Steve and Berg, Insoo Kim. In E. Neukrug (Ed.), *The Sage encyclopedia of theory in counseling and psychotherapy* (Vol. 1, pp. 275–277). Thousand Oaks, CA: Sage.

Piercy, F. P., Sprenkle, D. H., & Wetchler, J. L. (1996). *Family therapy sourcebook* (2nd ed.). New York, NY: Guilford.

Pieterse. A. L., Evans, S. A., Risner-Butner, A., Collins, N. M., & Mason, L. B. (2009). Multicultural competence and social justice training in counseling psychology and counselor education: A review and analysis of a sample of multicultural course syllabi. *The Counseling Psychologist, 37*, 93–115. doi: 10.1177/0011000008319986

Pirodsky, D. M., & Cohn, J. S. (1992). *Clinical primer of psychopharmacology* (2nd ed.). New York, NY: McGraw-Hill.

Polcin, D. L. (2006). Reexamining confrontation and motivational interviewing. *Addictive Disorders and Their Treatment, 54*(4), 201–209. doi: 10.1097 /01.adt.0000205048.44129.6a

Polster, E., & Polster, M. (1973). *Gestalt therapy integrated: Contours of theory and practice*. New York, NY: Brunner /Mazel.

Ponterotto, J. G., Casas, J. M., Suzuki, L.A., & Alexander, C. M. (Eds.) (2010). *Handbook of multicultural counseling* (3rd ed.). Thousand Oaks, CA: Sage.

Ponton, R., & Duba, J. (2009). The "ACA Code of Ethics": Articulating counseling's professional covenant. *Journal of Counseling & Development, 87*, 117–121. doi: 10.1002/j.1556-6678.2009.tb00557.x

Pope, M. (2008). Culturally appropriate counseling considerations for lesbian and gay clients. In P. B. Pedersen, J. G. Draguns, W. J. Lonner, & J. E. Trimble (Eds.), *Counseling across cultures* (6th ed., pp. 201–222). Thousand Oaks, CA: Sage.

Pope, M., & Sveinsdottir, M. (2005). Frank, we hardly knew ye: The very personal side of Frank Parsons. *Journal of Counseling and Development, 83*, 105–115. doi: 10.1002/j.1556-6678.2005.tb00585.x

Pope, R. L., Reynolds, A. L., & Mueller, J. A. (2014). *Creating multicultural change on campus.* San Francisco, CA: John Wiley & Sons.

Popple, P. R., & Leighninger, L. (2011). *Social work, social welfare, and American society* (8th ed.). Upper Saddle River, NJ: Pearson.

Posthuma, B. W. (2002). *Small groups in counseling and therapy: Process and leadership* (4th ed.). Boston, MA: Allyn & Bacon.

Pottick, K. J. (1988). Jane Addams revisited: Practice theory and social economics. *Social Work with Groups, 11*, 11–26. doi: 10.1300/J009v11n04_04

Prescott, H. M. (2008). College mental health since the early twentieth century. *Harvard Review of Psychiatry, 16*, 258–266. doi: 10.1080/10673220802277771

Preston, J. D., O'Neal, J. H., & Talaga, M. C. (2013). *Handbook of clinical psychopharmacology for therapists* (7th ed.). Oakland, CA: New Harbinger Publications.

Prieto, L. R., & Scheel, K. R. (2002). Using case documentation to strengthen counselor trainees' case conceptualization skills. *Journal of Counseling and Development, 81*, 11–21.

Proudlock, S., & Wellman, N. (2011). Solution-focused groups: The results look promising. *Counselling Psychology Review, 26*(3), 45–55.

PsychCorp. (2014a). *Harrington-O-Shea Career Decision-Making System Revised.* Retrieved from http://www.pearsonassessments.com/HAIWEB/Cultures/en-us/Productdetail.htm?Pid=PAa12633&Mode=summary

PsychCorp. (2014b). *Career Assessment Inventory—The Enhanced Version.* Retrieved from http://www.pearsonassessments.com/tests/cai_e.htm

Psychological Assessment Resources (PAR) (2013). *Self-directed search.* Retrieved from http://www.self-directed-search.com/default.aspx

Puig, A., Baggs, A., Mixon, K., Park, Y. M. Kim, B. Y., & Lee, S. M. (2012). Relationship between job burnout and personal wellness in mental health professionals. *Journal of Employment Counseling, 49,* 98–109. doi: 10.1002/j.2161-1920.2012.00010.x

Pullan, M. (2010). Student support services for millennial undergraduates. *Journal of Educational Technology Systems, 38*, 235–251. doi: 10.2190/ET.38.2.k

Puma, M., Bell, S., Cook, R., Heid, C., Shapiro, G., Broene, P., & Jenkins, F. (2010). *Head Start impact study. Final report.* Retrieved from ERIC database (ED507845)

Pusateri, C. G., & Headley, J. A. (2015). Feminist therapy. In E. Neukrug (Ed.), *The Sage encyclopedia of theory in counseling and psychotherapy* (Vol. 1, pp. 414–418). Thousand Oaks, CA: Sage Publishing.

Quinlen, D. W. (2014). The perfect resume: *Resumes that work in the new economy.* Roseburg, OR: Cold Spring Press.

Rankin, L. (2013). *Mind over medicine: Scientific proof that you can heal yourself.* Carlsbad, CA: Hay House.

Rasmussen, C., & Johnson, G. (2008, May). *The ripple effect of Virginia Tech: Assessing the nationwide impact on campus safety and security policy and practice.* Minneapolis, MN: Midwestern Higher Education Compact.

Ratner, H., George, E., & Iveson, C. (2012). Solution-focused brief therapy: 100 key points and techniques. New York, NY: Routledge.

Ratts, M. J. (2009). Social justice counseling: Toward the development of a fifth force among counseling paradigms. *Journal of Humanistic Counseling, Education, and Development, 48*(2), 160–172. doi: 10.1002/j.2161-1939.2009.tb00076.x

Ratts, M. J. (2011). Multiculturalism and social justice: Two sides of the same coin. *Journal of Multicultural Counseling and Development, 39*(1), 24–37. doi: 10.1002/j.2161-1912.2011.tb00137.x

Ratts, M. J., DeKruyf, L., & Chen-Hayes, S. F. (2007). The ACA Advocacy Competencies: A social justice advocacy framework for professional school counselors. *Professional School Counseling, 11*, 90–97.

Raya, P. (2010). Female genital mutilation and the perpetuation of multigenerational trauma. *Journal of Psychohistory, 37*(4), 297–325.

Rayle, A. D., & Adams, J. R. (2008). An exploration of 21st-century school counselors' daily work activities. *Journal of School Counseling, 5.* Retrieved from http://files.eric.ed.gov/fulltext/EJ901169.pdf

Rayle, A., Chee, C., & Sand, J. (2006). Honoring their way: Counseling American Indian women. *Journal of Multicultural Counseling and Development, 34*(2), 66–80. doi: 10.1002/j.2161-1912.2006.tb00028.x

Rehfuss, M. C., Gambrell, C. E., & Meyer, D. (2012). Counselors' perceived person-environment fit and career satisfaction. *Career Development Quarterly, 60*(2), 145–151. doi: 0.1002/j.2161-0045.2012.00012.x

Remley, T. P., & Herlihy, B. (2014). *Ethical, legal, and professional issues in counseling* (4th ed.). Boston, MA: Pearson.

Remley, T. P., Herlihy, B., & Herlihy, S. B. (1997). The U.S. Supreme Court decision in *Jaffe v. Redmond*: Implications for counselors. *Journal of Counseling and Development, 75*, 213–218.

Remley, T. P., Hermann, W. C., & Huey, W. C. (2003). Chapter 5: Records. In T. P. Remley, M. A. Hermann, & W. C. Huey (Eds.), *Ethical and legal issues in school counseling* (2nd ed., pp. 223–238. Alexandria, VA: American School Counselor Association.

Rentz, A. L. (2004). Student affairs: An historical perspective. In F. J. D. MacKinnon (Ed.), *Rentz's student affairs practice in higher education* (3rd ed., pp. 27–57). Springfield, IL: Charles C. Thomas.

Rentz, A. L., & Howard-Hamilton, M. (2011). Student affairs: An historical perspective. In N. Zhang (Ed.), *Rentz's student affairs practice in higher education* (4th ed., pp. 30–62). Springfield, IL: Charles C. Thomas.

Rice, R. (2015). Narrative therapy. In E. Neukrug (Ed.), *The Sage encyclopedia of theory in counseling and psychotherapy* (Vol. 2, pp. 695–700). Thousand Oaks, CA: Sage.

Richardson, M., Abraham, C., & Bond, R. (2012). Psychological correlates of university students' academic performance: A systematic review and meta-analysis. *Psychological Bulletin, 138*, 353–387. doi: 10.1037/a0026838

Riding the . . . (2006, October). Riding the underground railroad: Insoo Kim Berg talks about the origins and future of the solution-focused approach. *Solution News, 2*(3), 3 – 6.

Ridley, C. R., Mollen, D., & Kelly, S. M. (2011). Beyond microskills: Toward a model of counseling competence *The Counseling Psychologist, 39*, 825–864. doi: 10.1177/0011000010378440

Rinaldi, A. P. (2013). Prescriptive authority and counseling psychology: Implications for practitioners. *The Counseling Psychologist, 41*, 123–1228. doi: 10.1177/0011000012461956

Ripley, J., Jackson, L., Tatum, R., & Davis, E. (2007). A developmental model of supervisee religious and spiritual development. *Journal of Psychology and Christianity, 26*(4), 298–306.

Ritter, J.A., Vakalahi, H. F. O., & Kiernan-Stern, M. (2009). *101 careers in social work*. New York, NY: Springer Publishing.

Riva, M., & Erickson Cornish, J. A. (2008). Group supervision practices at psychology predoctoral internship programs: 15 years later. *Training and Education in Professional Psychology, 2*(1), 18–25. doi: 10.1037/1931-3918.2.1.18

Robinson, B. A. (2014). Female genital mutilation (FGM) in Africa, the Middle East, and the Far East. Retrieved from http://www.religioustolerance.org/fem_cirm1.htm

Robinson, D. S., Rickels, K., & Yocca, F. D. (2009). Buspirone and gepirone. In A. F. Schatzberg & C. B. Nemeroff (Eds.), *Textbook of psychopharmacology* (4th ed., pp. 487–502). Washington, DC: American Psychiatric Press.

Rochefort, D.A. (1984). Origins of the "third psychiatric revolution": The Community Mental Health Centers Act of 1963. *Journal of Health Politics, Policy, and Law, 9*(1), 1–30. doi: 10.1215/03616878-9-1-1

Rockwell, P. J., & Rothney, W. M. (1961). Some social ideas of pioneers in the guidance movement. *Personnel and Guidance Journal, 40*, 349–354. doi: 10.1002/j.2164-4918.1961.tb02117.x

Roe, A. (1956). *The psychology of occupations*. New York, NY: Wiley.

Roe, A., & Siegelman, M. (1964). *The origin of interests*. APGA Inquiry Studies No. 1. Washington, DC: American Personnel and Guidance Association.

Rogers, C. R. (1942). *Counseling and psychotherapy: New concepts in practice*. Boston, MA: Houghton Mifflin.

Rogers, C. R. (1951). *Client-centered therapy: Its current practice, implications, and theory*. Boston, MA: Houghton Mifflin.

Rogers, C. R. (1957). The necessary and sufficient conditions of therapeutic personality change. *Journal of Consulting Psychology, 21*, 95–103. doi: 10.1037/h0045357

Rogers, C. R. (1959). A theory of therapy, personality and interpersonal relationships as developed in the client-centered framework. In S. Koch (Ed.), *Psychology: A study of science,* Vol. 3, Formulations of the person and the social context (pp. 184–256). New York, NY: McGraw-Hill.

Rogers, C. R. (1970). *Carl Rogers on encounter groups*. New York, NY: Harper & Row.

Rogers, C. R. (1980). *A way of being*. Boston, MA: Houghton Mifflin.

Rogers, C. R. (1989a). A client-centered/person-centered approach to therapy. In H. Kirschenbaum & V. L. Henderson (Eds.), *The Carl Rogers reader* (pp. 135–152). Boston, MA: Houghton Mifflin. (Original work published 1986)

Rogers, C. R. (1989b). A therapist's view of the good life: The fully functioning person. In H. Kirschenbaum & V. Henderson (Eds.), *The Carl Rogers reader* (pp. 409–419). Boston, MA: Houghton Mifflin. (Original work published 1961)

Rogers, C. R. (1989c). Ellen West and loneliness. In H. Kirschenbaum & V. L. Henderson (Eds.), *The Carl Rogers reader* (pp. 157–167). Boston, MA: Houghton Mifflin. (Original work published in 1961)

Rosaldo, R. (1993). *Culture and truth: The remaking of social analysis*. Boston, MA: Beacon Press.

Rosenhan, T. (1973). On being sane in insane places. *Science, 179*(19), 250–258. doi: 10.1126/science.179.4070.250

Rosenthal, H. (Ed.). (2011a). *Favorite counseling and therapy techniques.* New York, NY: Routledge.

Rosenthal, H. (Ed.). (2011b). *Favorite counseling and therapy homework assignments.* New York, NY: Routledge.

Routh, D. K. (2000). Clinical psychology: History of the field. In A. E. Kazdin (Ed.), *Encyclopedia of psychology* (Vol. 2, pp. 113–118). New York, NY: Oxford University Press.

Royse, D., Thyer, B. A., & Padgett, D. K., (2010). *Program evaluation: An introduction* (5th ed.) Belmont, CA: Wadsworth.

Roysircar, G. (2008). Response to "social privilege, social justice, and group counseling: An inquiry": Social privilege: counselors' competence with systemically determined inequalities. *Journal for Specialists in Group Work, 33,* 377–384. doi: 10.1080/01933920802424456

Roysircar, G., Arredondo, P., Fuertes, J. N., Ponterotto, J. G., & Toporek, R. L. (Eds.). (2003). *Multicultural counseling competencies 2003.* Alexandria, VA: Association for Multicultural Counseling and Development.

Rudes, J., & Guterman, J. T. (2007). The value of social constructionism for the counseling profession: A reply to Hansen. *Journal of Counseling and Development, 85,* 387–392.

Rudow, H. (2013, January 9). Resolution of EMU case confirms ACA code of ethics, counseling profession's stance against client discrimination. *Counseling Today.* Retrieved from http://ct.counseling.org/2013/01/resolution-of -emu-case-confirms-aca-code-of-ethics-counseling -professions-stance-against-client-discrimination/

Rutkow, L. Vernick, J. S., Wissow, L. S., Kaufmann, C. N., Hodge, J. G., (2011). Prescribing authority during emergencies. *Journal of Legal Medicine, 32,* 249–260. doi: 10.1080/01947648.2011.600154

Ryan, J. J. (2008). Intelligence. In S. F. Davis, & W. Buskit (Eds.), *21st-century psychology: A reference handbook* (Vol. 1, pp. 413–421). Thousand Oaks, CA: Sage Publications.

Sabnani, H. B., Ponterotto, J. G., & Borodovsky, L. G. (1991). White racial identity development and cross-cultural counselor training: A stage model. *The Counseling Psychologist, 19*(1), 76–102. doi: 10.1177/0011000091191007

Sabshin, M. (1990). Turning points in twentieth-century American psychiatry. *American Journal of Psychiatry, 147,* 1267–1274.

Safransky, R. J. (2010, December 14). Civil Rights Act of 1964. *Law and Higher Education.* Retrieved from http:// lawhighereducation.org/29-civil-rights-act-of-1964.html

Salary.com. (2014). *Counselor–Higher ed. salaries.* Retrieved July 5, 2014, from http://www1.salary.com/Counselor -Higher-Ed-Salary.html

Sampson, J. P. (1995). *Computerassisted testing in counseling and therapy.* Retrieved from ERIC database (ED 391983)

Sandhu, D. S. (2000). Alienated students: Counseling strategies to curb school violence. *Professional School Counseling, 4,* 81–85.

Santiago-Rivera, A. L. (2009). Allen Ivey: Pioneer in counseling theory and practice, and crusader for multiculturalism and social justice. *The Counseling Psychologist, 31*(1), 67–92.

Santrock, J. W. (2013). *Life-span development* (14th ed.). Boston, MA: McGraw Hill.

Santrock, J. W. (2014). *A topical approach to life-span development* (5th ed.). Boston, MA: McGraw Hill.

Saravi, F. (2007). The elusive search for a "gay gene." In D. S. Sergio (Ed.), *Tall tales about the mind and brain: Separating fact from fiction* (pp. 461–477). New York, NY: Oxford University Press.

Satir, V. (1967). *Conjoint family therapy.* Palo Alto, CA: Science and Behavior Books.

Satir, V. (1972a). *Peoplemaking.* Palo Alto, CA: Science and Behavior Books.

Satir, V. (1972b). Family systems and approaches to family therapy. In G. D. Erickson & T. P. Hogan (Eds.), *Family therapy: An introduction to theory and technique* (2nd ed., pp. 211–225). Pacific Grove, CA: Brooks/Cole. (Original work published 1967)

Saunders, J. L., Barros-Bailey, M., Rudman, R., Dew, D., & Garcia, J. (2007). Ethical complaints and violations in rehabilitation counseling: An analysis of Commission on Rehabilitation Counselor Certification data. *Rehabilitation Counseling Bulletin, 51*(1), 7–13, doi: 10.1177 /00343552070510010301

Scaife, J. (2008). *Supervision in clinical practices: A practitioner's guide* (2nd ed.). New York, NY: Routledge.

Scarborough, J. L., & Culbreth, J. R. (2008). Examining discrepancies between actual and preferred practice of school counselors. *Journal of Counseling & Development, 86,* 446–459. doi: 10.1002 /j.1556-6678.2008.tb00533.x

Schatzberg, A. F., & Nemeroff, C. B. (Eds.). (2009). *The American Psychiatric Publishing textbook of psychopharmacology* (4th ed.). Washington, DC: American Psychiatric Press.

Schein, E. H. (1999). *Process consultation revisited: Building the helping relationship.* Reading, MA: Addison-Wesley.

Schein, E. H. (2013). *Humble inquiry: The gentle art of asking instead of telling.* San Francisco, CA: Berrett-Koehler.

Schinka, J. A. (2012). *Mental status checklist-adult.* Lutz, FL: Psychological Assessment Resources.

Schmidt, J. J. (2010). *The elementary/middle school counselor's survival guide* (3rd ed.). San Francisco, CA: Jossey-Bass.

Schmidt, J. J. (2013). *Counseling in schools: Comprehensive programs of responsive services for all students* (6th ed.). Boston, MA: Pearson.

Schmidt, L. D. (2000). Counseling psychology: History of the field. In A. E. Kazdin (Ed.), *Encyclopedia of psychology* (Vol. 2, pp. 317–320). New York, NY: Oxford University Press.

Schneider, W., & Bullock, M. (2009*). Human development from early childhood to early adulthood: Findings from a 20-year longitudinal study.* New York, NY: Psychology Press.

Schultheiss, D. E. P. (2007). The emergence of a relational cultural paradigm for vocational psychology. *International Journal for Educational and Vocational Guidance, 7,* 191–201. doi: 0.1007/s10775-007-9123-7

Schweiger, W. K., Henderson, D. A., McCaskill, K., Clawson, T., & Collins, D. R. (2012). *Counselor preparation: Programs, faculty, trends* (13th ed.). New York, NY: Routledge.

Schweiger, W. K., Henderson, D., Clawson, T., Collins, D., & Nuckolls, M. (2008). *Counselor preparation: Programs, faculty, trends.* (12th ed.) New York, NY: Routledge.

Schwitzer, A. M., & Rubin, L. (2012). Diagnosis and treatment planning skills for mental health professionals: A popular culture casebook approach. Thousand Oaks, CA: Sage.

Schwitzer, A., MacDonald, K. E., & Dickinson, P. (2008). Using pop culture characters in clinical training and supervision. In L C. Rubin (Ed.), *Popular culture in counseling, psychotherapy, and play-based interventions* (pp. 315–342). New York, NY: Spring Publishing.

Scoville, E., & Newman, J. S. (2009, May). A very brief history of credentialing. *ACP Hospitalist.* Retrieved from http://www.acphospitalist.org/archives/2009/05/newman.htm

Scribner, R., Ackleh, A. S., Fitzpatrick, B. G., Jacquez, G., Thibodeaux, J. J., Rommel, R., & Simonsen, N. (2009). A systems approach to college drinking: Development of a deterministic model for testing alcohol control policies. *Journal of Studies on Alcohol and Drugs, 70*(5), 805–821.

Scriven, M. (1996). Types of evaluation and types of evaluator. *Evaluation Practice, 17*(2), 151–161.

Scriven, M. S. (1967). *The methodology of evaluation* (American Educational Research Association Monograph Series on Curriculum Evaluation, No. 1). Chicago, IL: Rand NcNally.

Sears, R., Rudisill, J., & Mason-Sears, C. (2006). *Consultation skills for mental health professionals.* Hoboken, NJ: John Wiley.

Sears, S. (2005). Large group guidance: Curriculum development and instruction. In C. Sink (Ed.) *Contemporary school counseling: Theory, research, and practice* (pp. 189–213). Boston, MA: Lahaska Press.

Seligman, L. (1999). Twenty years of diagnosis and the DSM. *Journal of Mental Health Counseling, 21,* 229–239.

Seligman, L. (2004). *Diagnosis and treatment planning in counseling* (3rd ed.). New York, NY: Kluwer Academic/Plenum Press.

Seligman, M. E. P., Ernst, R. M., Gilham, J., Reivich, K., & Linkins, M. (2009). Positive education: Positive psychology and classroom interventions. *Oxford Review of Education, 35*(3), 293–311. doi: 10.1080/ 03054980902934563

Senge, P. (2006). *The fifth discipline: The art and practice of the learning organization* (rev. ed.). New York, NY: Doubleday.

Seto, A., Young, S., Becker, K., & Kiselica, M. (2006). Application of the triad training model in a multicultural counseling course. *Counselor Education and Supervision, 45*(4), 304–318.

Severy, L. (2011). Career services. In N. Zhang (Ed.), *Rentz's student affairs practice in higher education* (4th ed., pp.119–150). Springfield, IL: Charles C. Thomas.

Sewell, H. (2009). *Working with ethnicity, race, and culture in mental health.* Philadelphia, PA: Jessica Kingsley Publishers.

Shadish, W. R., Cook, T. D., & Campbell, D. T. (2002). *Experimental and quasi-experimental designs for generalized causal inference.* Boston, MA: Houghton Mifflin.

Shallcross, L. (2009, November). Counseling profession reaches the big 50. *Counseling Today.* Retrieved from http://ct.counseling.org/2009/12/counseling-profession-reaches-the-big-5-0/

Shane, L., (2012, June 27). A matter of degrees: VA finally opens doors to licensed counselors. *Starts and Stripes.* Retrieved from http://www.stripes.com/news/a-matter-of-degrees-va-finally-opens-doors-to-licensed-counselors-1.181475

Sharf, R. S. (2013). *Applying career development theory to counseling* (6th ed.). Belmont, CA: Brooks/Cole.

Sharfstein, S. S. (2000). What happened to community mental health? *Psychiatric Services, 51,* 616–620.

Shaw, B. M., Bayne, H., & Lorelle, S. (2012). A constructivist perspective for integrating spirituality into counselor training. *Counselor Education and Supervision, 51,* 270–280.

Sheehan, D., & Raj, B. A. (2009). Benzodiazepines. In A. F. Schatzberg & C. B. Nemeroff (Eds.), *Textbook of psychopharmacology* (4th ed., pp. 465–486). Washington, DC: American Psychiatric Press.

Sheehy, G. (2006). *Passages: Predictable crises of adult life.* New York, NY: Bantam Books. (Original work published 1976)

Sheridan, E. P., Matarazzo, J. D., & Nelson, P. D. (1995). Accreditation of psychology's graduate professional education and training programs: An historical perspective. *Professional Psychology, Research, and Practice, 26,* 386–392. doi: 10.1037/0735-7028.26.4.386

Sherman, R. (1999). Family therapy: The art of integration. In R. E. Watts & J. Carlson (Eds.), *Intervention and strategies in counseling and psychotherapy* (pp. 101–134). Philadelphia, PA: Taylor and Francis.

Shorter, E. (2013). Psychiatry and fads: Why is this field different from all other fields? *Canadian Journal of Psychiatry, 58,* 555–559.

Shuford, B. C. (2011). Multicultural affairs. In N. Zhang (Ed.), *Rentz's student affairs practice in higher education* (4th ed., pp. 245–280). Springfield, IL: Charles C. Thomas.

Singh, A. A., & Salazar, C. F. (2010a). The roots of social justice in group work. *Journal of Specialists in Group Work, 35*(2), 97–104. doi: 10.1080/01933921003706048

Singh, A. A., & Salazar, C. F. (Eds.). (2010b). Social justice issues in group work, part I [special issue]. *Journal of Specialists in Group Work, 35*(2). doi: 10.1080/01933921003706048

Sink, C. A., & Stroh, H. R. (2003). Raising achievement test scores of early elementary school students through comprehensive school counseling programs. *Professional School Counseling, 6,* 350–364.

Sink, C. A., Akos, P., Turnbull, R. J., & Mvududu, M. (2008). An investigation of comprehensive school counseling programs and academic achievement in Washington state middle schools. *Professional School Counseling, 12,* 43–53. doi: 10.5330/PSC.n.2010-12.43

Sizer, N. (1872). *What to do, and why; and how to educate each man for his proper work: Describing seventy-five trades and professions, and the talents and temperaments required for each.* New York, NY: Mason, Baker, & Bratt.

Skinner, B. F. (1938). *The behavior of organisms: An experimental analysis.* New York, NY: Appleton-Century.

Skinner, B. F. (1971). *Beyond freedom and dignity.* New York, NY: Knopf.

Skynner, A. C. R. (1976). *Systems of marital and family psychotherapy.* New York, NY: Brunner/Mazel.

Skynner, A. C. R. (1981). An open-systems, group-analytic approach to family therapy. In A. S. Gurman & D. P. Kniskern (Eds.), *Handbook of family therapy* (pp. 39–84). New York, NY: Brunner/Mazel.

Sloan, J. J., & Fisher, B. S. (2011). *The dark side of the ivory tower: Campus crime as a social problem.* New York, NY: Cambridge University Press.

Smart, J. (2009). Counseling individuals with disabilities. In I. Marini & M. A. Stebnicki (Eds.), *The professional counselor's desk reference* (pp. 639–646). New York, NY: Springer.

Smith, H. B., & Robinson, G. (1995). Mental health counseling: past, present, and future. *Journal of Counseling and Development, 74,* 158–162. doi: 10.1002/j.1556-6978.2012.00020.x

Smith, J., Amrhein, P., Brooks, A., Carpenter, K., Levin, D., Schreiber, E., . . . Nunes, E. (2007). Providing live supervision via teleconferencing improves acquisition of motivational interviewing skills after workshop attendance. *American Journal of Drug and Alcohol Abuse, 33*(1), 163–168. doi: 10.1080/00952990601091150

Smith, L., C., & Shin, R. Q. (2008). Social privilege, social justice, and group counseling: An inquiry. *Journal of Specialists in Group Counseling, 33,* 351–366. doi: 10.1080/01933920802424415

Snow, K. (2013). The importance of advocacy and advocacy competencies in human service professions. *Journal of Human Services, 33,* 5–16.

Social Security Administration. (n.d.). *Asian Americans and Pacific Islanders.* Retrieved from http://www.ssa.gov/people/aapi/

Sokal, M. M. (1992). Origins and early years of the American Psychological Association, 1890–1906. *American Psychologist, 47,* 111–122. doi: 10.1037/0003-066X.47.2.111

Solomon, M. (1918). The increasing importance of the biological viewpoint in psychopathology and psychiatry. *Journal of Abnormal Psychology, 13,* 168–171. doi: 10.1037/h0070702

Sommers-Flanagan, J., & Sommers-Flanagan, R. (2014). *Clinical interviewing* (5th ed.). Hoboken, NJ: John Wiley & Sons.

Somody, C., Henderson, P., Cook, K., & Zambrano, E. (2008). A working system of school counselor supervision. *Professional School Counseling, 12*(1), 22–33. doi: 10.5330/PSC.n.2010-12.22

Southern, J. A., Erford, B. T., Vernon, A., & Davis-Gage, D. (2011). The value of group work: Functional group models and historical perspective. In B. T. Erford (Ed.), *Group work: Processes and applications* (pp. 1–19). New York, NY: Pearson.

Spillman, L. (2007). Culture. In G. Ritzer (Ed.) *Blackwell encyclopedia of sociology.* Retrieved from www.blackwellreference.com/subscriber/tocnode?id=g9781405124331_chunk_g97814051243319_ss1-183

Spokane, A. R., Luchetta, E. J., & Richwine, M. H. (2002). Holland's theory of personalities in work environments. In D. Brown (Ed.), *Career choice and development* (4th ed., pp. 373–426). New York, NY: John Wiley and Sons.

Spruill, D. A., & Benshoff, J. M. (2000). Developing a personal theory of counseling: A theory building model for counselor trainees. *Counselor Education and Supervision, 40,* 70–80. doi: 10.1002/j.1556-6978.2000.tb01800.x

Stark-Rose, R. M., Livingston-Sacin, T. M., Merchant, N., & Finley, A. C. (2012). Group counseling with united states racial minority groups: A 25-year content analysis. *Journal for Specialists in Group Work, 37,* 277–296.

Stearns, S. C., Allal, N., & Mace, R. (2008). Life history, theory, and human development. In C. Crawford & D. Krebs (Eds.), *Foundations of evolutionary psychology* (pp. 47–70). New York, NY: Taylor & Francis.

Steinem, G. (1992). *Revolution from within: A book on self-esteem.* Boston, MA: Little, Brown.

Stenzel, C. L., & Rupert, P. A. (2004). Psychologists' use of touch in individual psychotherapy. *Psychotherapy: Theory, Research, Practice, Training, 41*, 332–345. doi: 10.10370033-3204.41.3.332

Sterner, W. (2009). Influence of the supervisory working alliance on supervisee work satisfaction and work-related stress. *Journal of Mental Health Counseling, 31*(3), 249–263.

Stickle, F., & Onedera, J. (2006). Teaching gerontology in counselor education. *Educational Gerontology, 32*, 247–259. doi: 10.1080/03601270500493974

Stinchfield, T., Hill, N. R., & Kleist, D. M. (2007). The reflective model of triadic supervision: Defining an emerging modality. *Counselor Education and Supervision, 46*(3), 172–183. doi: 10.1002/j.1556-6978.2007.tb00023.x

Stoltenberg, C. D. (2005). Enhancing professional competence through developmental approaches to supervision. *American Psychologist, 60*(8), 857–864. doi: 10.1037/0003-066X.60.8.85

Stoltenberg, C. D., & McNeil, B. W. (2010). *IDM supervision: An integrative developmental model of supervising counselors and therapists* (3rd ed.). New York, NY: Routledge.

Stone, C. B. (2013). *School counseling principles: Ethics and law* (3rd ed.). Alexandria, VA: American School Counselor Association.

Stone, G. L., & Archer, J. (1990). College and university counseling centers in the 1990s: Challenges and limits. *The Counseling Psychologist, 18*, 539–607. doi: 10.1177/0011000090184001

Strauss, A., & Corbin, J. (1990). Basics of *qualitative research: Grounded theory procedures and techniques.* Newbury Park, CA: Sage.

Strong, T., & Nielsen, K. (2008). Constructive conversations: Revisiting selected developments with clients and counsellors. *Counselling & Psychotherapy Research, 8*, 253–260. doi.org/10.1080/14733140802355841

Strong, T., & Zeman, D. (2010). Dialogic considerations of confrontation as a counseling activity: An examination of Allen Ivey's use of confronting as a microskill. *Journal of Counseling & Development, 88*, 332–339. doi.org/10.1002/j.1556-6678.2010.tb00030.x

Stroup, A. L., & Manderscheid, R. W. (1988). The development of the state mental hospital system in the United States: 1840–1890, *Journal of the Washington Academy of the Sciences, 78*: 59–68.

Substance Abuse and Mental Health Services Administration (SAMHSA) (2010). *Homelessness Resource Center.* Retrieved from http://homeless.samhsa.gov/Resource/View.aspx?id=48800

Substance Abuse and Mental Health Services Administration (SAMHSA) (2013). *Tips for talking with and helping children and youth cope after a disaster or traumatic event: A guide for parent, carergivers,* and teachers. Retrieved from http://store.samhsa.gov/shin/content//SMA12-4732/SMA12-4732.pdf

Substance Abuse and Mental Health Services Administration (SAMHSA) (n.d.). *Behavioral health treatment service locater.* Retrieved from http://findtreatment.samhsa.gov/

Sue, D., & Lam, A. G. (2002). Cultural and demographic diversity. In J. C. Norcross (Ed.), *Psychotherapy relations that work: Therapist contributions and responsiveness to patients* (pp. 401–420). New York, NY: Oxford University Press.

Sue, D. W. (1992). The challenge of multiculturalism: The road less traveled. *American Counselor, 1*(1), 6–15.

Sue, D. W. (2010). *Microaggressions in everyday life: Race, gender, and sexual orientation.* New York, NY: Wiley.

Sue, D. W., & Sue, D. (2013). *Counseling the culturally diverse* (6th ed.). Hoboken, NJ: John Wiley and Sons.

Sue, D. W., & Torino, G. C. (2005). Racial-cultural competences: Awareness, knowledge, and skills. In Carter, R. T. (Ed.), *Handbook of racial-cultural psychology and counseling: Theory and research* (pp. 3–18). Hoboken, NJ: Wiley.

Sue, D. W., Arredondo, P., & McDavis, R. (1992). Multicultural counseling competencies and standards: A call to the profession. *Journal of Counseling and Development, 70*, 477–486. doi: 10.1002/j.2161-1912.1992.tb00563.x

Sun, A. (2012). Helping homeless individuals with co-occurring disorders: The four components. *Social Work, 57*(1), 23–37. doi: 10.1093/sw/swr008

Sun, K. (2013). *Correctional counseling: A cognitive growth perspective.* Burlington, MA: Jones and Bartlett Learning.

Super, D. E. (1953). A theory of vocational development. *American Psychologist, 8*(2), 185–190. doi: 10.1037/h0056046

Super, D. E. (1957). *The psychology of careers.* New York, NY: Harper & Row.

Super, D. E. (1976). *Career education and the meaning of work.* Monographs on career education. Washington, DC: Office of Career Education, U.S. Dept. of Education.

Super, D. E. (1990). A life-span, life-space approach to career development. In D. Brown, L. Brooks, & Associates (Eds.), *Career choice and development: Applying contemporary theories to practice* (2nd ed.). San Francisco, CA: Jossey-Bass.

Super, D. E., & Hall, D. T. (1978). Career development: Person, position, and process. *Counseling Psychologist, 1,* 2–9.

Super, D. E., Savickas, M. L., & Super, C. M. (1996). Life-span, life-space approach to careers. In D. Brown, L. Brooks, & Associates (Eds.), *Career choice and development* (3rd ed. pp. 121–178). San Francisco, CA: Jossey-Bass.

Suzuki, L. A., Kugler, J. F., & Aguiar, L. J. (2005). Assessment practices in racial-cultural psychology. In R. T. Carter (Ed.), *Handbook of racial-cultural psychology and counseling: Theory and research* (Vol. 2, pp. 297–315). Hoboken, NJ: John Wiley.

Swanson, J. L., & Schneider, M. (2013). Minnesota theory of work adjustment. In S. D. Brown & R. W. Lent (Eds.), *Career development and counseling: Putting theory and research to work* (pp. 29–54). Hoboken, NJ: Wiley.

Sweeney, T. (2009). *Adlerian counseling and pyschotherapy: A practitioner's approach* (5th ed.). New York, NY: Routledge.

Sweeney, T. J. (1991). Counselor credentialing: Purpose and origin. In F. O. Bradley (Ed.), *Credentialing in counseling* (pp. 81–85). Alexandria, VA: Association for Counselor Education and Supervision.

Sweeney, T. J. (1992). CACREP: Precursors, promises, and prospects. *Journal of Counseling and Development, 70*(6), 667–672. doi: 10.1002/j.1556-6676.1992.tb02143.x

Swenson, L. C. (1997). *Psychology and law for the helping professions* (2nd ed.). Pacific Grove, CA: Brooks/Cole.

Szasz, T. (1961). *The myth of mental illness.* New York, NY: Paul B. Hoeber.

Szasz, T. (1970). *Ideology and insanity: Essays on the psychiatric dehumanization of man.* New York, NY: Anchor Books.

Szasz, T. (1995). The healing word: Its past, present, and future. In J. K. Zeig (Ed.), *The evolution of psychotherapy: The third conference.* New York, NY: Brunner/Mazel.

Szasz, T. (Speaker) (1990). *A conversation with an officially documented schizophrenic patient* (Cassette Recording No. PC289-W9AD). Phoenix, AZ: The Milton H. Erickson Foundation.

Szymanski, D. (2013). Counseling lesbian, gay, bisexual, and transgendered clients. In G. J. McAuliffe (Ed.), *Culturally alert counseling: A comprehensive introduction* (2nd ed., pp. 415–554). Thousand Oaks, CA: Sage Publications.

Thelin, J. R., & Gasman, M. (2011). Historical overview of American higher education. In J. H. Schuh, S. R. Jones, S. R. Harper, et al. (Eds.), *Student services: A handbook for the profession* (5th ed., pp. 3–23). San Francisco, CA: John Wiley & Sons.

Thomas, C. M., & Martin, V. (2006). Group work: Elderly people and their caregivers. In D. Capuzzi & D. R. Gross (Eds.), *Introduction to group work* (4th ed., pp. 483–513). Denver, CO: Love.

Thomason, T. C. (2010). The trend toward evidence-based practice and the future of psychotherapy. *American Journal of Psychotherapy, 64*(1), 29–38.

Thompson, B. (1995). *Inappropriate statistical practices in counseling research: Three pointers for readers of research literature.* Retrieved from ERIC database (ED 392990)

Thompson, C. L., & Henderson, D. A. (2010). *Counseling children* (8th ed.). Pacific Grove, CA: Cengage.

Thornton, R. (1996). Population: Precontact to present. In F. E. Hoxie (Ed.), *Encyclopedia of North American Indians* (pp. 500–502). New York, NY: Houghton Mifflin.

Thyer, B. A. (2006). It is time to rename the DSM. *Ethical Human Psychology and Psychiatry, 8,* 61–67. doi: 10.1891/ehpp.8.1.61

Todd, J., & Bohart, A. C. (2006). *Foundations of clinical and counseling psychology* (4th ed.). Long Grove, IL: Waveland Press.

Tomm, K. (1998). A question of perspectives. *Journal of Marital and Family Therapy, 24*(4), 409–413.

Toporek, R. L., & Lewis, J. A., & Crethar, H. C. (2009). Promoting systemic change through the ACA advocacy competencies. *Journal of Counseling and Development, 87,* 260–268. doi: 10.1002/j.1556-6678.2009.tb00105.x

The Top 10: The most influential therapists of the past quarter-century. (2007). *Psychotherapy Networker, 31*(2), Retrieved from http://www.psychotherapynetworker.org/404

Treatment Advocacy Center. (2014). *No room at the inn: Trends and consequences of closing public psychiatric hospitals.* Retrieved from http://tacreports.org/bed-study #whatsneeded

Trepal, H. C., Wester, K. L., & Notestine, L. (2013). Counseling men and women: Considering gender and sex. In G. J. McAuliffe (Ed.), *Culturally alert counseling: A comprehensive introduction* (2nd ed., pp. 383–414). Thousand Oaks, CA: Sage Publications.

Trotzer, J. P. (2013). *The counselor and the group: Integrating theory, training, and practice* (4th ed.). New York, NY: Routledge.

Truax, C. B., & Mitchell, K. M. (1961). Research on certain therapist interpersonal skills in relation to process and outcome. In A. E. Bergin & S. L. Garfield (Eds.), *Handbook of psychotherapy and behavior change: An empirical analysis* (3rd ed.). New York, NY: Wiley.

Tsering, G. T. (2005). *The four noble truths: The foundation of Buddhist thought* (Vol. 1). Somerville, MA: Wisdom Publications.

Tuckman, B. W. (1965). Developmental sequence in small groups. *Psychological Bulletin, 63,* 384–399. doi: 10.1037/h0022100

Tuckman, B. W., & Jensen, M. A. C. (1977). Stages of small-group development revisited. *Group and Organization Management, 2*, 419–427. doi: 10.1177/105960117700200404

Turkewitz, J. (2014, June 10). A fight as U.S. girls face genital cutting abroad. *The New York Times.* Retrieved from http://www.nytimes.com/2014/06/11/us/a-fight-as-us-girls-face-genital-cutting-abroad.html

Turkington, C. (1985). Analysts sued for barring non-MDs. *APA Monitor, 16*(5), 2.

Turner, L. H., & West, R. (2013). *Perspectives on family communication* (4th ed.). Boston, MA: McGraw-Hill.

Turner, S. M., DeMers, S. T., Fox, H. R., & Reed. G. M. (2001). APA's guidelines for test user qualifications: An executive summary. *American Psychologist, 56*(12), 1099–1113. doi: 10.1037/0003-066X.56.12.1099

Tyler, L. E. (1969). *The work of the counselor* (3rd ed.). Englewood Cliffs, NJ: Prentice Hall.

U. S. Environmental Protection Agency (2011). U.S. *Environmental and Pacific Islander—primer.* Retrieved from http://www.epa.gov/aapi/primer.htm

U.S. Department of Labor (2014–2015b). *Occupational outlook handbook: Mental health counselors and marriage and family therapists.* Retrieved from http://www.bls.gov/ooh/community-and-social-service/mental-health-counselors-and-marriage-and-family-therapists.htm

U.S. Census Bureau (2006). *We the people: American Indians and Alaska Natives in the United States.* Retrieved from http://www.census.gov/prod/2006pubs/censr-28.pdf

U.S. Census Bureau (2008). *An older, more diverse nation by midcentury.* Retrieved from http://www.census.gov/newsroom/releases/archives/population/cb08-123.html

U.S. Census Bureau (2009a). *Annual estimates of the resident population by sex, race, and Hispanic origin for the United States: April 1, 2000 to July 1, 2009* (NC-EST2009-03). Retrieved from http://www.census.gov/popest/national/asrh/NC-EST2009-srh.html

U.S. Census Bureau (2009b). *Income, poverty, and health insurance coverage in the United States: 2008.* Retrieved from http://www.census.gov/prod/2009pubs/p60-236.pdf

U.S. Census Bureau (2011). *The older population: 2010: 2010 census briefs.* Retrieved from http://www.census.gov/prod/cen2010/briefs/c2010br-09.pdf

U.S. Census Bureau (2012). *Nearly 1 in 5 people have a disability in the U.S., Census Bureau reports.* Retrieved from https://www.census.gov/newsroom/releases/archives/miscellaneous/cb12-134.html

U.S. Census Bureau (2013). *U.S. Census Bureau news: Hispanic Heritage Month 2013.* Retrieved from http://www.census.gov/newsroom/releases/pdf/cb13ff-19_hispanicheritage.pdf

U.S. Census Bureau (2014a). *U.S. Census Bureau projections show a slower-growing, older, more diverse nation a half century from now.* Retrieved from http://www.census.gov/newsroom/releases/archives/population/cb12-243.html

U.S. Census Bureau (2014b). *State and county quickfacts.* Retrieved from http://quickfacts.census.gov/qfd/states/00000.html

U.S. Department of Education (2001). *Elementary and secondary education act (No Child Left Behind).* Retrieved from http://www2.ed.gov/policy/elsec/leg/esea02/beginning.html#sec1

U.S. Department of Education (2007). *Carl D. Perkins Career and Technical Education Act of 2006.* Retrieved from http://www2.ed.gov/policy/sectech/leg/perkins/index.html?exp=7.

U.S. Department of Education (2012). *Public elementary and secondary school student enrollment and staff counts from the common core of data: School year 2010–2011.* Retrieved from http://nces.ed.gov/pubs2012/2012327.pdf

U.S. Department of Education (2014a). ESEA flexibility. Retrieved from http://www2.ed.gov/policy/elsec/guid/esea-flexibility/index.html

U.S. Department of Education (2014b). *Family Education Rights and Privacy Act (FERPA).* Retrieved from http://www2.ed.gov/policy/gen/guid/fpco/ferpa/index.html

U.S. Department of Education (n.d). *Building the legacy: IDEA 2004.* Retrieved from http://idea.ed.gov/

U.S. Department of Health and Human Services (2001). *Mental health: Culture, race, and ethnicity: A supplement to mental health: A report to the Surgeon General.* Retrieved from http://download.ncadi.samhsa.gov/ken/pdf/SMA-01-3613/sma-01-3613.pdf

U.S. Department of Health and Human Services (2006a). *Fact sheet: Your rights under Section 504 of the Rehabilitation Act.* Retrieved from http://www.hhs.gov/ocr/504.html

U.S. Department of Health and Human Services (2006b). *State regulation of residential facilities for children with mental illness.* Retrieved from http://www.samhsa.gov/News/NewsReleases/residfacilchildrenFinal.pdf

U.S. Department of Health and Human Services (2014a). *Complementary, alternative, or integrative health: What's in a name?* Retrieved from http://nccam.nih.gov/health/whatiscam

U.S. Department of Health and Human Services (n.d.). *Understanding health information privacy.* Retrieved from http://www.hhs.gov/ocr/privacy/hipaa/understanding/index.html

U.S. Department of Housing and Urban Development (2013). *The 2013 annual homeless assessment report (AHAR) to Congress.* Retrieved from https://www.onecpd.info/resources/documents/ahar-2013-part1.pdf

U.S. Department of Justice (2011). *Freedom of Information Act guide.* Retrieved from http://www.foia.gov/about.html

U.S. Department of Justice. (2012) *2012 hate crime statistics: Incidents, offenses, victims, and known offenders.* Retrieved from http://www.fbi.gov/about-us/cjis/ucr/hate-crime /2012/tables-and-data-declarations/1tabledatadecpdf /table_1_incidents_offenses_victims_and_known _offenders_by_bias_motivation_2012.xls

U.S. Department of Justice (2013). *What is FOIA?* Retrieved from http://www.foia.gov/

U.S. Department of Justice (2014). *Hate crime victimization, 2004–2012 statistical tables.* Retrieved from http://www .bjs.gov/content/pub/pdf/hcv0412st.pdf

U.S. Department of Justice (n.d.). *Information and technical assistance on the Americans with Disabilities Act.* Retrieved from http://www.ada.gov/

U.S. Department of Labor (2014). *Occupational outlook handbook, 2014 edition.* Retrieved from http://www.bls.gov/ooh/

U.S. Department of Labor (2015). *Occupational outlook handbook, 2014–2015 edition.* St. Paul, MN: JIST Publishing.

U.S. Equal Employment Commission (n.d.). *ADA enforcement guidance: Preemployment disability-related questions and medical examinations.* Retrieved from http://www .eeoc.gov/policy/docs/medfin5.pdf

UNAIDS (2013). *Global report: UNAIDS report on the global AIDS epidemic: 2013.* Retrieved from http://www.unaids .org/en/media/unaids/contentassets/documents /epidemiology/2013/gr2013/UNAIDS_Global_Report _2013_en.pdf

Urofsky, R., Bobby, C. L., & Ritchie, M. (Eds.). (2013). CACREP: 30 years of quality assurance in counselor education [special section]. *Journal of Counseling and Development, 91.*

Urofsky, R., Engels, D., & Engebretson, K. (2008). Kitchener's principle ethics: Implications for counseling practice and research. *Counseling and Values, 53*(1), 67–78. doi: 10.1002/j.2161-007X.2009.tb00114.x

Vaillant, G. E. (2003). *Aging well: Surprising guideposts to a happier life from the landmark Harvard study of adult development.* Boston, MA: Little, Brown, & Company.

Valpar. (2014). *Sigi3: Education and career planning software for the Web.* Retrieved from http://www.valparint.com /sigi3.htm

van Deurzen, E. (2002). *Existential counseling and psychotherapy in practice* (2nd ed.). London, UK: Sage Publications.

Van Rooyen, H., Durrheim, K., & Lindegger, G. (2011). Advice-giving difficulties in voluntary counselling and testing: A distinctly moral activity. *AIDS Care, 23,* 281–286. doi: 10.1080/09540121.2010.507755

Van Velsor, P., & Orozco, G. L. (2007). Involving low-income parents in the schools: Community-centric strategies for school counselors. *Professional School Counseling, 11,* 17–24.

Vander Kolk, C. J. (1990). *Introduction to group counseling and psychotherapy.* Prospect Heights, IL: Waveland Press.

Vasquez, M. J. T., Bingham, R. P., & .Barnett, J. E. (2008). Psychotherapy termination: Clinical and ethical responsibilities. *Journal of Clinical Psychology 64,* 653–665. doi: 10.1002/jclp.20478

Vera, E. M., Buhin, L. & Shin, R. Q. (2006). The pursuit of social justice and the elimination of racism. In M. G. Constantine & D. W. Sue (Eds.), *Addressing racism: Facilitating cultural competence in mental health and educational settings* (pp. 87–103). Hoboken, NJ: Wiley.

Verbruggen, M., & Sels, L. (2010). Social-cognitive factors affecting clients' career and life satisfaction after counseling. *Journal of Career Assessment, 18*(1), 3–15.

Verny, T. R. (1974). *Inside groups: A practical guide to encounter groups and group therapy.* New York, NY: McGraw Hill.

Vespia, K. M. (2007). A national survey of small college counseling centers: Successes, issues, and challenges. *Journal of College Student Psychotherapy, 22*(1), 17–40. doi: 10.1300/J035v22n01_03

Videbeck, S. L. (2014). *Psychiatric mental health nursing* (5th ed.). Philadelphia, PA: Wolters Kluwer/Lippincott, Williams, & Wilkins.

Virginia Board of Counseling (2013). *Laws governing counseling.* Retrieved from http://www.dhp.virginia.gov /counseling/counseling_laws_regs.htm

Virginia Code (2009). *Communications between physicians and patients.* Retrieved from http://leg1.state.va.us/cgi-bin /legp504.exe?091+ful+CHAP0714

Virginia School Counselor Association (2008). *Virginia professional school counseling program manual.* Yorktown, VA: Author.

von Bertalanffy, L. (1934). *Modern theories of development: An introduction to theoretical biology.* London, UK: Oxford University Press.

von Bertalanffy, L. (1968). *General systems theory.* New York, NY: Braziller.

Von Gizycki, C. (2013, July 25). APRN prescribing law: A state-by-state summary. Retrieved from http://www .medscape.com/viewarticle/440315

Waachter, A. (2004). To "create a conversation that is a little bit different." In N. M. Lambert, I. Hylander, & J. H. Sandoval (Eds.), *Consultee-centered consultation: Improving the quality of professional services in schools and community organizations* (pp. 323–337). Mahwah, NJ: Lawrence Erlbaum.

Wakefield, J. C. (2013). DSM-5: An overview of changes and controversies. *Clinical Social Work Journal, 41,* 139–154. doi: 10.1007/s10615-014-0445-2

Walsh, J. (2000). *Clinical case management with persons having mental illness: A relationship-based perspective.* Belmont, CA: Brooks/Cole.

Walsh, P. G., Currier, G., Shah, M. N., Lyness, J. M., & Friedman, B. (2008). Psychiatric emergency services for the U. S. elderly: 2008 and beyond. *American Journal of Geriatric Psychiatry, 16*(9), 706–707. doi: 10.1097/JGP.0b013e31817e73c7

Walsh, R., & Dasenbrook, N. (2009). Contracting strategies with managed care and other agencies. In I. Marini & M. A. Stebnicki (Eds.), *The professional counselor's desk reference* (pp. 79–87). New York, NY: Springer.

Walsh, R., & Dasenbrook, N. (2010). Managed care update. *Counseling Today, 52*(9), 16–17.

Wampold, B. E. (2010a). *The basics of psychotherapy: An introduction to theory and practice.* Washington, DC: American Psychological Association.

Wampold, B. E. (2010b). *The great psychotherapy debate: Models, methods, and findings.* Mahwah, NJ: Lawrence Erlbaum Associates.

Wampold, B. E. (2010c). The research evidence for common factors models: A historically situated perspective. In B. L. Duncan, S. D. Miller, B. E. Wampold, & M A. Hubble (Eds.), *The heart and soul of change* (2nd ed., pp. 49–82). Washington, DC: American Psychological Association.

Wampold, B. E., & Budge, S. L. (2012). The relationship—and its relationship to the common and specific factors in psychotherapy. The *Counseling Psychologist, 40,* 601–623. doi: 10.1177/0011000011432709

Ward, B. W., Dahlamer, J. M., Galinsky, A. M., & Joesti, S. S. (2014, July 15). *Sexual orientation and health among U.S. adults: National Health Interview Survey, 2013. National Health Statistics Reports, 77.* Hyattsville, MD: National Center for Health Statistics.

Ward, D. E. (2004). The challenge of defining techniques in group work. *Journal for Specialists in Group Work, 29,* 155–158. doi: 10.1080/01933920490437925

Ward, D. E. (2007). The evidence mounts: Group work is effective. *Journal for Specialists in Group Work, 32,* 207–209. doi: 10.1080/01933920701431719

Watson, J. B. (1925). *Behaviorism.* Chicago, IL: University of Chicago Press.

Watson, J. B., & Raynor, R. (1920). Conditioned emotional reactions. *Journal of Experimental Psychology, 3,* 1–14. doi: 10.1037/h0069608

Watson, R. (1968). *The great psychologists from Aristotle to Freud.* Philadelphia, PA: Lippincott.

Watts, G. A. (1994). Frank Parsons: Promoter of a progressive era. *Journal of Career Development, 20*(4), 265–286. doi: 10.1007/BF02106300

Watts, R. E. (1996). Could it be that Adler influenced Rogers? *Journal of Humanistic Education and Development, 34,* 165–170. doi: 10.1002/j.2164-4683.1996.tb00342.x

Watts, R. E., & Holden, J. M. (1994). Why continue to use "fictional finalism?" *Individual Psychology, 50,* 161–163.

Watts, R. E., & Pietrzak, D. (2000). Adlerian "encouragement" and the therapeutic process of -solution-focused brief therapy. *Journal of Counseling and Development, 78,* 442–447. doi: 10.1002/j.1556-6676.2000.tb01927.x

Watzlawick, P., Beavin, J. H., & Jackson, D. D. (1967). *Pragmatics of human communication: A study of interactional patterns, pathologies, and paradoxes.* New York, NY: Norton.

Watzlawick, P., Weakland, J. H., & Fisch, R. (1974). *Change; Principles of problem formation and problem resolution.* New York, NY: Norton.

Weishaar, M. E. (1993). *Aaron T. Beck.* Thousand Oaks, CA: Sage Publications.

Weissmann, G. (2008). Citizen Pinel and the madman at Bellevue. *Journal of the Federation of American Societies for Experimental Biology. 22,* 1289–1293. doi: 10.1096/fj.08-0501ufm

Welfel, E. R. (2013). *Ethics in counseling and psychotherapy: Standards, research, and emerging issues* (5th ed.). Belmont, CA: Cengage.

Wertheimer, M. (2012). *A brief history of psychology* (5th ed.). New York, NY: Taylor & Francis Group.

West, J. D., Hosie, T. W., & Mackey, J. A. (1987). Employment and roles of counselors in mental health agencies. *Journal of Counseling and Development, 66,* 135–138. doi: 10.1002/j.1556-6676.1987.tb00818.x

Westbrook, F. D., Kandell, J. J., Kirkland, S. E., Phillips, P. E., Regan, A. M., Medvene, A., & Oslin, Y. D. (1993). University campus consultation: Opportunities and limitations. *Journal of Counseling and Development, 71,* 684–688. doi.org/10.1002/j.1556-6676.1993.tb02260.x

Wester, K. L., Borders, L. D. Boul, S., & Horton, E. (2013). Research quality: Critique of quantitative articles in the *Journal of Counseling & Development. Journal of Counseling and Development, 91*(3), 280–290.

Wexler, D. B. (2009). *Men in therapy: New approaches for effective treatment.* New York, NY: W. W. Norton.

Wheeler, A. M. N., & Bertram, B. (2012). *The counselor and the law: A guide to legal and ethical practice* (6th ed.). Alexandria, VA: American Counseling Association.

Whipple, E. G., & O'Neil, K. B. (2011). Student activities. In N. Zhang (Ed.), *Rentz's student affairs practice in higher education* (4th ed., pp. 359–395). Springfield, IL: Charles C. Thomas.

Whiston, S. C. (1996). Accountability through action research: Research methods for practitioners. *Journal of Counseling and Development, 74,* 616–623.

Whiston, S. C., & Coker, J. K. (2000). Reconstructing clinical training: Implications from research. *Counselor Education and Supervision, 39,* 228–253.

Whitaker, C. (1976). The hindrance of theory in clinical work. In P. J. Guerin (Ed.), *Family therapy* (pp. 154–164). New York, NY: Gardner Press.

Whitaker, R. (2010). *Anatomy of an epidemic: Magic bullets, psychiatric drugs, and the astonishing rise of mental illness.* New York, NY: Random House.

White, B. (2007). Student rights: From in loco parentis to sine parentibus and back again? Understanding the Family Education Rights and Privacy Act in higher education. *Brigham Young University Education and Law Journal, 2,* 321–350.

White, E. R., & Lindhorst, M. J. (2011). Academic advising. In N. Zhang (Ed.), *Rentz's student affairs practice in higher education* (4th ed., pp. 96–118). Springfield, IL: Charles C. Thomas.

The White House (n.d.a). *Higher education.* Retrieved from http://www.whitehouse.gov/issues/education/higher-education

The White House (n.d.b). *Reforming No Child Left Behind.* Retrieved from http://www.whitehouse.gov/issues/education/k-12/reforming-no-child-left-behind

White, M. (1993). *Narrative therapy using a reflective team* [video]. Alexandria, VA: American Counseling Association.

White, M. (1995). *Re-authoring lives: Interviews and essays.* Adelaide, South Australia: Dulwich Centre Publications.

White, M., & Epston, D. (1990). *Narrative means to therapeutic ends.* New York, NY: Norton.

Whitfield, H., Venable, R., & Broussard, S. (2010). Are client-counselor ethnic/racial matches associated with successful rehabilitation outcomes? *Rehabilitation Counseling Bulletin, 53*(2), 96–105. doi: 10.1177/0034355209338526

Whitman, J. S., Glosoff, H. L., Kocet, M. M., & Tarvydas, V. (2006). *ACA in the news: Ethical issues related to conversion or reparative therapy.* Retrieved from http://www.counseling.org/PressRoom/NewsReleases.aspx?AGuid=b68aba97-2f08-40c2-a400-0630765f72f4

Whitman, J. S., Glosoff, H. L., Kocet, M. M., Tarvydas, V. (2013). *Ethical issues related to conversion or reparative therapy.* Retrieved from http://www.counseling.org/news/news-release-archives/2013/01/16/ethical-issues-related-to-conversion-or-reparative-therapy

Widick, C. (1977). The Perry scheme: A foundation for developmental practice. *The Counseling Psychologist, 6*(4), 35–38. doi: 10.1177/001100007700600415

Wiger, D. E. (2009). *The clinical documentation sourcebook: The complete paperwork resource for your mental health practice* (4th ed.). Hoboken, NJ: John Wiley & Sons.

Wilcoxon, S. A., Remley, T. P., Gladding, S., & Huber, C. H. (2012). *Ethical, legal, and professional issues in the practice of marriage and family therapy* (5th ed.). Upper Saddle River, NJ: Pearson.

Williams, S. (2013). *Mental health service utilization among African American emerging adults* (Unpublished doctoral dissertation). Washington University, St. Louis, MO.

Williamson, E. G. (1950). *Counseling adolescents.* New York, NY: McGraw-Hill.

Williamson, E. G. (1958). Value orientation in counseling. *Personnel and Guidance Journal, 37,* 520–528. doi: 10.1002/j.2164-4918.1958.tb01107.x

Williamson, E. G. (1964). An historical perspective of the vocational guidance movement. *Personnel and Guidance Journal, 42,* 854–859. doi: 10.1002/j.2164-4918.1964.tb04743.x

Williamson, E. G., & Darley, J. G. (1937). *Student personnel work: An outline of clinical procedures.* New York, NY: McGraw-Hill.

Willig, C. (2011). The ethics of interpretation. *Existential Analysis: Journal of the Society For Existential Analysis, 22,* 255–271.

Wilson, F. R., & Newmeyer, M. D. (2008). A standards-based inventory for assessing perceived importance of and confidence in using ASGW's core group work skills. *Journal of Specialists in Group Work, 33,* 270–289. doi: 10.1080/01933920802196146

Wilson, F. R., Rapin, L. S., & Haley-Banez, L. (2004). How teaching group can be guided by foundational documents: Best practice guidelines, diversity principles, training standards. *Journal for Specialists in Group Work, 29,* 19–29. doi: 10.1080/01933920490275321

Winslade, J. M., & Monk, G. D. (2007). *Narrative counseling in schools: Powerful and brief* (2nd ed.). Thousand Oaks, CA: Corwin Press.

Winston, R. B. (2003). Counseling and helping skills. In S. R. Komives & D. B. Woodward (Eds.), *Student services: A handbook for the profession* (4th ed., pp. 484–506). San Francisco, CA: Jossey-Bass.

Woititz, J. G. (2002). *The complete ACOA sourcebook: Adult children of alcoholics at home, at work, and in love.* Deerfield Beach, FL: Health Communications.

Wolf, A., & Schwartz, E. K. (1972). Psychoanalysis in groups. In H. I. Kaplan & B. J. Sadock (Eds.), *The origins of group psychoanalysis* (pp. 41–100). New York, NY: Jason Aronson.

Wolf, A., Schwartz, E. K., McCarty, G. J., & Goldberg, I. A. (1972). Psychoanalysis in groups: Comparison with other group therapies. In C. J. Sager & H. S. Kaplan

(Eds.), *Progress in group and family therapy* (pp. 47–53). New York, NY: Brunner/Mazel.

Wolfgang, C. H. (2008). *Solving discipline and classroom management problems: Methods and models for today's teachers* (7h ed.). New York, NY: John Wiley & Sons.

Wolpe, J. (1958). *Psychotherapy by reciprocal inhibition.* Stanford, CA: Stanford University Press.

Wolpe, J. (1969). *The practice of behavior therapy.* New York, NY: Pergamon Press.

Wolpe, J., & Lazarus, A. A. (1966). *Behavior therapy techniques: A guide to the treatment of neuroses.* New York, NY: Pergamon Press.

Wong, D. F. K. (2006). *Clinical case management for people with mental illness: A biopsychosocial vulnerability-stress model.* Binghamton, NY: Haworth Press.

Wong, P., & Buckner, J. (2008). Multiracial student services come of age: The state of multiracial student services in higher education in the United States. *New Directions for Student Services, 123,* 43–41. doi: 10.1002/ss

World Health Organization (2013). *Mental health and older adults.* Retrieved from http://www.who.int/mediacentre/factsheets/fs381/en/

World Health Organization (2014). *Female genital mutilation.* Retrieved from http://www.who.int/mediacentre/factsheets/fs241/en/

Worthington, R., Soth-McNett, A., & Moreno, M. V. (2007). Multicultural counseling competencies research: A 20-year content analysis. *Journal of Counseling Psychology, 54*(4), 351–361. doi: 10.1037/0022-0167.54.4.351

Wubbolding, R. (2000). *Reality therapy for the 21st century.* Philadelphia, Pa: Brunner-Routledge.

Wubbolding, R. (2010). *Reality therapy: Monograph psychotherapy series.* Washington, DC: American Psychological Association.

Wubbolding, R. E. (2011). *Reality therapy.* Washington, DC: American Psychological Association.

Wubbolding, R., & Brickell, J. (1999). *Counseling with reality therapy.* Oxon, UK: Speechmark Publishing Ltd.

Yalom, I. D. (1980). *Existential psychotherapy.* New York, NY: Basic Books.

Yalom, I. D. (2005). *The theory and practice of group psychotherapy* (5th ed.). New York, NY: Basic Books.

Yarhouse, M. A. (2003). Working with families affected by HIV/AIDS. *The American Journal of Family Therapy, 31,* 125–137. doi: 10.1080/01926180301124

Yonteff, G. M. (1976). Theory of Gestalt therapy. In C. Hatcher & P. Himelstein (Eds.), *The handbook of Gestalt therapy* (pp. 213–221). New York, NY: Jason Aronson.

Younggren, J. A., & Harris, E. A. (2008). Can you keep a secret? Confidentiality in psychotherapy. *Journal of Clinical Psychology, 64,* 589–600.

Zalaquett, C. P., & Ivey. A. E. (2015). Developmental counseling and therapy: Theory and brain-based practice. In E. Neukrug (Ed.), *The Sage encyclopedia of theory in counseling and psychotherapy* (Vol. 1, pp. 283–288). Thousand Oaks, CA: Sage.

Zalaquett, C. P., Fuerth, K. M., Stein, C., Ivey, A. E., & Ivey, M. (2008). Reframing the "DSM-IV-TR" from a multicultural/social justice perspective. *Journal of Counseling & Development, 86,* 364–371. doi: 10.1002/j.1556-6678.2008.tb00521.x

Zeisel, E. (2009). Affect education and the development of the interpersonal ego in modern group psychoanalysis. *International Journal of Group Psychotherapy, 59*(3), 421–432. doi: 10.1521/ijgp.2009.59.3.421

Zhang, N. (Ed.) (2011). *Rentz's student affairs practice in higher education* (4th ed). Springfield, IL: Charles C. Thomas.

Zhang, N., & Brandel, I. W., & McCoy. (2011). Counseling centers. In N. Zhang (Ed.), *Rentz's student affairs practice in higher education* (4th ed., pp. 151–195). Springfield, IL: Charles C. Thomas.

Zuckerman, E. L. (2008). *The paper office: Forms, guidelines, and resources to make your practice work ethically, legally, and profitably* (4th ed.). New York, NY: Guilford.

Zunker, V. G. (2012). *Career counseling: A holistic approach* (8th ed.). Belmont, CA: Cengage.

Zur, O. (2007). *Boundaries in psychotherapy: Ethical and clinical explorations.* Washington, DC: American Psychological Association.

Zur, O. (2009). Therapist self-disclosure: Standard of care, ethical considerations, and therapeutic context. In A. Bloomgarden, & R. B. Mennuit (Eds.), *Psychotherapist revealed: Therapists speak about self-disclosure in psychotherapy* (pp. 31–51). New York, NY: Taylor and Francis Group.

Zuroff, D. C., Kelly, A. C., Leybman, M. J., Blatt, S. J., & Wampold, B. E. (2010). Between-therapist and within-therapist differences in the quality of the therapeutic relationship: effects on maladjustment and self-critical perfectionism. *Journal of Clinical Psychology, 66,* 681–697. doi: 10.1002/jclp.20683

Zwelling, S. S. (1990). *Quest for a cure: The public hospital in Williamsburg, Virginia, 1773–1885.* Williamsburg, VA: The Colonial Williamsburg Foundation.

Zytowski, D. G. (1972). Four hundred years before Parsons. *Personnel and Guidance Journal, 50,* 443–450. doi: 10.1002/j.2164-4918.1972.tb03910.x

Author Index

Subject Index